P9-AEU-677

BRAIN LATERALIZATION IN CHILDREN

BRAIN LATERALIZATION IN CHILDREN

DEVELOPMENTAL IMPLICATIONS

Edited by

DENNIS L. MOLFESE

Southern Illinois University at Carbondale

SIDNEY J. SEGALOWITZ

Brock University

THE GUILFORD PRESS

New York London

To Tori, David & Peter, and Jane, Ed, Elysia & Christopher

A Division of Guilford Publications Inc.
72 Spring Street, New York, N.Y. 10012

Printed in the United States of America

Last digit is print number: 9 8 7 6 5 4 3 2 1

LIBRARY OF CONGRESS CATALOGING-IN-PUBLICATION DATA

Brain lateralization in children: developmental implications / edited by Dennis L. Molfese, Sidney J. Segalowitz.
p. cm.
Includes bibliographies and index.
ISBN 0-89862-719-2
1. Cerebral dominance. 2. Brain—Growth. 3. Laterality.
I. Molfese, Dennis L. II. Segalowitz, Sidney J.
[DNLM: 1. Brain—physiology. 2. Child development—physiology.
3. Cognition—in infancy & childhood. WL 335 D489]
QP385-5.D48 1988
152.3′35—dc19
DNLM/DLC 88-11269
for Library of Congress CIP

Contributors

DOROTHY M. ARAM, PhD, Rainbow Babies and Childrens Hospital, Cleveland, Ohio

CATHERINE T. BEST, PhD, Department of Psychology, Wesleyan University, Middletown, Connecticut

JACQUELINE C. BETZ, MA, Department of Psychology, Southern Illinois University at Carbondale, Carbondale, Illinois

ROGER A. BRUMBACK, MD, Division of Neuropathology, University of Oklahoma College of Medicine, Oklahoma City, Oklahoma

M. P. BRYDEN, PhD, Department of Psychology, University of Waterloo, Waterloo, Ontario, Canada

DOUGLAS F. CARLSON, MA, Department of Psychology, Michigan State University, East Lansing, Michigan

RICHARD J. DAVIDSON, PhD, Psychology Department, University of Wisconsin—Madison, Madison, Wisconsin

GERALDINE DAWSON, PhD, Child Clinical Psychology Program, Psychology Department, University of Washington, Seattle, Washington

VICTOR H. DENENBERG, PhD, Biobehavioral Sciences Graduate Degree Program and Department of Psychology, University of Connecticut—Storrs, Storrs, Connecticut

JOHN L. FISK, PhD, Henry Ford Hospital, Detroit, Michigan

NATHAN A. FOX, PhD, University of Maryland, College Park, Maryland

CHERYL GIBSON, PhD, E. C. Drury School for the Hearing Handicapped, Milton, Ontario, Canada

HAROLD W. GORDON, PhD, University of Pittsburgh School of Medicine, Pittsburgh, Pennsylvania

LAUREN JULIUS HARRIS, PhD, Department of Psychology and Neuroscience Program, Michigan State University, East Lansing, Michigan

MERRILL HISCOCK, PhD, Division of Psychology, University of Saskatchewan, Saskatoon, Saskatchewan, Canada

JOHN R. KERSHNER, PhD, Department of Special Education, Ontario Institute for Studies in Education, University of Toronto, Toronto, Ontario

DEBRA L. KIGAR, RT, Department of Psychiatry, McMaster University, Hamilton, Ontario, Canada

MARCEL KINSBOURNE, MD, Department of Behavioral Neurology, Eunice Kennedy Shriver Center, Waltham, Massachusetts, and Harvard Medical School, Boston, Massachusetts

JACQUELINE LIEDERMAN, PhD, Psychology Department, Boston University, Boston, Massachusetts

DENNIS L. MOLFESE, PhD, Department of Psychology, Southern Illinois University at Carbondale, Carbondale, Illinois

CHARLES NETLEY, PhD, Department of Psychology, Hospital for Sick Children, Toronto, Ontario, Canada

JOHN E. OBRZUT, PhD, Department of Educational Psychology, College of Education, University of Arizona, Tucson, Arizona

DONNA L. ORSINI, Department of Neuropsychology, Neuropsychiatric Institute, University of California, Los Angeles, Los Angeles, California

BYRON P. ROURKE, PhD, Department of Psychology, University of Windsor, Windsor, Ontario, Canada

JOANNE ROVET, PhD, Department of Psychology, Hospital for Sick Children, Toronto, Ontario, Canada

PAUL SATZ, PhD, Department of Neuropsychology, Neuropsychiatric Institute, University of California, Los Angeles, Los Angeles, California

SIDNEY J. SEGALOWITZ, PhD, Department of Psychology, Brock University, St. Catherines, Ontario, Canada

HENRY V. SOPER, PhD, Department of Neuropsychology, Neuropsychiatric Institute, University of California, Los Angeles, Los Angeles, California

GERALD TURKEWITZ, PhD, Department of Psychology and Graduate Center, Hunter College of the City University of New York, New York, New York, and Department of Pediatrics and Psychiatry, Albert Einstein College of Medicine, New York, New York

SANDRA F. WITELSON, PhD, Department of Psychiatry, McMaster University, Hamilton, Ontario, Canada

HARRY A. WHITAKER, PhD, The Neuropsychiatric Institute, Fargo, North Dakota

Preface

This book developed out of a conference on the Developmental Implications of Brain Lateralization held at Brock University in St. Catherines, Ontario, Canada, during May 1985. The meeting was held in part to celebrate the tenth anniversary of the first Brock conference on Language Development and Neurological Theory (May 1975). The 1975 Brock conference was held at a time when scientists were just beginning to recognize the existence of some types of early cerebral specialization in young infants. The papers presented then, consequently, were directed toward assessing whether such hemispheric differences were in fact present from birth or whether they emerged at some later point in infancy. By the time of the second meeting in 1985, however, the notion of early hemispheric specialization appeared to be widely accepted. The organizers hoped that this more recent meeting would offer an opportunity to critically examine the research on early lateralization and its relationship to cognitive and linguistic processes that had emerged since the time of the first Brock University conference. In addition, the 1985 meeting focused on the implications of such early hemispheric differences for later development. The questions considered by the conferees included such issues as: Are such early hemispheric differences important for normal development? Can they be used to predict long-term outcomes or disabilities, such as delayed language development or learning disabilities? Do children with abnormal patterns of lateralization develop normally? These same questions are treated in the present book.

The book itself contains 22 chapters, divided into five sections: (1) early developmental factors related to lateralization, (2) lateralization in normal development, (3) handedness and intellectual development, (4) lateralization and atypical development, and (5) lateralization in learning-disabled children. The first two sections and, indeed, part of the third review and evaluate theory and research concerned with normal developing populations of infants and children, whereas the final two sections attempt to determine the relationship between cerebral lateralization and atypical forms of development. The majority of the chapters provide a critical review of various methodologies used to study early hemispheric differences such as hand preferences, anatomical asymmetries, electrophysiological measures, dichotic listening techniques, and behavioral asymmetries.

Although, as the chapters in the book relate, a great deal of research concerned with early hemispheric asymmetries has in fact occurred during the past 15 years, it is all too evident that our knowledge of both the early organization of the brain for cognitive processes and the relationship of such organization to other aspects of development is still incredibly limited. It is obvious that we have only begun to scratch the surface in this new and exciting area. We hope that this book will serve as an additional springboard for further inroads into this area.

Contents

PART ONE

Early Developmental Factors Related to Lateralization

Functional asymmetries demonstrated by the two cerebral hemispheres have long interested researchers and practitioners in developmental psychology and developmental medicine. Whereas the left hemisphere had been known to be specially associated with language functions and therefore presumably could be related to models of language acquisition and the learning of reading skills, it was Lenneberg's 1967 volume *Biological Foundations of Language* that outlined for developmental psychologists an explicit relationship between language acquisition, brain maturation, and hemisphere specialization. He articulated the position current at that time: that the hemispheres are not specialized for cognitive functioning at birth, but begin to become so in the early years, coincident with the child's acquisition of language. An implication of this position was also that the two hemispheres are equipotential for cognitive functions at birth and gradually become less so as they take on specialized functions. Damage to either hemisphere during this time was expected to have little long-lasting effect on the acquisition of language. Support for this view was based on studies involving clinical populations who had lost the use of one hemisphere during this time period (Basser, 1962). In one case, Lenneberg (1967) argued that such work demonstrated that "in roughly half of the children with brain lesions sustained during the first two years of life, the onset of speech development is somewhat delayed; however the other half of this population begins to speak at the usual time. This distribution is the same for children with left hemisphere lesions as with right ones" (p. 151). Given that one could not predict systematically, on the basis of Basser's data, which intact hemisphere was able to support language functions following damage to the other during the early years of infancy and childhood, the equipotential model appeared to be a reasonable conclusion. In retrospect, however, it seems equally clear that the original data on which this notion was based were critically flawed. It is also evident that the issue of early lateralization had never been systematically addressed up to this time.

Within the next decade, however, these hypotheses were tested on numerous occasions, so that by 1977 there was good reason to doubt the main premises that the newborn's hemispheres are not specialized (Segalowitz & Gruber, 1977). Documentation of the existence of such asymmetries in the human infant and the development of measures to do so (Molfese, 1983; Segalowitz, 1983; Witelson, 1977, 1985) have made it clear that the hemispheres are specialized at birth (perhaps even more so than in the adult; see Molfese & Betz, Chapter 6, this volume). Nor are they entirely equipotential for cognitive functions (see Aram & Whitaker, Chapter 15, this volume). Given this descriptive function of lateralization, we can now fairly ask whether there are serious developmental implications of brain lateralization.

We have divided the book into several sections to deal with the relationship between brain lateralization and normal development, and between brain lateralization and atypical development. In this first section, we focus on the implications of hemispheric specialization for our understanding of brain ontogenesis and phylogenesis. This relationship is a two-way street. The authors of the chapters in this first section have reviewed ideas and data on physiological maturation of the brain (Best, Chapter 1; Witelson & Kigar, Chapter 2); phylogenetic development (Denenberg, Chapter 3); psychobiological epigenesis (Turkewitz, Chapter 4); and how these ideas can help us understand the phenomenon of hemisphere specialization. By a similar token, however, we can see the phenomenon of lateralization as a vehicle for understanding more general issues in the functional maturation of the brain by targeting key issues: Best discusses the evidence for a maturational gradient (right to left); Witelson and Kigar present the data on corpus callosum growth rates and the implications of these data for cognitive development.

The next two chapters concern the interplay between brain development and early experience. Denenberg discusses the functional hemispheric asymmetries that exist in other animals and how these asymmetries are influenced by early stimulation. Turkewitz, taking this issue further, presents an explicit model of the ontogenesis of human brain lateralization. He suggests a way to understand how the timing of brain growth interacts with experience to produce the hemispheric specialization that is usually found. This speculative model minimizes the amount of information that needs to be genetically coded, and therefore begs fewer questions.

The presentations in these two chapters implicitly touch on a more general issue in developmental psychology. An often unstated assumption of those working in the field is that brain organization is a preordained affair, that somehow the pattern of left/right distribution of cognitive representation is coded genetically, thereby relegating individual differences to genetic analysis. This may stem somewhat from the prejudice many psychologists have that explicitly biological traits probably are linked tightly to explicitly biological origins. Where brain lateralization has been tested, however, it presents difficulty with this. For example, various genetic models have been devised for handedness (Levy-Nagylaki; Annett; McManus), yet animal research suggests that it is by no means clear that a solely genetic model is appropriate. For example, Collins (1985) reports that although individual mice show a very consistent paw preference, the full range of left to right preference is found in a pure genetic strain. Even selective breeding within paw-preference subgroups yields offspring demonstrating the entire range.

What does seem to be transferred through reproduction is the strength of asymmetry. Bryden (1987) finds similar results with humans: that strength of asymmetry but not direction is related between generations. Given the lack of cross-generational data for measures of hemispheric specialization, it is difficult to conclude whether we should expect that differences in brain organization are genetically coded. Should we attribute biological states, in the null hypothesis, to deterministic genetic sources? Some might claim, for example, that biological epigenetic models are necessarily of the deterministic type—that biological epigenesis does not permit probabilistic influences, and therefore excludes any real role for the environment. But the history of developmental psychobiology from at least the 1960s is replete with complex interactions that argue for an environmental influence. The tuning of the visual system to experience is the best documented example (Greenough, 1986), but similar studies have been made of other sensory systems. To what extent we can extrapolate these notions to cortical representation of cognitive functions is yet to be seen (see Gibson, Chapter 22, this volume).

REFERENCES

Basser, L. S. (1962). Hemiplegia of early onset and the faculty of speech with special reference to the effects of hemispherectomy. *Brain, 85,* 427–460.

Bryden, M. P. (1987). Handedness and cerebral organization: Data from clinical and normal populations. In D. Ottoson (Ed.), *Duality and unity of the brain* (pp. 55–70). Houndmills, England: MacMillan.

Collins, R. L. (1985). On the inheritance of direction and degree of asymmetry. In S. D. Glick (Ed.), *Cerebral lateralization in nonhuman species* (pp. 41–71). New York: Academic Press.

Greenough, W. T. (1986). What's special about development? Thoughts on the bases of experience-sensitive synaptic plasticity. In W. T. Greenough & J. M. Juraska (Eds.), *Developmental neuropsychology* (pp. 387–408). New York: Academic Press.

Lenneberg, E. (1967). *Biological foundations of language.* New York: Wiley.

Molfese, D. L. (1983). Event related potentials and language processes. In A. W. K. Galliard & W. Ritter (Eds.), *Tutorials in ERP research—Endogenous components* (pp. 345–367). Amsterdam: North Holland–Elsevier.

Segalowitz, S. J. (1983). *Language function and brain organization.* New York: Academic Presss.

Segalowitz, S. J., & Gruber, F. A. (1977). *Language development and neurological theory.* New York: Academic Press.

Witelson, S. F. (1977). Early hemisphere specialization and interhemisphere plasticity. In S. J. Segalowitz & F. A. Gruber (Eds.), *Language development and neurological theory* (pp. 213–287). New York: Academic Press.

Witelson, S. F. (1985). On hemisphere specialization and cerebral plasticity from birth: Mark II. In C. T. Best (Ed.), *Hemispheric specialization and collaboration in the child* (pp. 33–85). New York: Academic Press.

1

The Emergence of Cerebral Asymmetries in Early Human Development: A Literature Review and a Neuroembryological Model

CATHERINE T. BEST
Wesleyan University

Ever since Broca's century-old discovery of cerebral asymmetries in human perceptual–cognitive functions, there has been speculation about the developmental emergence of those asymmetries. The basic question has been: Do the asymmetries first appear only at some point after birth, starting from an initial state of bilateral equivalence or symmetry at birth, or are the hemispheres instead functionally asymmetrical from the start? A related question is whether functional asymmetries can be traced to some lateral bias in the structural development of the hemispheres, such that one hemisphere matures in advance of the other. Thus, the term "emergence" in the title of this chapter might refer either to functional asymmetries in infants or to the embryological development of the hemispheres. An underlying assumption of this chapter is that the ontogeny of functional asymmetries is influenced by an asymmetry in the formation and physical maturation of the cerebral hemispheres. Both issues will be addressed in the following discussion, beginning with a review of behavioral evidence for perceptual–cognitive asymmetries in early infancy, and ending with a proposed model for a lateralizing gradient in the neuroembryological emergence of the cerebral hemispheres during prenatal development.

As for the development of functional asymmetries, Broca (1865) himself speculated that language becomes lateralized to the left hemisphere during language development (see Bever, 1978). Later, Samuel Orton (1937) expanded on this concept of "developmental lateralization" in his influential theory that dyslexic children suffer from a failure to developmentally establish cerebral dominance for language. More recently, Lenneberg (1967) further detailed the model of developmental change in lateralization of functions, proposing a critical period for language development, and hence for the progressive establishment of left-hemisphere language dominance, during the period between 2 years and puberty. More important for the present discussion, however, his model explicitly assumed that the child's cerebral hemispheres are equal in their capability to acquire language—a trait referred to as "equipotentiality"—until at least 2 years of age. In fact, the focus on language in theoretical discussions of those times, to the exclusion of other cognitive functions, led to the reasoning that since infants have not yet acquired language, they should not show any hemispheric specialization. Implicit in the equipotentiality concept has been the notion that the infant's hemispheres show functional symmetry, or lack of behavioral differentiation.

Since the mid-1970s, however, evidence of functional cerebral asymmetries in young infants has indicated that the assumption of functional symmetry between the hemispheres in early development cannot be correct. Generally, this literature suggests a pattern of functional cerebral asymmetries by at least 2 to 3 months of age, and possibly even before full-term birth, that is analogous to the adult pattern of left-hemisphere superiority for language-related functions and right-hemisphere superiority for music and holistic perception of patterns and faces. The next part of the chapter will focus on perceptual–cognitive asymmetries in infants (for discussion of motoric asymmetries in infants, see Chapter 4 by Turkewitz, this volume), and particularly on behavioral evidence (electrophysiological data are presented in Chapter 6 by Molfese and Betz, this volume).

FUNCTIONAL ASYMMETRIES IN INFANTS

Before the specific findings are reviewed here, some preliminary qualifications are necessary. Up to this point, many questions about infant hemispheric specialization remain unanswered. It is not yet known, for example, whether infant asymmetries are fundamental responses to certain stimulus properties or classes, such as the physical characteristics of speech versus nonspeech, or whether, instead, they reflect different processing styles, such as feature-analysis versus holistic processing, as has been proposed for adults. In addition, the behavioral studies are actually quite few in number. Moreover, they have focused overwhelmingly on auditory asymmetries, particularly for human speech. This is due in part to a strong theoretical bias toward assessing language-related functions, but it is also due to pragmatic constraints. The dichotic listening procedure is more obviously amenable to infant research than are the lateralized behavioral measures of asymmetries in other modalities (e.g., the requirements of the visual split-field tachistoscopic technique are more difficult to adapt to infants).

Nonauditory Asymmetries

Thus far only two behavioral studies of infant cognitive–perceptual asymmetries in other, nonauditory modalities have been conducted, both of which assessed right-hemisphere advantages for pattern recognition. One of these was inconclusive regarding functional asymmetries during infancy; the other is not yet published. In the first, Rose (1984) tested 1-, 2-, and 3-year-olds for a left-hand advantage (right-hemisphere superiority) in haptic perception of shapes. After blind, unimanual palpation of a three-dimensional nonsense shape, children were tested for cross-modal shape recognition on a visual preference task in which they saw a picture of the palpated object presented alongside a picture of a different-shaped object. Although all children showed preferences for the novel figure, and hence recognition memory for the palpated object, only the 2- and 3-year-olds showed a left-hand/right-hemisphere superiority. The 1-year-olds—the only infants in the study—failed to show a right-hemisphere advantage. As Rose argues, however, this cannot be taken as evidence for a lack of infant right-hemisphere specialization, because the visual test phase of the task involved bihemispheric, or nonlateralized, visual input. In fact, even for the older children the left-hand effects were rather small. Perhaps some other, more sensitive and completely lateralized test measure would detect tactile asymmetries in infants.

In the other nonauditory behavioral study, Witelson and Barrera (Witelson, 1981, personal communication) tested visual asymmetries in 3-month-olds. They presented the infants with side-by-side slides of two identical photographs, both of which were either of the infant's mother, or of a female stranger, or of a standard black-and-white checkerboard pattern. The infants showed a fixation-time preference for the left-side photo of the mother, as well as for the left-side checkerboard, suggesting greater activation of their right hemispheres. However, they did not show any side preference for the stranger. The authors' interpretation was that both mother and checkerboard constituted gestalt patterns to the infants, which they processed holistically, thus showing a right-hemisphere bias in activation. In contrast, the female stranger was not processed as a gestalt and thus not handled preferentially by the right hemisphere. This argument, at least with respect to the infants' responses to mother versus stranger, is consistent with developmental research on face recognition in children (Levine, 1985). Young children perceive unfamiliar faces in terms of salient features rather than holistically and show no hemispheric asymmetry for recognition of those faces. The same children, however, do perceive familiar faces holistically, as well as showing a right-hemisphere advantage for the familiar faces. Thus, the Witelson and Barrera results offer some suggestion of a right-hemisphere bias in holistic perception of faces (and patterns) by 3 months, which is compatible with the literature on visual asymmetries in adults. This suggestion, however, must be viewed as still tentative, given that it is based only on a single, unpublished finding.

Auditory Asymmetries

By comparison, the behavioral studies of auditory asymmetries have been more numerous, and have included assessments of both left- and right-hemisphere specialization in infants. The technique used is some modification of the dichotic listening procedure. In the first such study, reported at a conference held at Brock University in 1975, Anne Entus (1977) used a nonnutritive sucking measure with a dichotic habituation–dishabituation procedure. Two groups of infants, who averaged 2½ months in age, were tested for ear differences in discrimination either of musical notes played by different instruments, or of consonant differences in speech syllables. In the first phase of each test, the infants heard a rapidly repeated presentation of a dichotic pair of stimuli until they reached a criterion of habituation. At that point, the element in either the right or the left ear was changed to, respectively, a new music note or syllable, while the other ear continued to receive its original habituation stimulus. The infants in the speech condition showed a greater recovery of the sucking response when the syllable changed in the right ear (REA) than when it changed in the left, indicating left-hemisphere superiority. The music group showed the opposite pattern, a left-ear (LEA) or right-hemisphere advantage. However, Vargha-Khadem and Corballis (1979) subsequently failed to replicate with 2-month-olds the speech REA that Entus found, a point to which we will return later in the chapter. In this later study, the infants discriminated the speech syllable change equally well with both ears.

In a similar dichotic habituation study with 3-month-olds, Glanville, Best, and Levenson (1977) used the heart rate measure of a deceleratory orienting response, reflecting interested attention to a stimulus, in order to introduce a memory component to the task. Friedes (1977) has presented evidence that, in adults, memory retrieval is more strongly associated with dichotic ear asymmetries than is a simple input-processing dominance. Therefore, the intervals between presentations of the dichotic pairs in the Glanville *et al.* test were long enough ($M = 25$ sec) that the infants had to rely on short-term memory in order to learn the habituation pair and to recognize the stimulus change on the test trial. In each test block, the habituation pair was presented 9 times, and the stimulus change was then presented on the 10th and final trial. All infants received separate left- and right-ear discrimination test blocks each for speech syllables and for music notes. The results provided converging evidence with Entus's findings for an adultlike pattern among 3-month-olds of REA in response to speech syllable changes, and LEA in response to music changes (see Figure 1-1).

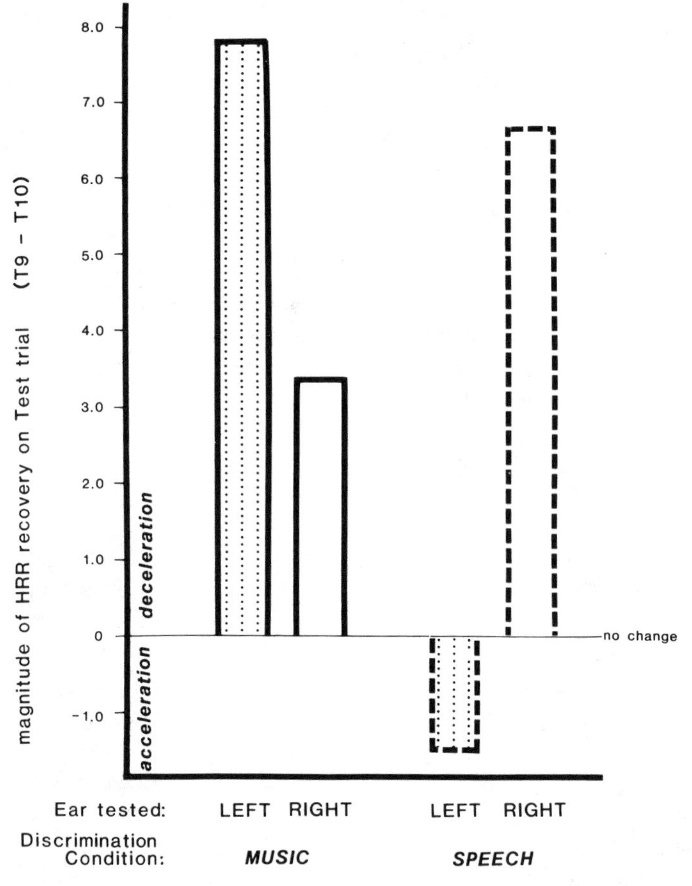

Figure 1-1. Ear differences in 3-month-olds' discrimination of speech syllables differing in initial consonant, and of music notes differing in instrument timbre. The task was a dichotic habituation–dishabituation task using heart rate deceleration as the response measure; represented here is the magnitude of dishabituation (cardiac deceleration) on the test trial (stimulus change in either right or left ear), relative to the cardiac response on the last habituation trial (trial 9). Redrawn from data reported in Glanville, Best, and Levenson (1977).

These first dichotic studies left several important questions unanswered, two of which were addressed by subsequent research with infants. First, there have been two attempts to obtain a better specification of the speech properties to which the infant's left hemisphere is preferentially responsive. Second, age changes in behavioral evidence of auditory cerebral asymmetries during infancy have been assessed.

THE BASIS OF LEFT-HEMISPHERE SPEECH SPECIALIZATION

For a more detailed understanding of the infant's left-hemisphere response to speech, Best (1978) used the dichotic heart rate habituation procedure to determine whether $3\frac{1}{2}$-month-olds show different patterns of ear asymmetries for vowel versus consonant discriminations. Several studies with adults had suggested that the right-ear speech perception advantage is greatest for consonant perception, whereas there is often a weaker or absent ear advantage for vowel perception (e.g., Darwin, 1971; Studdert-Kennedy & Shankweiler, 1970; Weiss & House, 1973). This pattern may be related to the fact that consonants

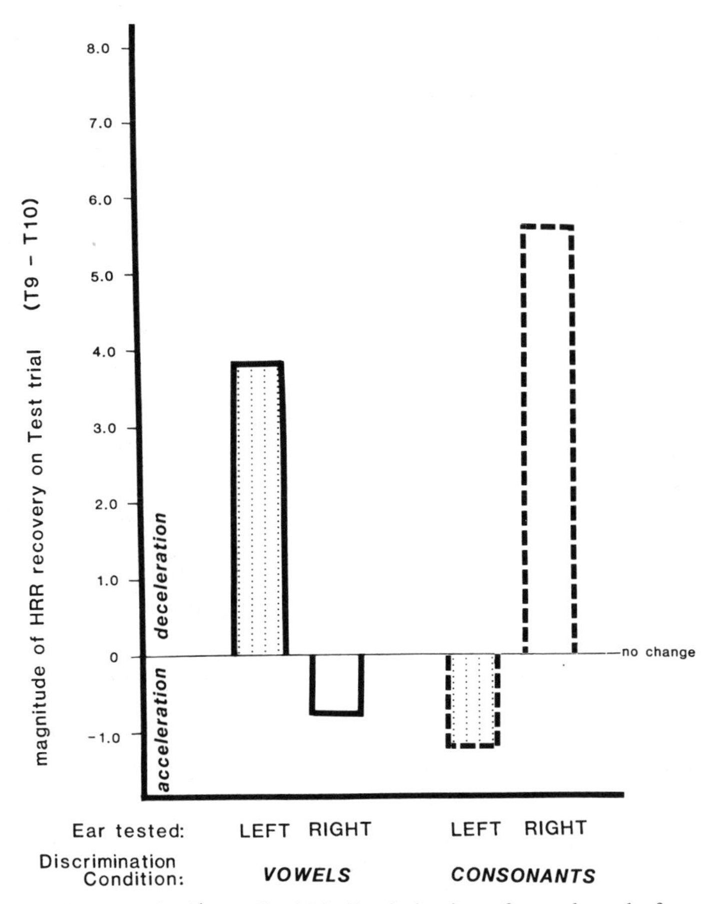

Figure 1-2. Ear differences in $3\frac{1}{2}$-month-olds' discrimination of vowels and of consonants in computer-synthesized syllables. The method and response measure are the same as described for Figure 1-1. Based on data presented in Best (1978).

involve rapidly changing acoustic properties, whereas vowels are associated with much more slowly changing, or even steady-state, acoustic properties (see Cutting, 1974; Schwartz & Tallal, 1980). Therefore, Best developed a set of computer-synthesized syllables that exaggerated the rapidly changing acoustic properties versus steady-state characteristics associated with consonants versus vowels. The results revealed a REA for discrimination among the exaggerated consonants, consistent both with the earlier infant studies and with adult findings. The infants, however, unlike adults, showed an LEA for steady-state vowel discrimination (see Figure 1-2).

These findings suggest that the infant's left hemisphere may be particularly responsive to rapidly changing acoustic information, whereas the right hemisphere is more responsive to steady-state spectral information. The vowel LEA is compatible with John Sidtis's (1980) findings of a right-hemisphere advantage in adults' perception of steady-state harmonic information. The lack of an adult ear advantage for vowels suggests that this steady-state information may be easily transferred across the corpus callosum; the left-ear advantage in infants may be due to the immaturity of their corpus callosa (see also Molfese, Freeman, & Palermo, 1975; Molfese & Molfese, 1985; Studdert-Kennedy & Shankweiler, 1980).

MacKain, Studdert-Kennedy, Spieker, and Stern (1983) further explored the nature of the infant's left-hemisphere specialization for speech perception, in a bimodal-matching study with 5- to 6-month-olds. The infants viewed two side-by-side synchronous videotapes of a woman repeating two different two-syllable nonsense words, while they simultaneously heard a synchronous audio recording (over a centrally located loudspeaker) that corresponded to one of the two video displays. Infants detected the cross-modal equivalence, as indicated by a looking preference for the film that matched the audio presentation, but only when the correct video was in the right-side video monitor. This finding implies selective left-hemisphere activation, and suggests a left-hemisphere specialization for perception of the common underlying articulatory pattern that produced the disparate information in the two sensory modalities.

Together, these two studies on cerebral asymmetries for the properties of speech suggest that the infant's left hemisphere may be specialized for recognizing articulatory patterns in speech, and particularly the rapid acoustic changes resulting from the dynamic articulatory gestures that produce consonant sounds. However, this still leaves open the question: Why the left hemisphere? One possibility is a lateralized gradient in the maturation of the two hemispheres.

LATERAL DIFFERENCES IN HEMISPHERE MATURATION?

If a lateralized developmental gradient exists, uncertainty still remains as to whether the asymmetry in speech perception would result from earlier or later development of the left hemisphere relative to the right. Broca (1865) proposed a left-to-right gradient to explain language lateralization (see Bever, 1978); Corballis and Morgan (1978) seconded the notion of a left–right gradient. However, Taylor (1969); Crowell, Jones, Kapuniai, and Nakagawa (1973); and Brown and Jaffe (1975) have argued for a right-to-left gradient, which is also suggested by recent embryological evidence that cortical fissures appear consistently earlier in the right than in the left fetal hemisphere (Dooling, Chi, & Gilles, 1983).

To test the possibility of early age changes in asymmetrical function, Best, Hoffman, and Glanville (1982) tested for ear asymmetries in memory-based discriminations of speech syllables versus music notes by 2-, 3-, and 4-month-old infants. The 3- and 4-month-olds replicated the earlier findings of a right-ear/left-hemisphere advantage for speech and a left-ear/right-hemisphere advantage for music. The 2-month-olds, however, showed only the LEA for music; they did not detect the speech syllable change in either ear (see Figure 1-3). These results suggest an increase in functional maturity of the left hemisphere sometime between 2 and 3 months of age, at least for auditory discriminations that depend on short-term memory capacities. Such a change in cortical maturity around 2 to 3 months of age is consistent with reports of widespread biobehavioral changes and maturation of cortical influences over behavior around that time (Emde & Robinson, 1979).

This finding may also help explain the negative report by Vargha-Khadem and Corballis (1979), which had failed to replicate Entus's (1977) findings of a speech REA in infants. Although their infant subjects discriminated the syllable change in both ears, discrimination under the rapid-stimulus presentation conditions used in the sucking habituation procedure clearly does not depend solely on cortical involvement, since Frances Graham and her colleagues (Graham, Leavitt, Strock, & Brown, 1978) have found similar speech discrimination in a 6-week-old anencephalic infant. The conclusion of Best *et al.* (1982) was that the speech-specialized function of the left hemisphere may be insufficiently mature at 2 months to control behavioral responses in a memory-dependent discrimination task. In contrast, the analogous right-hemisphere function appears sufficiently mature at that age to effect a LEA for memory-based music timbre discrimination, suggesting a right-to-left

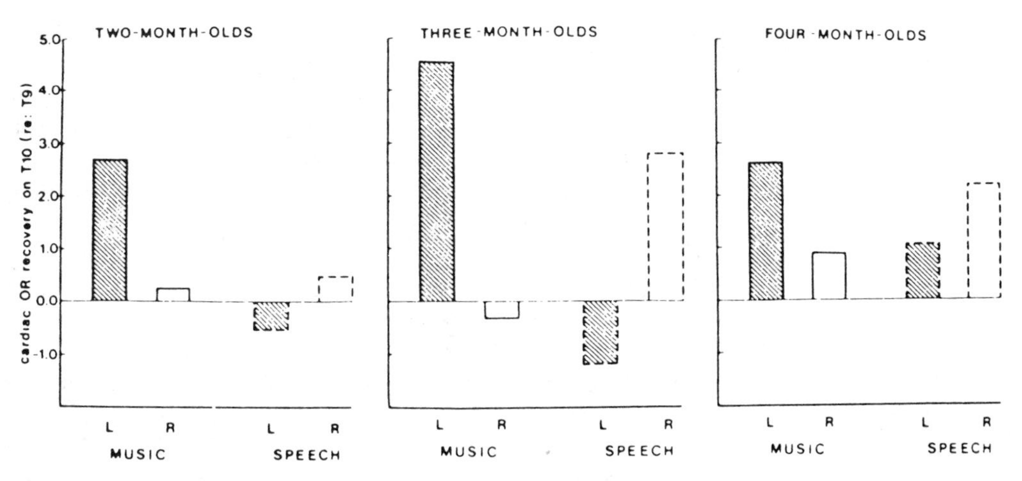

Figure 1-3. Age changes in ear differences for infants' discrimination of speech syllables and of musical timbre. Method and response measure are identical to the description of Figure 1-1. Reprinted with permission of the publisher from "Development of Infant Ear Asymmetries for Speech and Music" by C. T. Best, H. Hoffman, and B. B. Glanville, 1982, *Perception and Psychophysics, 31,* pp. 75–85. Copyright © 1982 by the Psychonomic Society.

gradient in the maturation of asymmetrical perceptual memory functions. This does not necessarily imply that cerebral lateralization itself develops out of an unlateralized substrate. Alternatively, cognitive and perceptual functions may mature developmentally at different rates, but within the context of a neural substrate that is already laterally specialized from the start (see Witelson, 1977, 1985; see also Kinsbourne, 1975).

If the latter view is correct, the question becomes: What is the source of this lateralized gradient in functional maturation? According to developmental biologists, morphologists, and particularly neuroembryologists, the patterns of embryological development are ultimately responsible for the structure and form of the adult organism, including the brain, at both the gross morphological level and the histological level. Given the basic neuropsychological assumption that variations in neuronal organization and development affect behavior and its development, then, fetal brain development should provide evidence of a lateralized developmental gradient. In the remainder of this chapter it will be argued that a right-to-left gradient in postnatal functional maturation parallels a similar gradient in the prenatal, embryologic development of the cerebral hemispheres.

PROPOSAL FOR A LATERALIZED GRADIENT IN NEUROEMBRYOLOGICAL DEVELOPMENT

Gross Morphological Asymmetries

The notion that morphological properties of the brain find their expression during embryogenesis can be traced back at least to the early neuroscientist Pernkopf (see Keller, 1942) and is consistent with general principles of contemporary theory in embryology and evolutionary biology. Thus, the patterns of morphological asymmetries found in adult brains should be attributable to embryological growth patterns. From a complementary perspective, we should be able to "read" adult asymmetries in brain structure as a record of the forces in embryological growth. Presented in the following pages is a working model of just this sort of interpretive view of the various structural asymmetries in the cerebral hemispheres that have been reported in the past 15 to 20 years.

The best known asymmetry found in the majority of right-handed adults' brains was first reported by Geschwind and Levitsky (1968) and was replicated and extended in numerous subsequent reports (e.g., Galaburda, 1984; Galaburda, LeMay, Kemper, & Geschwind, 1978; Galaburda, Sanides, & Geschwind, 1978). The left hemisphere shows a larger surface area of the planum temporale (see Figure 1-4), which incorporates the auditory association area known as Wernicke's area that is central to language comprehension. This asymmetry is found in the majority of infant (Witelson & Pallie, 1973) and fetal brains as well (Chi, Dooling, & Gilles, 1977; Wade, Clarke, & Hamm, 1975).

Another language-specialized area in the left hemisphere is Broca's area in the frontal lobe, encroaching on the Sylvian fissure. The size of this crucial speech production area is paradoxically smaller in the left hemisphere than in the right in the majority of both adult and fetal brains, if measured as the visible surface area, according to Wada, Clarke, and Hamm (1975). However, several reports suggested that this region is more deeply fissurated in the left hemisphere. Following up on this suggestion, Falzi and colleagues (Falzi, Perrone, & Vignolo, 1982) measured the cortical surface area in the regions corresponding to Broca's area, pars triangularis and pars opercularis, in both hemispheres, such that their measurements included the cortex buried inside the sulci. They found this anterior speech region to be larger on the left than the right in three-quarters of their cases, when "hidden cortex" inside the sulci was taken into account in this manner (see Figure 1-5), thus implicating greater fissuration on the left, a point to which we will later return.

Let us focus now on another set of morphological asymmetries reported by Marjorie LeMay (1976, 1977, 1984; LeMay & Geschwind, 1978, LeMay & Kido, 1978), which exist in the majority of adults, children, and fetuses, as well as in corresponding measurements of prehistoric human skulls (LeMay, 1976, 1984). The pattern is a wider and more protruding right frontal lobe, a characteristic referred to as right frontopetalia; there is a converse left-hemisphere bias in the posterior portion of the brain, where a left occipitopetalia (greater backward protrusion) is found along with a wider left occipital region. These patterns are illustrated in Figures 1-6, 1-7, 1-8, and 1-9. Notice that the left occipitopetalia is generally more striking than the right frontopetalia. These characteristics are reflected in gross volumetric measures of frontal and occipital regions (Weinberger, Luchins, Morihisa, & Wyatt, 1982; see Figure 1-10) and by corresponding asymmetries in the skull itself. As mentioned earlier, they are also evident in fetal brains (Figure 1-11) and skulls (Figure 1-12—note the positions of the bone plates before the fontanelles have closed).

MORPHOLOGIC ASYMMETRIES AS EVIDENCE OF A LATERALIZED NEUROEMBRYOLOGIC GRADIENT

The argument put forth in this chapter is that these morphological asymmetries can be read as a record of a right-to-left gradient in the embryological emergence of the cerebral hemispheres. This proposal depends on several considerations: First, the brain develops in a general anterior-to-posterior direction. Second, this general gradient is complicated by interaction with other developmental gradients, in the ventrodorsal and primary → secondary → tertiary dimensions.[1] Third, it assumes (on the basis of reasoning and some indirect evidence which will be presented later) that earlier onset in the formation and growth of a given region of telencephalon will strongly tend to result in a larger volume of that region (e.g., greater hemispheric width, but not necessarily a larger measurement of cortical surface area of gray matter), relative to the homologous contralateral region. This hypothesis

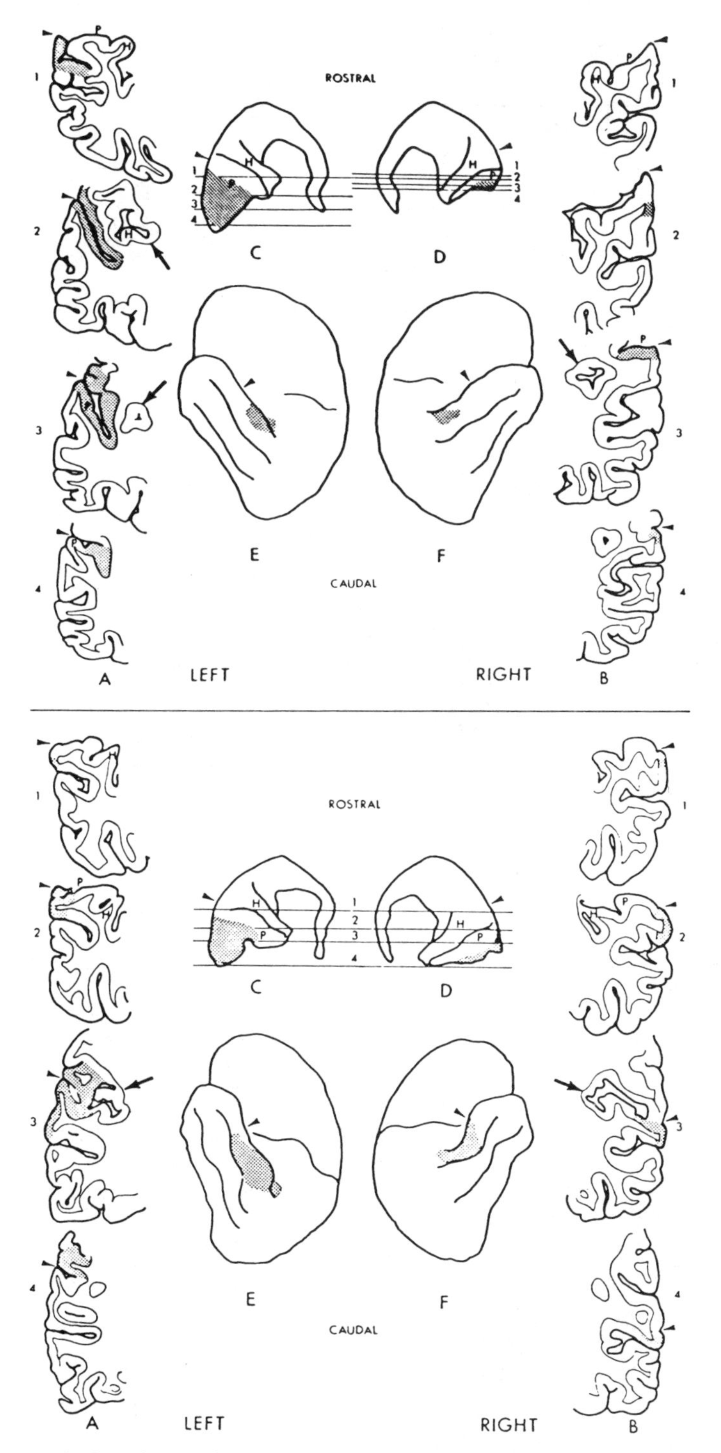

Figure 1-4. Anatomical analyses of two brains are shown here, illustrating the left-hemisphere bias in size of planum temporale. Coronal sections are shown in columns A and B; superior temporal plana in C and D showing planum temporale (P) and Heschl's gyrus (H); and lateral surfaces of brain showing area Tpt (shaded) in E and F. Arrowheads point to Sylvian fissures. Note large asymmetry in Tpt and P. Also note buried temporal cortex on coronal sections (arrows). Reprinted with permission of the senior author and publisher from "Cytoarchitectonic Left–Right Asymmetries in the Temporal Speech Region" by A. M. Galaburda, F. Sanides, and N. Geschwind, 1978, *Archives of Neurology, 35,* pp. 812–817. Copyright © 1978 by the American Medical Association.

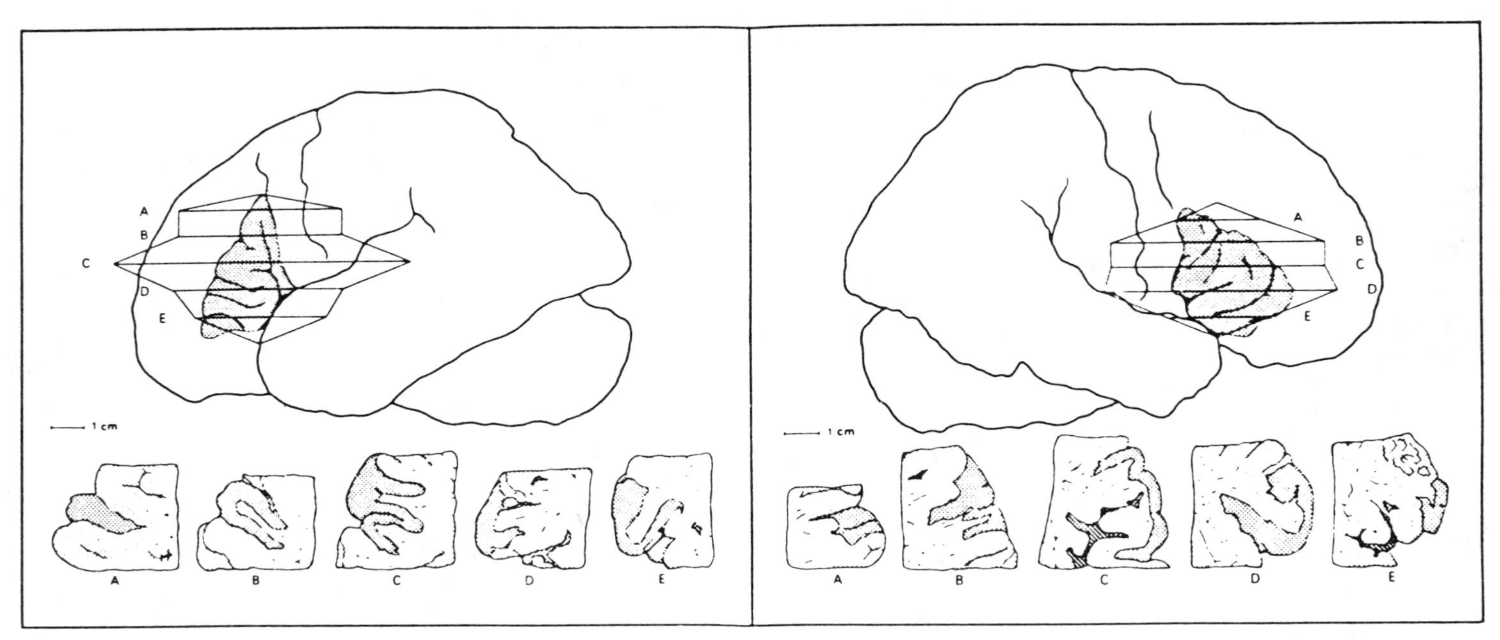

Figure 1-5. "Entire" anterior speech region (defined as pars opercularis and pars triangularis of the third frontal convolution), and its right-hemisphere homologue, shown here superimposed within the polygons on the surface of both hemispheres. The figure illustrates one of the 12 right-handed cases reported in Falzi, Perrone, and Vignolo (1982). The authors measured both the extrasulcal and intrasulcal cortex of these regions (the polygons superimposed on the hemispheres show the sections made in order to measure intrasulcal cortex). There was more *intra*sulcal cortex found in the left hemisphere in three-quarters of their cases, indicating greater fissuration on the left than on the right hemisphere. Reprinted with permission of the authors and publisher from "Right–Left Asymmetry in Anterior Speech Region" by G. Falzi, P. Perrone, and L. A. Vignolo, 1982, *Archives of Neurology, 39,* pp. 239–240. Copyright © 1982 by the American Medical Association.

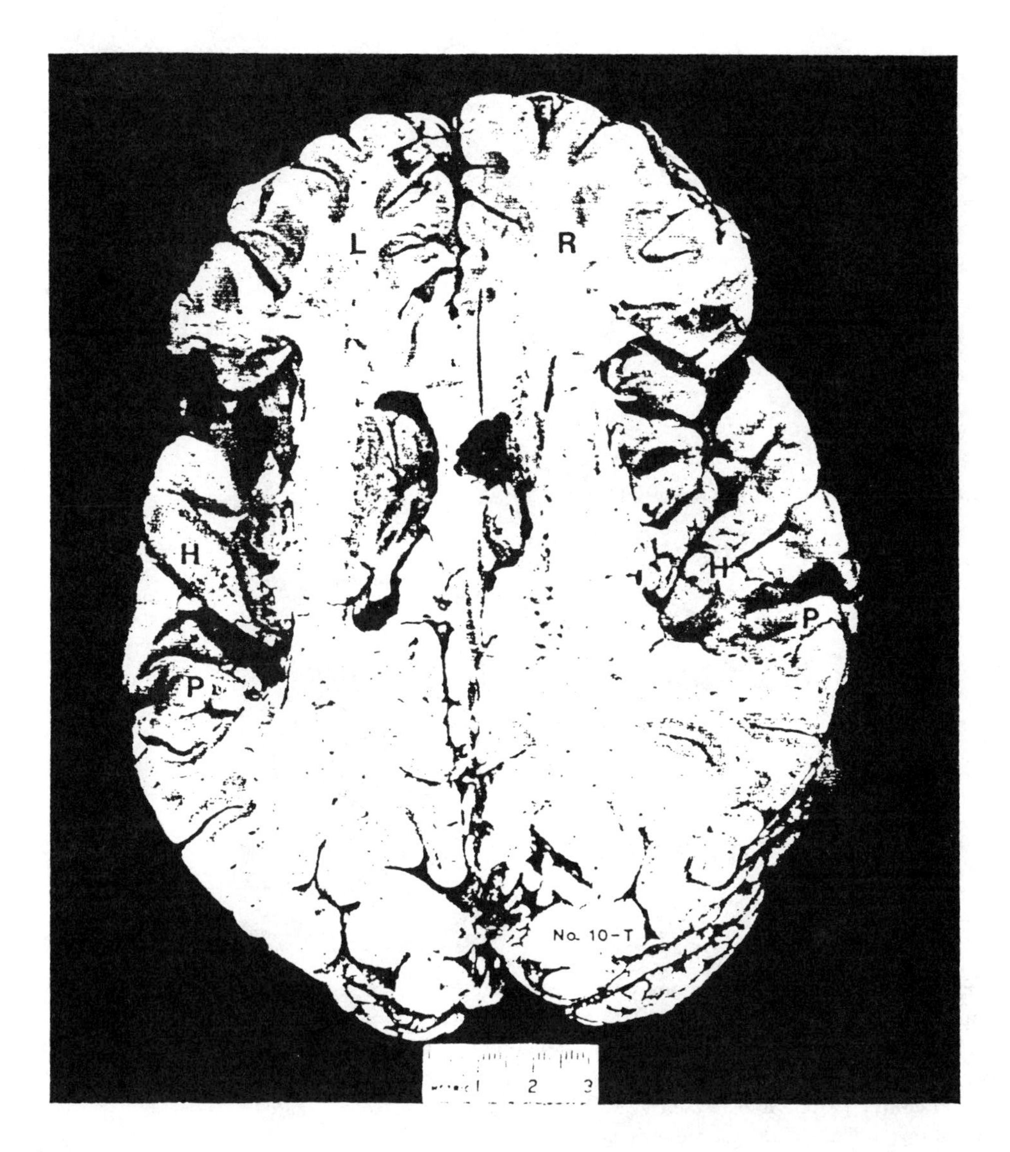

Figure 1-6. Horizontal section of an adult brain, exposing the plana temporale (P) and Heschl's gyri (H). Note both the larger planum on the left, and the right frontopetalia and left occipitopetalia. Reprinted with permission of the publisher from "Early Hemispheric Specialization and Interhemispheric Plasticity: An Empirical and Theoretical Review" by S. F. Witelson, 1977, *Annals of the New York Academy of Sciences, 299,* pp. 328–354. Copyright © 1977 by the New York Academy of Sciences.

of a right-to-left growth gradient is consistent with recent evidence that in fetal development, the major (primary-region) fissures appear 1 to 2 weeks earlier on the right hemisphere than on the left (Dooling, Chi, & Gilles, 1983).

The current proposal differs in one crucial respect from earlier proposals of a right-to-left or left-to-right gradient in brain growth. The earlier models assumed or implied that the earlier-maturing hemisphere would show advanced development over the other hemi-

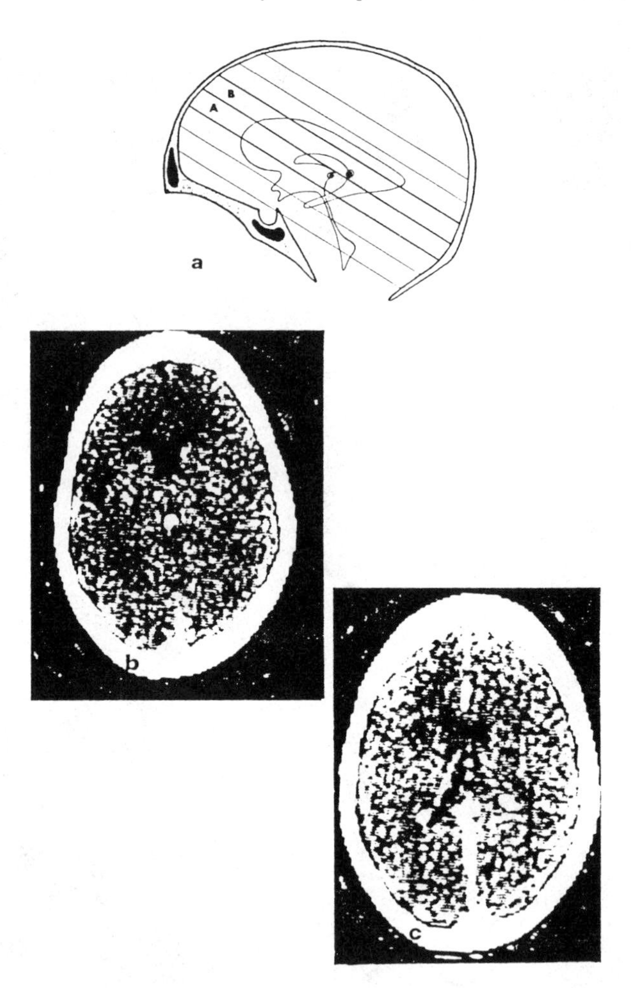

Figure 1-7. (a) Diagram of sections taken through the brain during routine examination by X-ray computerized axial tomography (CT). (b) CT scan though section A. (c) CT scan though section B. Note the left occipitopetalia and wider right frontal region. Reprinted with permission of the publisher from "Morphological Cerebral Asymmetries of Modern Man, Fossil Man, and Nonhuman Primate" by M. LeMay, 1976, *Annals of the New York Academy of Sciences, 280,* pp. 349–366. Copyright © 1976 by the New York Academy of Sciences.

sphere *throughout its extent.* If we combined that assumption with the assumption stated in the previous paragraph that there should be greater volume for earlier-emerging regions, the resulting prediction would be that the earlier-emerging hemisphere should end up larger overall, which is simply not the case. In fact, the simple-minded lateral gradients of earlier models would have to posit some sort of post hoc explanation (like Ptolemy's planetary epicycles) for the fact of larger right-hemisphere volume in the frontal regions but larger left-hemisphere volume in the posterior regions.

The present proposal refers to a dynamic, developmental gradient in the lateral right-to-left axis of the embryo; that is, it refers to a shift over time from right to left. The proposal also takes into account the fact that there are growth gradients along the other main axes of embryologic development—that is, that emergence of the hemispheres takes place *over time in three-dimensional space.* The right-to-left gradient is only one of several

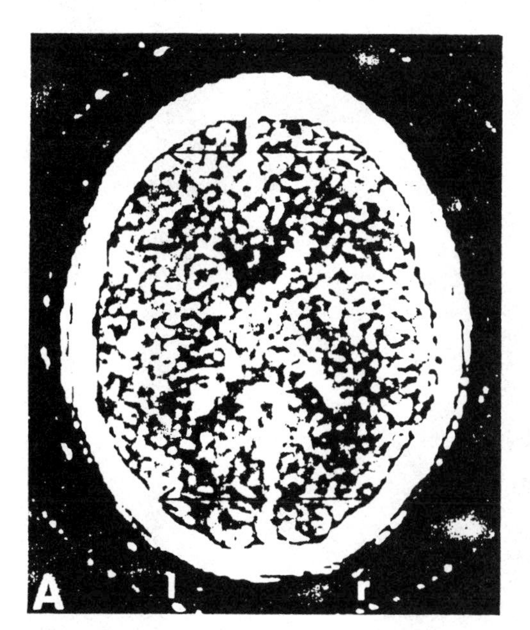

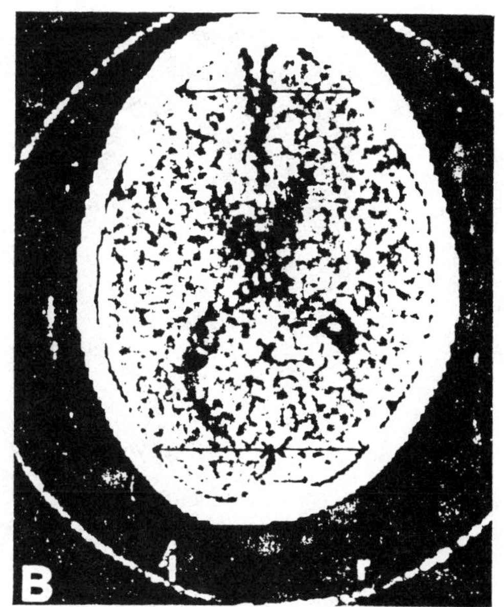

Figure 1-8. CT scans. The central arrows mark the interhemispheric region. Note the wider right frontal and left posterior parietal-occcipital areas. (a) Note the slight left occipitopetalia. (b) Note the left occipitopetalia and slight right frontopetalia (patient B has slightly enlarged ventricles). Reprinted with permission of the publisher from "Asymmetries of the Human Cerebral Hemispheres" by M. LeMay and N. Geschwind, 1978, in *Language Acquisition and Language Breakdown,* edited by A. Caramazza and E. B. Zurif, Baltimore, MD: Johns Hopkins University Press. Copyright © 1978 by Johns Hopkins University Press.

axial growth gradients, and its influence on morphological asymmetries can only be understood in the context of the other gradients. In other words, we need to conceptualize a *growth vector* cutting through at least three dimensions over time; this vector represents a *wave of leading growth activity*. There are actually three other developmental gradients that should be accounted for in this hypothesized growth vector (see Figure 1-13 for general reference on human fetal brain growth). The anterosposterior gradient refers to the general direction of growth from the frontal region toward the occipital region (e.g., Gilles, Leviton, & Dooling, 1983). This gradient, however, is complicated by a growth gradient that moves in the following direction: from primary motor and sensory zones to secondary association areas, and finally to tertiary association zones. This is important to keep in mind, because although the motor and premotor zones of the frontal lobe are early-emerging, the forward extension of the *pre*frontal area is one of the last developments of the hemispheres, and is a tertiary association area (e.g., Rabinowicz, 1979; Yakovlev & Lecours, 1967). The third developmental gradient to consider is the ventrodorsal gradient (Jacobson, 1978), from basal regions toward upper or superior regions. In hemispheric development, however, the ventrodorsal gradient is distorted by the fact that the hemispheres develop radially around the core of the basal ganglia and the insula (considered to be the basal or floor region of the hemisphere), moving in an inverted C-shaped direction, folding down and under around the back of the head and then turning forward to form, respectively, the occipital and temporal poles.

The resulting prediction of a three-dimensional growth vector starts with an earlier

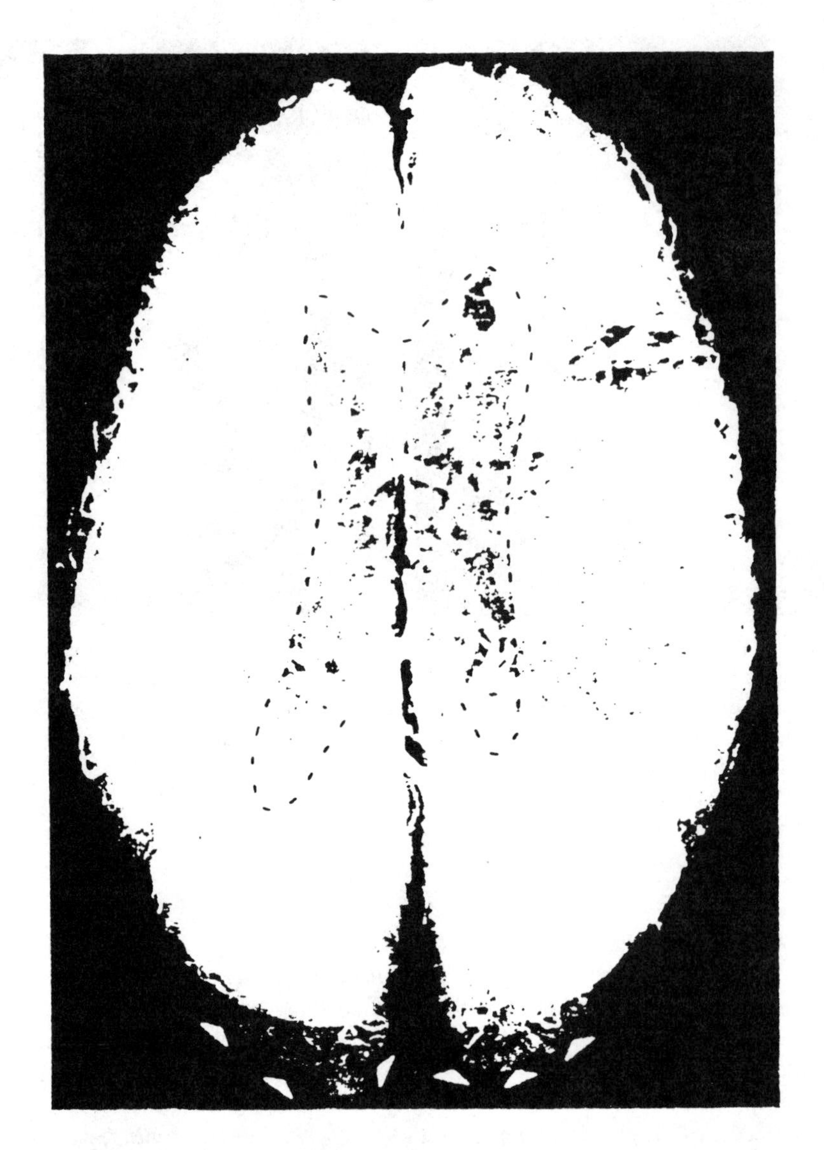

Figure 1-9. X-ray of a brain in which the blood vessels were injected with an opaque substance post-mortem. The tips of the occipital lobes are shown by white arrowheads. The ventricular outlines are shown by interrupted dark lines. The frontal and central portions of the right hemisphere are wider than those of the left. Note also the right frontopetalia and left occipitopetalia. Reprinted with permission of the publisher from "Morphological Cerebral Asymmetries of Modern Man, Fossil Man, and Nonhuman Primate" by M. LeMay, 1976, *Annals of the New York Academy of Sciences, 280,* pp. 349–366. Copyright © 1976 by the New York Academy of Sciences.

emergence of right primary motor (and premotor) and sensory regions that, at least initially, lie more frontal and ventral. With concurrent developmental shifts along all gradients, the advancing wave of the growth vector would then proceed toward *earlier* emergence of the *left* side for tertiary association regions (including Wernicke's area) that lie more dorsal and posterior (e.g., superior parietal), again at least initially (but recall the

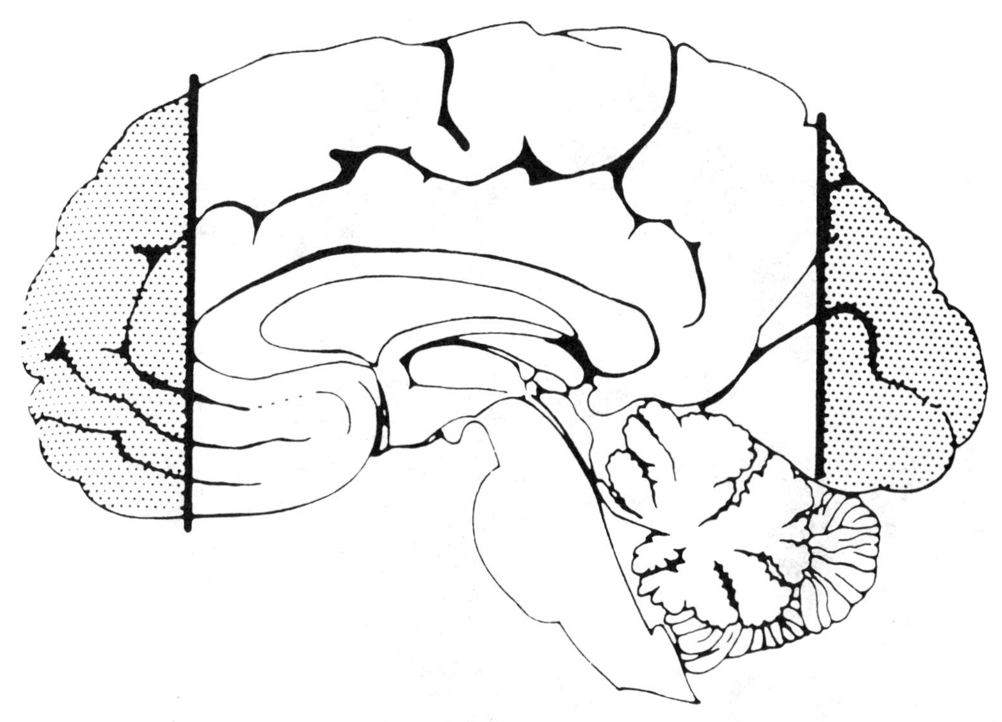

Figure 1-10. Sagittal section of the adult brain. Stipled areas were measured volumetically. The anterior region was larger on the right, and the posterior region was larger on the left, in the majority of brains studied (taken from the Yakovlev collection). Reprinted with permission of the publisher from "Asymmetrical Volumes of the Right and Left Frontal and Occipital Regions of the Human Brain" by D. R. Weinberger, D. J. Luchins, J. Morihisa, and R. J. Wyatt, 1982, *Annals of Neurology, 11,* pp. 97–100. Copyright © 1982 by Little, Brown and Company.

late and presumed leftward bias in protrusion of prefrontal regions). At some point midway between these extremes, growth should reach equilibrium between the two sides (possibly in secondary association areas).

The effect of this growth vector is a counterclockwise torque evident in the shape of the developing as well as the adult brain. This can only be illustrated here in two dimensions at a time. Figure 1-14 shows a brain viewed from above (from LeMay, 1976), to illustrate the combined influences of the anteroposterior and right–left gradients, producing a counterclockwise torque, as though some force had molded the brain with a fore-to-aft twist on the left, concurrent with an opposing twist on the right. The counterclockwise torque resulting from the combined effects of the ventrodorsal and right–left gradients is seen in coronal views of fetal brains (from Dooling, Chi, & Gilles, *1983*), as shown in Figure 1-15 (easiest to view in the 34-week brain at top).

The overall effect on the hemispheres is as though some force had twisted the left hemisphere rearward and dorsal, while twisting the right hemisphere forward and ventral. LeMay's (1984) observations of asymmetries in the positions and angles of the central (Rolandic) fissure and the Sylvian fissure are consistent with this image: The Rolandic fissure appears farther forward (and tilted more vertically) on the right hemisphere, even in fetal brains, whereas the Sylvian fissure slants more horizontally (i.e., lower) on the left, with a lower and more posterior endpoint (Sylvian point). The right Sylvian fissure angles more sharply upward and has a more anterior endpoint.

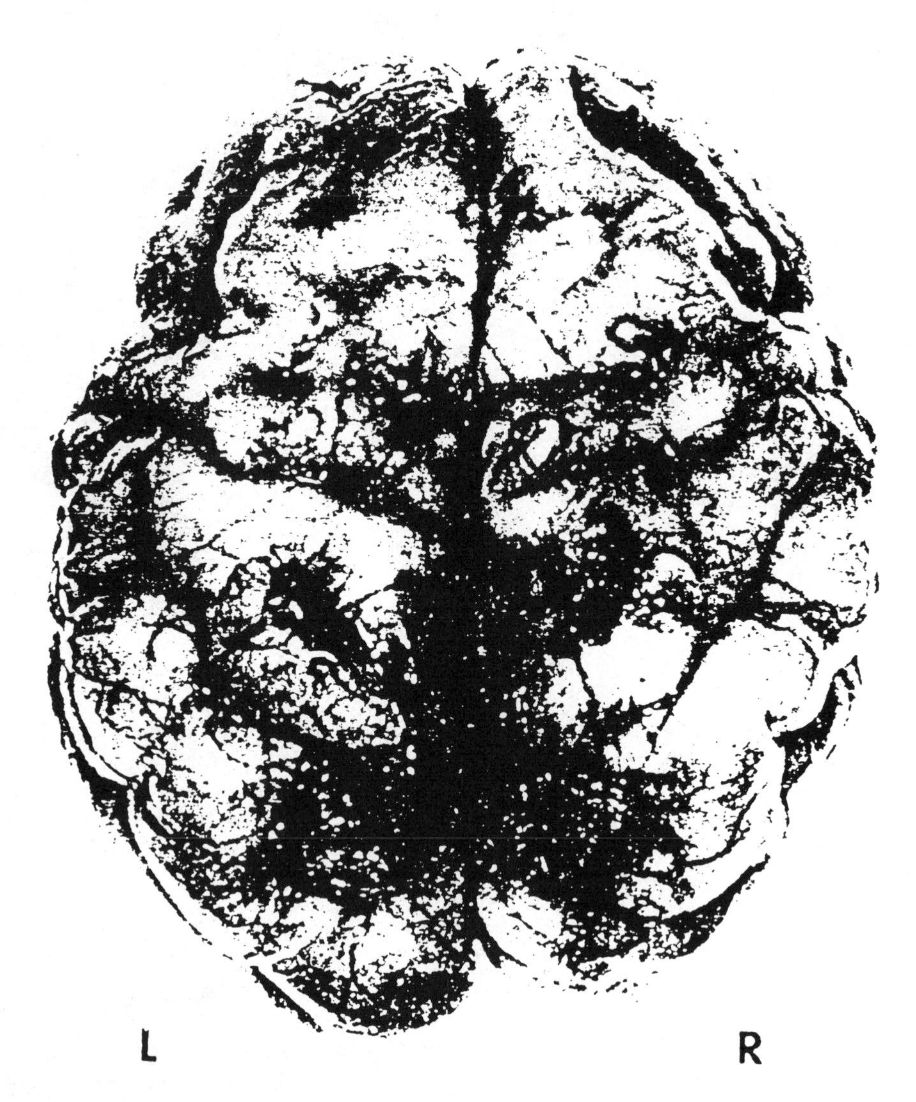

Figure 1-11. Photograph of superior surface of a 32-week-old fetal brain showing a slight right frontopetalia and a more striking left occipitopetalia. Reprinted with permission of the publisher from "Asymmetries of the Human Cerebral Hemispheres" by M. LeMay and N. Geschwind, 1978, in *Language Acquisition and Language Breakdown,* edited by A. Caramazza and E. B. Zurif, Baltimore, MD: Johns Hopkins University Press. Copyright © 1978 by Johns Hopkins University Press.

This model of embryological hemisphere development leads to several predictions. First, the gross morphological effect of earlier-emerging right frontal-motor regions may become attenuated by the later, *left*-biased growth of the tertiary association cortex in the prefrontal region. This would contrast with the convergence of the left-side bias for posterior regions and the left-side bias in the growth of the posterior tertiary association areas. The result should be a more striking left occipitopetalia than right frontopetalia, at least in adult brains. LeMay's (1976) data are in agreement with this pattern. Moreover, since the left-biased tertiary association areas are late to emerge in development, we should expect

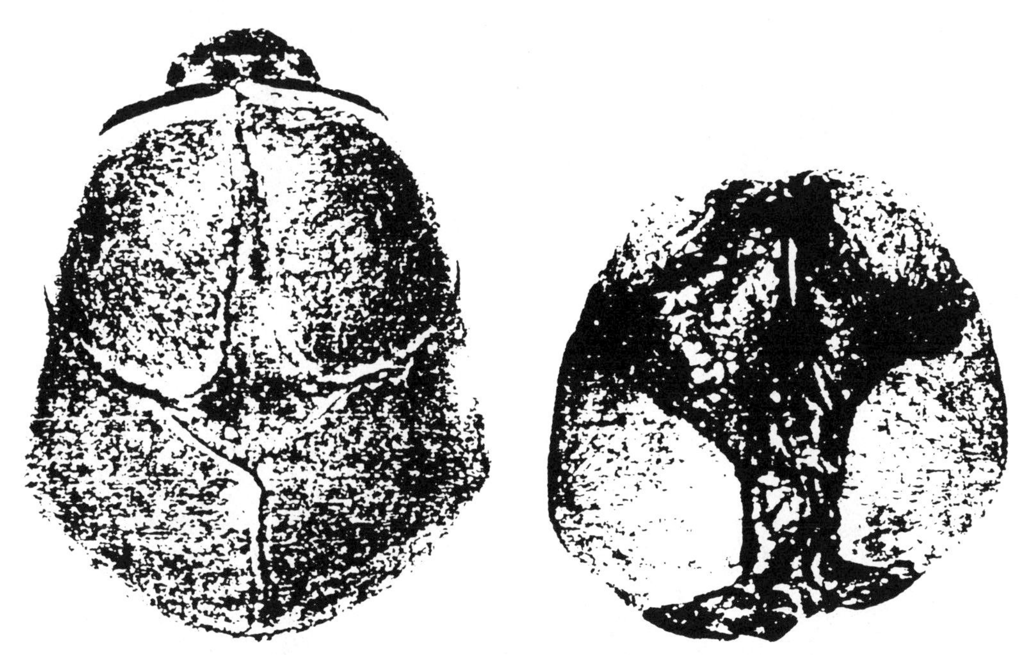

Figure 1-12. (a) Fetal skull. The bone over the right frontal region and the coronal suture, forehead, and lower rim of the orbit are farther forward than on the left side. The vault extends slightly more posteriorly on the left. (b) Upper surface of the skull of a young fetus. The fetus probably had hydrocephalus, but again note the forward position of the right frontal region, the posterior extension of the left hemisphere beyond the right, and the positions of the bony islands of the developing vault. Reprinted with permission of the publisher from "Radiological, Developmental, and Fossil Asymmetries" by M. LeMay, 1984, in *Cerebral Dominance: The Biological Foundations,* edited by N. Geschwind and A. M. Galaburda, Cambridge, MA: Harvard University Press. Copyright © 1984 by Harvard University Press.

to see *greater* evidence of right frontopetalia in fetuses than in adults, but *lesser* left occipitopetalia in fetuses than adults. Again, LeMay's data (1977) are in accord with these predictions. Also in accord is the Wada *et al.* (1975) finding of greater left-side bias in planum temporale among adult brains than among fetuses.

Another prediction is for a left-side bias in earlier emergence of tertiary sulci and gyri, in the tertiary association regions of prefrontal and posterior cortex. There are no data available on this possibility, because only primary sulci have been carefully mapped out on left versus right hemispheres in this manner (see Gilles, Leviton, & Dooling, 1983). In fact, the earlier right hemisphere appearance of fissures on the superior temporal surface actually refers to the formation of the transverse (Heschl's) gyrus, or primary auditory cortex, and not to the formation of Wernicke's association area (a tertiary area) itself (Dooling, Chi, & Gilles, 1983).

Effect of the Growth Vector on Neuronal Organization

The model also carries implications for asymmetries in neuronal organization of cortical areas, and hence for functional development and plasticity of the various regions on the two sides. The impact of the growth vector on neuronal organization must be understood

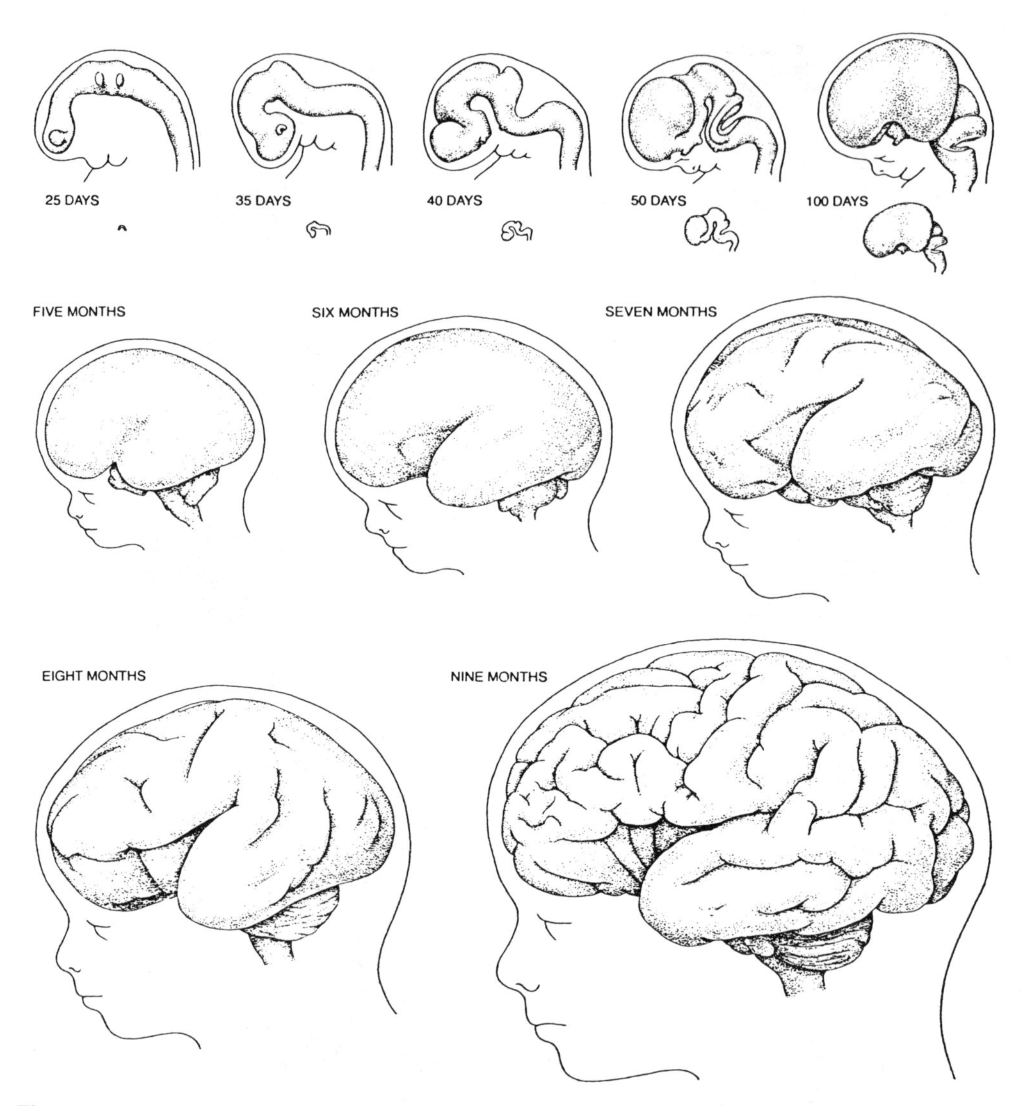

Figure 1-13. Developing human brain, seen from the left side in a succession of embryonic and fetal stages. The illustrations for the bottom two rows are approximately four-fifths life size, and drawn to scale. Those in the top row are enlarged to show structural details; the insets show four-fifths life size scale. Reprinted with permission of the publisher from "The Development of the Brain" by M. W. Cowan, 1979, *Scientific American, 241,* pp. 112–133. Copyright © 1979 by Scientific American, Inc. All rights reserved.

in the context of the sequential development of the six layers of neocortex and their differing contributions to the development of cortical fissuration and gyration, that is, the development of cortical folding. The five cortical layers that contain actual cell bodies of neurons develop in an inside-out sequence (Figure 1-16), with the cells of layer 6, the deepest inner layer, reaching their target positions and developing dendritic and axonal connections earliest (e.g., Rakic, 1980). The earliest-developing layers, 5 and 6, contain primarily efferent cells projecting to regions outside of cortex per se, and so give rise to long, myelinated axons, that is, subcortical white matter. Layer 4 is also directly associated with

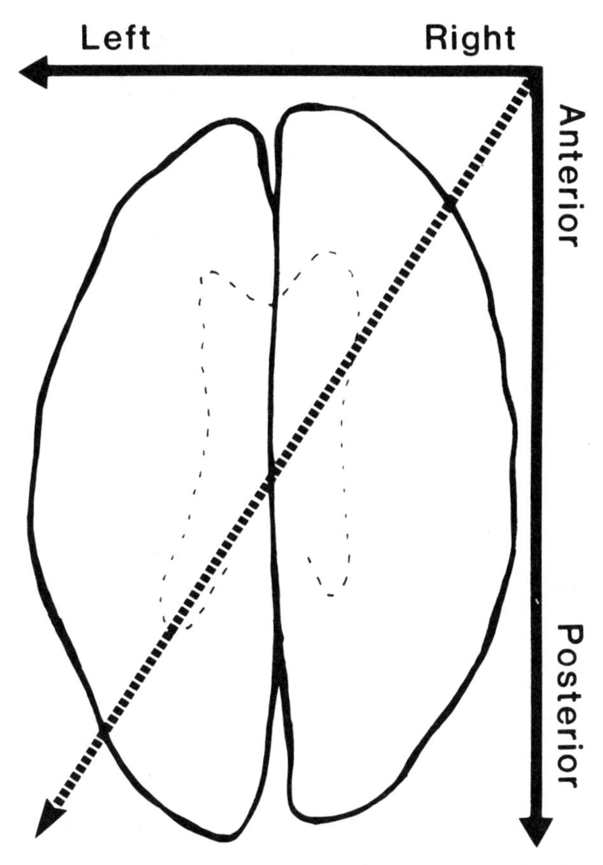

Figure 1-14. Schematic diagram of the proposed growth vector, proceeding from the right anterior to the left posterior region of the hemispheres. This diagram is a simplification of the vector, in that it shows only the left–right and anterior–posterior dimensions (it omits the primary → secondary → tertiary dimension and the ventral–dorsal dimension).

subcortical white matter, because in most regions of cortex it is the layer that receives initial, primary input from afferents to cortex. That is, its cells synapse with incoming long, myelinated axons that arise largely from subcortical areas or from other, relatively distant cortical regions. Thus, the lower layers 4, 5, and 6 of cortex contribute disproportionately to the "white matter" side of regional measurements of ratios of gray matter (aggregated neural cell bodies and short, unmyelinated axons within the cortical mantle itself) to white matter (subcortical myelinated axon bundles) (e.g., Gur *et al.,* 1980; Meyer *et al.,* 1978; McHenry *et al.,* 1978). For those areas with relatively higher proportions of subcortical white matter (low gray/white ratio), there should be a tendency toward greater width and/or volume than in areas with a higher gray/white ratio, given that white matter makes up more of the bulk of the width and volume of the hemispheres than does cortical gray matter.

Conversely, the cells of the most superficial cellular layer, layer 2, form latest. This latest-developing layer contains neurons that make predominantly local connections with

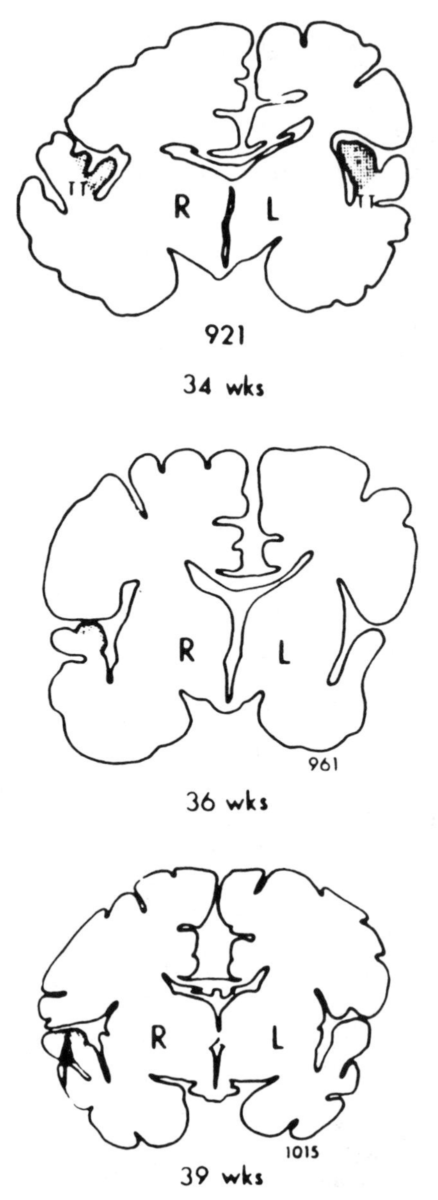

Figure 1-15. Tracings of photographs of sections in frontal plane of representative fetal brains of different gestational ages. Reprinted with permission of the publisher from *The Developing Human Brain* by F. H. Gilles, A. Leviton, and E. C. Dooling, 1983, Boston: John Wright, PSG. Copyright © 1983 by John Wright, PSG, Inc.

other cells lying within the nearby cortical layers. That is, it does not contribute substantially to subcortical white matter, and thereby contributes relatively more to cortical gray matter. Layer 3, which is next to last in development, also contributes more to gray matter than to subcortical white matter, in that its cells make mostly intracortical connections, including connections with the contralateral hemisphere via the corpus callosum. Thus, layers 2 and 3 contribute disproportionately to the gray matter side of the gray/white ratio. Furthermore, the late-developing, superficial layer 2 is primarily responsible for the process

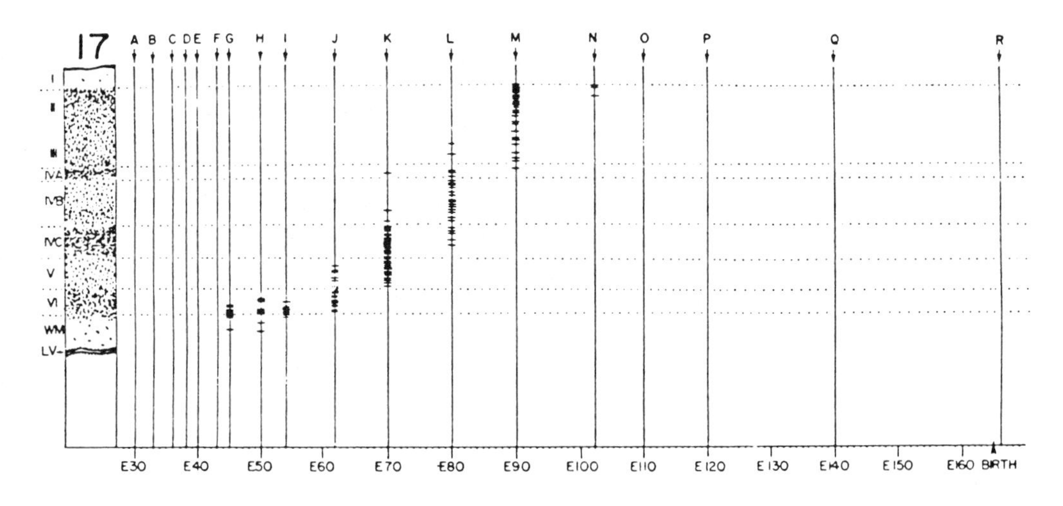

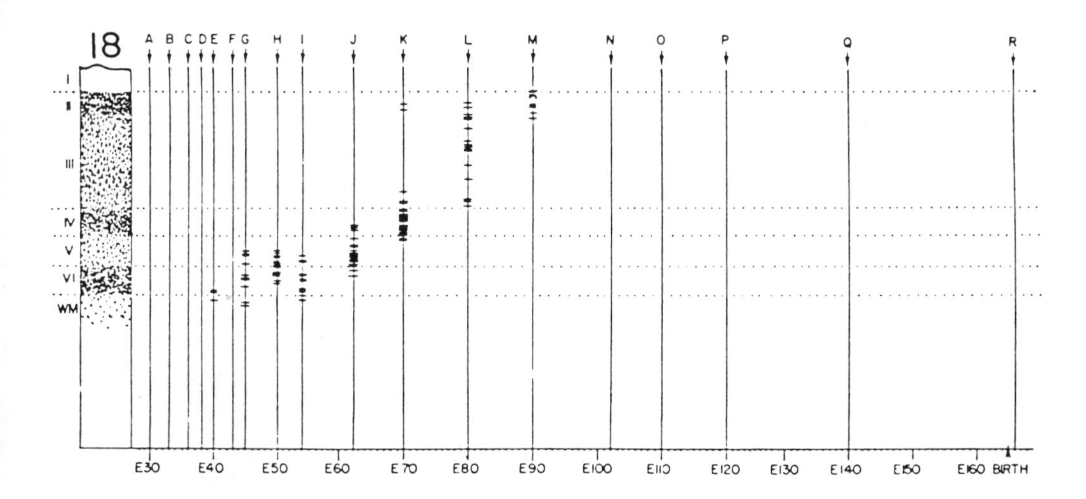

Figure 1-16. Diagrammatic representation of heavily labeled neurons in the visual cortex of juvenile monkeys that had been injected with [^{3}H]-TdR at selected embryonic days. The top picture shows Brodman's area 17, and the bottom shows area 18. On the left of each diagram is a drawing of cortex sections with cresyl-violet staining with Brodman's layers indicated in roman numerals. WM: white matter; LV: lateral ventricles. Embryonic days (E) are shown on the *X* axis, starting with the end of the first fetal month (E27) and ending at term (E165). The vertical lines represent the embryonic days on which subsets of the animals received a pulse of [^{3}H]-TdR. On each vertical line, short vertical markers indicate the positions of all heavily labeled neurons. Since [^{3}H]-TdR labels the cells undergoing mitosis at the time of injection, these diagrams indicate that cortex is built in inside-out order, with layer VI neurons generated earliest and layer II neurons latest. Reprinted with permission of the publisher from "Developmental Events Leading to Laminar and Areal Organization of the Neocortex" by P. Rakic, 1981, in *The Organization of the Cerebral Cortex,* edited by F. O. Schmitt, F. G. Worden, G. Adelman, & S. G. Dennis, Cambridge, MA: MIT Press. Copyright © 1981 by the Massachusetts Institute of Technology.

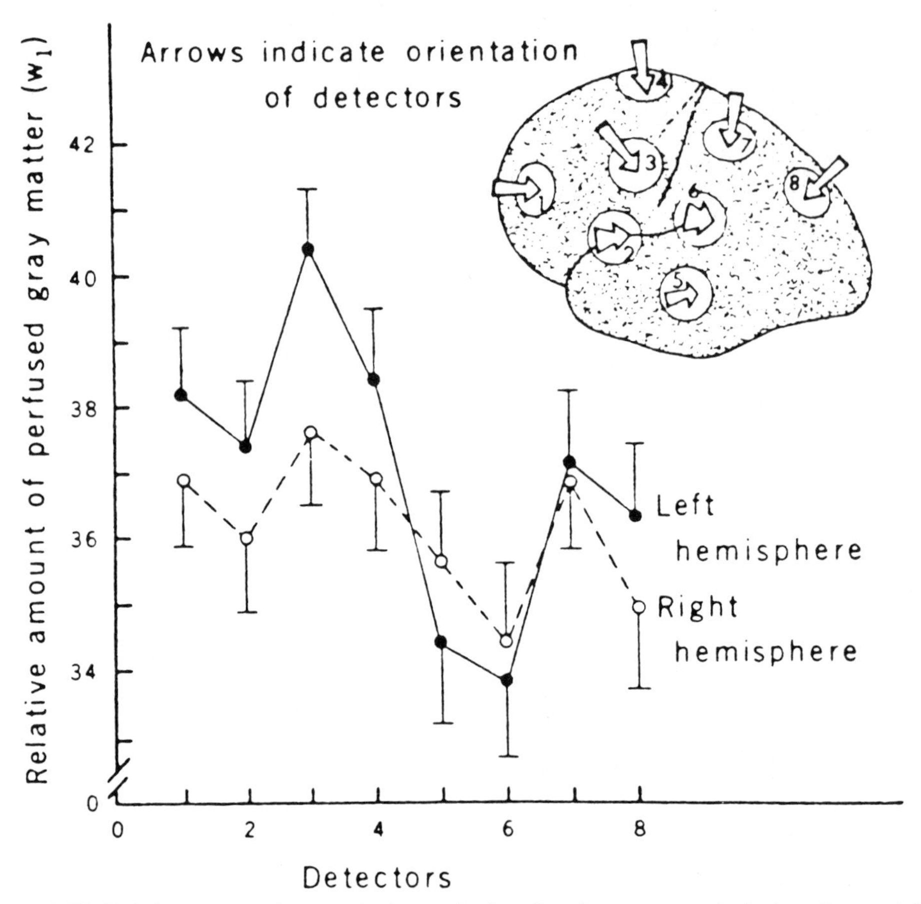

Figure 1-17. Relative amount (± standard errors) of perfused gray matter (w_1) plotted separately for 8 homologous regions in the left and right hemispheres. Reprinted with permission of the authors and publisher from "Differences in the Distribution of Gray and White Matter in Human Cerebral Hemispheres" by R. C. Gur, I. K. Packer, J. P. Hungerbuhler, M. Reivich, W. D. Obrist, W. S. Amarnek, & H. A. Sackeim, 1980, *Science, 207,* March 14, pp. 1226–1228, Copyright © 1980 by the American Association for the Advancement of Science.

of cortical fissuration and gyration, during the period of fetal ontogeny when that layer greatly expands in thickness relative to the lower layers, as a result of its developing dendritic processes and proliferation of glial support cells (Jacobson, 1978). Therefore, later development and higher gray/white ratios should be associated with deeper, denser fissuration but also with *lesser* width and volume in that area of the hemisphere, given the argument made in the previous paragraph.

The growth vector would be expected to have the following influence on the development of cortical gray and white matter: For earlier-developing cortical regions relatively greater growth emphasis would be seen in the earlier-emerging deeper cell layers, which should result in smaller ratios of gray matter to white matter and greater regional width/volume. Figure 1-17, taken from Gur and colleagues (1980), illustrates that indeed the gray/white ratio is smaller in the right hemisphere for at least the primary motor and sensory cortical regions. In contrast, later-maturing regions should reflect greater growth emphasis of the later-emerging, more superficial cortical layers, 2 and perhaps 3. This should yield smaller width and volume but a more deeply fissurated region with higher gray/white ratios, which may imply a somewhat higher degree of local intracortical organization of neuronal connections. In accordance, there is a higher gray/white ratio in the left hemisphere for motor, premotor, and primary sensory areas, (Gur *et al.,* 1980), consistent with Semmes's (1968) claim (based on her studies of somatosensory deficits in unilateral brain-damaged patients) that the left hemisphere is focally organized, whereas the right is diffusely organized. Correspondingly, it is those same areas in which LeMay (1976) found smaller hemispheric width on the left, and Meyer *et al.* (1978) measured a smaller volume on the left. Also, at least for the anterior speech area in the premotor region (Broca's area), there is deeper fissuration on the left (Falzi *et al.,* 1982).

Interestingly, and consistent with the predictions of the growth vector model, there is a higher gray/white ratio in the right hemisphere for tertiary association areas in posterior cortex (parietal association areas, numbered 5 and 6 in Figure 1-17). Recall the model's prediction that tertiary association areas in posterior cortex would emerge later in the right than in the left hemisphere. Also, in posterior regions, LeMay (1976) found lesser hemispheric width, and Meyer *et al.* (1978) found smaller volume, on the right side.

As for development of dendritic processes and of neuronal connections, the influence of the growth vector should be a bias toward later-emerging characteristics in the later-maturing regions of the cortex. Scheibel (1984) has thus far provided the only data revelant to this issue, and it appears to corroborate one part of the hypothesis. In layer 3 of the anterior speech region in the left hemisphere (LOP in Figure 1-18), the dendritic trees of the neurons show relatively greater elaboration of the later-emerging dendritic features, such as proportionally more higher-order branching points, than is true of the homologous region in the right hemisphere (ROP in Figure 1-18).

Implications for Functional Development

This morphological growth vector should also have implications for the development of perceptual and cognitive functions, and for asymmetrical patterns in developmental plasticity. Gross morphological asymmetries of the adult brain, both *in vivo* (Ratcliff, Dila, Taylor, Milner, 1980) and postmortem (Witelson, 1983), are associated, in fact, with at least some measures of functional asymmetries, notably speech lateralization and handedness. Development of regional functional maturity should proceed according to the same growth vector as already outlined for the morphological development of the hemispheres. Specifically, in the frontal motor and premotor regions, and in primary sensory regions, right-hemisphere functions should mature earlier than the left-hemisphere functions in homologous areas. This is supported by the Best *et al.* (1982) finding of a right-hemisphere advantage for memory-based discrimination of musical notes by 2 months, but no evidence of the homologous left-hemisphere ability for discrimination of speech syllables until 3 months (also compare the speech REA in Entus's $2\frac{1}{2}$-month-olds, 1977, with the lack thereof in Vargha-Khadem & Corballis's 2-month-olds, 1979).[2] Moreover, it is consistent with numerous reports in the language acquisition literature that children comprehend and produce the emotional intonational properties of language earlier than they comprehend and produce words and word combinations (e.g., Lewis, 1936). Research with both brain-damaged and neurologically intact adults indicates that the right hemisphere is specialized for affective, or emotional, prosodic aspects of spoken utterances both in perception (e.g., Haggard & Parkinson, 1971; Heilman, Scholes, & Watson, 1975; Ley & Bryden, 1982; Papanicolaou, Levin, Eisenberg, & Moore, 1983; Safer & Leventhal, 1977; Tucker, Watson, & Heilman,

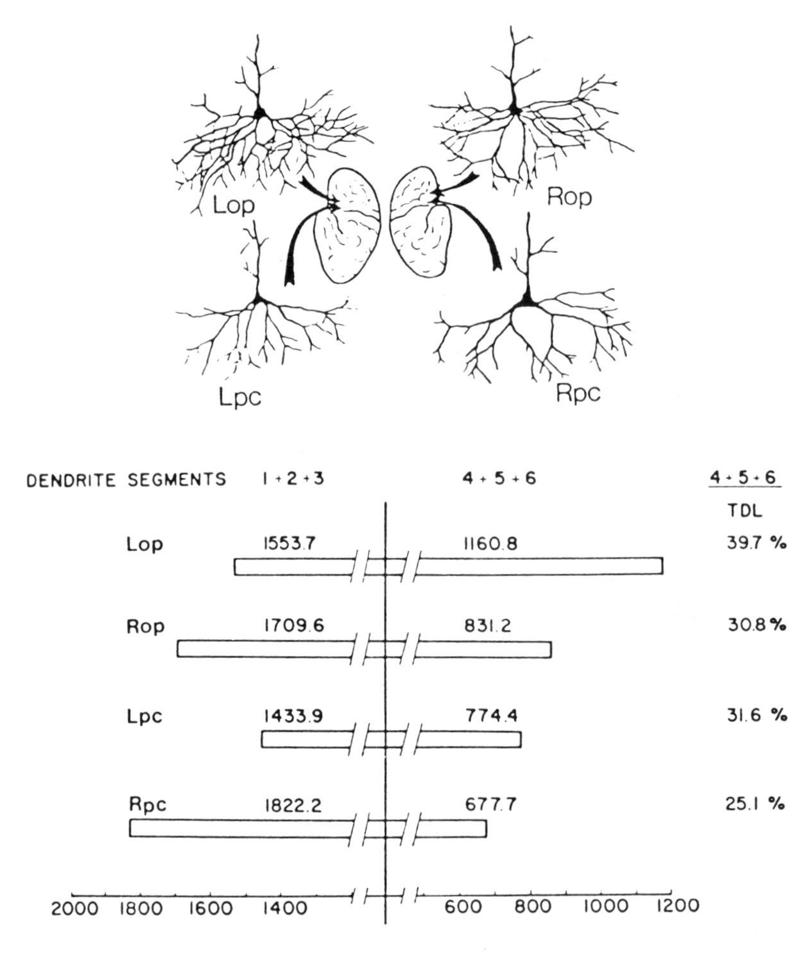

Figure 1-18. The top of the figure shows a somewhat schematicized drawing of typical dendritic ensembles from cells of the left and right frontal operculum and precentral regions in human cortex. Note the increased number of higher-order segments in left operculum (Lop) compared to the other three areas, and the relatively greater length of second- and third-order branches in the right operculum (Rop) and right precentral (Rpc) areas. The bottom of the figure shows dendritic length and proportion of the dendritic ensemble made up of lower-order (1,2,3) and higher-order (4,5,6) dendritic segments in left opercular (Lop), left precentral (Lpc), right opercular (Rop), and right precentral (Rpc) areas. The column of figures on the extreme right shows the percentage of total dendritic length (Tdl) occupied by higher-order dendrites in each region. Reprinted with permission of the publisher from "A Dendritic Correlate of Human Speech" by A. B. Scheibel, 1984, in *Cerebral Dominance: The Biological Foundations,* edited by N. Geschwind and A. Galaburda, Cambridge, MA: Harvard University Press. Copyright © 1984 by Harvard University Press.

1976; Wechsler, 1973) and in production (e.g., Benowitz *et al.*, 1983; Kent & Rosenbeck, 1982; Ross, 1981, 1984; Ross & Mesulam, 1979; Tucker *et al.*, 1976). In addition, according to the neuroembryological principle that later-maturing brain structures generally show greater functional plasticity than do earlier-maturing structures (Jacobson, 1978), the relative degree of plasticity of various cortical regions should be inversely correlated with their rate of maturation.

The proposed pattern of asymmetry in functional development should correspond to a greater plasticity of the later-maturing left frontal-motor, premotor, and primary sensory regions, relative to the plasticity of the homologous right-hemisphere regions. Conversely, there should be later development and greater plasticity on the right relative to the left side for posterior tertiary association area functions. Unfortunately, there are no published data relevant to this issue. Moreover, it will be difficult, to say the least, to match right- and left-hemisphere skills in terms of cortical areas involved, as well as for level of cognitive complexity and/or difficulty, in order to compare their development in normal children and their plasticity in brain-damaged children. For example, one might wish to compare the development and plasticity of reading ability, which depends on a tertiary association region of the left hemisphere in adults (angular gyrus), versus that of complex spatial and face-recognition abilities, which depend in adults on right tertiary association areas (parietal and inferotemporal). In our society, normal children begin reading around 6 years of age but do not develop the ability to solve complex mazes, or a right-hemisphere configurational-processing superiority for recognition of unfamiliar faces, until about 10 years of age (e.g., Kohn & Dennis, 1974; Levine, 1985). If we could assume that the criteria of comparability were met by these findings, the model would then predict greater ability of the *right* hemisphere to acquire reading skills, relative to the left hemisphere's ability to acquire spatial/facial skills, following early unilateral damage. However, there are several inherent problems. The comparability of cognitive levels for these skills is uncertain. The onset ages may be, at least in part, artifacts of our educational system. Finally, acquisition of a skill may call on different cortical regions in the child than those that underlie the execution of the already-acquired skill in the adult (see Kirk, 1985).

INDIVIDUAL DIFFERENCES IN FUNCTIONAL ASYMMETRIES

The growth vector is very likely influenced by hormonal and genetic factors, given the current understanding in neuroembryology that developmental gradients involve some sort of gradient(s) in biochemical influences on the prenatal guidance of neuronal migration and development of neuronal connections (Jacobson, 1978; Sperry, 1963. The possibility of hormonal influences on growth gradients may aid our understanding of the development of sex differences in brain organization and cognitive functions (see also Chapter 14 by Netley & Rovet, this volume), which may be mediated by sex differences in maturation rates (see Newcombe & Bandura, 1983; Waber, 1976, 1977; but see also Rovet, 1983; Waber, Mann, Merola, & Moylan, 1985).[3] These sex differences are most apparent in the extreme cases of sexual anomalies, such as Turner syndrome (XO). Turner syndrome is associated with large deficits in spatial abilities (e.g., Waber, 1979), an increase in the rate of prenatal development (Netley & Rovet, 1981), and maldevelopment of tertiary association areas in the right hemisphere (Christensen & Nielsen, 1981). Sex differences in brain organization and function are also apparent in anomalies such as supernumerary-X syndrome (XXX and XXY), which is linked with low verbal relative to spatial abilities, and slow prenatal growth rates (Netley & Rovet, Chapter 14, this volume; Netley & Rovet, 1981, 1982, 1983; Rovet & Netley, 1983).

Hormonal and genetic influences on the growth vector may also be involved in heritable learning disorders. For example, Galaburda and colleagues (Galaburda & Eidelberg, 1982; Galaburda & Kemper, 1979; Galaburda, Rosen, Sherman, & Assal, 1986; Galaburda, Sherman, Rosen, Aboitiz, & Geschwind, 1985; Kemper, 1984) found symmetrical plana temporale in the brains of all four male dyslexics and the one female dyslexic that they have studied postmortem. The same brains showed abnormalities in cortical neuronal organization, which predominated in the left-hemisphere perisylvian regions. The nature of the latter abnormalities led them to posit a neuroembryological disturbance in the prenatal migration of neurons during mid-gestation. Hormonal/genetic effects on the growth vector may be particularly relevant to understanding observed sex and handedness biases in the incidence of learning disabilities, for example, the suggestion that testosterone's effect on brain development forms the basis for the higher incidence of learning disabilities among males and left-handers (Geschwind & Behan, 1982, 1984; Marx, 1982).

CONCLUSION

What of the original question: Is the pattern of cerebral asymmetry developmentally invariant, or do functional asymmetries develop? Whether we refer to evidence of functional and/or structural asymmetries, even in very early development the extant data support "developmental invariance" (see also Kinsbourne, 1975; Witelson, 1985). Yet this does not necessarily imply that *nothing* is changing or developing. The timeless constancy of cerebral asymmetries coexists with continuous developmental change at many levels. Lateralized perceptual and cognitive functions *do* undergo developmental change (e.g., the child's language and spatial skills change both qualitatively and quantitatively); plasticity of function also undergoes developmental change (see Witelson, 1985); and the cerebral hemispheres supporting these abilities undergo change themselves (e.g., increases in dendritic arborization, neuronal connections, neurotransmitter functions, glial support cells, and myelinization).

According to developmental biology, change and constancy are codeterminants of developmental growth in a biological system. The structural and functional properties of the two cerebral hemispheres do change developmentally, but always in different manners because they develop within the context of an ever-present lateralization of functions, which is continuous with a lateralized gradient of neuronal differentiation and maturation. The argument presented in this chapter is that the normal direction of this lateralizing gradient is from right to left, and that it interacts with gradients in the other main axes of embryologic development to result in a three-dimensional diagonal growth vector from right frontal-motor and primary sensory areas to left-posterior and tertiary association areas. This growth pattern has implications for hemispheric and regional differences in gross morphology and neuronal organization, as well as for differences in plasticity and in maturation of perceptual and cognitive functions.

ACKNOWLEDGMENT

This work has profited from discussions with numerous colleagues and students. I am particularly grateful for discussions with, and careful critiques by, Marcel Kinsbourne, Donald Shankweiler, Ursula Kirk, and Marshall Gladstone.

NOTES

1. There is also a general mediolateral gradient, but Jacobson (1978) states that it is less consistent than the other gradients; that is, in numerous regions it reverses to a lateromedial gradient, or else there is no obvious gradient in either direction along this dimension. Furthermore, it is difficult to conceptualize a vector of greater than three dimensions cutting through time without using some visualization aid such as computer animation modeling. Therefore, the mediolateral dimension will not be considered further in this discussion of the proposed model for hemispheric growth.

2. This is not meant to imply that music discrimination depends on *frontal* cortex in the right hemisphere. Presumably it would rely, in part, on primary auditory cortex (Heschl's gyrus) in the right hemisphere (see Shankweiler, 1966); the growth vector model does assume rightward bias in development of primary sensory areas. Indeed, a double Heschl's gyrus is more often encountered in the right hemisphere than in the left (Geschwind & Levitsky, 1968; but see also Witelson & Pallie, 1973). In addition, recall that the experimental paradigm required that the infants use short-term memory in order to make their discriminations. Short-term memory ability is largely dependent on the hippocampus, an early-emerging, ventrally located structure within the telencephalic hemispheres (Gilles, Leviton, & Dooling, 1983). Thus, the growth vector model would also predict a rightward bias in hippocampal maturation.

3. The effect of sex differentiation on the growth vector may also be related to sex differences in morphological asymmetries for other body parts, such as the hands and feet (Levy & Levy, 1978; Means & Walters, 1982); the latter asymmetries, in turn, appear to be traceable to prenatal development (Mittwoch, 1977).

REFERENCES

Benowitz, L. I., Bear, D. M., Rosenthal, R., Mesulam, M. M., Zaidel, E., & Sperry, R. W. (1983). Hemispheric specialization and nonverbal communication. *Cortex, 19,* 5–12.

Best, C. T. (1978). *The role of consonant and vowel acoustic features in infant cerebral asymmetries for speech perception.* Unpublished doctoral dissertation, Michigan State University.

Best, C. T., Hoffman, H., & Glanville, B. B. (1982). Development of infant ear asymmetries for speech and music. *Perception and Psychophysics, 31,* 75–85.

Bever, T. G. (1978). Broca and Lashley were right: Cerebral dominance is an accident of growth. In D. Caplan (Ed.), *Biological studies of mental processes* (pp. 186–230). Cambridge, MA: MIT Press.

Broca, P. (1865). Sur la faculté du langage articulé. *Bulletin of Social Anthropology, 6,* 493–494.

Brown, J. W., & Jaffe, J. (1975). Note: Hypothesis on cerebral dominance. *Neuropsychologia, 13,* 107–110.

Chi, F. G., Dooling, E. C., & Gilles, F. H. (1977). Left–right asymmetries of the temporal speech areas of the human fetus. *Archives of Neurology, 34,* 346–348.

Christensen, A-L., & Nielsen, J. (1981). A neuropsychological investigation of 17 women with Turner's syndrome. In W. Schmid & J. Nielsen (Eds.), *Human behavior and genetics* (pp. 151–166). Amsterdam: Elsevier/North-Holland.

Corballis, M. C., & Morgan, M. J. (1978). On the biological basis of human laterality: I. Evidence for a maturational left–right gradient. *The Behavioral and Brain Sciences, 2,* 261–267.

Cowan, M. W. (1979). The development of the brain. *Scientific American, 241,* 112–133.

Crowell, D. H., Jones, R. H., Kapuniai, L. E., & Nakagawa, J. K. (1973). Unilateral cortical activity in newborn humans: An early index of cerebral dominance? *Science, 180,* 205–208.

Cutting, J. E. (1974). Two left hemisphere mechanisms in speech perception. *Perception and Psychophysics, 16,* 601–612.

Darwin, C. J. (1971). Ear differences in the recall of fricatives and vowels. *Quarterly Journal of Experimental Psychology, 23,* 46–62.

Dooling, E. C., Chi, J. G., & Gilles, F. H. (1983). Telencephalic development: Changing gyral patterns. In F. H. Gilles, A. Leviton, & E. C. Dooling (Eds.), *The developing human brain: Growth and epidemiologic neuropathy* (pp. 94–104). Boston: John Wright, PSG.

Emde, R. N., & Robinson, J. (1979). The first two months: Recent research in developmental psychobiology and the changing view of the newborn. In J. Noshpitz & J. Call (Eds.), *Handbook of child psychiatry:* 1. *Development.* New York: Basic Books.

Entus, A. K. (1977). Hemispheric asymmetry in processing of dichotically presented speech and nonspeech sounds by infants. In S. Segalowitz & F. A. Gruber (Eds.), *Language development and neurological theory* (pp. 63–73). New York: Academic Press.

Falzi, G., Perrone, P., & Vignolo, L. A. (1982). Right–left asymmetry in anterior speech region. *Archives of Neurology, 39,* 239–240.

Friedes, D. (1977). Do dichotic listening procedures measure lateralization of information processing or retrieval strategy? *Perception and Psychophysics, 21,* 259–263.

Galaburda, A. M. (1984). Anatomical asymmetries. In N. Geschwind & A. M. Galaburda (Eds.), *Cerebral dominance: The biological foundations* (pp. 11–25). Cambridge, MA: Harvard University Press.

Galaburda, A. M., & Eidelberg, D. (1982). Symmetry and asymmetry in the human posterior thalamus: II. Thalamic lesions in a case of developmental dyslexia. *Archives of Neurology, 39,* 333–336.

Galaburda, A. M., & Kemper, T. L. (1979). Cytoarchitectonic abnormalities in developmental dyslexia: A case study. *Annals of Neurology, 6,* 94–100.

Galaburda, A. M., LeMay, M., Kemper, T. L., & Geschwind, N. (1978). Right–left asymmetries in the brain. *Science, 199,* 852–856.

Galaburda, A. M., Rosen, G. D., Sherman, G. F., & Assal, F. (1986). Neuropathological findings in a woman with developmental dyslexia. *Annals of Neurology, 20,* 170.

Galaburda, A. M., Sanides, F., & Geschwind, N. (1978). Cytoarchitectonic left–right asymmetries in the temporal speech region. *Archives of Neurology, 35,* 812–817.

Galaburda, A. M., Sherman, G. F., Rosen, G. D., Aboitiz, F., & Geschwind, N. (1985). Developmental dyslexia: Four consecutive patients with cortical anomalies. *Annals of Neurology, 18,* 222–233.

Geschwind, N., & Behan, P. O. (1982). Left-handedness: Association with immune disease, migraine, and developmental learning disorder. *Proceedings of the National Academy of Science, 79,* 5079–5100.

Geschwind, N., & Behan, P. O. (1984). Laterality, hormones, and immunity. In N. Geschwind & A. M. Galaburda (Eds.), *Cerebral dominance: The biological foundations* (pp. 211–224). Cambridge, MA: Harvard University Press.

Geschwind, N., & Levitsky, W. (1968). Human brain: Left–right asymmetries in temporal speech region. *Science, 161,* 186–189.

Gilles, F. H., Leviton, A., & Dooling. E. C. (1983). *The developing human brain: Growth and epidemiologic neuropathology.* Boston: John Wright, PSG.

Glanville, B. B., Best, C. T., & Levenson, R. (1977). A cardiac measure of cerebral asymmetries in infant auditory perception. *Developmental Psychology, 13,* 54–59.

Graham, F. K., Leavitt, L. A., Strock, B. D., & Brown, J. W. (1978). Precocious cardiac orienting in a human anencephalic infant. *Science, 199,* 322–324.

Gur, R. C., Packer, I. K., Hungerbuhler, J. P, Reivich, M., Obrist, W. D., Amarnek, W. S., & Sackeim, H. A. (1980). Differences in the distribution of gray and white matter in human cerebral hemispheres. *Science, 207,* 1226–1228.

Haggard, M. P., & Parkinson, A. M. (1971). Stimulus and task factors as determinants of ear advantages. *Quarterly Journal of Experimental Psychology, 23,* 168–177.

Heilman, J. M., Scholes, R., & Watson, R. T. (1975). Auditory affective agnosia: Disturbed comprehension of affective speech. *Journal of Neurology, Neurosurgery and Psychiatry, 38,* 69–72.

Jacobson, M. (1978). *Developmental neurobiology.* New York: Plenum Press.

Keller, R. (1942). The asymmetry of the human body. *CIBA Symposium, 3,* 1126–1127.

Kemper, T. L. (1984). Asymmetrical lesions in dyslexia. In N. Geschwind & A. M. Galaburda (Eds.), *Cerebral dominance: The biological foundations* (pp. 75–89). Cambridge, MA: Harvard University Press.

Kent, R. D., & Rosenbeck, J. C. (1982). Prosodic disturbance and neurologic lesion. *Brain and Language, 15,* 259–291.

Kinsbourne, M. (1975). The ontogeny of cerebral dominance. *Annals of the New York Academy of Sciences, 263,* 244–250.

Kirk, V. (1985). Hemispheric contributions to the development of graphic skill. In C. T. Best (Ed.), *Hemispheric function and collaboration in the child* (pp. 193–228). New York: Academic Press.

Kohn, B., & Dennis, M. (1974). Selective impairments of visuospatial abilities in infantile hemiplegics after right cerebral hemi-decortication. *Neuropsychologia, 12,* 505–512.

LeMay, M. (1976). Morphological cerebral asymmetries of modern man, fossil man, and nonhuman primate. *Annals of the New York Academy of Science, 280,* 349–366.

LeMay, M. (1977). Asymmetries of the skull and handedness. *Journal of Neurological Science, 32,* 243–253.

LeMay, M. (1984). Radiological, developmental, and fossil asymmetries. In N. Geschwind & A. M. Galaburda (Eds.), *Cerebral dominance: The biological foundations* (pp. 26–42). Cambridge, MA: Harvard University Press.

LeMay, M., & Geschwind, N. (1978). Asymmetries of the human cerebral hemispheres. In A. Caramazza & E. B. Zurif (Eds.), *Language acquisition and language breakdown.* Baltimore, MD: Johns Hopkins Press, pp. 311–328.

LeMay, M., & Kido, D. K. (1978). Asymmetries of the cerebral hemispheres on computed tomograms. *Journal of Computer-Assisted Tomography, 2,* 471–476.

Lenneberg, E. H. (1967). *Biological foundations of language.* New York: Wiley.

Levine, S. C. (1985). Developmental changes in right hemisphere involvement in face perception. In C. T. Best (Ed.), *Hemispheric function and collaboration in the child* (pp. 157–191). New York: Academic Press.

Levy, J., & Levy, J. M. (1978). Human lateralization from head to foot: Sex-related factors. *Science, 200,* 1291–1292.

Lewis, M. M. (1936). *Infant speech: A study of the beginnings of language.* New York: Harcourt Brace.

Ley, R. G., & Bryden, M. P. (1982). A dissociation of right and left hemispheric effects for recognizing emotional tone and verbal content. *Brain and Cognition, 1,* 3–9.

MacKain, K. S., Studdert-Kennedy, M., Spieker, S., & Stern, D. (1983). Infant intermodal speech perception is a left hemisphere function. *Science, 219,* 1347–1349.

Marx, J. L. (1982). Autoimmunity in left-handers. *Science, 217,* 141–144.

McHenry, L. C., Merory, J., Bass, E., Stump, D. A., Williams, R., Witcofski, R., Howard, G., & Toole, J. F. (1978). $Xenon_{133}$ inhalation method for regional cerebral blood flow measurements: Normal values and test results. *Stroke, 9,* 393–399.

Means, L. W., & Walters, R. E. (1982). Sex, handedness and asymmetry of hand and foot length. *Neuropsychologia, 20,* 715–719.

Meyer, J. S., Ishihara, N., Deshmukh, V. D., Naritomi, H., Sakai, F., Hsu, M-C., & Pollack, P. (1978). Improved method for noninvasive measurement of regional cerebral blood flow by $Xenon_{133}$ inhalation: I. Description of method and normal values obtained in healthy volunteers. *Stroke, 9,* 195–205.

Mittwoch, U. (1977). To be born right is to be born male. *New Scientist, 73,* 74–76.

Molfese, D. L., Freeman, R. B., & Palermo, D. S. (1975). The ontogeny of brain lateralization for speech and nonspeech stimuli. *Brain and Language, 2,* 356–368.

Molfese, D., & Molfese, V. J. (1985). Electrophysiological indices of auditory discrimination in newborn infants: The basis for predicting later language development? *Infant Behavior and Development, 8,* 197–211.

Netley, C., & Rovet, J. (1981). *Prenatal growth rate and hemispheric organization.* Paper presented at meeting of the International Neuropsychology Society, Atlanta, GA, February.

Netley, C., & Rovet, J. (1982). Verbal deficits in children with 47,XXY and 47,XXX karyotypes: A descriptive and experimental study. *Brain and Language, 17,* 58–72.

Netley, C., & Rovet, J. (1983). Relationships among brain organization, maturation rate, and the development of verbal and nonverbal ability. In S. Segalowitz (Ed.), *Language functions and brain organization* (pp. 245–265). New York: Academic Press.

Newcombe, N., & Bandura, M. (1983). Effect of age of puberty on spatial ability in girls. *Developmental Psychology, 19,* 215–224.

Orton, S. T. (1937). *Reading, writing, and speech problems in children.* New York: W. W. Norton.

Papanicolaou, A. C., Levin, H. S., Eisenberg, H. M., & Moore, B. D. (1983). Evoked potential indices of selective hemispheric engagement in affective and phonetic tasks. *Neuropsychologia, 21,* 401–405.

Rabinowicz, T. (1979). The differentiate maturation of the human cerebral cortex. In F. Falkner & J. M. Tanner (Eds.), *Human Growth: Vol. 3. Neurobiology and nutrition* (pp. 97–123) New York: Plenum Press.

Rakic, P. (1980). Developmental events leading to laminar and areal organization of the neocortex. In F. O. Schmitt, F. G. Worden, G. Adelman, & S. G. Dennis (Eds.), *The organization of cerebral cortex* (pp. 7–28). Cambridge, MA: MIT Press.

Ratcliff, G., Dila, C., Taylor, L., & Milner, B. (1980). The morphological asymmetry of the hemispheres and cerebral dominance for speech: A possible relationship. *Brain and Language 11,* 87–88.

Rose, S. A. (1984). Developmental changes in hemispheric specialization for tactual processing in very young children: Evidence from cross-modal transfer. *Developmental Psychology, 20,* 568–574.

Ross, E. D. (1981). The aprosodias: Functional–anatomic organization of the affective components of language in the right hemisphere. *Archives of Neurology, 38,* 561–569.

Ross, E. D. (1984). Right hemisphere role in language, affective behavior and emotion. *Trends in Neuroscience,* 342–346.

Ross, E. D., & Mesulam, M. M. (1979). Dominant language functions of the right hemisphere: Prosody and emotional gesturing. *Archives of Neurology, 36,* 144–146.

Rovet, J. (1983). Cognitive and neuropsychological test performance of persons with abnormalities of adolescent development: A test of Waber's hypothesis. *Child Development, 54,* 941–950.

Rovet, J., & Netley, C. (1983). The triple-X chromosome syndrome in childhood: Recent empirical findings. *Child Development, 54,* 831–845.

Safer, M. A., & Leventhal, H. (1977). Ear differences in evaluating emotional tone of voice and of verbal content. *Journal of Experimental Psychology: Human Perception and Performance, 3,* 75–82.

Scheibel, A. B. (1984). A dendritic correlate of human speech. In N. Geschwind & A. M. Galaburda (Eds.), *Cerebral dominance: The biological foundations* (pp. 43–52). Cambridge, MA: Harvard University Press.

Schwartz, J., & Tallal, P. (1980). Rate of acoustic change may underlie hemispheric specialization for speech perception. *Science, 207,* 1380–1381.

Semmes, J. (1968). Hemispheric specialization: A possible clue to mechanism. *Neuropsychologia, 6,* 11–26.

Shankweiler, D. (1966). Effects of temporal-lobe damage on perception of dichotically presented melodies. *Journal of Comparative and Physiological Psychology, 62,* 115–119.

Sidtis, J. J. (1980). On the nature of the cortical function underlying right hemisphere auditory perception. *Neuropsychologia, 18,* 321–330.

Sperry, R. (1963). Chemoaffinity in the orderly growth of nerve fiber patterns and connections. *Proceedings of the National Academy of Science, 50,* 703–710.

Studdert-Kennedy, M., & Shankweiler, D. (1970). Hemispheric specialization for speech perception. *Journal of the Acoustical Society of America, 48,* 579–594.

Studdert-Kennedy, M., & Shankweiler, D. (1980). Hemispheric specialization for language processes. *Science, 211,* 960–961.

Taylor, D. C. (1969). Differential rates of cerebral maturation between sexes and between hemispheres. *Lancet, 2,* 140–142.

Tucker, D. M., Watson, R. G., & Heilman, K. M. (1976). Affective discrimination and evocation in patients with parietal disease. *Neurology, 26,* 354.

Vargha-Khadem, F., & Corballis, M. C. (1979). Cerebral asymmetry in infants. *Brain and Language, 8,* 1–9.

Waber, D. P. (1976). Sex differences in cognition: A function of maturation rate. *Science, 192,* 572–574.

Waber, D. P. (1977). Sex differences and rate of physical growth. *Developmental Psychology, 13,* 29–38.

Waber, D. P. (1979). Neuropsychological aspects of Turner syndrome. *Developmental Medicine and Child Neurology, 231,* 58–70.

Waber, D. P., Mann, M. B., Merola, J., & Moylan, P. M. (1985). Physical maturation rate and cognitive performance in early adolescence: A longitudinal examination. *Development Psychology, 21,* 666–681.

Wada, J. A., Clarke, R., & Hamm, A. (1975). Cerebral hemispheric asymmetry in humans. *Archives of Neurology, 32,* 239–246.

Wechsler, A. F. (1973). The effect of organic brain disease on recall of emotionally charged versus neutral narrative text. *Neurology, 23,* 130–135.

Weinberger, D. R., Luchins, D. J., Morihisa, J., & Wyatt, R. J. (1982). Asymmetrical volumes of the right and left frontal and occipital regions of the human brain. *Annals of Neurology, 11,* 97–100.

Weiss, M. S., & House, A. S. (1973). Perception of dichotically presented vowels. *Journal of the Accoustical Society of America, 53,* 51–53.

Witelson, S. F. (1977). Early hemispheric specialization and interhemispheric plasticity: An empirical and theoretical review. In S. Segalowitz & F. A. Gruber (Eds.), *Language development and neurological theory* (pp. 213–287). New York: Academic Press.

Witelson, S. F. (1983). Bumps on the brain: Neuroanatomical asymmetries as a basis for functional asymmetries. In S. Segalowitz (Ed.), *Language functions and brain organization* (pp. 117–144). New York: Academic Press.

Witelson, S. F. (1985). Hemisphere specialization from birth: Mark II. In C. T. Best (Ed.), *Hemispheric function and collaboration in the child* (pp. 33–85). New York: Academic Press.

Witelson, S. F., & Pallie, W. (1973). Left hemisphere specialization for language in the newborn: Neuroanatomical evidence of asymmetry. *Brain, 96,* 641–646.

Yakovlev, P. I. & Lecours, A. R. (1967). The myelogenetic cycles of regional maturation of the brain. In A. Minkowski (Ed.), *Regional development of the brain in early life* (pp. 3–70). Oxford: Blackwell.

2

Anatomical Development of the Corpus Callosum in Humans: A Review with Reference to Sex and Cognition

SANDRA F. WITELSON
DEBRA L. KIGAR
McMaster University, Hamilton, Ontario

The corpus callosum, the main fiber tract connecting the two cerebral hemispheres, undergoes marked growth in overall size during postnatal development. In humans, the area of the midsagittal surface more than triples its size over the life span (Rakic & Yakovlev, 1968). Recent experimental work in nonhuman species indicates that new callosal fibers do not emerge after an early postnatal period, but rather there is a marked elimination of fibers. These results suggest that in humans, also, the increase in overall callosal size is not due to an increase in fiber number (Innocenti, 1986). Myelination of callosal fibers begins at the end of the fetal period (Larroche & Amakawa, 1973), increases throughout childhood, and reaches a plateau by about 7 to 10 years of age (Yakovlev & Lecours, 1967). Yakovlev (1962) suggeted that myelination of fibers reflects the maturation of cortical regions and is associated with changes in behavior and in capacity for neural plasticity.

The specific functions of the callosum for behavior and its physiological mechanisms are not well established. The callosum may provide interhemispheric excitation or, additionally, interhemispheric inhibition (e.g., Dennis, 1976). At a general level, however, it is clear that the callosum is important for the functional integration of the two cerebral hemispheres (e.g., Leporé, Ptito, & Jasper, 1986) and likely for the manifestation of hemisphere functional specialization. Interference with the functioning of the callosum due to the presence of tumors or following neurosurgical procedures (such as commissurotomy or callosotomy) results in the dramatic "split-brain" or hemisphere disconnection phenomenon in which an individual's behavior or cognition appears to be based only on information presented to one or the other of the hemispheres, as if the person had two separate streams of awareness (Sperry, 1974).

Functional specialization of the hemispheres has been extensively investigated during development. The available data suggest that under normal conditions hemispheric specialization is unchanging during chronological development (see review in Witelson, 1987b). However, brain damage or the effects of extremely atypical environmental conditions may affect the pattern of lateralization of function. The presence of the corpus callosum appears important for the manifestation of this aspect of brain organization. Congenital absence or agenesis of the corpus callosum may be associated with atypical patterns of hemispheric specialization (e.g., Chiarello, 1980).

Patterns of hemispheric specialization vary among normal individuals, particularly in relation to hand prefernce and sex (see review in Bryden, 1982). The anatomy of the corpus callosum has also been reported to vary with differences in hand preference (Witelson, 1985a, 1986) and sex (Holloway & de Lacoste, 1986; Witelson, 1987a). As these same factors appear related to variation in hemispheric specialization and callosal anatomy, it is possible that individual differences in the structure of the callosum are related to variation in brain lateralization.

These interrelationships raise the question of whether variations in callosal anatomy and brain lateralization of function follow a similar developmental course. Brain lateralization is present in infancy, and sex differences in hemispheric specialization have been noted early in life (Witelson, 1977, 1987b). Although the corpus callosum, like the overall brain, increases in size with chronological age, it seems worthwhile to consider possible congruencies in developmental aspects of callosal growth, hemisphere specialization, and cognition. Such information could be relevant to the mechanisms of developmental changes and individual differences in cognition and in patterns of hemisphere specialization (Witelson & Swallow, 1987a).

This chapter reviews the literature concerning the anatomical measurement of the corpus callosum at various ages in development: gestation, infancy (from birth to 24 months) and childhood (from 2 to 18 years). The results of these studies are presented for comparison in tabular and graphic form. A synthesis of the results is attempted to obtain a general view of the anatomical development of the corpus callosum. The evidence for any individual differences, particularly sex differences, is considered. Possible relationships between developmental landmarks in callosal growth and in behavior and cognition in the maturing child are also considered. The paucity and large gaps in the available literature in this field will be evident. In spite of this, there is considerable congruency in the existing data, and they highlight what may be important issues and worthwhile areas for future research. A model of callosal growth is suggested in which there is a rapidly accelerating growth in the fetal period, a somewhat lower but constant rate of growth in the first two years, followed by a marked slowing of callosal growth during childhood until the adult size is reached; and no sex differences in overall callosal area. Some speculations are offered for the possible mechanisms underlying individual differences in callosal size.

OVERVIEW OF EMPIRICAL STUDIES

A computerized literature search was done using the National Library of Medicine Medline database. The main Medical Subject Headings (MeSH) used were: Corpus Callosum, Anatomy, and Histology, within the population of fetus, infant, child, and humans. Text words used were morphometry, morphology, and size; excluded text words were agenesis and Aicardi; done for the period 1966 to September 1987, for all languages. This resulted in 235 references, of which only a few were relevant to the anatomical measurement of the callosum during development. The literature reviewed in this chapter also included all papers published earlier than 1966, which were retrieved via the bibliographies in the papers from the literature search. In addition, all published abstracts that we could find were included.

All the studies dealing with the size of the human corpus callosum during development were reviewed. Variables of chronological age, sex and brain weight were noted where given. Table 2-1 presents a summary of findings divided into three age spans: fetuses, infants, and children. Hand preference may be another factor related to variation in size of the callosum (Witelson, 1985a, 1986), but no measures of motoric laterality have yet been recorded in any studies of the callosum in children. The available data may therefore be complicated by the contribution of this and other undocumented variables.

Bean (1906) conducted the earliest study of the anatomy of the human corpus cal-

Table 2-1. Summary of Studies of the Anatomy of the Corpus Callosum in Fetuses, Infants, and Children

			Sample			Brain weight[a]	Total corpus callosum		Splenium[b]	
				Age			Length	Area	Width	Area
Study	Method	n	Sex	$\bar{X}$	Min./max.	(g) $\bar{X}$	(mm) $\bar{X}$	(mm^2) $\bar{X}$	(mm) $\bar{X}$	(mm^2) $\bar{X}$
Fetuses										
Luttenberg, 1965	Paraffin-	3		11 wk	10/13			0.57[d]		2.02[e]
	embedded	4		15 wk	13/17			11.33		9.72
	midsagittal	3		22 wk	19/26			50.64		33.54
	sections	3		35 wk	30/40			153.03		
Rakic &	Celloidin-	8		23 wk	18/26		19.48[f]	29.80	1.91	
Yakovlev,	embedded	15		30 wk	27/34		27.82	51.91	2.56	
1968	midsagittal	20		38 wk	34/43		32.35	61.98	2.68	
	sections									
Baack,	Celloidin-	20	Male		Total	285		55.11	2.66	
de Lacoste-	embedded	18	Female		26/41	260		61.99	3.41*	
Utamsing, &	midsagittal									
Woodward,	sections									
1982	(Yakovlev									
(Abstract)	collection)[g]									
de Lacoste,	Celloidin-	8	Male	29 wk	26/32	215	28.36[h]	47.91	2.45	
Holloway, &	embedded	6	Female	29 wk	26/32	194	27.88	54.43	3.25*	
Woodward,	midsagittal	11	Male	37 wk	33/41	320	30.94	56.59	2.77	
1986	sections	7	Female	39 wk	33/41	327	31.71	69.55	3.55	
	(Yakovlev									
	collection)[g]									
Clarke,	Postmortem	12	Male					Total	No sex	No sex
Kraftsik,	midsagittal	15	Female					100–230	differ-	differ-
Innocenti, &	(formalin-								ence[i]	ence[j]
van der Loos,	fixed,									
1986	assumed)									
(Abstract)										

(continued)

Table 2-1 *(continued)*

Study	Method	Sample				Brain weight[a]	Total corpus callosum		Splenium[b]	
				Age			Length	Area	Width	Area
		n	Sex	$\bar{X}$	Min./max.	(g) $\bar{X}$	(mm) $\bar{X}$	(mm^2) $\bar{X}$	(mm) $\bar{X}$	(mm^2) $\bar{X}$
Infants and Children										
Bean, 1906[k]	Postmortem midsagittal drawings, (formalin-fixed)	7	Male	1! mo	0/24	702[m]		328.1		109.2[n]
		1	Female	1 mo		435		155.0		
		3	Male	12 yr	8/15	1,072		459.3		120.0
		1	Female	16 yr		840		613.0		155.0
Luttenberg, 1965	Paraffin-embedded midsagittal sections	2		4 mo	3/5			231.1[d]		51.1[e]
Rakic & Yakovlev, 1968	Celloidin-embedded midsagittal sections	4		11 mo	2/24		44.8[f]	147.9	4.0	
Bell & Variend, 1985	Postmortem midsagittal (formalin-fixed)	23	Male	4 mo	Total 0/24	625[p]	54.1	296.9	9.0	87.2
		14	Female	5 mo		624	52.6	270.9	8.1	72.8
		5	Male		3/12 yr	1,253	67.7	681.4	14.8	179.8
		2	Female	11 yr	7/14	930	70.4	552.5	9.5	150.5
Clarke, Kraftsik, Innocenti, & van der Loos, 1986 (Abstract)	Postmortem midsagittal (formalin-fixed, assumed)	11	Male		Total 0/24			Total Max. = 550[q]	No sex difference[i]	No sex difference[j]
		9	Female							

Note: The anatomical features are schematically represented in Figure 2-1.

*Indicates a statistically significant difference between the starred value and the one directly above it. No asterisk indicates no statistical difference. Level of significance used was .05.

[a]The fixed brain weight was used if both fresh and fixed weights were given. Mose studies do not indicate which weight measure was used.

[b]Splenial width was defined as the maximal dorsoventral width, and splenial area was defined in most of the studies as the posterior fifth region of the callosum (see Figure 2-1).

[c]Blank indicates no information available.

[d]Mean values for the callosal and splenial areas for each of the age subgroups in this study were calculated from raw data presented in Luttenberg (1965), Table 2, p. 139.

[e]Splenial area was defined in this study as the posterior third of the corpus callosum.

[f]Mean values for the callosal and splenial measurements for each of the age subgroups in this study were calculated from raw data presented in Tables 1 and 2, pp. 46–47 and p. 63.

[g]Though not stated in the report, the Yakovlev collection consists of celloidin-embedded brain sections.

[h]This measure differs from the length measures in other studies. It is the curved line from the tip of the rostrum to the tip of the splenium, with any line representing a width being perpendicular to it and bisected by it.

[i]Splenial width in this study was defined as the width of the splenium relative to the width of the posterior callosal body.

[j]Splenial area in this study was given only as splenial area relative to total callosal area.

[k]Bean's sample includes mainly ''Negro'' male infants and children, with only a few Caucasians.

[m]Mean values for all weight, callosal, and splenial measurements for each age group in this study were calculated from raw data presented in Bean (1906), Table 1, pp. 355–357.

[n]This measurement is based on only the six available cases.

[p]Bell and Variend did not report mean values separately for their groups of infants and children. However, they did give brain weight and callosal measurements (but not age) for each case, and did indicate that there were 7 cases (5 male, 2 female) older than 2 years of age. Based on these data presented in Bell and Variend (1985), Figures 2 through 5, pp. 144–146, we approximated the mean callosal values for the groups of children by assuming that those with the largest brain weights were the oldest.

[q]This value is the only measurement reported for this age group, and it is for an unknown number of 2-year-olds.

losum, which included the brain specimens of some infants and children within a large sample consisting mainly of adults. Bean was primarily concerned with neuroanatomical differences related to intelligence and race, but he also compared the sexes. The sample included only a few infants and children, with the majority being "Negro" males. Race may be a relevant variable in callosal size and morphology (Witelson & Kigar, 1987a). Bean, however, is the only author who reported the race of his cases.

Several decades later, Luttenberg (1965) presented data on overall callosal area and the packing density of callosal fibers throughout the callosum. A few years later, Rakic and Yakovlev (1968) published a report that includes the largest sample of fetal brains studied to date. They charted the gross morphological changes in the corpus callosum from fetal to adult life. Their measurements were made on celloidin-embedded brain sections. This embedding procedure results in greater shrinkage of tissue than formalin fixation alone (Van Buren & Borke, 1972), making it difficult to compare some measurements with other studies, most of which used only formalin-fixed tissue.

In 1982, Baack, de Lacoste-Utamsing, and Woodward presented a preliminary report of callosal size on a group of fetal brains in the first study of callosal size during development that addressed the issue of possible sex differences. Following the interest and controversy of possible sex differences in callosal size in adults (for review, see Witelson & Kigar, 1987a, 1987b), several studies followed that investigated possible sex differences in the developing callosum (Bell & Variend, 1985; Clarke, Kraftsik, Innocenti, & van der Loos, 1986; de Lacoste, Holloway, & Woodward, 1986).

Various linear and area measurements of callosal size were reported in the different studies. In this chapter, consideration of total size of the callosum deals mainly with area measurements rather than length or height, since area was found to be more sensitive to individual differences in callosal morphology than linear measures (Witelson & Kigar, 1987a). The main linear measures, however, are included in Table 2-1 for reference.

Most work has focused on the total callosum rather than on subdivisions. In the last decade, however, the splenium, the posterior bulbous region of the callosum, has been the subject of considerable study as to its function and anatomy in many species (Leporé *et al.*, 1986). The review of the work on the anatomy of the splenium in humans is also presented in Table 2-1. The anatomical features and dimensions of the callosum discussed in this chapter are schematically presented in Figure 2-1.

TOTAL CORPUS CALLOSUM: ABSOLUTE SIZE

Callosal size varies markedly with chronological age (see Table 2-1). It is essential, therefore, that age is matched as well as possible for any comparisons between studies. Other factors influencing callosal size are brain weight, sex, tissue-embedding procedures, and cause of death. These were usually specified in the individual reports. In the case of brain specimens from children, documented cause of death is essential in order to rule out cases with congenitally abnormal brain development. Other variables that could affect callosal size, such as body height, early nutrition, and the time interval between death and fixation of the brain, are not usually available in the reports.

The minimal criteria for a study to be included in the summarized data in Table 2-1 are information regarding chronological age, tissue fixation and embedding methods, and probable cause of death. Some of these studies, however, did not present the method by which their samples were selected.

In order to make maximal use of the data for the issue of the growth pattern of the

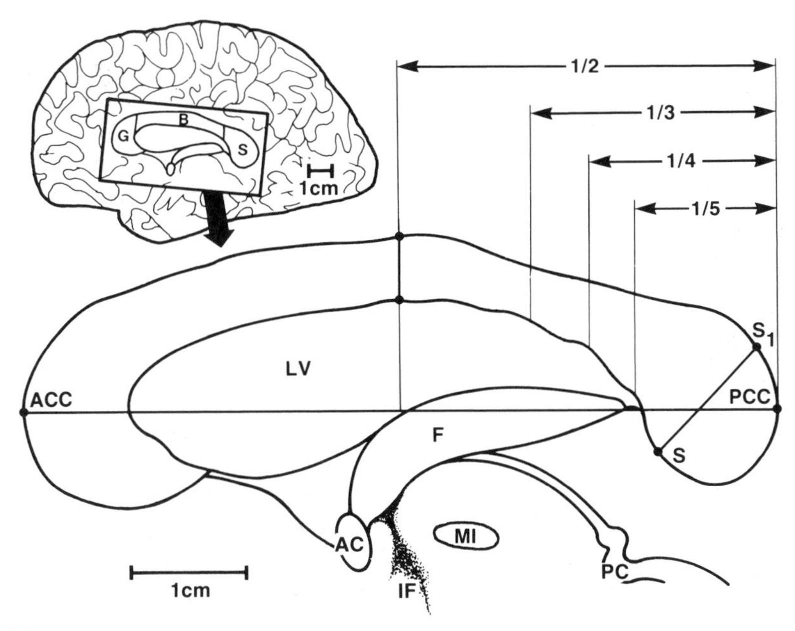

Figure 2-1. Schematic drawing of the corpus callosum of the brain of a human adult as seen in midsagittal view. The various measures and subdivisions referenced in Table 2-1 are shown. Abbreviations: G, genu; B, body; S, splenium; ACC and PCC, anteriormost and posteriormost points of the corpus callosum, respectively, which are joined to form the line of maximal length used to obtain geometric subdivisions of the callosum (anterior and posterior halves, and posterior one-third (referenced in Luttenberg, 1965; Witelson, 1987a), posterior quartile (referenced in Clarke *et al.*, 1986), and posterior one-fifth regions); AC, anterior commissure; F, fornix; IF, interventricular foramen; LV, lateral ventricle; MI, massa intermedia; PC, posterior commissure; S and S_1, points that are joined to form the line of maximal dorsoventral width of the splenium. Adapted from Witelson and Kigar (1987a).

callosum, in addition to reporting the mean values for the total groups for different studies in Table 2-1, where possible, we calculated mean values for age subgroups. Values for key groups that included only single cases are also presented in Table 2-1 and in subsequent figures, and are discussed in the text. In some studies, only the minimum and maximum callosal measurements were given, without the corresponding ages. In such situations, we made some assumptions in order to use the data to their fullest capacity, and the details are specified in the relevant sections.

Fetal Brains

The callosum of fetal brains was measured in five studies (Table 2-1). Three of the reports were based on subsets of the same collection of celloidin-embedded specimens. Our calculations for the mean callosal area for the groups of fetuses included in the common age interval of 26 to 43 weeks was almost identical in each study (58, 57, and 58 mm^2 for Baack *et al.*, 1982; de Lacoste *et al.*, 1986; and Rakic & Yakovlev, 1968, respectively). These values may be calculated from those presented in Table 2-1. The values are smaller than actual size because of the shrinkage caused by celloidin embedding.

Luttenberg (1965) studied a smaller sample of fetuses using paraffin-embedded material, which also has marked shrinkage. The mean callosal size for a subsample from this study, aged 19 to 40 weeks, was 102 mm^2, compared to 53 mm^2 for a similar age group (18 to 43 weeks) in the Rakic and Yakovlev study.

Two of the reports of fetal brains analyzed sex subgroups separately (Baack *et al.*, 1982; de Lacoste *et al.*, 1986). Mean callosal area of the female group tended to be larger than the male group in both studies, but the differences were not statistically significant.

Infant Brains

Measurements of callosal size were available for infants (birth to 24 months) in five studies. For a subgroup of 13 infants (male and female combined) varying in age from birth to 3 months, the mean callosal area was 213 mm^2 (Bell & Variend, 1985), only slightly less than the mean of 231 mm^2 for the two infant cases of 3 and 5 months in Luttenberg's (1965) study, athough the latter study involved paraffin embedding, which might be expected to yield smaller values. Bean's (1906) total infant group had a mean age of 9 months and a mean callosal area of 307 mm^2. These results show the increase of callosal size with age in infancy. Rakic and Yakovlev's (1968) infant group, which had a mean age of 11 months, had a mean callosal area of 148 mm^2; but again their study involved celloidin-embedded tissue, which would be expected to yield smaller values. The sample in the Clarke *et al.* (1986) study consisted of 20 infants, but the only value presented was 550 mm^2 for an unstated number of 2-year-olds. The mean callosal value for the two 2-year-olds in Bean's study was 465 mm^2.

Possible sex differences were considered in two studies, but statistical analyses showed no sex differences in either study (Bell & Variend, 1985; Clarke *et al.*, 1986). This was so even when differing age and brain weight were statistically controlled (Bell & Variend, 1985).

Children's Brains

For children aged 2 to 18 years, even fewer data are available. Bean's sample included 4 children who varied in age from 8 to 16 years (mean age = 13 years) and for whom callosal area varied from 420 to 613 mm^2, with a mean of 498 mm^2. Bell and Variend's total sample included 7 children who varied in age from 3 to 14 years. From the raw data given for callosal area, we approximated a mean value of 645 mm^2 and minimum and maximum values of 455 mm^2 and 853 mm^2 (for further details see Table 2-1). A noteworthy aspect of these observations is that there is little increase in callosal size after the age of 2 years.

Both Bean (1906) and Bell and Variend (1985) reported the sex of their cases in this age interval. However, Bean had only one female; Bell and Variend, two; and their ages were not comparable to those of the male cases, making any comparisons unreasonable.

To summarize, despite the many uncontrolled variables relevant to callosal size, the limited data available, and the major gaps in the data, the size of callosal area at various ages was found to be reasonably similar across studies. The callosum tends to increase in size with development, particularly in fetal and infant stages. No reliable sex differences were observed.

DEVELOPMENTAL COURSE OF ABSOLUTE CALLOSAL SIZE

The consistency in the data and the apparent trends in the developmental course of callosal size suggested that it would be reasonable and possibly fruitful to compare the studies graphically, as is done in Figure 2-2. This figure presents mean scores calculated for various age subgroups in each study, chosen in order to have subgroups comparable in age across studies and as comprehensive a developmental picture as possible.

Straight-line model regression analyses of callosal size on age were performed on the data in each study that had two or more data points within any age interval, as seen in Figure 2-2. The regression equations were used to plot the lines and are given in the figure legend. As can be seen in Figure 2-2, there is strong interstudy similarity. The slopes of the lines are similar for different studies within each of the fetal and infant periods. In the fetal period, the rate of growth is represented by rapidly accelerating lines with slopes of 1.2, 2.1, 5.9, 6.5, representing the callosal increase in area (mm^2) per week of fetal life (Clark *et al.*, 1986; de Lacoste *et al.*, 1986; Luttenberg, 1965; Rakic & Yakovlev, 1968; respectively). The first two studies are those that used celloidin-embedded tissue, and one might expect the slope of the lines reflecting rate of callosal growth to be less with material having greater shrinkage, which is the case. The mean values at different ages, particularly within the infant age interval, are very similar across different studies.

In the two studies using formalin-fixed or paraffin-embedded tissue, the increase in fetal callosal area varies from approximately 10 mm^2 per month near the end of the first trimester, to 20 mm^2 per month during the second and 30 mm^2 per month in the final trimester. The rate of growth is not constant during fetal life, and therefore growth of the callosum during this period is likely best represented by a curvilinear line as can be seen for the four data points for Luttenberg's study in Figure 2-2. However, a straight-line model was deemed adequate for the purposes of this chapter.

The picture of callosal growth during the first 2 years of postnatal life appears to be different from that during the fetal age interval. For the callosa of infants from birth to 24 months, the fitted lines have slopes of 14.4, 11.4, and 13.0 mm^2 per month (Bean, 1906; Bell & Variend, 1985; Luttenberg, 1965, respectively, all using formalin-fixed or paraffin-embedded material), and have a mean callosal growth of 13.1 mm^2 per month, or about 3.5 mm^2 per week, during infancy. This is a lower growth rate than in the middle or final stages of fetal life.

Callosal size in children aged 2 to 18 years has been reported in only two studies, and they include very small samples spanning this large age period. It can be seen from Figure 2-2 that the values of these two studies of children are similar to each other, similar to those in late infancy and only minimally smaller than the well-documented size of the callosum in adults. A review of individual differences in the adult callosum is given elsewhere (Witelson & Kigar, 1987a).

If the callosum were to continue growing from age 2 until 18 years of age at the same rate as it does in infancy (approximately 13 mm^2 per month), adult callosal size would end up 300% greater than is actually the case. One possible hypothetical model of callosal growth is that the callosum continues growing in childhood at the same rate as it does in infancy, and that the adult callosal size is reached between age 3 and 4 years, with no further overall growth. Another possible model is that soon after age 2, there is a marked decrease in the rate of callosal growth, with very slow growth occurring throughout childhood until the full adult size is reached, possibly by about age 10 years, when callosal myelination is completed (Yakovlev & Lecours, 1967). The lack of data on callosal size between age 2 years and maturity prevents selecting a particular model, although the latter

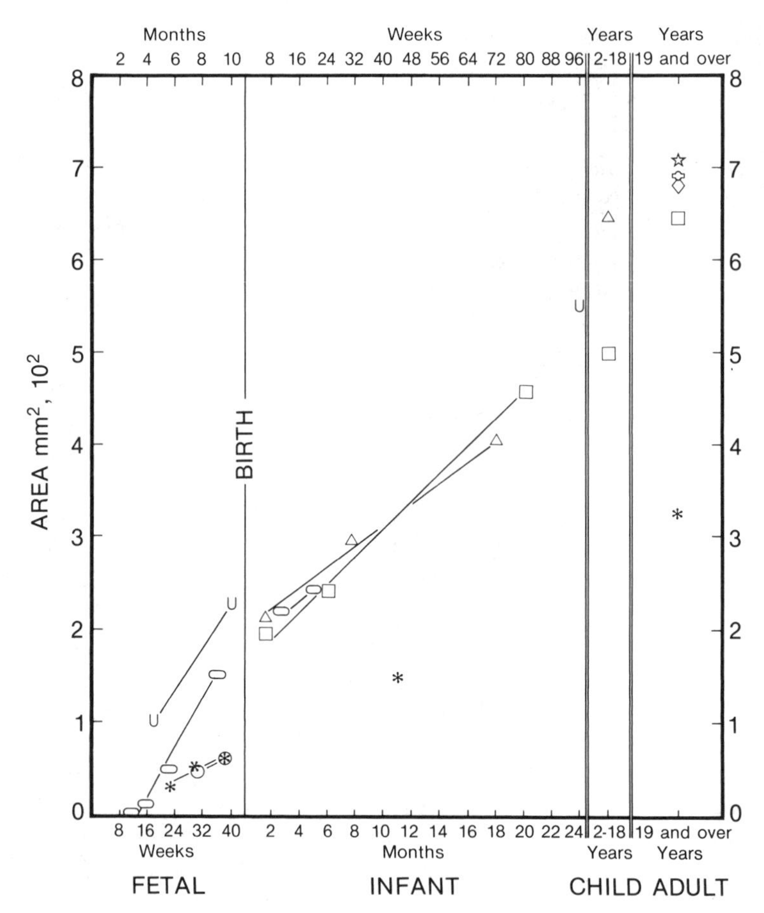

Figure 2-2. Total actual area of the corpus callosum over development. Most data points are mean values; a few are scores for individual cases. Most of these values may be compared to or calculated from those in Table 2-1, which also provides sample sizes and the minimum and maximum ages of the samples. The location of tick marks on the X-scale for fetal and infant age intervals corresponds to exactly the same time intervals (8 weeks or 2 months). In Bean's report, callosal size and age were presented for each case, which allowed the present authors to subdivide the total infant sample into three age groupings to match those of Bell and Variend, the only other study with subgroups in this age interval. For Bell and Variend's report, using the sample sizes given for several infant age subgroups, we organized the total sample into three age groupings based on given brain weights. In the report of Clarke *et al.*, no mean values, only the minimum and maximum callosal areas, were given for the fetal group. We approximated the ages of these extreme cases by using the ages of the youngest and oldest fetuses that underwent comparable callosal measurement in other studies. All studies of adults providing mean callosal values are plotted; a more complete review of callosal size in adults is presented elsewhere (Witelson & Kigar, 1987b).

Symbols	Regression equations (A = area in mm²)
□ Bean (1906)	Infant: A = 168.0 + 14.4 Age (mo)
△ Bell & Variend (1985)	Infant: A = 201.0 + 11.4 Age (mo)
∪ Clarke *et al.* (1986)	Fetus: A = −6.4 + 5.9 Age (wk)
○ De Lacoste *et al.* (1986)	Fetus: A = 15.6 + 1.2 Age (wk)
☆ De Lacoste-Utamsing & Holloway (1982)	
◇ Holloway & de Lacoste (1986)	
⊂⊃ Luttenberg (1965)	Fetus: A = −81.8 + 6.5 Age (wk)
	Infant: A = 179.0 + 13.0 Age (mo)
* Rakic & Yakovlev (1968)	Fetus: A = −16.1 + 2.1 Age (wk)
≎ Witelson (1985a)	

hypothesis of a marked early change with very slow growth during childhood is consistent with the developmental course of other neuroanatomical changes: callosal myelination, which begins at 39 weeks gestation (Larroche & Amakawa, 1973) and is complete by 7 to 10 years of age (Yakovlev & Lecours, 1967); synaptic density in some cortical areas, which reaches a maximum in the second year of life and then slowly declines between 2 and 16 years of age; neuronal density, which decreases dramatically from around birth to age one year, when it reaches a level similar to that of adults (Huttenlocher, 1984); and growth in brain size, which, after an initial growth spurt until about age 3 years, continues to increase slowly until, depending on sex, age 9 to 18 years (Dekaban, 1978). A subsequent section shows the constant ratio of callosal size to brain size throughout life (see Figure 2-4), which suggests that callosal size is tied to brain size and therefore must show rapid growth only until age 2 to 3 years, with very slow increase thereafter.

SEX AND CALLOSAL SIZE

Sex and Developmental Course of Absolute Callosal Size

Some studies measured the total callosum separately for each sex, as indicated in Table 2-1. These data are presented graphically in Figure 2-3 to help in consideration of the developmental course of callosal growth in males and females. Regression analyses were again used to fit straight lines to the data points. The regression equations are given in Figure 2-3. Only one study in each age interval included both sexes and at least data points for two age subgroups. The results suggest that the rate of growth of the callosum is similar for the two sexes during gestation and infancy. During fetal life, the fitted lines for callosal area for the one study (involving celloidin-embedded tissue) have slopes of 1.1 mm^2 per week (males) and 1.6 mm^2 per week (females.). In infancy, the one study with growth lines for each sex, using formalin-fixed tissue (Bell & Variend, 1985), yielded similar slopes for males and females, 11.4 and 12.3 mm^2 per month, respectively. Callosal growth during infancy was also available for males only in a second study (Bean, 1906), which was methodologically comparable to that of Bell and Variend; the observed slope of 13.2 was also very similar.

Overall callosal size during gestation appears to be slightly greater in females than in males, but the difference was not statistically significant (de Lacoste *et al.*, 1986). In infancy, males tend to have a larger corpus callosum, but the difference was not statistically significant (Bell & Variend, 1985). It is emphasized that there are few data points for children, and that these are based on small numbers of cases.

In the four studies to date that presented values for men and women separately, two studies (Bean, 1906; Witelson, 1985a) found no significant sex difference, with males tending to have a larger callosal area. In the two other reports, one study (de Lacoste-Utamsing & Holloway, 1982) found no difference in callosal area between the sexes, but a later study (Holloway & de Lacoste, 1986), unlike all the others, found the female group to have a significantly larger callosum. This study, however, was also atypical in that mean brain weight for the male group was very similar to that of the female group, which is not usually the case. This is even more unexpected, as the male group was younger in age than the female group. In addition, as can be seen in Figure 2-3, the values of the callosum are atypical: The male group of this study has the smallest mean value of all male adult subgroups, and their female group has the greatest value of all, suggesting that these samples may not be representative of the population. A detailed discussion of callosal size for

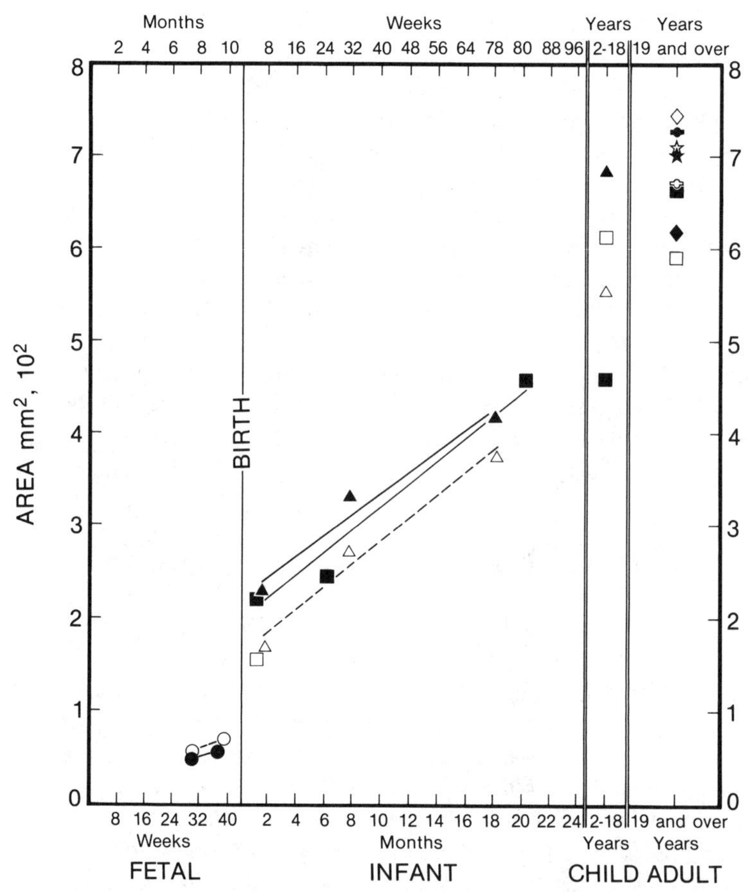

Figure 2-3. Total actual area of the corpus callosum over development for males and females. Most data points are mean values; a few are scores for individual cases. Most of these values may be compared to or calculated from those in Table 2-1, which also provides sample sizes and the minimum and maximum ages of the sample. The location of tick marks on the X-scale for fetal and infant age intervals corresponds to exactly the same time intervals (8 weeks or 2 months). In Bean's report, age, sex, and callosal size were presented for each case, which allowed the present authors to subdivide the male infant sample into three age groupings to match those of Bell and Variend, the only other study with subgroups in this age interval. For Bell and Variend's report, using the sample sizes given for several infant age subgroups, we organized the males and females into three age groupings based on given brain weights. All studies of adults providing mean callosal values for the sexes separately are plotted; a more complete review of callosal size for male and female adults is presented elsewhere (Witelson & Kigar, 1987b).

Symbols

Male: Closed symbols and solid lines.
Female: Open symbols and dotted lines.

■ □ Bean (1906)
▲ △ Bell & Variend (1985)
● ○ De Lacoste *et al.* (1986)
★ ☆ De Lacoste-Utamsing & Holloway (1982)
◆ ◇ Holloway & de Lacoste (1986)
⯐ ⯐ Witelson (1985a)

Regression equations (A = area in mm^2)

Infant male: $A = 188.0 + 13.2$ Age (mo)
Infant male: $A = 220.0 + 11.4$ Age (mo)
Infant female: $A = 160.0 + 12.3$ Age (mo)
Fetus male: $A = 15.4 + 1.1$ Age (wk)
Fetus female: $A = 7.6 + 1.6$ Age (wk)

the sexes separately in adults is presented elsewhere (Witelson & Kigar, 1987a, 1987b).

In sum, there is no reliable evidence of a sex difference in the absolute size of the overall callosum during fetal life, in infancy, or at maturity, nor in the rate of growth of the callosum.

Sex and Developmental Course of Relative Callosal Size

The data indicate no sex difference in actual callosal area or its growth curve during development. During development and at maturity, however, the sexes differ in brain size (Dekaban, 1978; Holloway, 1980), and it is thus possible that parts of the brain, such as the callosum, may be smaller if overall brain size is smaller. In a study of 42 brain specimens of adults, a statistically significant correlation ($r = .51$, $p < .001$) was found between brain weight and total callosal area (Witelson, 1985a). Therefore, consideration of total callosal area relative to total brain weight (relative callosal area) may reveal some differences in callosal size between groups of different sex and age for whom brain size differs. It is noted that the ratio score of relative callosal area may be only a crude approach to control for varying brain size. Other approaches, such as analyses of covariance with brain weight, volume, or some estimate of crotical surface as the covariate, may be more appropriate. For the purposes of this review, the mean ratio scores that are possible to calculate for the various studies may be adequate estimations.

In those studies that provided callosal measurements and brain weights separately for males and females, we calculated mean relative ratio scores if this was not already done by the original authors. In most reports, no statistical analyses were done. The observations are presented in Figure 2-4. As in Table 2-1 and Figures 2-2 and 2-3, a few data points represent individual values, although most are mean values. This was done to try to present as complete a developmental picture as possible.

If relative callosal area differs at various ages, either within or between age intervals, this would be represented by lines whose slope is not equal to zero and would suggest that the callosum and the brain are growing at different rates in that developmental stage. If relative callosal area over a developmental period does not change, this would be represented by a horizontal line (i.e., slope $= 0$) and would indicate a similar rate of growth of the callosum with respect to the brain.

Regression analyses were performed, where possible, for each study within each developmental phase. The equations are given in Figure 2-4. In the one study of fetuses (de Lacoste *et al.*, 1986), the female group tended to show a larger relative callosal area than males, but there were no statistical differences within either fetal age subgroup or the total group. Within the fetal period studied (third trimester), relative callosal area decreased with age. The slopes of the fitted lines for the ratio scores are similar for males and females (-0.007 and -0.005, respectively) and show a decrease in relative callosal area (mm^2/g brain weight) of 0.005 and 0.007 per fetal week. Comparison of this study with the one study of infants (Bell & Variend, 1985) suggested that relative callosal area appears greater after than before birth. This difference in ratio scores may be a function of different embedding techniques affecting actual callosal size differently, with brain weights not differentially affected.

In the infant period, the one study having both male and female subgroups (Bell & Variend, 1985) showed that, in contrast to the fetal period, males tended to have larger relative callosal areas, but no statistical analyses were available. Relative callosal area had

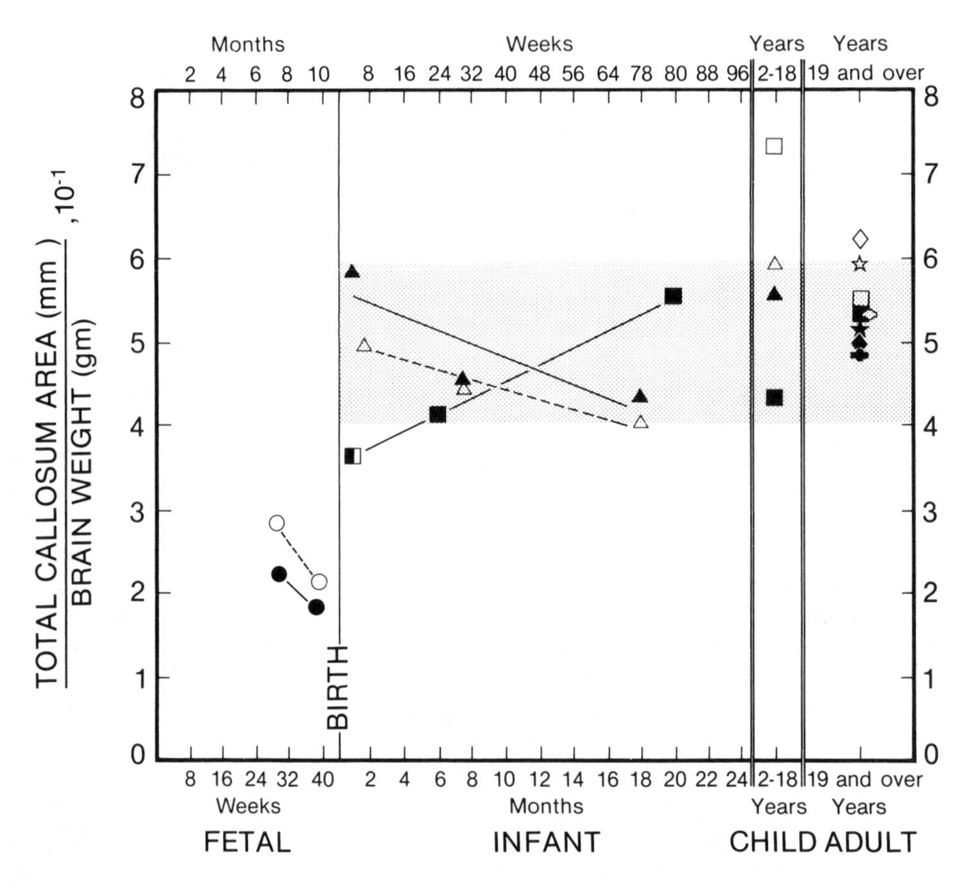

Figure 2-4. Callosal area relative to brain weight over development for males and females. Most data points are mean values; a few are scores for individual cases. All values were calculated from given callosal areas and brain weights as presented in Table 2-1, which also gives sample sizes and the minimum and maximum ages of the samples. Where possible, the mean of the ratio scores was calculated; otherwise the ratio of the means was calculated. The location of tick marks on the X-scale for fetal and infant age intervals corresponds to exactly the same time intervals (8 weeks or 2 months). The stippled area highlights the apparent stability in the ratio scores in postnatal life. In Bean's report, age, sex, brain weight, and callosal size were presented for each case in raw data form only. We subdivided the male infant sample into three age groupings to match those of Bell and Variend, the only other study with subgroups in this age interval. For Bell and Variend's report, using the sample sizes given for several infant age subgroups, we organized the males and females into three age groupings based on given brain weights. All studies of adults providing values for callosal area and brain weight for the sexes separately are plotted; further discussion of relative callosal size in male and female adults is given elsewhere (Witelson & Kigar, 1987b).

Symbols			Regression equations (A = area in mm^2)
Male: Closed symbols and solid lines.			
Female: Open symbols and dotted lines.			
■	□	Bean (1906)	Infant male: $A = .35 + .01$ Age (mo)
▲	△	Bell & Variend (1985)	Infant male: $A = .56 - .008$ Age (mo)
			Infant female: $A = .50 - .006$ Age (mo)
●	○	De Lacoste *et al.* (1986)	Fetus male: $A = .37 - .005$ Age (wk)
			Fetus female: $A = .48 - .007$ Age (wk)
★	☆	De Lacoste-Utamsing & Holloway (1982)	
◆	◇	Holloway & de Lacoste (1986)	
⬳	⬳	Witelson (1985a)	

similar slopes for the male and female subgroups (-0.008 and -0.006 mm^2 per gram per month, respectively). In contrast, the slope of the ratio scores for Bean's male infant group was $+0.01$ mm^2 per gram per month.

In children there is a suggestion of another reversal in the relationship between male and female relative callosal size, with females having greater values; but again no statistical analyses were available. The same trend continues in adult life, but here statistical analyses are available. The differences are not significant except in the de Lacoste *et al.* (1986) study which, as mentioned before, is based on samples that have atypical brain weight and atypical absolute callosal values. A detailed discussion of callosal size relative to brain size in men and women is presented elsewhere (Witelson & Kigar, 1987a, 1987b).

In sum, during fetal life, male and female callosa appear to be decreasing in relative size, compatible with brain growth exceeding callosal growth in that period. After birth and throughout childhood until maturity, there appears to be little change in relative callosal size, with almost all the values falling within a restricted range, denoted by a stippled area in Figure 2-4. Although there are few data, there appears to be a pattern and one may speculate about the underlying model of the developmental course. Usually one expects a constant or decreasing positive slope over chronological development. What appears to occur from birth throughout life is a horizontal or near horizontal line of relative callosal size. Such results suggest a close correspondence between size of the callosum as represented by area, and brain size as represented by brain weight. This situation is consistent with the observation of a correlation between callosal size and brain weight in middle age as reported by Witelson (1985a), and questions the results of a recent study of callosal size using magnetic resonance imaging, in which almost zero correlation was found between the scan measures of callosal area and brain size, and all other variables examined (Kertesz, Polk, Howell, & Black, 1987).

In fetuses, the relative callosal size of females tends to be larger than that of males; the opposite result appears for infants; and the trend appears to reverse again in the period from 2 years to maturity, in which females tend to show a larger callosum relative to brain size. Although the sex differences in relative callosal area may not be significant within any age interval, there is the suggestion of an interaction in callosal size between sex and age (before and after age 2 years). We suggest that such a reversal may occur in early childhood, the same period in which we suggested that growth in absolute size of the callosum slows markedly and the period in which it was found that a sex difference starts emerging in brain size (Dekaban, 1978).

Sex and Splenial Size

The posterior region of the callosum forms an expanded bulbous area posterior to the narrow end of the body of the callosum and is generally referred to as the splenium. No clear anatomical landmarks define the splenium from the body of the callosum, and thus it is often arbitrarily defined for measurement by geometrical definitions, such as the posterior one-fifth region of the callosum (see Figure 2-1).

The splenium has received considerable attention with respect to both anatomy and function (Leporé *et al.*, 1986). With the use of various experimental techniques, it has been demonstrated to include interhemispheric fibers from occipital prestriate and visual regions in the temporal lobe in rhesus monkeys (Pandya, Karol, & Heilbronn, 1971; Rockland & Pandya, 1986) and in humans (de Lacoste, Kirkpatrick, & Ross, 1985). The splenium shows considerable variation in shape as well as size, which may account for some of the inconsistencies in the deficits observed following commissurotomy (see Witelson, 1986).

Splenial size does not appear to vary with hand preference as do other callosal regions (Witelson, 1985a, 1986). As in the case of the total callosum, some variation in the anatomy of the splenium may be related to sex. The status of sex differences in the splenium in adults has received considerable attention recently. The results to date are inconsistent, however, with most studies finding no significant difference in actual or relative size of the splenium between men and women. A few studies are now available concerning the anatomy of the splenium during development.

FETAL BRAINS

There are three reports that measured splenial size in male and female fetal brains (see Table 2-1). In one (an abstract by Baack *et al.*, 1982), the female group was found to have a significantly greater maximal splenial width than the male group. In a later report (de Lacoste *et al.*, 1986), which may include some of the same cases as the 1982 abstract (no information on method of sample selection was given), the fetuses were separated into two age subgroups. A significant sex difference in splenial size was observed only for the younger fetuses (26 to 32 weeks). Area measurements of the splenium were not given in either report. This possible sex difference of callosal growth in fetal development is congruent with the course of another developmental feature of the callosum. Rakic and Yakovlev (1968) observed that the splenium undergoes the greatest portion of its prenatal growth before 26 weeks gestation, in contrast to the genu and body of the callosum which do not show a spurt in prenatal growth until after this age. The third study (Clarke *et al.*, 1986) examined both splenial width and area, but it is only in abstract form and does not provide the mean values for the anatomical measures or for fetal ages. However, the authors reported that there were no sex differences in either splenial measure.

INFANT BRAINS

Two studies (Bell & Variend, 1985; Clarke *et al.*, 1986) measured the splenium in infants, and neither found any significant sex difference for splenial width or area. Moreover, Bell and Variend statistically analyzed their results, controlling for varying chronological age and brain weight in the two sex groups, and found no significant sex difference.

CHILDREN'S BRAINS

Two studies measured the splenium in the brains of children aged 2 years and over. Clarke *et al.*, did not give the callosal measurements but reported that there was no statistical difference between male and female children for either splenial width or area. In the Bell and Variend study, the total number of children was only 5 males and 2 females, and no statistical analysis of a sex difference could be done for this age subgroup alone. For the total group of infants and children, however, a sex difference was found for splenial area, but not for splenial width. Males (birth to 12 years) had a significantly greater region than females (birth to 14 years). Analysis for the infant group by itself indicated no significant sex difference, suggesting that the 7 cases older than age 2 years contributed to the sex difference in the combined group. We approximated the mean values for the subgroups of male and female children from the data given in the original report, and found that the average splenial area was about 30 mm^2 greater in the males than the females (see Table 2-1).

ADULT BRAINS

Most of the studies with adults have found no significant difference between men and women in absolute splenial area (Bean, 1906; Demeter, Ringo, & Doty, 1985; Witelson,

1985a). One study (de Lacoste-Utamsing & Holloway, 1982) reported that females had a larger splenial area at the .08 level of probability, which was interpreted as a statistically significant level. Splenial area was not reported in a later study by the same authors (Holloway & de Lacoste, 1986). Clarke *et al.* (1986) reported a larger splenial region for females, but the measure they used, the posterior quartile region, was different than that used in the other studies comparing the sexes (see Figure 2-1). Width of the splenium was found to be greater in females than males in reports by de Lacoste and colleagues; by Clarke *et al.* (1986) who again used a different measure (splenial width relative to callosal body width); but not in the study by Demeter *et al.* (1985).

In an attempt to control for varying overall callosal size and brain size between the sexes and between different samples, we calculated the mean splenial area relative to mean total callosal area for all the studies of adults. The ratio scores tended to be very similar between males and females both within studies and between studies, except for the report by de Lacoste-Utamsing and Holloway (1982) in which the female group appeared different than in all other studies (see further discussion in Witelson & Kigar, 1987b). A recent study found a sex difference in the posterior trunk region (the isthmus: the posterior one-third minus posterior one-fifth region; see Figure 2-1). Both absolute isthmus area and area relative to total callosal area were larger in females than in males, particularly among consistent right-handers (Witelson, 1987a).

HYPOTHESIS OF DEVELOPMENTAL COURSE OF CALLOSAL GROWTH

A review of the available literature has led to the following hypothetical model of callosal growth. The major portion of growth of the callosum appears to be complete as early as age 2 years, by which time the callosum has reached a size close to that of minimal adult values. The growth may include three different developmental phases: (1) a fetal stage, in which there is rapidly accelerating growth; (2) a stage from birth to age 2 years, in which there is extensive growth, but at a lower rate than in fetal life, and in which, the rate of growth appears to be constant (approximately 13 mm^2 per month); and (3) a stage in early childhood (2 to 3 years of age) when the callosum either continues to grow as in infancy, reaching its peak by age 3 to 4 years with no further overall growth, or, perhaps more likely, has an abrupt change in its growth pattern at age 2 years, with a very slow rate of growth ensuing from then throughout childhood, slowly reaching the adult callosal size around mid-childhood. In addition, callosal size relative to brain size appears to be a constant ratio from birth throughout life, suggesting a close correspondence between callosal anatomy and brain size. In general, there does not appear to be any sex difference in absolute or relative size of the callosum in any stage of development. Females tend to have relatively larger callosa in fetal life, males tend to have relatively larger callosa in infancy, and females again tend to have relatively larger callosa in childhood and at maturity, suggesting a possible interaction of differential rates of brain and callosal growth over development in males and females.

This model must be considered very preliminary as it is based on minimal data. The review of the available data concerning the growth of the corpus callosum has revealed more gaps and questions than firm findings, but it has highlighted specific hypotheses that may be fruitful to pursue, and appears consistent with other aspects of physical growth.

The early rapid course of callosal growth and the hypothesized slowing of this growth after age 2 years closely parallel changes that occur in the growth of the whole brain.

There are two extensive studies of the developmental course of brain size in infants and children (Dekaban, 1978; Voigt & Pakkenberg, 1983). Brain weight increases rapidly during the first 3 postnatal years, then grows more slowly until maturity.

In the primary growth period before age 2 to 3 years, there is no difference in the brain weight between males and females. In contrast, after age 4 years, brain weight tends to be consistently larger in males than females by about 10% to 13%, although no statistical analyses were reported. Thus, some sex difference appears to emerge around age 3 to 4 years. Males continue to have larger brains than females throughout childhood and maturity, and their rates of growth in these periods and eventual decrease in size appear to be the same as for females (Dekaban, 1978).

This sex difference in brain size, which starts in childhood, cannot be simply attributed to differences in body height as is frequently done. Male and female children do not differ in body height until age 14 years. At that time, the difference occurs because females stop growing in height and males continue. This sex difference parallels that of brain size. Brain size stops increasing earlier in girls than boys. In females, the brain reaches adult size by about age 9 to 13 years, whereas in males, brain size continues to increase until about 14 to 18 years of age (Voigt & Pakkenberg, 1983).

This differential course of growth of the brain and body height may underlie the possible interaction of sex differences in relative callosal size with age, as seen in Figure 2-4 in this chapter. The larger relative callosal size in female than in male children and adults compared to infants may be related to the factors that the corpus callosum appears to increase in absolute area at the same rate for boys and girls during infancy, and possibly also in childhood; but, in contrast, around age 3 to 4 years, males start showing greater brain size, and brain growth continues longer in males than females. Such observations suggest that the trend of a sex difference in the developmental course of callosal growth, and the eventual sex differences in the magnitude of both brain weight and body height, may be influenced by a common developmental mechanism.

It is estimated from experimental work that new callosal fibers do not develop after the first few postnatal months in humans but, rather, that there is extensive elimination of callosal axons or axon collaterals before and soon after birth (Innocenti, 1986). Accordingly, it is likely that if individual differences in gross measures of the callosum reflect differences in fiber number, the differences are due not to growth of new fibers, but to differences in the loss of fibers in the regressive stages of neural development. Such changes could underlie the differences in callosal size observed between different hand preference groups (Witelson, 1986) or between the sexes (Witelson, 1987a), and may be related to differences in functional asymmetry. Such biological mechanisms begin to offer factors involved in the origin of functional lateralization in normal human development. At an even more speculative level, groups of individuals that have a higher incidence of left-handedness than in the general population, as has long been noted for developmental dyslexics (e.g., Orton, 1937) or for premature infants (e.g., O'Callaghan *et al.*, 1987) may, for some reason, undergo fewer regressive neural events, resulting in different neuroanatomical features and different cognitive features.

CALLOSAL GROWTH AND IMPLICATIONS FOR COGNITION

The brain and possibly the callosum change their growth pattern at approximately 2 to 3 years of age. Callosal growth may reflect myelination, which in turn may reflect maturational changes of the cortex related to dendritic growth and synaptogenesis. Thus, the developmental course of callosal growth may have repercussions on and also may be reflected in cognitive changes during development. A few examples follow of some developmental changes in cognition possibly related to the hypothesized callosal growth pattern and brain parameters it may reflect.

The second to third year of life has long been implicated as a possible pivotal year for cognitive and neurocognitive events. For example, brain damage sustained in the first year of life results in a different pattern of cognitive strengths and weaknesses than does brain damage suffered after one year of age. Damage before age one year is associated with generally lower overall IQ scores and with lower nonverbal than verbal abilities. After age one, however, overall IQ level is less affected and the pattern of deficits varies more with locus of the lesion (see reviews in Witelson, 1977, 1985b, 1987b).

These patterns of psychological sequelae are compatible with the general neural characteristic of decreasing neural plasticity with increasing chronological age, and an associated increasing manifestation of preprogrammed functional specificity of different parts of the brain. In one of the earliest theories of neuropsychological development, Lenneberg (1967) proposed that the manifestations of decreasing plasticity reflected an increase or development in hemispheric specialization. Few methods were then available to test hemispheric specialization directly in children. Although Lenneberg's model is logically possible, it is not logically necessary. And the increasing clinical and experimental evidence amassed in the last two decades supports the existence of hemispheric specialization, present from birth and unchanging over development (Witelson, 1987b). The general phenomenon of decreasing plasticity is sufficient to account for the different psychological sequelae to brain damage.

Several behavioral changes occur in the second year of life. In normal children, by about one year of age, hand preference begins to be stabilized (e.g., Michel & Harkins, 1986), and the emergence of hand preference in bimanual object manipulation appears to be correlated with the onset of the production of strings of dissimilar syllables (Ramsay, 1980).

In the model of callosal growth presented here, it was also suggested that callosal growth may slow markedly after age 2 and then continue slowly until the callosum reaches near adult size between ages 8 and 14 years. The slow growth of the callosum in childhood may represent some consolidation of cortical maturational changes.

Numerous psychological studies show that cortical maturational changes continue to occur during childhood. The transferability of cognitive functions to the opposite hemisphere after brain damage, which is a manifestation of the equipotential nature of the brain, continues to express itself, albeit less completely, during childhood. Some cases of brain damage sustained as late as 5 to 6 years of age have been documented to show a transfer of verbal functions (see Witelson, 1987b) and spatial functions (see Witelson & Swallow, 1987b) to the opposite hemisphere.

Changes in the accuracy or efficiency of interhemispheric communication of information occur during childhood. For example, 3-year-old children were found to have more difficulty comparing two tactile stimuli when each was presented to one hand only (each, by inference, mainly dependent on contralateral hemisphere processing) than when both were presented to the same hand (same hemisphere). No such difference on this task was observed for 5-year-olds (Galin, Johnstone, Nakell, & Herron, 1979). Similar results were obtained in a developmental study of interhemispheric transfer of information in which normal 5-year-old children showed less evidence of transfer between hemispheres on spatial and motor tasks than did older children (O'Leary, 1980). In a recent study (Potter & Graves, 1987) it was observed that tasks involving interhemispheric transfer of information within the tactile and motor systems, but not in the visual system, were performed less well by adults having consistent right-hand preference than by those having some left-hand preference. The authors suggested that their results may be related to greater overall callosal size and possibly more callosal fibers in non-consistent-right-handers than in consistent-right-handers, as suggested by Witelson (1985a). The hypothesis of callosal growth during childhood presented in this chapter would suggest specific hypotheses about developmental changes in performance on these tests of interhemispheric communication and related cognitive tasks.

Our model suggests that by about age 10 years, the callosum is close to adult size. Its myelination is also nearing completion (Yakovlev & Lecours, 1967). At this age, there are examples of qualitative changes in cognition. One such example may be taken from aspects of face perception. Before age 10 years, familiar faces show greater dependence on right-hemisphere processing, but only after age 10 have unfamiliar faces been observed to show this pattern of brain lateralization. Such results suggest that mediation of all faces mainly by the right hemisphere and, by inference, by a configurational strategy, becomes possible only by age 10 years. At about the same age, the recognition of inverted faces has been found to be more difficult than for younger children. Additionally, face perception in general shows a temporary decline around this age.

In another area of perception, children over age 10 were observed to perform better with bilateral (one stimulus to each hemisphere) than with unilateral input of different, conflicting visual stimuli to the hemispheres, whereas children younger than age 10 did not benefit from bilateral presentation (see review of these studies in Witelson & Swallow, 1987b). As a final example, children undergoing therapeutic transection of the corpus callosum before age 10 years were found to show less of a deficit in interhemispheric integration of tactile functions than were individuals with callosotomy done in later childhood (Lassonde, Sauerwein, Geoffroy, & Décarie, 1986).

After adolescence there is less change in brain and callosal size. Brain growth and myelination appear to have slowed to a plateau. Yakovlev and Lecours (1967) have suggested that cells, from which fully myelinated fibers emerge, are strongly committed to established neural networks resulting from maturation and learning. After adolescence, fewer qualitative changes in cognition may occur.

The possible correlation of brain changes, as indexed by callosal growth, with cognitive changes suggests that the measurement of the growth of the callosum after age 2 years until maturity may be important for further elucidation of neuroanatomical and psychological issues. In future work, it might prove fruitful to chart the growth of different regions of the callosum as indicators of possibly different maturational changes in different cortical regions. An extensive source is already available for such work: the Yakovlev collection (Kretschmann *et al.*, 1982). Such information could have implications for specific hypotheses of cognitive growth that might not be as evident without a neuroanatomical guide.

SUMMARY

This chapter reviews studies concerning the measurement of the corpus callosum during development in humans. The results of the studies were summarized in tabular and graphic form, with some statistical analyses performed on the data. In general, the results suggest the following model of callosal growth: a rapid and accelerating rate during gestation, followed by a lower but constant rate of growth during infancy, which in turn is followed by an even slower rate of callosal growth after age 2 years that continues until adult size is reached sometime in mid-childhood. There is no reliable evidence of sex differences in absolute or relative total callosal area in fetuses, infants, children, or adults. However, there may be an interaction of sex and developmental stage for callosal size relative to brain size. This interaction is consistent with the differential patterns observed for overall brain growth in males and females. Moreover, brain growth does not have the same developmental course as does body height. The overall pattern suggests that although the growth of the callosum, the brain, and the body follow different developmental courses, they may have a common antecedent mechanism.

Callosal growth may represent cortical changes and, accordingly, cognitive changes. The ages at which callosal growth patterns changed were considered in terms of cognitive development. Some possible cognitive changes associated with these ages were presented. The results of this review point to specific gaps in the knowledge of neuroanatomical development and suggest some specific neuropsychological hypotheses that may be worthwhile to pursue.

ACKNOWLEDGMENTS

The authors thank Professor Charles H. Goldsmith, Department of Clinical Epidemiology and Biostatistics, McMaster University, for statistical advice, and Diane Clews for typing the manuscripts. Preparation of this chapter was supported in part by NIH grant RO1-NS18954 awarded to SFW.

REFERENCES

Baack, J., de Lacoste-Utamsing, M. C., & Woodward, D. J. (1982). Sexual dimorphism in human fetal corpora callosa. *Society for Neuroscience Abstracts, 8,* No. 57.18.

Bean, R. B. (1906). Some racial peculiarities of the Negro brain. *American Journal of Anatomy, 5,* 353–432.

Bell, A. D., & Variend, S. (1985). Failure to demonstrate sexual dimorphism of the corpus callosum in childhood. *Journal of Anatomy, 143,* 143–147.

Bryden, M. P. (1982). *Laterality: Functional asymmetry in the intact brain.* Toronto: Academic Press.

Chiarello, C. (1980). A house divided? Cognitive functioning with callosal agenesis. *Brain and Language, 11,* 128–158.

Clarke, S., Kraftsik, R., Innocenti, G. M., & van der Loos, H. (1986). Sexual dimorphism and development of the human corpus callosum. *Neuroscience Letters, 26,* S 299. [Abstract.]

Dekaban, A. S. (with D. Sadowsky). (1978). Changes in brain weights during the span of human life: Relation of brain weights to body heights and body weights. *Annals of Neurology, 4,* 345–356.

de Lacoste, M. C., Holloway, R. L., & Woodward, D. J. (1986). Sex differences in the fetal human corpus callosum. *Human Neurobiology, 5,* 93–96.

de Lacoste, M. C., Kirkpatrick, J. B., & Ross, E. D. (1985). Topography of the human corpus callosum. *Journal of Neuropathology and Experimental Neurology, 44,* 578–591.

de Lacoste-Utamsing, C., & Holloway, R. L. (1982). Sexual dimorphism in the human corpus callosum. *Science, 216,* 1431–1432.

Demeter, S., Ringo, J., & Doty, R. W. (1985). Sexual dimorphism in the human corpus callosum? *Society for Neuroscience Abstracts, 11,* No. 254.12.

Dennis, M. (1976). Impaired sensory and motor differentiation with corpus callosum agenesis: A lack of callosal inhibition during ontogeny? *Neuropsychologia, 14,* 455–469.

Galin, D., Johnstone, J., Nakell, L., & Herron, J. (1979). Development of the capacity for tactile information transfer between hemispheres in normal children. *Science, 204,* 1330–1332.

Holloway, R. L. (1980). Within-species brain–body weight variability: A reexamination of the Danish data and other primate species. *American Journal of Physical Anthropology, 53,* 109–121.

Holloway, R. L., & de Lacoste, M. C. (1986). Sexual dimorphism in the human corpus callosum: An extension and replication study. *Human Neurobiology, 5,* 87–91.

Huttenlocher, P. R. (1984). Synapse elimination and plasticity in developing human cerebral cortex. *American Journal of Mental Deficiency, 88,* 488–496.

Innocenti, G. M. (1986). General organization of callosal connections in the cerebral cortex. In E. G. Jones & A. A. Peters (Eds.), *Cerebral cortex Vol. 5* (pp. 291–353). New York: Plenum.

Kertesz, A., Polk, M., Howell, J., & Black, S. E. (1987). Cerebral dominance, sex, and callosal size in MRI. *Neurology, 37,* 1385–1388.

Kretschmann, H-J., Kammradt, G. L., Cowart, E. C., Hopt, A., Krauthausen, I., Lange, H. W., & Sauer, B. (1982). The Yakovlev collection: A unique resource for brain research and the basis for a multinational data bank. *Journal für Hirnforschung, 23,* 647–656.

Larroche, J. C., & Amakawa, H. (1973). Glia of myelination and fat deposit during early myelogenesis. *Biology of the Neonate, 22,* 421–435.

Lassonde, M., Sauerwein, H., Geoffroy, G., & Décarie, M. (1986). Effects of early and late transection of the corpus callosum in children. *Brain, 109,* 953–967.

Lenneberg, E. H. (1967). *Biological foundations of language.* New York: Wiley.

Leporé, F., Ptito, M., & Jasper, H. H. (Eds.) (1986). *Two hemispheres, one brain: Functions of the corpus callosum. Neurology and Neurobiology, 17* (whole issue).

Luttenberg, J. (1965). Contribution to the fetal ontogenesis of the corpus callosum in man: II. *Folia Morphologica, 13,* 136–144.

Michel, G. F., & Harkins, D. A. (1986). Postural and lateral asymmetries in the ontogeny of handedness during infancy. *Developmental Psychobiology, 19,* 247–258.

O'Callaghan, M. J., Tudehope, D. I., Dugdale, A. E., Mohay, H., Burns, Y., & Cook, F. (1987). Handedness in children with birthweights below 1,000 g. *Lancet, 1,* 1155.

O'Leary, D. S. (1980). A developmental study of interhemispheric transfer in children aged five to ten. *Child Development, 51,* 743–750.

Orton, S. T. (1937). *Reading, writing and speech problems in children.* New York: Norton.

Pandya, D. N., Karol, E. A., & Heilbronn, D. (1971). A topographical distribution of interhemispheric projections in the corpus callosum of the Rhesus monkey. *Brain Research, 32,* 31–43.

Potter, S., & Graves, R. (1987). Interhemispheric transfer in consistent right-handers and mixed-handers. *Journal of Clinical and Experimental Neuropsychology, 9,* 24. [Abstract.]

Rakic, P., & Yakovlev, P. I. (1968). Development of the corpus callosum and cavum septi in man. *Journal of Comparative Neurology, 132,* 45–72.

Ramsay, D. S. (1980). Beginnings of bimanual handedness and speech in infants. *Infant Behavior and Development, 3,* 67–77.

Rockland, K. S., & Pandya, D. N. (1986). Topography of occipital lobe commissural connections in the Rhesus monkey. *Brain Research, 365,* 174–178.

Sperry, R. W. (1974). Lateral specialization in the surgically separated hemispheres. In F. O. Schmitt & F. G. Worden (Eds.), *The neurosciences third study program* (pp. 5–19). Cambridge, MA: MIT Press.

Van Buren, J. M., & Borke, R. C. (1972). *Variations and connections of the human thalamus: Vol. 1. The nuclei and cerebral connections of the human thalamus.* New York: Springer-Verlag.

Voigt, J., & Pakkenberg, H. (1983). Brain weight of Danish children: A forensic material. *Acta Anatomica, 116,* 290–301.

Witelson, S. F. (1977). Early hemisphere specialization and interhemisphere plasticity: An empirical and theoretical review. In S. Segalowitz & F. Gruber (Eds.), *Language development and neurological theory* (pp. 213–287). New York: Raven Press.

Witelson, S. F. (1985a). The brain connection: The corpus callosum is larger in left handers. *Science, 229,* 665–668.

Witelson, S. F. (1985b). On hemisphere specialization and cerebral plasticity from birth: Mark II. In C. Best (Ed.), *Hemispheric function and collaboration in the child* (pp. 33–85). New York: Academic Press.

Witelson, S. F. (1986). Wires of the mind: Anatomical variation in the corpus callosum in relation to hemispheric specialization and integration. In F. Leporé, M. Ptito, & H. H. Jasper (Eds.), *Two hemispheres, one brain: Functions of the corpus callosum. Neurology and Neurobiology, 17,* 117–138.

Witelson, S. F. (1987a). Hand preference and sex differences in the isthmus of the corpus callosum. *Society for Neuroscience Abstracts, 13,* 48.

Witelson, S. F. (1987b). Neurobiological aspects of language in children. *Child Development, 58,* 653–688.

Witelson, S. F., & Kigar, D. L. (1987a). Individual differences in the anatomy of the corpus callosum: Sex, hand preference, schizophrenia and hemisphere specialization. In A. Glass (Ed.), *Individual differences in hemisphere specialization.* NATO ASI Series, Life Sciences, *130* (pp. 55–91). New York: Plenum.

Witelson, S. F., & Kigar, D. L. (1987b). Neuroanatomical aspects of hemisphere specialization in humans. In

D. Ottoson (Ed.), *Duality and unity of the brain. Wenner-Gren International Symposium Series* (Vol. 47, pp. 466–495). Hampshire, England: MacMillan Press.

Witelson, S. F., & Swallow, J. A. (1987a). Individual differences in human brain function. *National Forum, 67,* 17–24.

Witelson, S. F., & Swallow, J. A. (1987b). Neuropsychological study of the development of spatial cognition. In J. Stiles-Davis, M. Kritchevsky, & U. Bellugi (Eds.), *Spatial cognition: Brain bases and development* (pp. 373–409). Hillsdale, NJ: Erlbaum.

Yakovlev, P. I. (1962). Morphological criteria of growth and maturation of the nervous system in man. *Research Publication of the Association for Nervous and Mental Disease, 39,* 3–46.

Yakovlev, P. I., & Lecours, A. (1967). The myelogenetic cycles of regional maturation of the brain. In A. Minkowski (Ed.), *Regional development of the brain in early life* (pp. 3–65). London: Blackwell.

3

Laterality in Animals: Brain and Behavioral Asymmetries and the Role of Early Experiences

VICTOR H. DENENBERG
University of Connecticut–Storrs

The purpose of this chapter is to review and discuss research showing that animals, like humans, have lateralized brains and that experiences in early life play a significant role in determining the nature and degree of this laterality. Since different forms of stimulation during early development can affect brain organization and hemispheric specialization, we take this as evidence to support the thesis that laterality follows a developmental course. (See Chapter 4 by Turkewitz, Chapter 5 by Hiscock, Chapter 6 by Molfese, Chapter 8 by Harris, and Chapter 21 by Obrzut, this volume.)

A concomitant of brain laterality is behavioral asymmetry. We will show that different behavioral processes are associated with one or the other hemisphere. The evidence we have indicates that the nature of brain lateralization and behavioral asymmetry in animals and in humans is remarkably similar, thus strongly suggesting an evolutionary history for this complex set of brain–behavior relationship, and that we have more in common with our animal ancestors than we might have suspected.

The next section describes some of the major findings that establish that animals are lateralized. This is followed by a more extensive discussion of the role of early experiences in affecting brain laterality and behavioral asymmetry. After this there is a discussion of some very recent findings involving the corpus callosum and its possible contribution to the process of lateralization. To assist the reader, a summary of the major findings discussed in the chapter is given in Table 3-1.

BRAIN LATERALITY IN ANIMALS: SOME EXAMPLES

Population versus Individual Laterality

Before discussing research findings, it is first necessary to distinguish between laterality of an individual animal and laterality for a population of animals. The first point to make is that virtually any animal that is studied will be found to have laterality biases. Thus, most mice have a favorite paw they use when reaching for food; rats will generally circle consistently in a clockwise or a counterclockwise direction when placed inside a small cylinder; male dogs typically lift the same leg when they urinate, and so forth. For the individual, behavioral asymmetry appears to be the rule rather than the exception.

Now suppose that approximately half the mice use their right paw to reach for food, whereas the other half use their left paw (Collins, 1977). In this instance, there is no evidence that the population is biased, since one would expect a 50:50 distribution to occur by chance. Such findings would not be of major interest however, because the lack of

Table 3-1. Summary of Research Findings

Species	Investigated	Findings	References
Mice	Paw preference	50:50 distributions found	Collins, 1977
Parrots	Foot preference	More than half the species studied used their left foot in manipulating food	Friedman & Davis, 1938; Rogers, 1980
Songbirds	Neural parts of song system	Left side of brain controls song production.	Lemon, 1973; Nottebohm, 1970, 1971, 1972, 1979; Nottebohm, Manning, & Nottebohm, 1979; Nottebohm & Nottebohm, 1976; Nottebohm, Stokes, & Leonard, 1976
Chicks	Visual discrimination, auditory habituation, attack, copulation	Left-brain dominance for visual discrimination and auditory habituation; right brain controls attack and copulation and is inhibited by left brain.	Howard, Rogers, & Boura, 1980; Rogers, 1980; Rogers & Anson, 1978
Irus macaques	Communication functions	Localized in left temporal lobe.	Dewson, 1977, 1978, 1979
Japanese macaques	Auditory discrimination of species-specific vocalizations	Ability to distinguish between different "coo" sounds better when heard by right ear and processed by left hemisphere.	Petersen, Beecher, Zoloth, Moody, & Stebbins, 1978
Japanese macaques	Audotory discrimination of species-specific vocalizations	Left superior temporal gyrus is predominant in this behavior.	Heffner & Heffner, 1984
Rat	Infantile stimulation	As adults they are less emotional and more exploratory; the hypothalamic–pituitary–adrenal axis is less reactive to novel stimuli and more reactive to distinctly noxious stimuli.	Campbell, Zarrow, & Denenberg, 1973; Denenberg, 1964, 1969, 1975, 1980, 1981; Denenberg & Zarrow, 1971; Hunt, 1979; Levine, 1969; Levine & Mullins, 1966; Newton & Levine, 1968; Zarrow, Campbell, & Denenberg, 1972; Zarrow, Philpott, Denenberg, & O'Connor, 1968
Rat	Environmental enrichment	Superior in problem-solving and perceptual tasks; greater weight and thickness of brain; changes in brain chemistry.	Bennett, 1976; Greenough, 1976; Hebb, 1949; Krech, Rosenzweig, & Bennett, 1962; Rosenzweig, 1971; Rosenzweig, Bennett, & Diamond, 1972
Rat	Environmental enrichment	Reduced emotionality.	Denenberg, 1969
Rat	Infantile stimulation, environmental enrichment, and unilateral neocortical lesion	Stimulation in early life induces brain laterality for open-field behavior.	Denenberg, Garbanati, Sherman, Yutzey, & Kaplan, 1978

Species	Investigated	Findings	References
Rat	Infantile stimulation and unilateral neocortical lesions	Animals have left position bias controlled by right hemisphere; infantile stimulation enhances bias.	Sherman, Garbanati, Rosen, Yutzey, & Denenberg, 1980
Rat	Infantile stimulation and unilateral neocortical lesions	Stimulated groups have taste aversion and muricide lateralized in right hemisphere.	Denenberg *et al.*, 1980; Garbanati *et al.*, 1983
Rat	Infantile stimulation and the corpus callosum	Right hemisphere killing response inhibited by left hemisphere through neural impulses sent via the corpus callosum.	Denenberg, Gall, Berrebi, & Yutzey, 1986
Rat	Selected cortical brain lesions and corpus callosum section	Major involvement of right parietal lobe in open-field behavior.	Crowne, Richardson, & Dawson, 1986
Rat	Infantile stimulation and corpus callosum parameters	Male callosa larger than female; stimulated males have largest callosum; sex differences larger for stimulated animals.	Berrebi *et al.*, 1986

asymmetry in the population is not an intellectually compelling or challenging subject (however, see Collins, 1981, for a very different perspective).

In contrast, we *are* intrigued to discover that most individuals in a population are biased in the same direction. The most obvious example is handedness in humans. We immediately ask why most people are right-handed, and we wonder why a small minority are left-handed (for a good discussion of left-handers, see Herron, 1980). A population bias virtually compels one to think in terms of long-term functional consequences. There must be important reasons that selection pressures forced a shift away from the expected 50:50 distribution.

Tool use has been one of the favorite explanations offered for the heavy predominance of right-handers in all human populations studied so far. Since that sounds like a reasonable explanation, we are likely to accept it. It is known, however, that more than half the species of parrots studied are found to use their left foot when manipulating food (Friedman & Davis, 1938; Rogers, 1980). Yet, no obvious functional explanation can be offered for this finding. If we take a broad comparative perspective and wonder why nature has arranged for parrots to be left-footed and humans right-handed, the hypothesis about tool use loses some of its potency. Thus, one of the advantages of studying laterality in animals is that it forces us to move beyond an anthropocentric view of the world.

Only studies for which population laterality has been demonstrated will be discussed in this chapter.

Examples of Brain Laterality

This section will be limited to a brief review of findings involving birds and nonhuman primates. Many of the findings involving rodents will be discussed in the following section. For more extensive reviews see Denenberg (1981) and Walker (1980).

For many years it was thought that the human was the only species that had an asymmetrical brain and concomitant behavioral asymmetry. Then, in 1970 Nottebohm showed that songbirds had brain laterality for control of song. The syrinx (vocal apparatus) of chaffinches, canaries, and the white-crowned sparrow is activated by the left hypoglossal nerve, which is controlled by a nucleus called the hyperstriatum ventrale, pars caudale (HVc) located in the left forebrain (Lemon, 1973; Nottebohm, 1970, 1971, 1972; Nottebohm & Nottebohm, 1976; Nottebohm, Stokes, & Leonard, 1976). The key findings were (1) severing the left hypoglossal nerve caused most of the components of the song to disappear, (2) severing the right hypoglossus had only a minor effect on song production, (3) bilateral lesions of the HVc eliminated song production, (4) birds with lesions of the left HVc did sing, but the song lacked structure and included none or very few of the components observed prior to the surgery, and (5) a lesion of the right HVc had a much lesser effect upon singing.

The bird, like the human, has considerable brain plasticity. The right side of the brain does have the capability to control song, for, if the left hypoglossal nerve is severed early in life in chaffinches or canaries, a normal song is still produced via the right hypoglossus and the right HVc. However, a similar operation in adulthood upon the chaffinch results in permanent song loss (Nottebohm, 1979)—which appears to be similar, in principle, to what is known about human speech.

The canary has some interesting differences. Unlike chaffinches, canaries learn a new song repertoire every year. Thus, if the left hypoglossal nerve is severed or if the left HVc is lesioned in adult canaries, they lose their song for the remainder of that season, but they learn a new set of songs the next season (Nottebohm, Manning, & Nottebohm, 1979).

The newborn chick has also been found to have a lateralized brain. The approach taken by Rogers and Anson (1978) was to inactivate a hemisphere by the injection of cycloheximide. Since there is complete crossover of the visual fibers in the chick at the optic chiasm, they were able to control input of visual stimuli to a hemisphere by occluding one eye. In these studies, control animals received injections of saline in one or both hemispheres.

They tested the chicks for visual discrimination by requiring them to search for starter crumbs scattered randomly on a Plexiglas floor in which small pebbles were embedded. A test for auditory habituation was devised by presenting a banging sound while the birds were feeding and measuring the number of presentations until the birds no longer responded to the sound. Chicks with cycloheximide injections into their left forebrain were significantly impaired in visual discrimination learning and auditory habituation.

These findings, as well as Nottebohm's studies, may be interpreted as examples of left-hemisphere dominance for song production, visual discrimination, and auditory habituation. A particular hemisphere is considered dominant for a behavior when there is reduction or disappearance of that behavior following (1) a hemispheric lesion, or (2) interruption of the neural pathway from a sense organ to that hemisphere, and (3) there are no effects when the opposite hemisphere is lesioned. However, when a lesion results in an increase in the behavior, or in the appearance of a new behavior, it is not possible to interpret such findings as the result of hemispheric dominance. Instead, one must invoke an inhibitory mechanism and conclude that one hemisphere is acting to inhibit the behavioral response of the other hemisphere.

Evidence for such an inhibitory process was found in other studies by Rogers (1980; Howard, Rogers, & Boura, 1980). In separate tests she showed that chicks with injections of cycloheximide in their left forebrains had significantly higher scores for attack and copulation than did controls or those with injections in their right forebrain, whereas the latter two groups did not differ from each other. From these findings we draw the inference that these behaviors are activated in the right hemisphere and are under inhibitory control of the left. When the left was inactivated by the cycloheximide injection, its inhibitory control was removed, with a resulting increase in attack and copulation.

Several studies have presented evidence that in primates the left hemisphere is preferentially involved in communicative functions. Dewson (1977, 1978, 1979) studied Irus macaques using an auditory task involving a delayed response. He found that a lesion of the lateral cortex of the left temporal lobe interfered with task performance. By means of a behavioral paradigm, Peterson, Beecher, Zoloth, Moody, and Stebbins (1978) also showed a preferential involvement of the left hemisphere. They trained Japanese macaques to discriminate between two classes of "coo" sounds that are commonly used when the animals are engaged in social interactions. The monkeys did a better job of discriminating when the sounds were played into the right ear than when they were played into the left ear. Since information from the ear goes primarily to the contralateral hemisphere, this is evidence that the left hemisphere is more competent to make discriminations of species-specific relevant communications.

Heffner and Heffner (1984) combined the procedures used by Dewson and Peterson *et al.* Japanese macaques were trained to discriminate between two species-specific coo vocalizations in a conditioned avoidance task. After training, 5 monkeys received unilateral temporal lobe ablations that included all of the left primary and secondary auditory cortex, 5 others received unilateral lesions that included all of the right primary and secondary auditory cortex, and 1 monkey received a unilateral lesion of the left superior temporal gyrus that spared part of the auditory cortex. They were retested in the conditioned avoidance task. Following this, the animals received similar lesions in the other hemisphere and were retested for conditioned avoidance.

Ablating the left, but not the right, superior temporal gyrus resulted in an initial deficit in the conditioning task. Removal of the homologous area in the other hemisphere totally abolished the conditioned discrimination. Neither unilateral nor bilateral lesions of cortex dorsal to and sparing the auditory cortex had any effect on the conditioned discrimination. The authors conclude that "the perception of species-specific vocalizations by Japanese macaques is mediated in the superior temporal gyrus. Furthermore, the left temporal lobe seems to play a predominant role in this perception" (p. 76). This conclusion confirms the prediction made by Denenberg several years earlier that "ablating the left superior temporal gyrus should abolish the Japanese monkeys' ability to make communicatively relevant discriminations" (Denenberg, 1981, p. 9).

EARLY EXPERIENCES, BRAIN LATERALITY, AND BEHAVIORAL ASYMMETRY IN THE RAT

Background

For the past 30 years I have been studying the effects of early experiences on later behavioral and biological processes in animals. The rat, mouse, and rabbit have been the three species investigated. Several techniques have been used to stimulate infant animals; the most frequently used is called "handling" (Denenberg, 1977). The cages of pregnant animals are inspected every day. When a litter is born, the pups are removed, sexed, and reduced to 8, generally 4 males and 4 females. A coin is flipped to determine whether the litter is to be handled or a nonhandled control. If it is to be handled, the pups are placed singly into one-gallon cans partially filled with shavings and left there for 3 minutes. They are then returned to their nest cage. This procedure is repeated daily from Day 1 through Day 20. All pups are weaned on Day 21.

Pups assigned to the nonhandled treatment are immediately returned to their nest cage and are not disturbed thereafter until weaning. Food and water are supplied via a hopper and bottle attached to the outside of the front door of the cage.

Handling has multiple effects on the offspring, involving behavioral, physiological, biochemical, and morphological parameters (Denenberg, 1969, 1975, 1980, 1981; Hunt, 1979; Newton & Levine, 1968). A general conclusion is that handling makes the rat less emotional and more exploratory, and that it modifies the hypothalamic–pituitary–adrenal axis (Campbell, Zarrow, & Denenberg, 1973; Denenberg, 1964; Denenberg & Zarrow, 1971; Levine, 1969; Levine & Mullins, 1966; Zarrow, Campbell, & Denenberg, 1972; Zarrow, Philpott, Denenberg, & O'Connor, 1968).

When weaned, littermates are placed into standard laboratory cages or into an enriched environment. The latter consists of large cages identical in physical dimensions to the units used by the Berkeley group (Rosenzweig, Bennett, & Diamond, 1972) for their environmental complexity condition. Each cage contains food, water, a shelf on the back wall for the animals to climb, and a variety of "playthings." Twelve rats occupy this unit from 21 until approximately 50 days of age. Animals reared in such an environment are superior in problem-solving and perceptual tasks. They also show differences in the weight, thickness, and chemistry of the brain (Bennett, 1976; Greenough, 1976; Hebb, 1949; Krech, Rosenzweig, & Bennett, 1962; Rosenzweig, 1971; Rosenzweig *et al.*, 1972). In addition, exposure to this environment reduces the animal's emotionality (Denenberg, 1969).

Effects of Early Experiences on Brain–Behavior Asymmetry

In these experiments our procedure has been to take four adult male littermates and randomly assign them to one of four surgical procedures: a left or right neocortical ablation, sham surgery, or no surgery. In all of our experiments we have never found a difference between the sham and the no-surgery animals, and these groups have always been pooled.

OPEN-FIELD ACTIVITY

In our first study some litters of rats were handled in infancy, while others were nonhandled controls (Denenberg *et al.*, 1978). After weaning at 21 days these groups were split, with some going into enriched environments while others were placed into standard laboratory cages. At 50 days the rats in the enriched environment were removed and put into standard laboratory cages. At approximately 135 days the rats were subjected to brain surgery as described earlier. They were tested for 4 days in the open field starting around 165 days and their activity measured.

Rats without extra handling stimulation in infancy showed no evidence of laterality, regardless of their postweaning enrichment experiences. In contrast, the handled groups were lateralized. The findings differed as an interactive function of handling and enrichment. For those handled rats not receiving enrichment experience after weaning, a right neocortical ablation in adulthood resulted in significantly more activity in the open field than in equivalent rats given a left hemispherectomy. For the groups that were jointly handled and enriched, the opposite pattern was obtained: Those with a right neocortical ablation were significantly less active than those with a left ablation.

A partial replication and extension of our findings has recently been reported by Crowne,

Richardson, and Dawson (1987). They showed that a lesion of the right parietal cortex, especially after section of the corpus callosum, brought about a significant increase in open-field activity. Their results are consistent with ours in showing a right-hemisphere involvement, and go beyond what we have done by isolating the effect to parietal cortex.

The finding that early experiences induce laterality for open-field activity was difficult to interpret because of the factorial complexity of open-field performance. The activity score has been found to load on both an emotionality factor and an exploratory factor (Whimbey & Denenberg, 1967a, 1967b). We carried out several additional studies to try to determine which behavioral dimension or dimensions were being lateralized by our early stimulation procedures.

LEFT–RIGHT SPATIAL CHOICE

To examine exploration, which is an aspect of spatial behavior, we recorded whether rats went right or left when leaving the starting square in the open field. The subjects were rats that had been handled or not disturbed in infancy, followed by brain surgery in adulthood (Sherman, Garbanati, Rosen, Yutzey, & Denenberg, 1980). Those handled in infancy, with an intact brain, had a significant leftward bias. Intact control rats were not biased, but when the two lesion groups were compared, those with an intact right hemisphere had a greater magnitude of response to the left than did those with an intact left hemisphere to the right. Thus, in both the handled and nonhandled groups there was evidence that the right hemisphere was preferentially involved in making a spatial choice. This experiment also established that normal laboratory rats are lateralized for some behaviors (in this instance spatial choice), but to a much lesser extent than those given extra stimulation in infancy.

Camp, Robinson, and Becker (1984) have recently reported an independent confirmation of our basic findings.

Having found that an aspect of spatial behavior was lateralized, we then investigated affective behavior in two subsequent experiements.

TASTE AVERSION

Rats handled in infancy and nonhandled controls were given, when adult, a one-trial conditioned aversion experience, by pairing a pleasant novel-tasting substance (sweetened milk) with gastric upset caused by a lithium chloride injection. The animals were then given a right or a left neocortical lesion, or received sham surgery. After recovery from the operation, they were tested for retention of the avoidance response. There was no evidence of retention by the nonhandled controls, but all three handled groups differed significantly from each other: Those with a right neocortical lesion consumed the least amount of milk, thereby indicating the greatest retention of fear, followed by the group with only an intact left hemisphere. Those with a fully intact brain consumed the most milk (Denenberg *et al.*, 1980). These findings indicate that the right hemisphere is more sensitive to strong emotional stimuli. The next experiment confirms that conclusion.

MURICIDE

The second experiment studying emotional reactivity investigated muricide or mouse killing (Garbanati *et al.*, 1983). There is good evidence that emotional rats are more likely to kill mice than are nonemotional animals (see Garbanati *et al.* for a brief review of this literature). We obtained essentially the same findings as with taste aversion: Handled rats with only an intact right hemisphere had the greatest incidence of killing, thus reflecting heightened emotionality, whereas there were no differences among the nonhandled control animals.

CONTROL OF MURICIDE VIA AN INHIBITORY MECHANISM

In the muricide study described here handled rats with only an intact right hemisphere had a significantly higher incidence of killing than did animals with only an intact left hemisphere or those with a fully intact brain. Furthermore, the latter two groups did not differ from each other in rate of muricide. These findings suggest the hypothesis that in the intact animal the left hemisphere acts to inhibit the killing response of the right hemisphere. If this is true, and assuming that the inhibition is mediated transcortically, then severing the neural connections between the two hemispheres should eliminate this inhibition, thus resulting in an increase in mouse killing. We have recently carried out a study to test this prediction (Denenberg, Gall, Berrebi, & Yutzey, 1986).

There were two parts to the experiment. First, it was necessary to replicate the Garbanati *et al.* findings that nonhandled rats were not lateralized for mouse killing, whereas handled animals were, with the group having only an intact right hemisphere having the highest incidence of killing. Although the overall incidence of killing was less in this study, we did find essentially the same results: no significant differences among the nonhandled groups, regardless of brain lesion, whereas within the handled groups those with only an intact right hemisphere had a significantly higher incidence of muricide than did the other two groups.

Once we had established replicability of our original findings, the second part of the experiment was to test two predictions derived from the inhibition hypothesis. The first prediction concerned the handled group and states that splitting the brains of these animals by severing the corpus callosum will remove the left hemisphere's inhibitory control over the right hemisphere, thus resulting in a higher incidence of muricide. The second prediction, involving the nonhandled group, states that splitting the brains of these animals will not change the incidence of killing because there is no evidence from our lesion studies that either hemisphere is inhibiting the other. Both predictions were confirmed.

EARLY EXPERIENCES, BRAIN LATERALITY, AND THE CORPUS CALLOSUM

The studies summarized here lead to the question: How do early experiences exert their effect on the brain? The answer is unknown, but one line of thinking suggests that the corpus callosum plays a major role.

The immature brain has considerable plasticity, including the nature of its asymmetry. Our early experience studies and the effects of early brain lesions (e.g., a lesion to Broca's area) both speak to this issue. The corpus callosum is a late-maturing organ, with myelination occurring postnatally in the rat (Seggie & Berry, 1972) and the human (Davidson, 1978). Thus, it is a prime candidate for mediating the effects of hemispheric specialization. Several years ago I proposed two hypotheses about the corpus callosum. The first is:

> Homologous brain areas and their connecting callosal fibers must be intact at birth, and must remain intact throughout development, for lateralization to reach its maximum level. If there is either hemispheric damage or callosal damage, the brain will be less specialized with respect to hemispheric differences. (Denenberg, 1981, p. 18)

The principle underlying this hypothesis is that lateralization develops by competition between the hemispheres. This principle is applied, by analogy, from the work of Rakic (1977, 1979), who showed that the dorsal lateral geniculate nucleus (LGd) becomes differentiated as a function of competition. He concluded from his studies that competition is necessary for the development of the layers and also for the segregation of afferent connections in the LGd. More recently Rakic (1985) has shown that this principle of competition also occurs in cortex.

In addition to theory, there are also data supporting the concept that brain laterality develops via competition mediated through the corpus callosum. These data involve individuals who are born without a corpus callosum (a condition called agenesis). Saul and Sperry (1968) gave a 20-year-old agenesis patient a battery of tests on which split-brain patients were found to be impaired. They found that "On all the foregoing tests, the normal test scores of the agenesis patient contrasted sharply with the severely impaired performance of the commissurotomy patients" (p. 307). Saul and Gott (1973) state that "Recent studies of callosal agenesis report the absence of the severe cross-integrational deficits associated with surgical brain bisection . . ." (p. 443). They studied two agenesis patients and concluded that in both patients "behavioral compensation derives from each hemisphere becoming more self-sufficient through bilateralization of language . . ." (p. 443).

Jeeves (1979) and Milner and Jeeves (1979) have recently reviewed much of the material on agenesis in humans. In discussing visual perception, Milner and Jeeves state: "Unlike the 'split-brain' patients, subjects with total agenesis of the corpus callosum have been found able both to read words and to name drawn objects, when these stimuli were presented in the left half (or the right half) of the visual field" (p. 431). Later on they say, "Again, unlike the operated patients, acallosal subjects are generally able to cross-match correctly verbal material or non-verbal stimuli presented in opposite visual half-fields" (p. 431). They reach the same conclusions in their discussion of tactile and auditory perception. The important point here is that the lack of a corpus callosum appears to result in hemispheres that are redundant rather than specialized (i.e., lateralized), thus arguing that it is the presence of the callosum that allows specialization to occur via competition.

The first hypothesis is concerned with the corpus callosum as the key link in determining brain laterality, but does not deal with the effects of early experiences. That is the purpose of the second hypothesis, which states:

> Stimulation in early life acts to enhance the growth and development of the corpus callosum, just as stimulation of sensory systems leads to their growth and development. Based on this hypothesis and our earlier discussions, one would expect cross-sectional areas of callosal fiber tracts to be larger in handled animals. (Denenberg, 1981, p. 20)

The rationale for this hypothesis comes from the general finding that sensory systems that lack adequate and appropriate stimulation during early development will almost certainly be defective in later life. Restrictions in visual stimulation (von Senden, 1960; Wiesel & Hubel, 1965), tactile and proprioceptive experiences (Nissen, Chow, & Semmes, 1951), or general sensory stimulation (Melzack & Scott, 1957) in early life have been found to cause lasting sensory and perceptual defects. After reviewing this literature, Riesen (1961, p. 78) concluded: "The growth and maintenance of neural structures depend upon the adequacy of functional demands placed on them by stimulation."

We have recently tested this hypothesis by examining the corpus callosum of handled and nonhandled male and female rats (Berrebi *et al.*, 1987). The cross-sectional area of the callosum was largest in handled male rats, a finding that is consistent with the second hypothesis.

We also found a sex difference in callosal size favoring the male over the female. This latter finding is opposite to the findings with the human, where the female's callosum has been reported to be the larger (Baack, de Lacoste-Utamsing, & Woodward, 1982; Nasrallah *et al.*, 1985; Witelson, 1983). The issue is controversial, however, and two research groups (Demeter, Ringo, & Doty, 1985; Witelson, 1985) have failed to replicate the sex difference effect (see also Chapter 2 by Witelson and Kiger, this volume). If the effect does hold up, this raises interesting evolutionary questions as to why there is a reversal in callosal size as one ascends the phyletic scale, and where the reversal starts (with the primates?).

Finally, we obtained a sex × handling interaction: The difference between male and female callosa was much larger within those given handling stimulation in infancy. These findings have been replicated (Fitch, Berrebi, & Denenberg, 1987) and open up a new research area that will be explored for some time.

SUMMARY

Songbirds, chicks, rats, and nonhuman primates have been found to have brain laterality associated with behavioral asymmetries. The patterns of associations are remarkably similar to what is known about behavioral lateralization of the human brain, thus suggesting that brain lateralization has an evolutionary history (and not necessarily the same history for the two hemispheres).

Early experience studies show that when rats are given extra handling stimulation in infancy, their brains are lateralized, with emotional and spatial behaviors predominantly associated with the right hemisphere. Nonhandled rats also show some evidence of brain laterality, but to a much lesser extent than those that were handled. Data are presented showing that the left hemisphere is less emotional than the right and exerts inhibitory control over the right via the corpus callosum. Other findings indicate that within the right hemisphere it is the parietal cortex that is predominantly involved in emotional behaviors.

Finally, theoretical considerations and empirical findings on agenesis patients lead to the hypothesis that the corpus callosum plays a major role in the process of brain lateralization. A study done with rats on this topic did find that males given extra stimulation in infancy, and which are more lateralized, had a larger callosum than nonstimulated males.

REFERENCES

Baack, J., de Lacoste-Utamsing, C., & Woodward, D. J. (1982). Sexual dimorphism in human fetal corpora callosa. *Society for Neuroscience Abstracts, 8,* 213.

Berrebi, A. S., Fitch, R. H., Ralphe, D. L., Denenberg, J. O., Friedrich, V. L., Jr., & Denenberg, V. H. (1987). Corpus callosum: region-specific effects of sex, early experience and age. *Brain Research,* in press.

Bennett, E. L. (1976). Cerebral effects of differential experience and training. In M. R. Rosenzweig & E. L. Bennett (Eds.), *Neural mechanisms of learning and memory* (pp. 279–287). Cambridge, MA: MIT Press.

Camp, D. E., Robinson, T. E., & Becker, J. B. (1984). Sex differences in the effects of early experience on the development of behavioral and brain asymmetries in rats. *Physiology and Behavior, 33,* 433–439.

Campbell, P. S., Zarrow, M. X., & Denenberg, V. H. (1973). The effects of infantile stimulation upon hypo-

thalamic CRF levels following adrenectomy in the adult rat. *Proceedings for the Society of Experimental Biology and Medicine, 142,* 781–783.
Collins, R. (1977). Toward an admissible genetic model for the inheritance of the degree and direction of asymmetry. In S. Harnad, R. W. Doty, L. Goldstein, J. Jaynes, & G. Krauthamer (Eds.), *Lateralization in the nervous system* (pp. 137–150). New York: Academic Press.
Collins, R. (1981). On asymmetries exhibiting a near-equiprobable distribution of directions. *Behavioral and Brain Sciences, 4,* 23–24.
Crowne, D. P., Richardson, C. M., & Dawson, K. A. (1987). Lateralization of emotionality in right parietal cortex of the rat. *Behavioral Neuroscience, 101,* 134–138.
Davidson, R. J. (1978). Lateral specialization in the human brain: Speculations concerning its origin and development. *Behavioral and Brain Sciences, 1,* 291.
de Lacoste-Utamsing, C., & Holloway, R. L. (1982). Sexual dimorphism in the human corpus callosum. *Science, 216,* 1431–1432.
Demeter, S., Ringo, J., & Doty, R. W. (1985). Sexual dimorphism in the human corpus callosum. *Society for Neuroscience Abstracts, 11,* 868.
Denenberg, V. H. (1964). Critical periods, stimulus input, and emotional reactivity: A theory of infantile stimulation. *Psychological Review, 71,* 335–351.
Denenberg, V. H. (1969). The effects of early experiences. In E. S. E. Hafez (Ed.), *Behaviour of domestic animals* (pp. 95–130). London: Bailliere.
Denenberg, V. H. (1975). Effects of exposure to stressors in early life upon later behavioural and biological processes. In L. Levi (Ed.), *Society, stress, and disease: Childhood and adolescence* (pp. 269–281). New York: Oxford University Press.
Denenberg, V. H. (1977). Assessing the effects of early experience. In R. D. Myers (Ed.), *Methods of psychobiology* (Vol. III, pp. 127–147). New York: Academic Press.
Denenberg, V. H. (1980). General systems theory, brain organization, and early experiences. *American Journal of Physiology: Regulatory, Integrative, and Comparative Physiology, 238,* R3–R13.
Denenberg, V. H. (1981). Hemispheric laterality in animals and the effects of early experience. *Behavioral and Brain Sciences, 4,* 1–49.
Denenberg, V. H., Gall, J. S., Berrebi, A. S., & Yutzey, D. A. (1986). *Callosal mediation of cortical inhibition in the lateralized rat brain. Brain Research, 397,* 327–332.
Denenberg, V. H., Garbanati, J. Sherman, G., Yutzey, D. A., & Kaplan, R. (1978). Infantile stimulation induces brain laterality in rats. *Science, 201,* 1150–1151.
Denenberg, V. H., Hoffmann, M., Garbanati, J., Sherman, G. F., Rosen, G. D., & Yutzey, D. A. (1980). Handling in infancy, taste aversion, and brain laterality in rats. *Brain Research, 20,* 123–133.
Denenberg, V. H., & Zarrow, M. X. (1971). Effects of handling in infancy upon adult behavior and adrenocortical activity: Suggestions for a neuroendocrine mechanism. In D. N. Walcher & D. L. Peters (Eds.), *Early childhood: The development of self-regulatory mechanism* (pp. 39–64). New York: Academic Press.
Dewson, J. H., III. (1977). Preliminary evidence of hemispheric asymmetry of auditory function in monkeys. In S. Harnad, R. W. Doty, L. Goldstein, J. Jaynes, & G. Krauthamer (Eds.), *Lateralization in the nervous system* (pp. 63–71). New York: Academic Press.
Dewson, J. H., III. (1978). Some behavioral effects of removal of superior temporal cortex in the monkey. In D. Chivers & J. Herbert (Eds.), *Recent advances in primatology: Vol. 1. Behaviour* (pp. 763–768). London: Academic Press.
Dewson, J. H., III. (1979). Toward an animal model of auditory cognitive function. In C. L. Ludlow & M. E. Doran-Quinn (Eds.), *The neurological bases of language disorders in children: Methods and directions for research* (pp. 19–24). NINCDS Monograph No. 22. Washington, DC: U.S. Government Printing Office.
Fitch, R. H., Berrebi, A. S., & Denenberg, V. H. (1987). Corpus callosum: Masculinized via perinatal testosterone. *Society for Neurosceince Abstracts, 13,* 689.
Friedman, H., & Davis, M. (1938). "Left-handedness" in parrots. *Auk, 55,* 478–480.
Garbanati, J. A. Sherman, G. F., Rosen, G. D., Hofmann, M., Yutzey, D. A., & Denenberg, V. H. (1983). Handling in iinfancy, brain laterality and muricide in rats. *Behavioral Brain Research, 7,* 351–359.
Greenough, W. (1976). Enduring brain effects of differential exprience and training. In M. R. Rosenzweig & E. L. Bennett (Eds.), *Neural mechanisms of learning and memory* (pp. 255–278). Cambridge, MA.: MIT Press.
Hebb, D. O. (1949). *The organization of behavior.* New York: Wiley.
Heffner, H. E., & Heffner, R. S. (1984). Temporal lobe lesions and perception of species-specific vocalizations by macaques. *Science, 226,* 75–76.
Herron, J. (Ed.). (1980). *Neuropsychology of left-handedness.* New York: Academic Press.

Howard, K. J., Rogers, L. J., & Boura, L. A. (1980). Functional lateralization of the chicken forebrain revealed by use of intracranial glutamate. *Brain Research, 188,* 369–382.

Hunt, J. McV. (1979). Psychological development: Early experience. *Annual Review of Psychology, 30,* 103–143.

Jeeves, M. A. (1979). Some limits to interhemispheric integration in cases of callosal agenesis and partial commissurotomy. In I. S. Russell, M. W. van Hof, & G. Berlucchi (Eds.), *Structure and function of cerebral commissures* (pp. 449–474). London: Macmillan.

Krech, D., Rosenzweig, M. R., & Bennett, E. L. (1962). Relations between brain chemistry and problem-solving among rats raised in enriched or impoverished environments. *Journal of Comparative and Physiological Psychology, 55,* 801–807.

Lemon, R. E. (1973). Nervous control of the syrinx in white-throated sparrows *(Zonotrichia albicollis). Journal of Zoology, 171,* 131–140.

Levine, S. (1969). An endocrine theory of infantile stimulation. In A. Ambrose (Ed.), *Stimulation in early infancy* (pp. 45–55). London: Academic Press.

Levine, S., & Mullins, R. F., Jr. (1966). Hormonal influence on brain organization in infant rats. *Science, 152,* 1585–1592.

Melzack, R., & Scott, T. H. (1957). The effects of early experience on the response to pain. *Journal of Comparative and Physiological Psychology, 50,* 155–161.

Milner, A. D., & Jeeves, M. A. (1979). A review of behavioural studies of agenesis of the corpus callosum. In I. S. Russell, M. W. van Hof, & G. Berlucchi (Eds.), *Structure and function of cerebral commissures* (pp. 428–448). London: Macmillan.

Nasrallah, H. A., Andreasen, N. C., Olson, S. C., Coffman, J. A. Coffman, C. E., Dunn, V. D., & Ehrhardt, J. C. (1985). Absence of sexual dimorphism of the corpus callosum in schizophrenia: A magnetic resonance imaging study. *Society for Neuroscience Abstracts, 11,* 1308.

Newton, G., & Levine, S. (Eds.). (1968). *Early experience and behavior.* Springfield, IL: Thomas.

Nissen, H. W., Chow, K. L., & Semmes, J. (1951). Effects of restricted opportunity for tactual, kinesthetic, and manipulative experience on the behavior of a chimpanzee. *American Journal of Psychology, 64,* 485–507.

Nottebaum, F. (1970). Ontogeny of bird song. *Science, 167,* 950–956.

Nottebohm, F. (1971). Neural lateralization of vocal control in a passerine bird: I. Song. *Journal of Experimental Zoology, 177,* 229–262.

Nottebohm, F. (1972). Neural lateralization of vocal control in a passerine bird: II. Subsong, calls, and a theory of vocal learning. *Journal of Experimental Zoology, 179,* 35–50.

Nottebohm, F. (1979). Origins and mechanisms in the establishment of cerebral dominance. In M. Gazzaniga (Ed.), *Handbook of behavioral neurobiology* (pp. 295–344). New York: Plenum.

Nottebohm, F., Manning, E., & Nottebohm, M. E. (1979). Reversal of hypoglossal dominance in carnaries following unilateral syringeal denervation. *Journal of Comparative Physiology,* Series A, *134,* 227–240.

Nottebohm, F., & Nottebohm, M. E. (1976). Left hypoglossal dominance in the control of canary and white-crowned sparrow song. *Journal of Comparative Physiology, 108,* 171–192.

Nottebohm, F., Stokes, T. M., & Leonard, C. M. (1976). Central control of song in the canary, *Serinus canarius. Journal of Comparative Neurology, 165,* 457–486.

Petersen, M. R., Beecher, M. D., Zoloth, S. R., Moody, D. B., & Stebbins, W. C. (1978). Neural lateralization of species-specific vocalizations by Japanese macaques *(Macaca fuscata). Science, 202,* 324–327.

Rakic, P. (1977). Effects of prenatal unilateral eye enucleation on the formation of layers and retinal connections in the dorsal lateral genculate nucleus (LGd) of the rhesus monkey. *Society of Neuroscience Abstracts, 3,* 573.

Rakic, P. (1979). Genetic and epigenetic determinants of local neuronal circuits in the mammalian central nervous system. In F. O. Schmitt & F. G. Worden (Eds.), *Neurosciences: Fourth study program* (pp. 109–127). Cambridge, MA: MIT Press.

Rakic, P. (1985). Logistics of brain development. *Grass Foundation Lecture,* Dallas, TX: Society for Neuroscience.

Riesen, A. H. (1961). Stimulation as a requirement for growth and function in behavioral development. In D. W. Fiske & S. R. Maddi (Eds.), *Functions of varied experiences* (pp. 57–80). Homewood, IL: Dorsey Press.

Rogers, L. J. (1980). Lateralisation in the avian brain. *Bird Behaviour, 2,* 1–12.

Rogers, L. J., & Anson, J. M. (1978). Cycloheximide produces attentional persistence and slowed learning in chickens. *Pharmacology, Biochemistry and Behavior, 9,* 735–740.

Rosenzweig, M. R. (1971). Effects of environment on development of brain and behavior. In E. Tobach, L. R.

Aronson, & E. Shaw (Eds.), *The biopsychology of development* (pp. 303–342). New York: Academic Press.

Rosenzweig, M. R., Bennett, E. L., & Diamond, M. C. (1972). Brain changes in response to experience. *Scientific American, 226,* 22–29.

Saul, R. E., & Gott, P. S. (1973). Compensatory mechanisms in agenesis of the corpus callosum. *Neurology, 23,* 443.

Saul, R. E., & Sperry, R. W. (1968). Absence of commissurotomy symptoms with agenesis of the corpus callosum. *Neurology, 18,* 307.

Seggie, J., & Berry, M. (1972). Ontogeny of interhemispheric evoked potentials in the rat: Significance of myelination of the corpus callosum. *Experimental Neurology, 35,* 215–232.

Sherman, G. F., Garbanati, J. A., Rosen, G. D., Yutzey, D. A., & Denenberg, V. H. (1980). Brain and behavioral asymmetries for spatial preference in rats. *Brain Research, 192,* 61–67.

von Senden, M. (1960). *Space and sight.* Glencoe, IL: Free Press.

Walker, S. F. (1980). Lateralization of functions in the vertebrate brain: A review. *British Journal of Psychology, 71,* 329–367.

Whimbey, A. E., & Denenberg, V. H. (1967a). Experimental programming of life histories: The factor structure underlying experimentally created individual differences. *Behaviour, 29,* 296–314.

Whimbey, A. E., & Denenberg, V. H. (1967b). Two independent behavioral dimensions in open-field performance. *Journal of Comparative and Physiological Psychology, 63,* 500–504.

Wiesel, T. N., & Hubel, D. H. (1965). Extent of recovery from the effects of visual deprivation in kittens. *Journal of Neurophysiology, 28,* 1060–1072.

Witelson, S. F. (1983). The corpus callosum is larger in left handers. *Society for Neuroscience Abstracts, 9,* 917.

Witelson, S. F. (1985). The brain connection: The corpus callosum is larger in left-handers. *Science, 229,* 665–668.

Zarrow, M. X., Campbell, P. S., & Denenberg, V. H. (1972). Handling in infancy: Increased levels of the hypothalamic corticotropin releasing factor (CRF) following exposure to a novel situation. *Proceedings of the Society of Experimental Biology and Medicine, 141,* 356–358.

Zarrow, M. X., Philpott, J. E., Denenberg, V. H., & O'Connor, W. B. (1968). Localization of ^{14}C-4-corticosterone in a 2 day old rat and a consideration of the mechanismm involved in early handling. *Nature (London), 218,* 1264–1265.

4

A Prenatal Source for the Development of Hemispheric Specialization

GERALD TURKEWITZ
Hunter College of the City University of New York
and Albert Einstein College of Medicine

At this stage in the development of our understanding of brain function, there can be little doubt that by the time of birth or shortly thereafter, there are anatomical and functional differences between the two sides of the brain. This chapter deals with the source of these hemispheric differences in terms of the interaction between the timing of environmental and neural changes that occur during embryogenesis.

There is considerable evidence that at or shortly after birth, human infants are more responsive to speech presented to the right than to the left ear, and that the reverse is true with regard to nonspeech stimuli. Entus (1977), using a high-amplitude sucking procedure; Glanville, Best, and Levenson (1977), using a cardiac dishabituation procedure; and Hammer (1977), using a competition for response procedure have all found greater response to speech in the right and to noise or musie in the left ear of infants around birth. Segalowitz and Chapman (1980) have also reported a greater effect of speech on inhibiting tremors of the right than of the left side in a group of prematurely born infants. In addition, Molfese, Freeman, and Palermo (1975) have reported greater amplitude of cortical evoked potentials from the left than the right temporal lobe in response to speech, and the reverse pattern to music or pure tones. The extent, stability, and development of these asymmetries has been and continues to be a subject for considerable debate and discussion (see, for example, Chapter 1 by Best, Chapter 5 by Hiscock, and Chapter 13 by Liederman, this volume). Consideration of the mechanisms underlying the development of neonatal functional asymmetries, however, have barely been hinted at. It has been suggested that hemispheric specialization is genetically determined, and several models (Annett, 1973; Nagylaki & Levy, 1973) of the genetic transmission of specialization, particularly handedness, have been offered. None of these models, however, suggests the manner in which genetic factors would act to produce the observed functional asymmetries. Similarly, asymmetries of function have been related to anatomical asymmetries, but again there has been no specification of how anatomic asymmetry would translate into the particular functional asymmetries that have been found. Finally, although there have been a number of intriguing suggestions to the effect that hemispheric specialization is tied to rates of maturation and exposure to hormones (Levy, 1977; Rovet & Netley, 1982; Waber, 1976), the mechanisms whereby rates of development or age at exposure to gonadal hormones would influence hemispheric specialization have not been proffered.

PLAN OF THE CHAPTER

I suggest that there are systematic changes in the acoustic environment of the developing fetus and that these changes, in concert with changes in the relative state of development of the hemispheres, underlie the hemispheric specialization found at birth. In this chapter I will consider the nature of the acoustic environment and changes in its characteristics during fetal development. These changes will be related to concurrent changes in neural maturation, and a suggestion will be offered as to how the dynamic relationship between the acoustic environment and the nervous system could result in hemispheric specialization. I will have nothing to say concerning the determinants of the rate of neuroanatomical maturation. This silence on my part, however, does not reflect an acceptance of the view that the changes in neuroanatomy on which the proffered model is dependent are independent of the milieu in which the maturational changes occur.

The model I advance specifies that the nature of the acoustic environment undergoes changes during fetal development, but that these changes are not primarily driven by development within the fetus. Rate of development would therefore influence the relationship between the acoustic environment and the developing nervous system. Consequently, I will explore some of the implications of this model for understanding the effects of different rates of development on reported differences between individuals with respect to hemispheric specialization. In short, I will suggest (1) that the fetus is sensitive to its acoustic environment, (2) that there are systematic changes in the nature of this environment, (3) that there are differences in the rate of development of the two hemispheres, and (4) that the changes in acoustic environment and neurological substrate interact to produce the hemispheric specialization in function that appears to characterize even very early stages of human development. It is my thesis that the timing of changes in these systems in relation to each other is fundamental to the observed outcomes.

With this in mind, I will first discuss evidence that the fetus is responsive to its acoustic environment. Next I will describe likely changes in the acoustic environment of the developing fetus. This will be followed by a consideration of changes in the relative developmental status of the two hemispheres and the way in which changes in the acoustic environment, in concert with changes in structural asymmetry, could give rise to hemispheric specialization for processing speech at or around birth. Finally, I will consider the implications of this view for understanding sex differences in hemispheric specialization and some potential consequences of premature birth for such specialization.

FETAL RESPONSIVENESS TO THE ACOUSTIC ENVIRONMENT

There is a considerable body of evidence in the literature on animal development indicating that exposure to auditory input *in ovo* or *in utero* plays a role in the normal development of responsiveness to various components of the auditory environment. There is also a growing body of evidence that the same is true for the human infant. Some of the most elegant and detailed descriptions of the effects of prenatal experience on postnatal auditory responsiveness have been provided by Gottlieb (1981), who studied the response of newly hatched ducklings to the maternal call of their own and other species. In the ordinary course of events, when a "naïve" duckling is simultaneously presented with the call of its own species and that of another species, it responds by moving toward the source of the call of its own species. Gottlieb was able to show that this preference, as well as preferences for specific components of the call, was a function of the duckling's exposure to its own vocalizations and those of its siblings while still in the egg. Thus, by isolating the duck embryo from its siblings and temporarily devocalizing the embryo, Gottlieb was able to eliminate the species-typical preference and to modify preferences for various components of the call by manipulating the age of devocalization. Other birds have also been shown to exhibit preferences for auditory stimuli experienced prenatally. For example, chicks approach a tone to which they have been exposed during the last third of incubation more than a tone to which they have not been exposed (Grier, Counter, & Shearer, 1967); similarly, 4-hour-old Japanese quail chicks exhibit preferences for whichever of two tones they were exposed to 5 days earlier, while still in the egg (Lien, 1976). There are even suggestions that prenatal exposure is more potent that is postnatal exposure; thus, gull chicks exposed to one call prenatally and another postnatally prefer the prenatally presented call when tested 42 hours after the last prenatal exposure (Impekoven & Gold, 1973).

Data indicating effects of prenatal exposure on postnatal auditory responsiveness is not limited to birds. Thus, when fetal lambs were exposed either to a sequence of bleats or to a telephone signal and music during the last fifth of gestation, heart rate acceleration, which is considered to reflect arousal, occurred in response to the novel sounds, and deceleration, which is considered to represent an orienting response (Graham & Clifton, 1966) occurred to the previously presented sounds (Vince, Armitage, Walser, & Reader, 1982). Similarly, when fetal guinea pigs were exposed to the call of game bantam hen chicks each day for the last 2 or 3 weeks of their 68-day gestation period, they showed less cardiac deceleration when exposed to these sounds postnatally than did a group of control guinea pigs. Furthermore, continued presentation led to a diminution in deceleration in the controls but to no change in the prenatally exposed guinea pigs (Vince, 1979), suggesting that those sounds were already familiar to the exposed group on their initial postnatal exposure but only became familiar to the control animals during the course of postnatal testing.

Of greatest relevance to my point are the findings that prenatal exposure to maternal speech influences the infant's response to the mother's voice. DeCasper and Fifer (1980) found that changes in the sucking pattern of 1- to 3-day-old infants could be reinforced by exposure to the mother's voice, but not to that of another woman. This effect was, if anything, stronger in 1- than in 3-day-old infants, suggesting that it was not a consequence of postnatal experience. Furthermore, infants did not prefer their father's voice to that of another male even when they had had experience with their father's voice postnatally (DeCasper & Prescott, 1984).

A recent study (Panneton & DeCasper, 1984) has found that infants will also alter their sucking patterns to hear intrauterine heartbeat sounds. The most direct evidence that prenatal experience influences postnatal auditory responsiveness is provided by a study by DeCasper and Spence (1986). In this study, pregnant women read aloud to their fetuses during the last 5 weeks of gestation. The mothers read the same story twice a day for about 6 minutes, hence providing a total exposure of approximately 3 hours. Within 3 days after birth, the infants were placed in a choice situation in which production of a particular sucking pattern produced a tape recording of the mother reading either the old or a new story. During the course of testing, responses that produced the old story increased in frequency, whereas those that produced the new story remained relatively constant. Furthermore, other infants who were tested with a different mother reading the two stories also preferred the old story. Control infants who were given no prenatal exposure showed no differential response to the stories. These data indicate that the fetus heard the story and that the experience affected the infant's later response to it. In that the effect was seen even when the story was read postnatally by another woman, the data indicate that prenatal influences are not restricted to the recognition of voices alone, but also contribute to the infant's response to other, as yet unspecified, aspects of speech. Indeed, the effects of intrauterine acoustic stimulation on postnatal auditory responsiveness are not limited to the effects of exposure to speech. For example, Salk (1962) found that neonates cried considerably less while exposed to recorded heartbeat sounds than did infants not presented with the heartbeat sounds, and that this effect was specific to heartbeat sounds. In addition, a recent study by DeCasper and Sigafoos (1983) indicated that newborns would alter their sucking patterns to hear intrauterine heartbeat sounds.

CHARACTERISTICS OF THE UTERINE ACOUSTIC ENVIRONMENT

I believe that it is not accidental that the demonstrations of prenatal influences on responsiveness to auditory stimulation have involved intrauterine heartbeat sounds and maternal speech. It is my contention that characteristics of the uterine environment make both heartbeat sounds and speech salient, but at different times during gestation. Using a model of a slowly inflating balloon to characterize the development of the uterus during pregnancy makes it clear that the acoustic conduction properties of the uterus would undergo marked changes during the course of pregnancy. Early in pregnancy, while still relatively deflated, the uterus would be a poor transmitter of externally produced sounds because of the relative thickness and flaccidity of the uterine wall. Therefore, at this stage of development, the intrauterine acoustic environment would be likely to have a relatively high proportion of internally generated sounds (e.g., heartbeat and gastrointestinal noises) and a relatively low proportion of externally generated sounds. Later in development, when the uterine walls become thinner and tauter, externally generated sounds would be amplified rather than damped, so that the mix of internally and externally generated sounds would shift in the direction of an increased proportion of externally generated sounds. This shift would increase the incidence of speech sounds transmitted to the uterus by airborne conduction. It seems likely, therefore, that the acoustic environment of the fetus undergoes changes during the course of fetal development; early stages of fetal development would take place in an acoustic environment characterized by a relatively high incidence of internal noises, including both the fetus's own and its mother's heartbeat sounds, whereas later stages of development would occur in an environment in which maternal speech was considerably more prevalent and salient.

In addition to the general enhancement of speech sounds, maternal speech would become uniquely salient by virtue of the fact that it has access to the uterus by two routes. That is, in addition to airborne conduction, maternal speech is transmitted to the uterus via conduction along the vertebral column. Finally, maternal speech would be distinctive in having multimodal attributes associated with it. For example, because of the diaphragmatic movements accompanying speaking, there would be pressure changes in the fluids of the uterus associated with maternal speech. Thus, the fetus would be receiving tactile and possibly vestibular stimulation in conjunction with maternal speech, which might further serve to enhance its salience. Furthermore, the temporal contiguity between airborne and bone conduction components of maternal speech would provide a mechanism for producing the kind of unique effects that airborne maternal speech has been found to have for neonates. That is, temporal contiguity could give rise to the development of equivalence between airborne and spinal column–conducted maternal speech. In considering the characteristics of maternal speech, it is worth noting that in the previously described DeCasper and Prescott (1984) study, fathers' voices, even when they had been experienced postnatally, and presumably prenatally as well, had no special reinforcing properties for neonates.

Although it is understandably but unfortunately the case that intrauterine recording of sound has been restricted to the later portion of pregnancy, the evidence that is available supports the view that maternal speech would be particularly salient during the later period of gestation.

Recordings from inside the uterus after rupture of the amniotic sac indicate that at this stage of pregnancy human speech penetrates the uterus. Although externally generated speech was attenuated, the maternal voice was clearly transmitted (Querleu & Renard, 1981).

PRENATAL AUDITORY FUNCTIONING

The evidence is fairly clear that maternal speech is a prominent aspect of the acoustic environment of the fetus in the period near term. In addition to the previously cited evidence concerning the effects of prenatal auditory stimulation, which strongly suggests that the acoustic system is functional prenatally, there is independent evidence that the auditory system of the human fetus is functional well before birth. Birnholz and Benacerraf (1983), using an ultrasound imaging technique, found blink startle responses in fetuses when 0.5 second sound pulses with peaks at 250 and 850 Hz were applied to the maternal abdomen of fetuses who were as young as 24 weeks post conception. Twenty-six-week-old fetuses were found to increase their heart rate in response to a 1-second 3,000 Hz tone of 110 dB, SPL (Wedenberg, 1965). Similar increases in heart rate have been reported to 100 dB, 500 and 4,000-Hz tones presented to 30-week-old fetuses (Murphy & Smyth, 1962). Heart rate and movement responses were recorded from 38- to 42-week-old fetuses in response to tones ranging between 550 and 4,000 Hz when presented with an intrauterine SPL of 55 to 90 dB (Grimwade, Walker, Bartlett, Gordon, & Wood, 1971). In some of these studies, contact between speaker and maternal skin was prevented, and the pregnant women wore earphones through which a broad-band masking noise was presented which prevented them from hearing the sounds which were stimulating their fetuses. This control increased the likelihood that the fetal response was due to acoustic stimulation of the fetus rather than to a vibrotactile stimulus or to the maternal response.

ANATOMIC HETEROCHRONY

The way in which I think these data fit together to explain hemispheric differences in the processing of speech and nonspeech at or around birth is dependent on there being a form of anatomical heterochrony, that is, differential rates of development of the two hemispheres. Galaburda (1984) has indicated that such heterochrony is in fact characteristic of the development of the temporal lobes, with convolution of the right temporal lobe taking place earlier than that of the left, although ultimately the left temporal lobe reaches greater size and complexity.

Since convolution results in increased surface area, the degree of convolution can be used as a reasonable index of developmental status, with a greater degree of convolution representing more advanced development of the hemisphere. Although Galaburda (1984) provides evidence for a change during development in the hemisphere that is more advanced, the available evidence does not permit specification of when the shift occurs. In addition, although factors previously discussed make it clear that during fetal development there are changes in the characteristics of the uterine acoustic environment, available evidence does not enable any determination of when these changes occur.

ESTABLISHMENT OF HEMISPHERIC SPECIALIZATION

In my view, during the stage when the acoustic environment is dominated by noises, the right hemisphere is likely to be more advanced, whereas later in development, when maternal speech is salient, the left hemisphere is likely to be more advanced. My thesis is that because noise is prevalent during the period when the right hemisphere is more advanced, that hemisphere becomes specialized in dealing with noise. That is, all else being equal, the more advanced hemisphere would have priority in dealing with classes of input or information for which there was not an already established specialization. When maternal speech becomes the salient component of the fetal acoustic environment, two factors operate to generate left-hemisphere specialization with regard to processing this type of information. First, at this stage of development all else is not equal, and the previously developed right-hemisphere specialization for noise would assist in the establishment of the left-hemisphere specialization for maternal speech. That is, as the uterine environment still contains noise, even during the period when speech is achieving salience, it is likely that the right hemisphere will be engaged in processing the noise as a result of its previously described specialization for dealing with this type of input. As a consequence, the left hemisphere will be more available for processing speech and thus will have a competitive advantage in developing a specialization for dealing with this type of information. Additionally, during this period the more advanced state of development of the left hemisphere would further serve to ensure that it, rather than the right hemisphere, would become specialized for dealing with maternal speech and, through a process of generalization, with speech in general. This view suggests, first, that only relatively early-occurring events would interfere with or disrupt the establishment of the right-hemisphere specialization for noise, whereas both early- and late-occurring events could affect the development of the left-hemisphere specialization for speech. (Early events would affect the left-hemisphere specialization indirectly by reducing the right-hemisphere specialization for noise.) Second, as it is suggested that the left-hemisphere specialization for speech is a result of the generalization of the fetal specialization for maternal speech, a bigger left–right difference would be expected to maternal than to other speech at the time of birth.

Several aspects of this position require clarification. Although I am postulating several developmentally unique events associated with fetal development as fundamental contributors to the development of hemispheric specialization, I do not believe these to be the sole determinants of such specialization, nor do I believe that, once established, a particular specialization is immutable. I do, however, believe that the development of a particular specialization will affect subsequent hemispheric specialization in ways that are likely to reduce the probability of developmental shifts in specialization.

OTHER FACTORS

In addition to the previously discussed changes in acoustic environment and heterochronic development of the hemispheres, there are aspects of fetal and neonatal behavior that are likely to contribute to and result in elaboration of the developing specializations. The newborn infant shows a marked propensity to lie with its head turned to the right (Gesell & Ames, 1947; Michel, 1981; Turkewitz & Birch, 1971; Turkewitz, Gordon, & Birch, 1965), and there is evidence from observations of premature infants that this postural asymmetry develops between 32 and 39 weeks postconception (Gardner, Lewkowicz, & Turkewitz, 1977). Although the complexities of acoustic propagation in the uterus make it difficult to specify the manner in which sounds from different sources would be differentially distributed within the uterus, such a postural preference, coinciding with more limited fetal motility toward the later portion of gestation, would be likely to result in differential exposure of the two ears to different aspects of the fetal acoustic environment. Such differential exposure is likely to accentuate developmental differences in the nature of the acoustic environment.

IMPLICATIONS FOR DIFFERENCES BETWEEN SUBPOPULATIONS

To the extent that the concordances between the characteristics of the acoustic environment and the state of development of the hemispheres would determine establishment of at least certain aspects of hemispheric specialization, alteration in either of these would influence such specialization. In that it is generally accepted that females develop more rapidly than males, it is possible that some of the apparent differences between the sexes with regard to hemispheric specialization may have their origins in the different times relative to nervous system organization at which changes in the nature of the acoustic environment occur. That is, for females, in keeping with their generally accelerated maturation, more advanced development of the left than of the right hemisphere might be characteristic of the later portion of the period in which noise is more salient than speech in the uterine environment. This might dilute the specialization for noise. Inasmuch as one of the proposed mechanisms for the establishment of the left-hemisphere specialization for speech is the prior elaboration of a right-hemisphere specialization for noise, the reduced specialization for noise would also result in a reduced specialization for speech. The proposed model would therefore account for the generally higher level of bilateralization reported to obtain for females than for males (Springer & Deutsch, 1985).

This view would also help to provide a mechanism to account for the differences in brain organization identified in faster- and slower-maturing fetuses like those discussed by Netley and Rovet, 1983; (Chapter 14, this volume) and would have implications for the hemispheric organization of prematurely born infants as well. That is, in that the faster-developing fetuses would have made the transition to more advanced organization of the left hemisphere at a time when their acoustic environment had a less conspicuous maternal speech component, their hemispheric specialization for speech should be influenced. Unfortunately, until more detailed information about the specific timing of changes in the acoustic environment and changes in the rates of development of the two hemispheres becomes available, it is impossible to specify the direction of effect on the hemispheric specialization.

In the case of prematurely born infants, however, some relatively specific predictions can be made even in the absence of more detailed information about timing. Thus, since the early stages of acoustic environment will be more common to full and preterm infants than are later acoustic environments, we could anticipate greater effects of prematurity on left-hemisphere specialization for speech than on right-hemisphere specialization for noise, a presumably earlier-occurring specialization. These predictions remain to be examined. Other predictions are also rather straightforward. Thus, it would be predicted that infants born to mute mothers would exhibit typical or enhanced right-hemisphere specialization for noise, but reduced or no left-hemisphere specialization for speech.

It is obvious that this position is now, at best, a provocative one. Because it is testable in some of the ways suggested, however, it may provide an avenue for increasing our understanding of the basis for hemispheric specialization.

ACKNOWLEDGMENTS

I thank the following colleagues for their valuable suggestions on an earlier draft of this chapter: Wendy Eisner, Darlene Devenny, Katherine Lawson, Gilbert Gottlieb, Holly Ruff, Timothy Johnston, and Anthony DeCasper.

Portions of this chapter were prepared while I was a visiting professor at the University of North Carolina at Greensboro.

REFERENCES

Annett, M. A. (1973). Handedness in families. *Annals of Human Genetics* (London), *37*, 93–105.

Birnholz, J. C., & Benacerraf, B. R. (1983). The development of human fetal hearing. *Science, 222*, 516–518.

DeCasper, A. J., & Fifer, W. P. (1980). Of human bonding: Newborns prefer their mothers' voices. *Science, 208*, 1174–1176.

DeCasper, A. J., & Prescott, P. (1984). Human newborns perception of male voices: Preference, discrimination and reinforcing value. *Developmental Psychobiology, 17*, 481–491.

DeCasper, A. J., & Sigafoos, A. D. (1983). The intrauterine heartbeat: A potent reinforcer for newborns. *Infant Behavior and Development, 6*, 19–25.

DeCasper, A. J., & Spence, M. J. (1986). Prenatal maternal speech influences newborns' perception of speech sounds. *Infant Behavior and Development, 9*, 133–150.

Entus, A. K. (1977). Hemispheric asymmetry in processing of dichotically presented speech and nonspeech stimuli by infants. In S. J. Segalowitz & F. Gruber (Eds.), *Language development and neurological theory* (pp. 64–73). New York: Academic Press.

Galaburda, A. M. (1984). Anatomical asymmetries. In N. Geschwind & A. M. Galaburda, (Eds.), *Cerebral dominance: The biological foundations* (pp. 11–25). Cambridge, MA: Harvard University Press.

Gardner, J., Lewkowicz, D., & Turkewitz, G. (1977). Development of postural asymmetry in premature human infants. *Development Psychobiology, 10*, 471–480.

Gesell, A., & Ames, L. B. (1947). The development of handedness. *Journal of Genetic Psychology, 70*, 155–175.

Glanville, B. B., Best, C. T., & Levenson, R. (1977). A cardiac measure of cerebral asymmetries in infant auditory perception. *Developmental Psychology, 13*, 54–59.

Gottlieb, G. (1981). Early experience in species-specific perceptual development. In R. N. Aslin, J. R. Alberts, & M. R. Peterson (Eds.), *Development of perception, audition, somatic perception and the chemical sense* (Vol. 1) New York: Academic Press.

Graham, F. K., & Clifton, R. K. (1966). Heart rate change as a component of the orienting response. *Psychological Bulletin, 65*, 305–320.

Grier, J. B., Counter, S. A., & Shearer, W. M. (1967). Prenatal auditory imprinting in chickens. *Science, 155*, 1692–1693.

Grimwade, J. C., Walker, D. W., Bartlett, M., Gordon, S. & Wood, C. (1971). Human fetal heart rate change and movement in response to sound and vibration. *American Journal of Obstetrics and Gynecology, 109*, 86–90.

Hammer, M. (1977). Lateral differences in the newborn infant's response to speech and noise stimuli. *Dissertation Abstracts International, 38*, 1439B.

Impekoven, M., & Gold, P. S. (1973). Prenatal origins of parent–young interactions in birds. In G. Gottlieb (Ed.), *Behavioral embryology*. New York: Academic Press.

Levy, J. (1977). The origins of lateral asymmetry. In S. Harnad, R. W. Doty, L. Goldstein, J. Jaynes, & G. Krauthamer (Eds.), *Lateralization in the nervous system* (pp. 195–209) New York: Academic Press.

Lien, J. (1976). Auditory stimulation of coturnix embryos (Coturnix coturnix japonica) and its later effect on auditory preferences. *Behavioral Biology, 17*, 231–235.

Michel, G. F. (1981). Right handedness: A consequence of infant supine head orientation preference? *Science, 212*, 685–687.

Molfese, D. L., Freeman, R. B., & Palermo, D. S. (1975). The ontogeny of brain lateralization for speech and nonspeech stimuli. *Brain and Language, 2*, 356–368.

Murphy, K. P., & Smyth, C. M. (1962). Responses of fetuses to auditory stimulation. *Lancet, 1*, 972–973.

Nagylaki, T., & Levy, J. (1973). The sound of one paw clapping is not sound. *Behavior Genetics, 3*, 279–292.

Netley, C., & Rovet, J. (1983). Relationships among brain organization, maturation rate, and the development of verbal and nonverbal ability. In S. J. Segalowitz (Ed.), *Language functions and brain organization* (pp. 245–266). New York: Academic Press.

Netley, C., & Rovet, J. (1988). The development of cognition and personality in X aneuploids and other subject groups. Chapter 14, this volume.

Panneton, R. K., & DeCasper, A. J. (1984). *Newborns prefer intrauterine heartbeat sounds to male voices.* Paper presented at the International Conference on Infant Studies, New York, April.

Querleu, D., & Renard, X. (1981). Les perceptions du foetus humain. *Medical Hygiene, 39,* 2102–2110.

Rovet, J., & Netley, C. (1982). Processing deficits in Turner syndrome. *Developmental Psychology, 18,* 77–94.

Salk, L. (1962). Mothers' heartbeat as an imprinting stimulus. *Transactions of the New York Academy of Sciences, 24,* 753–763.

Segalowitz, S. J., & Chapman, J. G. (1980). Cerebral asymmetry for speech in neonates: A behavioral measure. *Brain and Language. 9,* 281–288.

Springer, S. P., & Deutsch, G. (1985). *Left brain right brain* (rev. ed). New York: Freeman.

Turkewitz, G., & Birch, H. G. (1971). Neurobehavioral organization of the human newborn. In J. Hellmuth (Ed.), *Exceptional infant* (Vol. 2, pp. 24–40). New York: Brunner/Mazel.

Turkewitz, G., Gordon, E. W., & Birch, H. G. (1965). Head-turning in the human neonate: Spontaneous patterns. *Journal of Genetic Psychology, 107,* 143–158.

Vince, M. A. (1979). Postnatal effects of prenatal sound stimulation in the guinea pig. *Animal Behavior, 27,* 908–918.

Vince, M. A., Armitage, S. E., Walser, E. S., & Reader, M. (1982). Postnatal consequences of prenatal sound stimulation in the sheep. *Behavior, 81,* 128–139.

Waber, D. (1976). Sex differences in cognition: A function of maturation rate. *Science, 192,* 572–574.

Wedenberg, E. (1965). Prenatal tests of hearing. *Acta Otolaryngology, 206,* 27–32.

PART TWO

Lateralization in Normal Development

Although the research outlined throughout this book strongly supports the position that lateralization of brain functions exists from early infancy, it is clear that such a view is a fairly recent one. The equipotentiality view of Lenneberg (1967) was still widely believed throughout the 1970s. The Segalowitz and Gruber (1977) volume reviewed for the first time what was then ground-breaking work indicating that brain lateralization was more dynamic and present in various forms at an earlier age than previously believed. The chapters in this section continued that earlier work. As Hiscock notes in Chapter 5, his chapter builds on the literature reviewed by Sandra Witelson in the Segalowitz and Gruber (1977) volume. Whereas Witelson was able to describe in a single chapter the majority of studies that used behavioral as well as psychophysiological measures to study early hemispheric differences, Hiscock was faced with a more formidable task given the tremendous increase in studies of early laterality during the 10-year period following Witelson's work. Consequently, Hiscock decided to limit his coverage to studies of behavioral laterality in normal children between 2 and 12 years of age within the context of dichotic listening studies, visual half-field presentations, tactile and haptic perception, and concurrent task interference. Even so, his chapter still includes over 100 additional studies beyond those reviewed by Witelson. As other chapter authors in this book have done, Hiscock also points out what he sees as the strengths and weaknesses of these procedures and attempts to put this work within the broader perspective of studies of cognitive growth and laterality.

Whereas Hiscock confines his comments concerning lateral differences to selected behavioral techniques, other chapters included in this section develop the theme of psychophysiological measures and early hemispheric differences. Chapter 6 by Molfese and Betz outlines the evoked potential studies from 1972 involving infants and children, which document the presence of hemispheric differences from birth and track their development into the preschool and adult years. Molfese and Betz note that the research in this area appeared to develop from studies that simply attempted to determine whether any type of hemispheric differences were present at birth to studies that attempted to study in more detailed form the nature of these differences (see also the review by Hahn, 1987). The articles reviewed here support the view that there are different types of lateralization for different perceptual and linguistic abilities and that these patterns of lateralization develop at different rates and times.

Psychophysiological measures used to study hemispheric differences are also reviewed in Chapter 7 by Davidson and Fox on cerebral asymmetry and emotion. They review the EEG research investigating emotional factors in infants and adults, noting individual and developmental differences related to differential hemispheric responding to emotion-evoking stimuli. These findings introduce a welcome addition to the literature on neuropsychological development. Traditionally, brain lateralization studies have focused virtually exclusively on cognitive functions, especially language and visuospatial processing. For the infant, however, the information of highest importance, and the infant's reactions to it are in what adults would call the domain of emotion. Whether this distinction between cognition and emotion makes sense when discussing infant development is another issue. But it is clear that these socioemotional functions are at least as important for the child's healthy development as are the traditional cognitive concerns of neuropsychology, and are probably more so. There is recent interest in the psychobiological origins of temperament, with many implications for the understanding of long-term development. It is interesting that the two streams both focus on the approach–avoidance issue. It is intriguing to consider how these two psychobiological/socioemotional links may relate to each other.

In Chapter 8, Harris attempts to address how such findings of early hemispheric differences can relate to educational training. Harris argues that efforts to apply findings from the neuropsychology literature to education have failed thus far because the issues have been grossly oversimplified within both the educational and scientific communities. Harris concludes that although such applications are still premature and although educators must await further developments in the neuropsychology domain, there is currently no shortage (and there probably will never be one) of those who will use neuropsychological data to support their models of learning and development.

Finally, Dr. Gordon's chapter focuses on the cognitive profiles of the normal developing child. By measuring the child's performance on a variety of specialized skills normally associated with the left (verbosequential skills) or right hemisphere (visuospatial skills), Gordon constructs a description of individual differences that may be related to brain function. These data are certainly relevant to attempts to explain performance in individuals who have reading difficulties.

REFERENCES

Hahn, W. K. (1987). Cerebral lateralization of function: From infancy through childhood. *Psychological Bulletin, 101,* 376–392.

Lenneberg, E. (1967). *Biological foundations of language.* New York: Wiley.

Segalowitz, S. J., & Gruber, F. (1977). *Language development and neurological theory.* New York: Academic Press.

5

Behavioral Asymmetries in Normal Children

MERRILL HISCOCK
University of Saskatchewan

The publication in 1977 of Segalowitz and Gruber's *Language Development and Neurological Theory* was a milestone in the growth of knowledge about the functional organization of the immature brain. At that time a new wave of neuropsychological research, which had its origins in the split-brain and dichotic listening studies of the 1960s, had begun to impinge on developmental issues in psychology and linguistics. Various investigators, using techniques borrowed from adult studies and adapted for infants and young children, were making discoveries that ran counter to venerable doctrines such as equipotentiality of the cerebral hemispheres and progressive lateralization.

The new findings were tentative. Some would be undermined by subsequent findings or methodological criticism; others would be accepted only as first approximations to a more complex reality (see Kinsbourne & Hiscock, 1983b). But it was clear in 1977 that knowledge about the neurological basis of cognitive and linguistic development was undergoing rapid change.

The impetus for much of this research can be credited to the availability of techniques and technologies—commissurotomy, hemispherectomy, the Wada test, evoked potential recording, spectral analysis of EEG—that provide information about brain structure or brain physiology. Yet, no evidence was more prominent in the 1970s than that from noninvasive behavioral studies. The Segalowitz and Gruber (1977) volume contained chapters on auditory asymmetry in infants, infants' manual specialization, ear asymmetries in children from various clinical populations, and the relationship of perceptual laterality to linguistic experience. In other chapters, Witelson (1977b) reviewed a vast literature dealing with various kinds of behavioral laterality in children, and Kinsbourne and Hiscock (1977) used evidence of early behavioral asymmetry to argue that precursors of cerebral dominance for language are present from birth.

The present chapter updates Witelson's (1977b) review of the literature on behavioral laterality in normal children. For several reasons, however, it is not just a summary of the laterality studies that have accrued since Witelson's review. Although recent studies are emphasized, studies from the 1960s and early 1970s are also covered. To disregard the earlier studies would be to isolate the more recent studies from their antecedents and thus to make the chapter unintelligible to readers unfamiliar with the earlier literature. Nevertheless, coverage is selective. Because the laterality literature has grown rapidly during the past decade, a truly comprehensive review in a single chapter is no longer feasible. Consequently, coverage will be restricted to four major methods: (1) dichotic listening, (2) visual half-field presentation, (3) tactile and haptic perception, and (4) concurrent-task interference. There will be no coverage of interhemispheric transfer, hand preference, manual skill, lateral gaze, or torque (the direction in which children draw circles). Attention will be focused on the age range of approximately 2 to 12 years. This means that studies of behavioral asymmetry in infants are excluded from consideration, as are those studies that address Waber's (1977) hypothesis about the timing of puberty and its significance for lateralization of higher mental functions.

The chapter is divided into four parts. The first section contains a brief review of the basic issues in laterality research with children and a description of the ways in which those issues are shifting with the accumulation of additional evidence. It also contains an appraisal of behavioral laterality as a source of evidence about hemispheric specialization. This initial section provides a backdrop against which the empirical work can be examined. The second section summarizes the evidence derived from each of the four experimental paradigms chosen for examination, as well as some of the methodological problems associated with each of those paradigms. The third section is devoted to a discussion of certain general problems that affect various laterality methods. These are problems that, until they are resolved, will continue to limit the value of behavioral laterality methods in developmental research. The final section is a short essay on the future of laterality research with children.

BACKGROUND

The Basic Issues

Of what theoretical value is information about hemispheric specialization in the brain of the infant or young child? To answer this question, one might begin by considering hemispheric specialization in the adult brain and its assumed implications for behavior. There is a tradition of regarding the lateralized brain as the end point of phylogenetic and ontogenetic progression (see Kinsbourne & Hiscock, 1983b). The argument is straightforward: Humans have lateralized brains but other species do not; adult humans have lateralized brains but immature humans do not. Thus, brain lateralization is thought to be correlated with degree of behavioral complexity. The principles of hemispheric equipotentiality and progressive lateralization complement this tradition. It is asserted that the left and right hemispheres of the infant are equally suitable substrates for language acquisition but that language representation subsequently becomes increasingly lateralized to the left hemisphere. These two principles, which were supported by a sparse literature concerning childhood aphasia (e.g., Basser, 1962), formed an important part of Lenneberg's (1967) influential account of the biological basis of language development.

Individual differences in the development of cognitive skills can be readily understood in terms of this putative relationship between degree of behavioral refinement and degree of cerebral lateralization. Not only are younger children claimed to be less lateralized than older children (Lenneberg, 1967), but, within an age group, disabled learners are thought to be less lateralized than their more able peers (Bakker, 1973; McFie, 1952; Orton, 1937; Satz & Sparrow, 1970). The putative correspondence between laterality and skill has even been extrapolated to social class differences (Geffner & Hochberg, 1971). Against this background, findings of neuroanatomical, electrophysiological, and behavioral asymmetry in infants and young children were problematical. Proponents of equipotentiality and progressive lateralization could still find comfort in the clinical evidence regarding childhood aphasia (Hécaen, 1976), but even that support became unconvincing in the face of logical and empirical challenges (Carter, Hohenegger, & Satz, 1982; Kinsbourne & Hiscock, 1977; Krashen, 1973; Woods & Teuber, 1978).

The doctrines of equipotentiality and progressive lateralization did not die easily. Indeed, they did not die at all but merely became transformed by their proponents so as to fit a new set of boundary conditions. If one could no longer claim that the brain is functionally symmetrical at the time of initial language acquisition, perhaps symmetry could nonetheless be demonstrated at an earlier age. It was proposed that some functions become lateralized before others, perhaps as a manifestation of a maturational gradient favoring the left side (Corballis & Morgan, 1978).

Accounts of early lateralization carry with them certain implications for recovery of function following unilateral damage and for right-hemisphere language capacity at different stages of development. It is not difficult, however, to reconcile early lateralization and equipotentiality (Witelson, 1977b). According to Corballis and Morgan's (1978) gradient model, for example, early lateralization is compatible with normal language development following left-sided damage. Even if specialization of the left brain takes place very early in development, the right side, by virtue of its relative immaturity and lack of specialization, retains the capacity to subserve language if the left side is subsequently damaged.

Similarly, the evidence of early lateralization would seem at first to constrain hypotheses about age-related differences and individual differences. If the brains of prelinguistic infants are functionally asymmetric, it seems implausible to propose that older children—for example, preschoolers or school-age children with learning disabilities—have no hemispheric specialization at all. The principle of progressive lateralization can be salvaged, however, by invoking the concept of degree of lateralization. Moscovitch (1977) pointed out that the evidence of early differences between the hemispheres "does not deny the possibility that some of the differences found in infancy may become more pronounced or that new differences may emerge as the child matures" (p. 196). If degree of lateralization normally increases as the child grows older, then delayed linguistic and cognitive development could once again be attributed to incomplete lateralization.

In short, although the evidence of early brain lateralization ultimately demands a reassessment of some fundamental assumptions about the relation of lateralization to behavior, the initial effect of this evidence was to raise questions about the *timing* and the *degree* of hemispheric specialization. What is the earliest age at which asymmetries can be measured? Does the degree of lateralization increase with age? Are developmental disabilities associated with a diminished degree of lateralization? Laterality methods have played a particularly important role in addressing these questions.

Shifting Priorities

More than a decade ago, as noted in Segalowitz and Gruber's preface to their 1977 book, there were signs of increasing sophistication among investigators studying the development of hemispheric specialization: "The question has changed from 'When does cerebral specialization begin?' to 'How does the nature of the specialization change as the child grows?' " (p. xiii). Moscovitch (1977) emphasized the importance of specifying the behaviors in question. He suggested that, even though phonetic and phonological processing appears to be lateralized very early in life, the lateralization of higher level linguistic functions may occur at a later stage of development (Porter & Berlin, 1975). Kinsbourne and Hiscock (1977) described some precursors of language lateralization and suggested that the brain may be lateralized for a skill before that skill can be expressed. Although the viewpoint of Kinsbourne and Hiscock was quite different from that of Moscovitch, there was agreement that any credible account of developmental change (or lack of change) in hemispheric specialization for a particular behavior must consider developmental changes in the behavior itself.

If priorities have shifted from descriptive questions about the timing and degree of lateralization to questions of what it is that is lateralized, this shift has been accompanied by a trend that might be called a retreat into methodology. The early studies were characterized by generally uncritical application of new and poorly understood methods, such as dichotic listening. Asymmetrical performance was attributed to hemispheric specialization; symmetrical performance was attributed to lack of such specialization. Differences among stimuli and tasks were often disregarded. Inconsistent findings, however, soon forced investigators to recognize that factors other than hemispheric specialization were contributing to the outcome of laterality studies. Porter and Berlin (1975) attempted to resolve a conflict regarding the development of dichotic ear asymmetry by arguing that different dichotic stimuli require different levels of processing and therefore yield different developmental patterns. Satz (1976) summarized the hopelessly inconsistent findings from dichotic and tachistoscopic studies of learning-disabled children, and pointed out that the problem was compounded by a similar lack of consistency for the normal control subjects in those studies. In another paper, Satz (1977) used Bayesian calculations to demonstrate that, when laterality tasks are used to infer language lateralization, the classification accuracy typically achieved is insufficient to allow meaningful prediction of an individual's speech representation.

Why Study Behavior?

Behavioral laterality measures have numerous shortcomings in addition to those noted here, and many of those shortcomings will be discussed in the subsequent sections of this chapter. The shortcomings already mentioned, however, are sufficient to raise a question about the usefulness of these behavioral techniques. Is the continued study of behavioral laterality justified in this era of rapid technological advance?

Perhaps the best way of defending behavioral methods is to point out the limitations of the various alternatives. This is not difficult to do, as a troublesome dilemma lies at the heart of research in neuropsychology. This dilemma may be understood as a negative correlation between the power of an investigative technique and the generalizability of results based on that technique. If one chooses to study diseased or damaged brains in order to acquire information about the functional organization of healthy brains, then relatively powerful techniques may be exploited. But the applicability of these techniques, which involve either invasive procedures or the study of deficits in brain-injured patients, is usually limited to people whose brain functioning is likely to be unrepresentative of brain functioning in the general population. Findings that characterize one clinical population may conflict not only with findings from normal individuals but also with findings from other clinical populations. As illustrated by the disagreement between aphasia researchers and commissurotomy researchers with respect to right-hemispheric language functions (Sperry, 1982; Whitaker & Ojemann, 1977), results obtained with one method and one clinical population may differ considerably from results obtained with another method and another population.

Admittedly, the other horn of the dilemma may be even more problematical: If one chooses to study the functioning of the normal human brain, then one is compelled by ethical and humanitarian constraints to rely on indirect and sometimes inadequate measures. Generalizability of findings may not be a major problem, but the validity of the methods is often suspect. Nonetheless, if the choice is between using poor methods and using no methods at all, then the inadequacies of the noninvasive measures are more readily tolerated. The wide applicability of these methods, as well as the lack of clearly superior alternatives, provides incentive for investigators to continue using laterality methods while attempting to increase their validity. In time, other noninvasive measures, such as the recording of cortical evoked potentials, or minimally invasive procedures, such as positron emission tomography (PET scanning), may prove to be so far superior to laterality measures that the latter will disappear from the literature. Until such time, there is a great need for valid behavioral measures of laterality and for converging evidence from various methods of assessing cerebral lateralization.

THE EVIDENCE

Dichotic Listening Studies

Dichotic listening is admirably suited for developmental studies. It requires neither reading nor writing; stimuli familiar to 2- and 3-year olds are readily available; the response may be as simple as "yes" or "no"; and memory demands can be reduced to a low level. For these reasons, as well as the relative simplicity and low cost of the technique, several investigators have chosen dichotic listening as a means of studying laterality in normal children of different ages.

Table 5-1 summarizes the various studies in which dichotic listening methods have been applied to normal children. The studies are ordered according to the year of publication. As can be seen from casual inspection of the table, these studies differ from each other with respect to numerous stimulus and task factors. For expository purposes, the studies will be divided into those employing the standard free-report methodology and those employing other approaches.

FREE-REPORT STUDIES

Beginning with Kimura's (1961) demonstration that the dichotic listening ear asymmetry indicates the cerebral lateralization of language, it has become standard practice to administer dichotic listening tests with free-report instructions. The subject is told to report all signals heard irrespective of the ear in which they are heard or the order in which they arrive. Even though this procedure tends to confound hemispheric asymmetry with nonstructural factors such as attentional bias, order of report, and output competition (see Bryden, 1978), relatively few investigators have abandoned the free-report procedure in favor of better controlled paradigms. In the adult literature, some of the confounds inherent in the free-report task have been minimized by substituting single dichotic pairs of perceptually difficult material—such as consonant–vowel (CV) nonsense syllables (Studdert-Kennedy & Shankweiler, 1970) or rhymed words (Wexler & Halwes, 1983)—for lists of digit-name or word pairs. Although use of single pairs of stimuli seems to ameliorate some of the problems associated with lists of stimuli (Hiscock & Stewart, 1984), even the single pairs of stimuli are susceptible to attentional biases under some circumstances (Bryden, Munhall, & Allard, 1983; Mackay & Hiscock, 1986). Moreover, perceptually difficult and meaningless speech sounds are not ideal for use with children.

Most studies of children, even very young children, have yielded a significant right-ear advantage (REA) for the perception of linguistic stimuli. Using words as stimuli, investigators have demonstrated right-ear superiority in children as young as $2\frac{1}{2}$ or 3 years (Bever, 1971; Gilbert & Climan, 1974; Harper & Kraft, 1986; Ingram, 1975; Kamptner, Kraft, & Harper, 1984; Kraft, 1984; Nagafuchi, 1970; Piazza, 1977; Yeni-Komshian &

Table 5-1. Summary of Dichotic Listening Studies

Study	Subjects	Stimuli	Response	Score	Results
Kimura, 1963	120 right-handed boys & girls (B & G) aged 4–9 years	1, 2, and 3 pairs of digit names	Free recall, verbal report	Number correct per ear	REA for all age and sex groups, except 7- and 9-year-old girls
Kimura, 1967	140 B & G aged 5–8 years. Low to middle socioeconomic level.	1, 2, and 3 pairs of digit names	Free recall, verbal report	Number correct per ear	All age and sex groups showed REA, with the exception of 5-year-old boys.
Inglis & Sykes, 1967	120 B & G aged 5–10 years	1, 2, and 3 pairs of digit names	Free recall, verbal report	Number correct per ear	RE recall was better than LE recall for 6- and 9-year-old children for 3 digit pairs. No significant REA in 16 of 18 age group × list length comparisons.
Bryden, 1970	234 B & G aged 7, 9, and 11 years. 152 right-handers and 82 left-handers.	2 and 3 pairs of digit names	Free recall, verbal report	Side of greater accuracy	Overall REA. Frequency of REA increased with age. Greater percentage of right-handers showed REA (64% vs. 45–53% for maternal and familial left-handers). Relative frequency of REA increased with age for right-handers and decreased for left-handers. When corrected for order of report, both right and left-handers showed an overall REA.
Knox & Kimura, 1970	Expt. 1: 80 right-handed B & G aged 5, 6, 7, 8 years	1, 2, and 3 pairs of digit names	Free recall, verbal report	Number correct per ear	All age and sex groups showed REA.
		Environmental sounds	Verbal identification	Number correct per ear	LEA for environmental sounds at all ages
	Expt. 2: 120 right-handed B & G aged 5, 6, 7 years	Concrete nouns	Nonverbal, pointing to pictures	Number correct per ear	All age and sex groups showed REA.
		Concrete nouns	Nonverbal, placing objects on pictures	Number correct per ear	All age and sex groups showed REA.
		Animal sounds	Verbal identification	Number correct per ear	No ear effect
	Expt. 3: 36 right-handed B & G aged 7, 8 years	Concrete nouns	Pointing to pictures and placing objects on pictures using both right and left hands	Number correct per ear	All age and sex groups showed REA, but no effect for hand used for reporting choice.
Nagafuchi, 1970	80 normal B & G aged 3–6 years	Sets of 1 pair of 2- and 3-syllable words	Free recall, verbal report	Number correct per ear	All age and sex groups showed REA, except 4- and 6-year-old girls.

Geffner & Hochberg, 1971	208 low and middle socioeconomic level right-handed B & G aged 4, 5, 6, 7 years	Pairs of digit names	Free recall, verbal report	Number correct per ear	REA for middle but not low socioeconomic level (SEL) children. For the low SEL group, 4-, 5-, and 6-year-olds failed to show REA.
Bever, 1971	195 B & G aged 2.5–5.5 years	2 pairs of animal names	Picking up toy animals corresponding to the dichotically presented animal names	Number correct per ear	Approximately 65% of children chose more RE stimuli than LE stimuli.
Satz, Rardin, & Ross, 1971 (control group for an LD sample)	20 boys, 2 age groups: 7–8 and 11–12 years	3 pairs of digit names per trial	Free recall, verbal report	Percentage correct per ear	Both age groups showed REA.
Somers & Taylor, 1972	10 B & G, aged 5–6 years. Control group for 10 language-disordered children	Pairs of phonetically similar words	Free recall, verbal report	Number correct per ear	All 10 Ss showed a REA.
		2 and 3 pairs of digit names	Free recall, verbal report	Number correct per ear	All 10 Ss showed a REA.
Berlin, Hughes, Lowe-Bell, & Berlin, 1973	150 B & G aged 5, 7, 9, 11, 13 years	Pairs of CV syllables	Free recall, verbal report; 5-year-olds made a written response, while 7- to 13-year-olds responded orally.	Number correct per ear, single correct trials only	Overall REA. No developmental change in ear advantage. Percentage of Ss in the 5-, 7-, 9-, and 11-year-old groups showing REA were: 53.3%, 70%, 77%, and 70%, respectively.
Goodglass, 1973	109 B & G aged 5.5–12 years	High frequency CVC word pairs 1: competition between initial consonants of words (gate–date) 2: competition between medial vowel (pole–pool) 3: competition between both initial consonant and medial vowel (dead–bad)	Free recall, verbal report	Number of consonants and vowels correct per ear	Overall REA No developmental change in ear advantage For consonants, REA for 7-, 8-, and 11-year-olds. For vowels, REA at all ages except 6 and 11.
Dorman & Geffner, 1974	52 low and middle SEL, right-handed B & G. Two groups: black children and white. Age range 6–6.8 years.	Pairs of CV syllables	Free recall, verbal report	$[(R-L)/(R+L)] \times 100$	All groups showed REA.

(continued)

Table 5-1 *(continued)*

Study	Subjects	Stimuli	Response	Score	Results
Satz, Bakker, Teunisson, Goebel, & Van der Vlugt, 1975	198 B & G, aged 5, 6, 7, 9, and 11 years. 7–11 year-olds were all right-handed; of 5- and 6-year-olds, 74% and 88% were right-handed, respectively.	4 pairs of digit names (Dutch language)	Free recall, verbal report	Number correct per ear	REA found for 9- and 11-year-olds.
Ingram, 1975	84 right-handed B & G aged 3, 4, 5 years, from a variety of socioeconomic backgrounds	Word pairs	Nonverbal, pointing to pictures and placing objects on pictures	Percentage correct per ear	Overall REA No developmental change in ear advantage
Yeni-Komshian, Isenberg, & Goldberg, 1975	38 B & G, aged 10–15 years (good readers and poor readers)	3 pairs of digit names	Ordered verbal report, with signals from the specified ear reported first. Report order reversed midway through expt.	Number correct per ear	Overall REA. No difference between groups in EA.
Geffner & Dorman, 1976	44 right-handed B & G from low and middle SEL backgrounds, aged 4 years	Pairs of CV syllables	Free recall, verbal report	$[(R-L)/(R+L)] \times 100$	Only male low and middle SEL groups showed REA.
Borowy & Goebel, 1976	120 B & G, aged 5, 7, 9, 11 years. Half of S were black, half were white. Grouped on the basis of SEL.	3 pairs of digit names	Free recall, verbal report	Number correct per ear	REA for all age, sex, race groups. No developmental change in ear advantage.
Geffen, 1976	40 right-handed B & G, two groups with mean ages 7.5 and 10.8 years	Pairs of one-syllable common nouns consisting of three stimulus types: target words, noise words, and irrelevant words	Right-ear targets and left-ear targets were identified by pushing buttons with the right and left hands, respectively.	Hit rates, false positive rates, and reaction time (RT)	Hit rate: more RE than LE targets detected (25% more for RE). No developmental change in ear advantage. RT: R faster than L.
Witelson, 1977c	156 B & 68 G. Boys aged 6–14 years, grouped into quartiles. Data for girls collapsed across age.	Pairs of digit names	Free recall, verbal report	Number correct per ear	Boys showed overall REA. No developmental change in ear advantage. Girls showed overall REA.

Piazza, 1977	72 right-handed B & G, aged 3, 4, 5 years	Expt. 1: Monosyllabic word pairs Expt. 2: Environmental sounds	One half of Ss were required to name stimuli that they heard, the other half were required to put a finger on pictures.	Number correct per ear	Overall REA for words and overall LEA for environmental sounds. No developmental change in either ear advantage.
Hiscock & Kinsbourne, 1977	42 right-handed B & G, aged 3, 4, 5 years	Pairs of digit names	S required to identify digit from the attended ear. Pre- and postcuing conditions.	Number of digits correct and number of intrusion errors per ear	REA for correct identifications. More RE intrusions in the LEM condition than LE intrusions in the REM condition. No developmental change in ear advantage.
Kinsbourne & Hiscock, 1977	Study 1: 150 right-handed B & G, aged 3–12 years	3 pairs of digit names per trial	Free recall, verbal report	Number correct per ear	Overall REA. No developmental change in ear advantage. 63% of children in Grade 2 and below showed REA; 70% of children in Grade 3 and above showed REA.
	Study 2: 20 B & G, aged 3–5 years	Pairs of digit names	S required to say whether a target digit was heard	Number of misses per ear	Overall REA. More left-ear than right-ear targets missed.
	Study 3: 16 right-handed B & G, aged 3.5 to 3.9 years	Pairs of digit names	S required to identify digit from the attended ear, which was designated prior to a block of 12 trials	Number of digits correct and number of intrusion errors per ear	REA for correct identifications. More RE intrusions in LEM condition than LE intrusions in REM condition.
Schulman-Galambos, 1977	186 right-handed, socioeconomically privileged children from K to G5, and 18 college students	3 pairs of one-syllable words	Free recall, verbal report	Percentage correct per ear; number correct per ear; phi coefficient	Overall REA. No developmental change in ear advantage.
Witelson, 1977a	156 right-handed boys, average age 10.5 years Controls for LD group	Sets of digit pairs, list length(s) not specified	Free recall, verbal report	Number correct per ear	REA
Geffen, 1978	48 right-handed B & G, aged 6.5, 8.8, 10.8 years	1, 2, 3, and 4 pairs of digit names	Ordered unilateral recall, verbal report. Recall was precued to either the left or the right ear.	Number recalled in correct order per ear. Intrusion errors.	REA for number of digits recalled. REA for intrusion errors from unattended ear. No developmental change in ear advantage. Ear differences increased with number of digits to be recalled.

(*continued*)

Table 5-1 *(continued)*

Study	Subjects	Stimuli	Response	Score	Results
Bryden & Allard, 1978	72 right-handed B & G, aged 7–12 years	2 and 3 pairs of digit names	Free recall, verbal report	Number correct per ear	REA for all three grades (G2, G4, G6). No interaction with age or sex.
				Side of greater accuracy	A majority of children performed better at the right ear at all grade levels, but this result only reached significance for the G6 group.
Geffen & Sexton, 1978	24 right-handed B & G, aged 7.25 and 10.8 years	Word pairs: one-syllable nouns. Three stimulus conditions: Two inputs could differ in terms of (1) ear of input, (2) type of voice (male or female), (3) both (1) & (2). Three kinds of words used: target words, noise words (sharing 2 phonemes with target), and irrelevant words.	Identification of a target word by a button press. Two conditions: focused and divided attention.	Percentage of designated target and noise words receiving responses (hits and false alarms). These data were used to calculate d′ and β	Focused attention: Overall sensitivity to the attended channel increased with age. No information regarding ear advantage. Divided attention: RE targets were selected more readily than LE targets. No developmental change in ear advantage.
Bakker, Van der Vlugt, & Claushuis, 1978	250 B & G, aged 5.2, 6.1, 7.2, 8.0, & 9.9 years. All subjects were tested and retested in 2 sessions 1 week apart.	2, 3, and 4 pairs of digit names	Free recall, verbal report	Number correct per ear	Reliability of different list lengths and of ear advantage was assessed. (1) 78.2% of Ss preserved their initial ear preference (84.4% of REAs and 56.6% of LEAs). Performance on the longest list was most reliable, followed by 2- and 3-digit lists.
Geffen & Wale, 1979	Expt. 1: 32 right-handed B & G, aged 7.4 and 9.8 years (G3 and G5)	Expt. 1: 3 pairs of digit names, one of each pair spoken in a male voice, one in a female voice.	Free recall, ordered verbal report of digits spoken by the attended voice. Subjects attended to the male or female voice in four conditions in which each voice: (1) remained on one channel, (2) switched on the 2nd or 3rd digit, or (3)	Number correct per ear and number of intrusion errors per ear	Expts. 1 and 2: REA for number of digits correct. More intrusion errors during LE monitoring than RE monitoring. REA for number correct and intrusion errors increased with presentation rate in 7-year-olds but decreased in 9-year-olds. No developmental change in ear advantage at the slower presentation rate (1 digit

			alternated between channels.		pair per sec). The REA decreased with age at the faster presentation rate (2 digit pairs per sec).
	Expt. 2: 32 right-handed B & G, aged 7.9 and 9.8 years (G3 and G5)	Same as Expt. 1, but rate of stimulus presentation was doubled.	Same as Expt.1	Same as Expt. 1	
Hynd, Obrzut, Weed, & Hynd, 1979	40 B & 8 G. Two groups: 8.3 years and 10.5 years. 43 right-handed and 5 left-handed. Control group for an LD experimental group.	Pairs of CV syllables	Free recall, verbal report	Number correct per ear	Overall REA. No developmental change in ear advantage.
Sexton & Geffen, 1979	Expt. 1: 36 right-handed B & G, aged 7, 11 & 20 years	Word pairs	Selective monitoring of one ear with response to target word heard at either ear. Identification of target word by a button press, indicating ear of origin (i.e., right or left ear = right or left button).	Hit and error rates	Expt. 1: Significant age × channel × attended ear interaction for hit rate reflected relative inability of 7-year-olds to focus attention on left ear.
	Expt. 2: 36 right-handed B & G, aged 7, 11 & 20 years	Same as Expt. 1	Same as Expt. 1 except responses made only to target word at attended ear		Expt. 2: REA for hit rate. No developmental change in ear advantage.
Bakker, Hoefkens, & Van Der Vlugt, 1979	Two samples: (1) 15 G & 22 B followed 1972–1977, aged 6.3 & 6.2 years respectively. (2) 11 G & 17 B followed 1971–1977, aged 6.6 & 6.5 years respectively	4 pairs of digit names	Free recall, verbal report	Number correct per ear	Sample 1: REA at all ages (K, G1, G2, G5). No developmental change in ear advantage. Sample 2: REA at all ages (K, G2, G3, G6). No developmental change in ear advantage. For both samples, correlations between ear differences were greatest for contiguous years.
Hiscock & Kinsbourne, 1980a	155 right-handed B & G, aged 3–12 years	1, 2, 3, & 4 pairs of digit names	Selective listening at each ear on successive blocks of trials, verbal report	Number correct per ear; RE and LE intrusion errors	Overall REA for correct responses. More intrusion errors from RE than from LE. No developmental change in ear advantage. Ear differences increased

(continued)

Table 5-1 *(continued)*

Study	Subjects	Stimuli	Response	Score	Results
					with number of digits to be recalled.
Obrzut, Hynd, Obrzut, & Leitgeb, 1980	48 right-handed B & G, aged 8, 9.5, & 11 years	Pairs of CV syllables	Free recall, verbal report	Number correct per ear	Overall REA. No developmental change in ear advantage.
				Mean percentage of error	Overall REA. No developmental change in ear advantage.
Caplan & Kinsbourne, 1981	105 B & G, aged 6–12 years. Three grade levels: G1–2, G3–4, & G5–6	Pairs of CV syllables	Free recall, verbal report	$(R-L)/(R+L)$	Overall REA. REA greater in males than in females. No developmental change in ear advantage.
Obrzut, Hynd, Obrzut, & Pirozzolo, 1981	32 right-handed children. Two age groups: 10.4–13.2 & 7.4–10.4 years.	Pairs of CV syllables	Selective listening procedure with 3 conditions: (1) free recall, (2) report from the RE, (3) report from the LE on successive blocks of trials, verbal report	Mean number of CV's recalled at each ear	REA for both age levels. No developmental change in ear advantage. REA maintained when attention was focused on the left ear. No increase in REA, relative to free report, when attention was focused on right ear.
Bryson, Mononen, & Yu, 1980	Expt. 1: 60 right-handed Chinese B & G, aged 4.2, 7.1, & 10.3 years	1, 2, and 3 pairs of Chinese digits spoken by a native Chinese speaker	Free recall, verbal report	Number correct per ear	REA for 7- and 10-year-olds. Only females in the youngest group showed REA.
	Expt. 2: Second group of B & G aged 4 years	Same as Expt. 1 except that the trials were self-paced (rather than scheduled with an intertrial interval of 5 seconds as in Expt. 1).	Same as Expt. 1	Same as Expt. 1	Overall REA
Kraft, 1981	80 right-handed males, aged 7.25 and 11.1 years. Ss were divided into groups along two dimensions of handedness: (1) right-handed vs. ambidextrous; (2) familial sinistral versus familial dextral.	1, 2, and 3 digit pairs; nonsense syllables (CVs), and environmental sounds	Free recall, verbal report for digits and nonsense syllables; pointing to a multiple-choice array for environmental sounds.	Laterality coefficient: f	Younger subjects had larger overall laterality coefficient scores. The familial dextral group showed REA for both the syllable and digit tasks, and LEA for the environmental sounds task; the familial sinistral group showed no significant differences across tasks.

Eling, Marshall, & Van Galen, 1981	80 B & G, aged 8, 10, 12, & 16 years. All right-handed. Followed longitudinally for 2 years.	Dichotically presented words. Two tasks: (1) Category monitoring: Ss had to identify exemplars of a particular category. (2) Rhyme monitoring: Ss had to indicate if either dichotic stimulus rhymed with a target word.	Yes/no button press to presence of target category or rhyme word on either channel. Reaction time recorded.	Number correct per ear. Choice RT.	RT was shorter to target words presented to the right ear channel across tasks. Overall REA for correct "yes" responses. REA smaller for category than rhyme monitoring. No developmental change in ear advantage.
Bryden & Allard, 1981	Expt. 1: 96 B & G from K, G2, G4, & G6, all right-handed.	3 types of stimuli: 2, 3, & 4 pairs of numbers; CV pairs; rhyming words pairs	Free recall, verbal report. For CV and word pairs, Ss were told to report only the single item of which they were more certain.	Number correct per ear	REA at all three grade levels for all types of stimuli. No developmental change in ear advantage. REA was greatest for 4-pair lists.
	Expt. 2: 60 right-handed B & G from G2, G4, G6	Rhyming word pairs; nonrhyming words; pairs of familiar environmental sounds	Rhyming words: Verbal report. Ss were told to report only the single item of which they were more certain. Nonrhyming words: Verbal report. Selective LE and RE monitoring on successive blocks of trials. Reporting of word from attended ear only. Environmental sounds: Verbal identification. Ss were told to report first the sound of which they were more certain.	Number correct per ear	Rhyming words: Overall REA. No developmental change in ear advantage. Nonrhyming words: Overall REA. No developmental change in ear advantage. Boys showed greater REA than girls. Environmental sounds: Only the oldest group tended to show LEA.
Davidoff, Done, & Scully, 1981	98 high and low SEL B & G, aged 6.4, 8.4, & 10.6 years	Pairs of CVs; 3 and 4 pairs of mixed letters and digit names	Free recall, verbal report	Number correct at each ear	CV's: Overall REA. All age groups showed REA except the low-SEL 6-year-olds. 3 dichotic pairs: Overall REA. No developmental change in ear advantage. 4 dichotic pairs: REA across all age levels. No developmental change in ear advantage.

(continued)

Table 5-1 *(continued)*

Study	Subjects	Stimuli	Response	Score	Results
Hiscock & Bergstrom, 1982	72 right-handed B & G, aged 6.7, 7.9, & 9.0 years	3 pairs of monosyllabic digit names	Free recall, verbal report Two selective listening conditions: Immediate switching and delayed (1 week) switching	Number correct per ear. Number of intrusion errors at each ear.	Overall REA. More RE intrusions in LE monitoring condition than LE intrusions in RE monitoring condition. No developmental change in ear advantage. Percentage of children showing REA remained constant across grade levels. No REA in children listening to the LE first.
Lewandowski, 1982	48 B & G, aged 8.7, 11.1, 13.2, and 15.0 years (92% strongly right-handed)	3 pairs of 1-syllable words	Free recall, verbal report	(R − L)/(R + L)	REA for each of the three youngest age groups. No developmental change in ear advantage.
Yeni-Komshian & Paul-Brown, 1982	36 right-handed B & G, aged 3, 4, & 5 years	CVC word pairs differing in initial stop consonant and middle vowel.	Free recall, verbal report	Percentage correct at each ear	Overall REA. No developmental change in ear advantage.
Fennell, Satz, & Morris, 1983	This study includes normal and children at-risk for reading problems. 184 boys followed longitudinally from kindergarten to G5.	3 pairs of digit names	Free recall, verbal report	Number correct per ear Percentage of Ss showing REA	Right-handers showed REA at all 3 testing sessions. Nonlinear change in REA (REA greatest at G2). Left-handers failed to show REA until G5. By G2 the majority of left- and right-handers showed REA.
Gordon, 1983	64 B & G (G3 & G4) and 64 B & G (G7 & G8). Four handedness groups: right- and left-handers with and without familial sinistrality.	Pairs of CVs	Free recall, written report. Ss were required to write a number corresponding to the CVs heard.	Number correct per ear (data for males and females analyzed separately).	Males showed REA. No developmental change in ear advantage. Females showed overall REA. Ear × age interaction showed that young females exhibited REA, whereas older females did not.
Larsen & Hakonsen, 1983	33 right-handed B & G aged 8–17 years. Control group for a study with blind children.	CVC concrete nouns	Free recall, verbal report	(R − L)/(R + L)	Overall REA
Morris, Bakker, Satz, & Van der Vlugt, 1984	Two samples followed longitudinally, one Dutch and one from Florida. Both consisted of right-handed males. In each	Dutch: 4 pairs of digit names Florida: 3 pairs of digit names	Free recall, verbal report	Number correct per ear	3 of the 4 samples showed overall REA. No samples had significant REA at all 3 testing sessions. Percentage of Ss showing REA, (RE − LE) > 1, varied across

	country, two subsamples, one year apart, were followed from kindergarten to G5.				samples and testing sessions from 40% to 94%. Between 41% and 64% of Ss shifted ear preference at least once.
Bissell & Clark, 1984	60 right-handed B & G. Two groups aged 5–6 and 11–12 years.	Pairs of CV syllables	Free recall, verbal report	Number correct per ear R/L	Overall REA. No developmental change in ear advantage.
Saxby & Bryden, 1984	95 right-handed B & G, aged 9–10 & 13–14 years.	Verbal phrases spoken with 4 different emotional intonations (happy, sad, angry, neutral). Two tasks: (1) Emotional task required judgments of dichotically presented phrases that varied in emotional tone. (2) Verbal task required judgments based on the verbal content of a phrase.	Verbal same/different response	Lambda Total number of correct "same" judgments for the verbal and emotional tasks	LEA for the emotional judgment task, REA for the verbal task. No developmental change in ear advantage. Magnitude of EA was greater for girls.
		In both conditions, Ss were required to compare a target (attended) sentence with a binaurally presented comparison sentence.			
Larsen, 1984	63 right-handed and 91 left-handed B & G aged 9–11, 12–13, & 14–15 years	Pairs of CVC words (mainly high-frequency concrete nouns)	Free recall, verbal report	$[(R-L)/(R+L)] \times 100$ Phi coefficient used to determine statistical significance of each S's EA. Percentage of Ss showing REA per group	Right-handers: Magnitude of EA decreased with increasing age for those 50 Ss who showed REA. Percentage of Ss showing REA increased with age. Percentage of Ss showing statistically significant REA decreased with age. Left-handers: Magnitude of EA decreased with increasing age. Percentage of Ss showing EA did not increase with age.
Kamptner, Kraft, & Harper, 1984	42 B & G, divided into two age groups: (1) 30–48 mo; (2) 49–66 mo. 27 Ss were right-handed, 15 non-right-handed.	1, 2, & 3 pairs of digit names	Free recall, verbal report	Number correct per ear	Overall REA. No developmental change in ear advantage.
Kraft, 1984	155 B & G aged 29–64 mo. All subjects were	1, 2, & 3 pairs of digit names; environmental	Digits: Free recall, verbal report	Number correct per ear Laterality coefficient: f	Digit names: Overall REA. No developmental change in ear advantage.

(*continued*)

Table 5-1 *(continued)*

Study	Subjects	Stimuli	Response	Score	Results
	grouped on the basis of familial handedness and hand preference.	and human nonverbal sounds	Other stimuli: choosing the appropriate pictures from a visual array depicting the dichotically presented environmental sounds and two distractors.	Lateral difference scores (laterality coefficient for digits minus laterality coefficient for others sounds)	Environmental sounds: No EA Only familial dextral children showed significant difference between EA for digits and EA for other sounds.
Van Duyne, Gargiulo, & Gonter, 1984	192 right-handed B & G aged 5.6, 6.7, 7.6, & 9.5 years	2, 3, & 4 word pairs, presented at three different rates (120, 160, & 180 words per minute)	Free recall, verbal report	Number correct per ear	Overall REA. All groups showed REA except G4 males at the lowest presentation rate, G1 females at 120 and 160 words per minute, and G4 females at 160 words per minute. For males, RE recall tended to increase with rate. RE was more sensitive to rate change than LE.
Lokker & Morais, 1985	13 B & G aged 21–31.5 months. Divided according to parental handedness.	5 disyllabic French animal names	Children were required to choose toys corresponding to the dichotically presented words.	Lateral coefficient: f	Right-handed parental group showed REA. Left-handed parental group showed a trend toward LEA.
Obrzut, Obrzut, Bryden, & Bartels, 1985	14 male and 2 female Ss, aged 7.7–12.1 years (control group for an LD sample).	Pairs of CV syllables	Three conditions: free recall; REM; LEM. Verbal report in all conditions.	Number correct per ear	REA across all 3 attention conditions
Hassler & Birbaumer, 1986	120 B & G aged 9–14 years were tested 3 times with 1 year intervening each time. Divided into 3 groups on the basis of scores on Wing's Tests of Musical Intelligence. Group 1 consisted of children who had high scores and demonstrated	3 pairs of 1-syllable German words	Free recall, verbal report	Number correct per ear	Session 1: No overall EA Session 2: Overall REA. REA significant for 3 of 6 sex × musical ability groups Session 3: Overall REA. REA significant for 4 of 6 sex × musical ability groups.

	an ability to compose or improvise; group 2 only had high scores; group 3 Ss were nonmusician controls. Handedness was mixed, with 101 right-handers and 19 left-handers.				
Obrzut, Boliek, & Obrzut, 1986	12 right-handed B & G aged 10.5 years (control group for LD sample).	Pairs of CV syllables; word pairs; melodies; and 3 pairs of digit names	Three conditions: free recall; REM and LEM. For the nonverbal stimuli, subjects pointed to pictures to indicate choice. All other responses were verbal.	Mean percentage correct per ear	CVs: Overall REA Words: Free recall: REA REM: REA LEM: Increase in LE and decrease in RE accuracy Digits: Free recall: REA REM: REA LEM: LEA Melodies: Free recall: LEA REM: REA LEM: LEA
Harper & Kraft, 1986	29 B & G, aged 35–65 months	1, 2, & 3 pairs of digit names. Two testing sessions, 7–9 days apart.	Free recall, verbal report	R – L Phi coefficient Lambda statistic Laterality coefficient (f)	Two-thirds of the sample showed REA at each testing session; 89% showed the same EA across testing sessions. Of children with a stable EA, 71% had REA and 29% LEA. Overall, the most reliable laterality indices were R – L and the phi coefficient.

Abbreviations: B & G (boys and girls); CCC (consonant trigram); CV (consonant–vowel syllable); CVC (consonant–vowel–consonant word); EA (ear advantage); Expt. (experiment); G (grade); L (left); R (right); LD (learning-disabled); LE (left ear); RE (right ear); LEA (left-ear advantage); REA (right-ear advantage); LEM (left-ear monitoring); REM (right-ear monitoring); LH (left hand); RH (right hand); LVF (left visual half-field); RVF (right visual half-field); RT (reaction time); S (subject); SEL (socioeconomic level); VF or VHF (visual half-field).

Paul-Brown, 1982). Although Lokker and Morais (1985) failed to find a significant ear difference in a sample of 26 children between the ages of 21 and 36 months, they did find a significant REA in the 18 children whose parents were right-handed. Insofar as children below the age of 2 years are very difficult, perhaps impossible, to test, it may be concluded that the REA for words is found in the youngest children that can be tested.

Demonstration of a REA in even younger children awaits development of an appropriate experimental paradigm. At present there remains a gap between auditory studies with infants (Best, Hoffman, & Glanville, 1982; Entus, 1977; Glanville, Best, & Levenson, 1977; Vargha-Khadem & Corballis, 1979), which employ habituation–dishabituation paradigms, and those with young children, which employ methods similar to those used with adults.

Despite one failure to find an ear difference in infants (Vargha-Khadem & Corballis, 1979) and despite the lack of information about children between infancy and the age of 2 years, most of the available evidence points to the early development of auditory asymmetries. A notable exception is the suggestion of delayed onset of the REA in children of relatively low socioeconomic level. Kimura (1967) reported that, in two samples of children from lower- and middle-class socioeconomic backgrounds, 5-year-old boys failed to show a significant REA on a dichotic digit-names task even though girls of the same age, as well as older children of both sexes, did show the expected ear difference. Since Kimura (1963) previously had found significant REAs in 4- and 5-year-old boys of higher socioeconomic status, her failure to find comparable ear asymmetries in 5-year-old boys from lower- and middle-class backgrounds raised the possibility that the development of auditory laterality might be delayed in certain populations of children. This possibility was supported by Geffner and Hochberg's (1971) failure to find a significant REA for dichotic digit names in 4-, 5-, and 6-year-olds from lower socioeconomic backgrounds. However, since children's socioeconomic level did not influence ear asymmetry in two subsequent studies in which CV stimuli were used (Dorman & Geffner, 1974; Geffner & Dorman, 1976), the earlier positive findings were dismissed as artifacts of "task difficulty and motivational variables" (Dorman & Geffner, 1974). The socioeconomic class effect is also contradicted by other findings of significant REAs in young children irrespective of socioeconomic background (Borowy & Goebel, 1976; Davidoff, Done, & Scully, 1981; Knox & Kimura, 1970).

More controversial than the age at which ear asymmetry begins is the question of whether the early REA for linguistic stimuli increases in magnitude with increasing age. On this topic the evidence has been somewhat unclear, although most studies indicate a comparable degree of asymmetry among different age groups. In her initial dichotic listening study of children, Kimura (1963) found a significant REA for digit names at each age level between 4 and 9 years. Although no statistical test was performed to ascertain the significance of age-related changes in the magnitude of the REA, the mean scores do not indicate any developmental increase in the size of the REA. In fact Kimura (1963) commented that the difference between ears was smaller among the older children than among the younger children, an outcome that she attributed to a restriction of range at the higher performance levels achieved by the older children. Many other dichotic listening studies of children, all of which employed linguistic stimuli and free-report instructions, failed to reveal a significant age-related change in the magnitude of the REA (Berlin, Hughes, Lowe-Bell, & Berlin, 1973; Bissell & Clark, 1984; Borowy & Goebel, 1976; Bryden & Allard, 1981; Goodglass, 1973; Gordon, 1983; Hynd & Obrzut, 1977; Hynd, Obrzut, Weed, & Hynd, 1979; Kamptner *et al.*, 1984; Kinsbourne & Hiscock, 1977; Knox & Kimura, 1970; Mirabile, Porter, Hughes, & Berlin, 1978; Obrzut, Hynd, Obrzut, & Leitgeb, 1980; Obrzut,

Hynd, Obrzut, & Pirozzolo, 1981; Schulman-Galambos, 1977; Van Duyne, Gargiulo, & Gonter, 1984).

Two typical sets of findings are shown in Figure 5-1. In one of these studies (Kinsbourne & Hiscock, 1977), strings of dichotic digit names were presented to 155 right-handed children between the ages of 3 and 12 years. In the other study (Berlin *et al.*, 1973), consonant–vowel (CV) nonsense syllables were presented to 150 right-handed children of ages 5, 7, 9, 11, and 13 years. Even though the stimulus material differed quite markedly between studies, the results were remarkably similar. Both studies yielded: (1) an overall REA, (2) an age-related increase in overall performance, and (3) no indication of an age-related change in degree of asymmetry.

A few other findings, however, suggest that children's REA for verbal material might become either more frequent or more pronounced with increasing age (Bryden, 1970; Bryden & Allard, 1978; Larsen, 1984; Satz, Bakker, Teunissen, Goebel, & Van der Vlugt, 1975). Probably the most influential of these is the Satz *et al.* (1975) study, from which the authors concluded that "the ear asymmetry, regardless of its age of onset, does undergo major changes after five years of age" (p. 184). Satz *et al.* administered dichotic pairs of Dutch-language digit names, four pairs per trial, to 190 schoolchildren. Using comparisons of linear models as a means of analyzing their data, Satz *et al.* found that the magnitude of the REA increased significantly from 5 to 11 years. Post hoc tests indicated that the REA was not statistically significant in children under the age of 9 years.

Satz *et al.* (1975) argued that at least some of the previous failures to find age-related increases in the magnitude of ear asymmetry (e.g., Kimura, 1963) can be attributed to ceiling effects, that is, to older children's tendency to perform well with both ears, thus limiting the range of possible differences between the ears. Ironically, as acknowledged by Satz *et al.*, their own use of lengthy strings of stimuli may have caused a floor effect among the younger children that might have restricted the magnitude of the REA at the youngest age levels. In addition, an idiosyncrasy of sampling may have contributed to the pattern of results obtained by Satz *et al.* Although all of their 7-, 9-, and 11-year-olds were right-handed, only 81% of their 5- and 6-year-olds were right-handed. It has been reported, at least for adults, that the REA is reduced in samples of left-handers (Bryden, 1983).

It is unfortunate that every dichotic listening study cited so far used a cross-sectional design, in that such studies do not provide direct information about developmental patterns. Differences among age groups may stem not only from true age-related changes but also from the vagaries of subject selection. Although longitudinal studies are not without problems, longitudinal designs are probably more powerful than cross-sectional designs for tracing the developmental course of the dichotic listening ear asymmetry. Clearly, the two kinds of design can complement each other.

Three longitudinal studies have appeared in the literature since 1978. In the first of these studies (Bakker, Hoefkens, & Van der Vlugt, 1979), two relatively small samples of right-handed schoolchildren ($N = 27$ and $N = 28$, respectively) were administered a dichotic digit-names test on four occasions over a period of 5 years. The average age of children in both samples at the time of initial testing was 6 years. The findings were similar for both groups of children: a significant age-related increase in overall performance, a significant REA, and no significant interaction between age and ear. These results are of special interest not only because of the longitudinal design but also because the dichotic stimuli were identical to those used by Satz *et al.* (1975) in the cross-sectional study that showed a developmental increase in the magnitude of REA.

The second longitudinal study was that of Fennell, Satz, and Morris (1983), who administered a somewhat different dichotic digit-names test on three occasions to 208 boys,

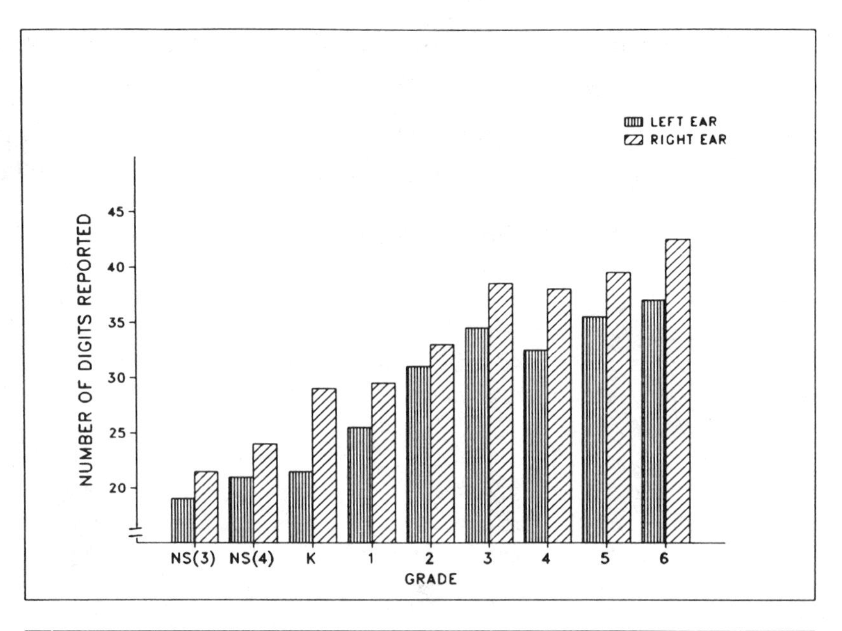

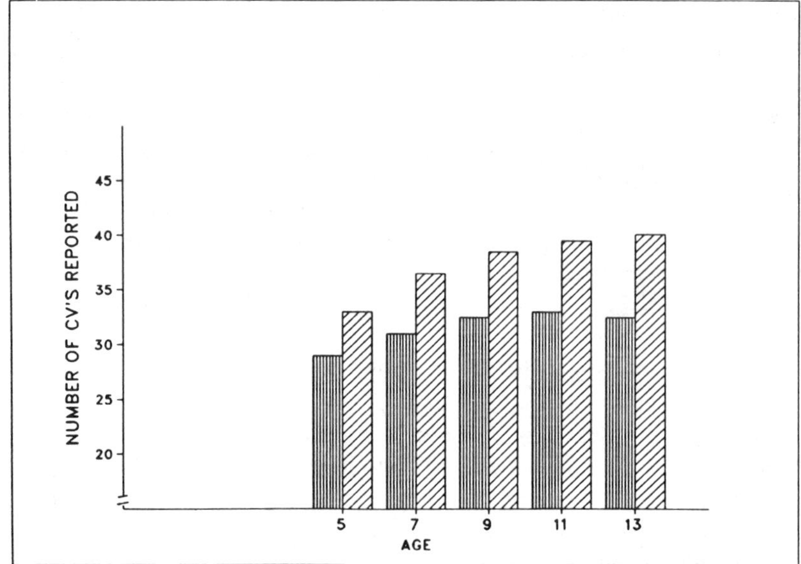

Figure 5-1. Mean number of verbal stimuli reported from the left and right ears as a function of grade level (age). The top panel shows the number of dichotic digit names reported by children between the ages of 3 and 12 years, and the bottom panel shows the number of consonant–vowel nonsense syllables (CVs) reported by children between the ages of 5 and 13 years. The upper graph is adapted by permission from "Does Cerebral Dominance Develop?" by M. Kinsbourne and M. Hiscock, 1977, in *Language Development and Neurological Theory,* edited by S. J. Segalowitz and F. A. Gruber, New York: Academic Press, p. 178. Copyright © 1977 by Academic Press, Inc. The lower graph is adapted by permission from "Dichotic Right Ear Advantage in Children 5 to 13" by C. I. Berlin, L. F. Hughes, S. S. Lowe-Bell, and H. L. Berlin, 1973, *Cortex, 9,* p. 397. Copyright © 1973 by Masson Italia Periodici.

half of whom had been identified as children at risk for developing reading problems. Analysis of data for the 184 right-handers yielded the usual main effects for grade level (kindergarten, Grade 2, and Grade 5) and ear. Although there was also a significant grade-level × ear interaction, it apparently reflected a nonlinear change such that the greatest REA was obtained from the Grade 2 testing. Developmental changes in the ear asymmetry of the 28 left-handers were not statistically significant.

The third longitudinal study (Morris, Bakker, Satz, & Van der Vlugt, 1984) was a composite of data collected by Satz and his colleagues in Florida and by Bakker and his colleagues in the Netherlands. Consequently, the data are partially redundant with data reported by Bakker *et al.* (1979) and by Fennell *et al.* (1983). Morris *et al.*, after defining two samples of Dutch boys and two samples of American boys, analyzed the dichotic listening performance of each sample at each of three grade levels from kindergarten to Grade 5 or 6. Of the 12 mean ear-difference scores obtained from this analysis, all but one favored the right ear, but only 7 of the 11 REAs were statistically significant. Moreover, the developmental patterns for the different samples bore little resemblance to each other. The authors concluded that "using the various types of analyses utilized in the literature, we could find support for all of the major hypotheses regarding the developmental patterns of [dichotic listening] performance" (p. 64).

Relatively little attention has been devoted to the study of children's ear asymmetry for nonverbal material. Infant studies suggest an early left-ear advantage (LEA) for music perception (Best *et al.*, 1982; Entus, 1977; Glanville *et al.*, 1977), but this has not been tested in studies of older children. Moreover, studies of adults suggest that the question of ear asymmetry for music may not have a simple answer. Since different components of music seem to contribute differentially to ear asymmetry (see Bryden, 1982b; Gates & Bradshaw, 1977), the pattern of ear asymmetry across the childhood years for any one aspect of music, such as discrimination of melodic patterns, may not represent the developmental pattern for another aspect, such as discrimination of rhythms.

The available information about children's ear asymmetry for nonverbal material pertains to environmental sounds. Knox and Kimura (1970) reported a significant LEA for environmental sounds in children between the ages of 5 and 8 years. There was no increase in the magnitude of the LEA across this age range. Piazza (1977) obtained similar results for 3-, 4-, and 5-year-olds. Nonetheless, the findings are not unanimous: Knox and Kimura (1970) failed to find a significant ear difference for animal sounds (in a sample of children who showed a significant LEA for other environmental sounds), and Bryden and Allard (1981) failed to find a significant ear difference for environmental sounds in a sample of 60 right-handed children from grades 2, 4, and 6. Although Kraft (1981, 1982, 1984) has found significant LEAs for environmental sounds among subgroups of children, none of his three studies yielded a significant overall LEA.

SIGNAL DETECTION AND SELECTIVE LISTENING STUDIES

Morris *et al.* (1984), in discussing the general state of dichotic listening research with children, reluctantly concluded that the free-recall paradigm does not provide the necessary control over various parameters of the task or strategies of the subject. These authors pointed to certain selective listening methods (Geffen, 1978; Hiscock & Kinsbourne, 1977) as promising alternatives to the free-report technique. Although it is unlikely that any method will prove to be a panacea, the results thus far with selective listening methods, as well as with signal detection methods, are encouraging. Selective listening, or focused attention, entails monitoring one ear in a dichotic listening task and reporting signals only from that ear. Signal detection entails listening for a single target that may occur at either ear.

Unambiguous listening asymmetries in preschool children were found in a signal detection study and two selective listening studies by Kinsbourne and his associates (see Kinsbourne & Hiscock, 1977). In the detection study, children between the ages of 3 and 5 years listened for a target that could be present at either ear as a member of a pair of dichotic digit names. The average number of misses was 3.2 (out of a possible 6) when the signal was at the left ear, as compared with 2.2 when the signal was at the right ear. In the first of the selective listening experiments, 3-year-olds monitored one ear for 12 trials and then switched attention to the opposite ear for another 12 trials. The task was to report only the digit name occurring at the attended ear on each trial. This experiment yielded a marked difference between the proportion of digits correctly identified at the right ear (67%) and at the left ear (26%). The other selective listening experiment also yielded a strong REA for digit names, the magnitude of which remained approximately constant across the age range of 3 to 5 years (Hiscock & Kinsbourne, 1977).

A more extensive series of selective listening and signal detection studies has been conducted with school-age children (Eling, Marshall, & van Galen, 1981; Geffen, 1976, 1978; Geffen & Sexton, 1978; Geffen & Wale, 1979; Hiscock & Bergstrom, 1982; Hiscock & Chipuer, in preparation; Hiscock & Kinsbourne, 1980a; Saxby & Bryden, 1984; Sexton & Geffen, 1979). Although these studies differ from each other in many respects, the results are consistent on the question of developmental change in ear asymmetry. In no instance is there evidence of an age-related increase in the magnitude of ear asymmetry. The ability to attend selectively to one ear, however, improves substantially during childhood, and this may produce an age-related *decline* in the magnitude of the REA under certain circumstances—for example, when multiple rapid shifts of attention are demanded (Geffen & Wale, 1979) or when the child's processing capacity is heavily taxed by having to respond to both the attended and unattended signals (Sexton & Geffen, 1979). Younger children, being able to allocate attention effectively in demanding tasks, revert to responding according to their "involuntary perceptual asymmetry" (Geffen & Wale, 1979, p. 145), thus showing an exaggerated REA.

With the exception of tasks that exceed the attentional capacity of young children, thus producing REAs that decline with increasing age, signal detection and selective listening methods yield a constant asymmetry across the childhood years. Geffen (1978), for example, who instructed children to report digit names only from the specified ear, found no significant change in the magnitude of the REA across the age range of 6 to 10 years. Overall performance improved with increasing age, and the REA increased as the list length increased from 1 to 4 pairs per trial, but the REA did not change with age. In a study with similar stimuli and procedures, Hiscock and Kinsbourne (1980a) duplicated Geffen's findings with a sample of 155 children between the ages of 3 and 12 years. Neither correct responses nor intrusion errors from the unattended ear revealed a significant change in asymmetry over this broad age range.

One of the most definitive selective listening studies is that of Saxby and Bryden (1984), who found that ear asymmetry for sentences varied according to task demands such that an emotional task yielded a significant LEA and a verbal task yielded a significant REA. Children attended to either the left or the right ear as brief dichotic sentences were presented, and attempted to judge whether the sentence from the attended ear matched a binaurally presented comparison sentence. In the emotional task, the matching was to be based on tone of voice (happy, sad, angry, or neutral) and, in the verbal task, on verbal content. Not only did the investigators find the expected dissociation in laterality between verbal and emotional tasks, but they also found the laterality patterns for the respective tasks to be very similar among their three age groups, which spanned the range of 5 to 14 years. There was no indication of an age-related increase in asymmetry for either task.

The Saxby and Bryden (1984) study is particularly noteworthy for three reasons. First, the LEA for emotional information and the REA for verbal information were found in the same sample of children. Second, the differential laterality patterns were obtained with the same stimulus material: Only task demands differentiated the verbal condition from the emotional condition. Third, the use of focused attention instructions makes it unlikely that children simply allocated attention differentially during the verbal and emotional tasks.

CONCLUSIONS

Dichotic listening, on the whole, has proved to be a useful technique for the developmentalist. It has yielded reasonably consistent answers to the most basic questions about auditory laterality in children, that is, to questions about the initial emergence of ear asymmetry and its subsequent developmental course. The REA for linguistic material is a robust phenomenon that is readily demonstrated in school-age children. An LEA for nonverbal stimuli, though more difficult to elicit, can also be demonstrated. Not only do similar asymmetries exist in preschool children, but these asymmetries may be particularly marked in preschool children if the dichotic listening task is modified so as to minimize extraneous variables and to match the processing capacity of the young child. Occasional reports of developmental change notwithstanding, the preponderance of evidence available at present suggests that auditory laterality develops early in life and neither increases nor decreases during childhood.

The dichotic listening method has been less successful when judged against more stringent criteria. More difficult questions—questions about mechanisms underlying asymmetric perception and developmental changes in these mechanisms—remain to be answered. With the availability of paradigms capable of isolating various components of ear asymmetry (allocation of attention, selection of inputs, rejection of competing inputs, short-term storage, order of report, etc.), researchers have means of addressing questions concerning mechanisms. Much empirical work, however, remains to be done.

Dichotic listening is also disappointing to those researchers interested in making inferences about the hemispheric specialization of the individual child. Dichotic listening, along with other laterality methods, may not be sufficiently reliable or valid to justify such inferences. These limitations will be discussed in the section entitled "General Problems."

Visual Half-Field Studies

Much of the adult laterality literature is devoted to studies of visual perception in which stimuli are presented briefly to the left or right visual half-field, or to both half-fields simultaneously, via a tachistoscope or cathode ray tube. Visual half-field (VHF) studies are favored over other laterality methods in one important aspect—in having a relatively clear-cut anatomical and physiological rationale. In the auditory, somatosensory, and motor systems, the crossed pathways are thought to be quantitatively superior to the uncrossed pathways (Kimura, 1961; Witelson, 1977b; Zaidel, 1983), but the exact degree of superiority is difficult to specify and is presumably subject to variation among individuals (Blumstein, Goodglass, & Tartter, 1975; Levy & Reid, 1978). In the primate visual system, input from either half-field is conducted exclusively to the primary visual cortex of the contralateral hemisphere. The lateralization of visual input is not relative but absolute.

Admittedly, this conceptual advantage of the VHF method is mitigated by the bilateral availability of the information in cortical regions outside the primary visual cortex, presumably due to transcallosal communication (Marzi, 1986), and by ambiguities regarding the locus of further processing (Zaidel, 1983). Nonetheless, the unilateral nature of the initial visual input is well established.

Unfortunately, VHF studies have been characterized by numerous methodological complexities and inconsistent findings (Beaumont, 1982b; Bradshaw, Nettleton, & Taylor, 1981; Bryden, 1982b; Hardyck, 1983, 1986; Sergent, 1986; White, 1969, 1972). In the absence of consistent laterality effects among adults, it is difficult to interpret developmental changes in children's laterality. Moreover, since preschool children seldom can read, only nonverbal stimuli are feasible for use with very young children. Despite these limitations, several tachistoscopic studies of children's laterality have appeared in the neuropsychological literature. These studies are summarized in Table 5-2.

Tachistoscopic studies are not readily grouped into a small number of categories on the basis of one salient aspect of methodology. The numerous potentially critical variations of stimulus, task, and response mode necessitate a multidimensional taxonomy. For the purpose of this discussion, however, VHF studies with children will simply be dichotomized according to the nominal category of the stimuli, that is, according to whether nonverbal or verbal stimuli were used.

STUDIES WITH NONVERBAL STIMULI

Many of the VHF studies with children have employed pictures of faces as stimuli with the expectation that early right-hemispheric specialization for face recognition would manifest itself as a left visual half-field superiority. In the first of these studies, Marcel and Rajan (1975) found that 7-year-old children required shorter exposure durations to recognize faces in the left visual half-field (LVF) than in the right visual half-field (RVF). This indication of an early LVF advantage for face recognition was supported by Young and Ellis (1976), who presented pictures of a face to either the left or the right visual half-field or at fixation and asked 5-, 7-, and 11-year-old children to say whether the face seen on each trial matched a comparison face shown subsequently. There was a significant advantage for the LVF over the RVF, but no significant interaction between age and visual half-field. Young and Ellis concluded that "lateralisation of visual information processing is well advanced by age 5" (p. 497). This conclusion is substantiated by several other studies yielding an LVF superiority for face recognition in children and showing no age-related increase in the magnitude of the asymmetry (Broman, 1978; Turkewitz & Ross-Kossak, 1984; Young & Bion, 1980, 1981). Broman (1978), in fact, found that the LVF advantage was significant in 7- and 10-year-olds but not in older subjects. Two other studies, however, yielded no evidence of LVF superiority for face recognition in 7- and 8-year-olds, although the effect was found in older children (Leehey, 1978, as summarized by Carey, Diamond, & Woods, 1980; Reynolds & Jeeves, 1978b).

Other tasks have failed to yield a significant LVF superiority at any age. When children were required to match faces on the basis of emotional expression (Saxby & Bryden, 1985), there was no significant asymmetry in any of three age groups ranging from 6 to 14 years. When 3- and 4-year-old children were required to determine whether a face presented to either the left or the right visual half-field was that of a female or a male (Jones & Anuza, 1982), there was a significant RVF advantage for male subjects and no significant asymmetry for female subjects. This was precisely the pattern of results obtained by Jones (1979, 1980) when he used the same paradigm with right-handed adults.

Table 5-2. Summary of Visual Half-Field Studies

Study	Subjects	Stimuli	Response	Score	Results
Forgays, 1953	144 males and females in G2–10 and 3 college years	3- or 4-letter words. Unilateral presentation.	Recognition. Verbal report.	Number of words recognized in each VHF	RVF superiority only for older subjects; no RVF for G2–G7
Braine, 1968	Hebrew-speaking males and females in G3, G5, G7, and college	Task 1: Families of 4-sided figures for which a distinguishing feature was oriented to the left, right, top, and bottom. Unilateral presentation.	Ss selected the figure presented from a multiple-choice sheet containing all the figures of a particular family.	Number of figures recognized in each VHF	Children in G5 showed more errors in the LVF.
	Hebrew-speaking males and females in G5, G7, and college	Task 2: A row of 8 circles, 4 in each VHF. On each trial, 2 or 3 of the circles (at least one in each VHF) appeared filled with dark ink.	Ss pointed to a card on which 8 circles were represented to indicate which had appeared filled on a given trial.	Order of report	Children in G5 reported more often from R to L. The G7 group showed no preference, but the college-age group tended to report L to R.
				Number of errors for each VHF.	College students made more errors in RVF (although the difference between VHFs did not reach significance). The G7 children showed slightly more errors in LVF, while the G5 children made significantly more errors in LVF.
McKeever & Huling, 1970	10 G7 children	Common 4-letter nouns. Unilateral presentation.	Recognition. Verbal report.	Number of words recognized in each VHF	RVF superiority
Miller, 1971	Expt. 1: 36 males and females, ages 8.0, 11.9, & 20.2 years	Displays divided into 4 quadrants containing 8 or 16 letters and subtending 3 or 5 degrees of visual angle.	Ss were required to indicate the quadrant in which the letter O appeared. Written response.	Number of letters recognized and localized in each quadrant	Accuracy was greatest for targets in the upper quadrants for the G6 children and college students. RVF superiority. No developmental change in VF superiority.
	Expt. 2: Same as Expt. 1	Same as Expt. 1 except that stimuli were presented using four different exposure durations (25, 75, 125, & 175 msec)	Same as Expt. 1.	Same as Expt. 1	Greater recognition accuracy for stimuli falling in the upper and R quadrants of the display

(continued)

Table 5-2 (*continued*)

Study	Subjects	Stimuli	Response	Score	Results
Jeeves, 1972	10 right-handed and 10 left-handed boys, age range 9.5–11.4 years	Point sources of light falling on the right or left nasal or temporal retina	Ss held two Morse keys down; when the stimulus appeared, they released the keys	RT	Reaction time of right-handed children was shorter for left nasal and right temporal retinal stimulation, i.e., for stimuli in LVF. Left-handed children showed no VHF superiority.
Miller, 1973	88 males and females in G1, G3, G6 and college, aged 6.5, 8.5, 11.5, & 18.5 years	Displays of approximately 400 letters in which the target letter O appeared on each trial. Displays were divided into 4 quadrants. Distance of the target from fixation and stimulus exposure time were also varied.	Ss were required to report the quadrant in which the target letter appeared. Written response	Number of responses for each quadrant	RVF superiority for the two youngest age groups. Hemifield differences were greatest when the target was nearest to fixation. The RVF advantage appeared at all stimulus exposure durations for the youngest group; at all but the longest duration for the G3 children; and at the two shortest durations for G6 children
Miller & Turner, 1973	60 males & females in G2, G4, G6, and college	4- and 5-letter words presented at 3 exposure durations. Unilateral presentation.	Verbal report	Number of correct responses from each VHF at each exposure duration	Accuracy increased across grade level. RVF superiority for all groups except G2 children
Olson, 1973	Expt. 1: 50 B & G aged 7, 8, 9, 10, 11 years	3- and 4-letter nouns. Unilateral and bilateral presentation.	Verbal report	Number of correct responses from each VHF	RVF superiority for word recognition (greater for bilateral presentation). No sex or age effects.
	Expt. 2: 43 B & G aged 8–13 years; classified as poor readers	Same as Expt. 1	Same as Expt. 1	Same as Expt. 1	Similar RVF superiority to Expt. 1, except not present for 8–9 year-olds
Marcel, Katz & Smith, 1974	20 B and 20 G, aged 7.5–8.6 years, classified as good or poor readers	40 5-letter words. Unilateral presentation, followed by a bilateral mask.	Verbal report: Words or letters	Number of words and letters correctly reported from each VHF	RVF superiority (greater for good readers). Greater VF asymmetry for boys than girls. Larger RVF effect for letters than words
Marcel & Rajan, 1975	20 B and 20 G, aged 7–9 years, classified as good or poor readers	40 5-letter words. 20 photographs of faces. Unilateral presentation, followed by a bilateral mask.	Words: Verbal report. Faces: Pointing to one of two faces shown after each trial	Words: Number of words and letters correctly reported from each VHF Faces: Criterion exposure duration (recognition ''threshold'')	Words: RVF superiority; greater asymmetry for good readers. Faces: LVF superiority

Turner & Miller, 1975	Expt. 1: 60 right-handed males and females in G1, G2, G3, G4, and college	3-letter words presented vertically or horizontally. Unilateral presentation.	Recognition. Verbal report.	Proportion of words recognized in each VHF	Overall RVF superiority
	Expt. 2: Same as Expt. 1	Random shapes and line drawings of common objects. Unilateral presentation.	Recognition. Verbal report.	Proportion of shapes or drawings recognized in each VHF	Overall LVF superiority for both types of stimuli. No developmental change in VF superiority.
	Expt. 3: Same as Expt. 1	Same as Expt. 1	Subjects were required to choose target stimuli from among alternatives, rather than simply identifying them.	Proportion of words recognized correctly in each VHF	No VF differences
	Expt. 4: Same as Expt. 1	Same as Expt. 1 except that stimulus presentation was followed by a dark field rather than a light field	Same as Expt. 1	Same as Expt. 1	No VF differences
	Expt. 5: 45 right-handed males and females in G2, G4, and college	4- and 5-letter words presented at three different exposure durations	Same as Expt. 1	Same as Expt. 1	RVF superiority at all grade levels for 5-letter words; RVF superiority for 4-letter words only for the oldest group. Differences between RVF and LVF accuracy increased with age.
Yeni-Komshian, Isenberg, & Goldberg, 1975	38 B & G, aged 10–15 years (good readers and poor readers)	Numerals and words. Unilateral presentation. 5 sequential presentations per trial with 1st, 3rd and 5th stimulus in either LVF or RVF, and 2nd and 4th stimulus at midline. Words were vertically oriented.	Recognition. Verbal report.	Number of numerals or words recognized in each VHF	Overall RVF superiority for numerals only. No VF difference for either numerals or words for the good readers. Poor readers showed RVF advantage for both categories of stimuli.
Carmon, Nachshon, & Starinsky, 1975	192 right-handed B & G aged 6, 8, 10, & 12 years	Single Hebrew letters; 2-letter Hebrew words; 2-digit numbers; 4-digit numbers. Unilateral and bilateral presentation.	Recognition. Verbal report.	Percentage correct responses for each VHF	Overall RVF advantage for words and digits. The youngest age group showed a LVF advantage for single letters. The RVF superiority appeared at age 10.

(continued)

Table 5-2 *(continued)*

Study	Subjects	Stimuli	Response	Score	Results
Aaron & Handley, 1975	57 right-handed boys aged 5–7 years, grouped on the basis of directional response tendency (left to right: right to left, or unsystematic) in free field viewing	Letters and shapes. Unilateral presentation.	Pointing to a visual array containing the stimulus and its mirror image.	Number of correct identifications in each VHF	Difference in asymmetry for letters and shapes found only for right-to-left group, which showed RVF advantage for letters and LVF advantage for shapes.
Schaller & Dziadosz, 1976	28 right-handed B & G aged 4.5 & 9 years	Arrays of 35 open circles. For each presentation one circle contained a horizontal or a vertical bar. The target bar appeared in different VHFs and vertical positions relative to fixation.	Ss pointed to a representation of a horizontal or vertical bar to indicate the orientation of the target bar.	Percentage correct at each of 35 different positions	Younger Ss showed no asymmetry; older Ss were most accurate in the top right quadrant of array.
Young & Ellis, 1976	42 right-handed B & G aged 5.7, 7.7, & 11.8 years	Pictures of faces presented in the right & left VHFs and at fixation	Same/different matching. Verbal report	Number of errors at each stimulus position	Overall LVF superiority No developmental change in VHF superiority
Barroso, 1976	150 right-handed B & G aged 6.4, 8.5, 9.6, 10.4, & 12.5 years	Line drawings of common objects. Two tasks: (1) *Verbal:* The name of one stimulus was presented aurally and an identical or different stimulus was presented to the RVF or LVF. Unilateral presentation. (2) *Nonverbal:* Same and different pairs of stimuli presented to the RVF or LVF. Unilateral presentation.	Same/different matching. Verbal report	RT	RVF superiority for verbal task and LVF superiority for nonverbal task for the two oldest age groups. No differences in RT across visual fields and tasks for the 6-, 8-, & 9-year-olds.
Witelson, 1977a	156 right-handed boys, average age 10.5 years (normal controls for LD group)	Unilateral presentation of pairs of human figures	Same/different matching. Verbal report.	Number of correct responses from each VHF	LVF superiority

Witelson, 1977c	85 boys, aged 6–7, 8–9, 10–11, & 12–14 years	Pairs of identical or different human figures presented vertically in the RVF or LVF. Unilateral presentation.	Same/different matching. Verbal report.	Number of correct matches in each VHF	Overall LVF superiority
	83 boys aged 6–7, 8–9, 10–11, & 12–14 years	Pairs of identical or different letters presented vertically in the RVF or LVF. Unilateral presentation.	Same/different matching. Verbal report.	Number of correct matches in each VHF	RVF superiority only for the youngest boys
Kershner, Thomae, & Callaway, 1977	86 right-handed B & G, aged 5.5–6.5 years	Triads of horizontally oriented digits. Bilateral presentation. Prior to stimulus onset a nonverbal stimulus (triangle, square, asterisk) or a verbal stimulus (digit) appeared at fixation.	Ss were required to name the digit or point to a display containing the form presented at fixation, after which they reported the digits they had seen.	Number of digits recalled from each VHF	When a nonverbal stimulus appeared at fixation, there was LVF superiority for digit recall; when a verbal stimulus appeared at fixation, there was RVF superiority for digit recall.
Broman, 1978	60 right-handed boys aged 7, 10, & 13 years and 20 adults, aged 18–30 years	Faces and pairs of letters arranged vertically. Unilateral presentation. Monocular viewing.	Ss moved a rocker switch to indicate that the face or letter pair was a member of the positive set (as designated by the experimenter).	RT and accuracy for stimuli presented in each VHF	RTs were faster for faces presented in the LVF for children aged 7 and 10 years but not for older children or adults. For letters there was LVF superiority for the youngest age group only.
Gross, Rothenberg, Schottenfeld, & Drake, 1978	15 normal B & G, aged 10–13.5 years. Control group for reading-disabled group	Single letters presented at threshold & suprathreshold. Unilateral presentation. Monocular viewing.	Verbal report	Duration threshold for identification (62% accuracy)	Duration threshold slightly longer for LVF
Young & Bion, 1979	60 right-handed B & G aged 5.8, 7.8, & 11.3 years	Randomly generated collections of 2, 3, 4, 5, or 6 dots. Unilateral presentation.	Ss required to enumerate the dots for each stimulus presented. Verbal response.	Accuracy for stimuli presented in each VHF RT for stimuli presented in each VHF	Accuracy: Overall LVF superiority. Boys showed a stronger LVF than girls. RT: Overall LVF superiority
Tomlinson-Keasey, Kelly, & Burton, 1978	154 right-handed males and females aged 8.6, 13.2, & 27.8 years	3-, 4-, & 5-letter high-imagery word pairs and picture pairs. Pairs of stimuli were projected sequentially to the same	Same/different matching. Manual response (button press).	RT for stimuli presented in each VHF	RT was faster for matched stimuli presented in the RVF for the two oldest age groups. This effect was greater for word stimuli. RT was faster for unmatched

(*continued*)

Table 5-2 (*continued*)

Study	Subjects	Stimuli	Response	Score	Results
		VHF. Unilateral presentation.			stimuli presented in the LVF. This difference was greatest for the oldest age group.
Reynolds & Jeeves, 1978a	36 females, aged 7–8, 13–14 and 18–20 years. Two of the Ss in the youngest group were left-handed.	The letters A, K, F, or R presented one at a time to the LVF or RVF. Unilateral presentation. Monocular viewing.	Subjects pressed one response key to indicate identification of F or R; another response key to indicate identification of other letters.	RT for stimuli presented in each VHF	The two older age groups showed RVF superiority on the task. The youngest group showed a similar trend, which did not reach significance.
Reynolds & Jeeves, 1978b	36 females, aged 7–8, 13–14, & 18–20 years. Two of the Ss in the youngest group were left-handed.	Four faces presented one at a time to the RVF or LVF. Unilateral presentation. Monocular viewing.	Go–no go procedure in which Ss were required to press a button in response to only two of the four faces.	RT for stimuli presented in each VHF	LVF superiority for the two older age groups
Butler & Miller, 1979	96 right-handed B & G, aged 7.1, 8.1, 9.0, & 10.2 years	English words and zero- to third-order approximations of English pseudowords 3 and 5 letters long. Unilateral presentation.	Recognition. Written response.	Mean number of letters identified in each VHF	RVF superiority for identification of letters for all but the youngest children. The youngest age group showed LVF superiority.
Carter & Kinsbourne, 1979	98 right-handed B & G aged 5.5, 6.5, 9.3, & 12.3 years	Triads of horizontally arranged digits. Bilateral presentation. Onset of digits was preceded by verbal (digit) or nonverbal (geometric shape) stimulus appearing at fixation.	Ss were required to name the digit or point to a display containing the shape presented at fixation, after which they reported the digits they had seen.	Phi coefficient	When the fixation stimulus was a digit, there was RVF superiority for digit recall. When the fixation stimulus was a geometric shape, there was LVF superiority for digit recall. The effects of the spatial fixation stimulus lasted over a period of several days for male subjects. No developmental change in VHF superiority for female Ss. The eldest male Ss showed significantly higher phi values than the younger males.
Silverberg, Bentin, Gaziel, Obler, & Albert, 1979	72 right-handed B & G, in G7, G9, & G11, aged 12–13, 14–15, and 16–17 years. Subjects in G7 had 2 years of English instruction; those in G11	24 Hebrew and 24 English three-letter concrete nouns. Unilateral presentation.	Prior to each group of four trials, a word was designated as the target. Ss pressed a microswitch upon seeing the target word in either VHF.	RT for stimuli presented in each VHF	Overall RVF superiority for Hebrew words. A trend toward LVF superiority for English words shifted to RVF superiority for students in their sixth year of English instruction.

	had 6 years of English instruction.				
Tomlinson-Keasey & Kelly, 1979	110 right-handed university and G7 students	Combinations of words (3, 4, & 5 letter high-imagery nouns) and pictures presented either simultaneously or sequentially. Unilateral presentation.	Same/different matching. Manual button press.	RT for stimuli presented in each VHF	Overall RVF superiority for sequential word–word pairs for both age groups. RVF superiority for sequential picture–picture pairs only for the adult group. Overall RVF superiority for picture–word sequential combinations. LVF superiority for simultaneously presented picture–picture pairs only in adults. Overall RVF for simultaneously presented picture–word combinations.
Young & Bion, 1980	96 right-handed B & G, aged 7, 10, & 13 years	Expt. 1: Upright and inverted faces presented at two levels of difficulty. Bilateral presentation.	Subjects pointed to a visual array of four faces in order to choose the two presented stimuli.	Proportion of upright and inverted faces correctly identified in each VHF	Overall LVF superiority for identification of upright faces
	96 right-handed B & G, aged 7, 10, & 13 years	Expt. 2: Same as Expt. 1 except that the pool of stimulus faces was larger. Bilateral presentation.	Same as Expt. 1	Same as Expt. 1	LVF superiority for identifying upright faces only for male subjects
Grant, 1980	120 predominantly right-handed B & G (9 left-handers), aged 5.6, 7.6, & 10.1 years	Achromatic and chromatic square color patches. Unilateral presentation. Monocular viewing.	Recognition. Verbal report.	(R − L)/(R + L)	LVF superiority for color naming for the youngest age group and for 10-year-old girls.
Garren, 1980	80 boys, aged 8–10 years, divided into four groups on the basis of reading age	4-letter lower-case words. Bilateral presentation.	Ss were required either to pronounce or to spell the presented words.	L − R	Normal reading group: RVF superiority for recall of words. The two poorest reading groups showed LVF advantage for word recall. The RVF superiority of Ss in the normal reading group differed significantly from the LVF superiority of the two poorest reading groups.
Ellis & Young, 1981	Expt. 1: 40 right-handed B & G, aged 8.0, 9.1, 10.2, & 10.9 years	20 three-letter concrete nouns. One word was underlined. Bilateral presentation.	Ss reported the underlined word first and then the other word.	Number of words reported from each VHF	RVF superiority for both first and second report. This advantage was greatest for second report. Drop in accuracy from first to second

(continued)

Table 5-2 *(continued)*

Study	Subjects	Stimuli	Response	Score	Results
					report for LVF presentation only.
	Expt. 2: 40 right-handed B & G, aged 8.1, 9.0, 10.1, & 11.0 years	Same as Expt. 1 except that 20 three-letter verbs were used as stimuli	Same as Expt. 1	Same as Expt. 1	Same as Expt. 1
Miller, 1981	120 right-handed males and females aged 7.7, 10.9, & 19.6 years	Capital letters and common four-letter words. Stimuli were presented singly or in pairs. Stimulus pairs were arranged vertically (unilateral presentation), horizontally (bilateral presentation), or diagonally (bilateral presentation).	Recognition. Verbal report	Number of letters and words correctly identified in each position	Letters: RVF superiority occurred only for vertically arranged two-letter arrays. Words: For the oldest group there was RVF superiority; for the middle group there was RVF superiority for single word and two-word vertical arrays.
Messina & Fogliani, 1981	64 right-handed B & G, aged 7 & 8 years	Geometric figures and words. Monocular presentation.	Recognition. Verbal report.	Perceptive thresholds (the stimulus presentation time above which the stimulus is reported)	No differences between the eyes for either of the stimuli. The design apparently entailed comparing left and right eyes but not LVF and RVF.
Grant, 1981	120 children, aged 5, 7, & 10 years, tested twice with one or two years intervening	Achromatic and chromatic square color patches. Unilateral presentation. Monocular viewing.	Recognition. Verbal report.	(R − L)/(R + L)	Only 10-year-olds showed LVF superiority for color naming, and only at the second testing session.
Lewandowski, 1982	48 B & G, aged 8.7, 11.1, 13.2, & 15.0 years (92% strongly right-handed)	Verbal task: Rows of 4 typed capital letters.	Recognition. Verbal report.	(R − L)/(R + L)	Verbal task: Overall RVF superiority. No developmental change in VHF superiority.
		Nonverbal task: Slanted lines Unilateral presentation	Matching from a visual array of 10 lines	(R − L)/(R + L)	Nonverbal task: No VHF differences
Jones & Anuza, 1982	27 B & G, aged 3.4 & 4.3 years.	Male and female faces. Unilateral presentation.	Ss were required to identify the faces as males or females.	Proportion of correct responses from each VHF	Boys showed RVF superiority at both age levels. No developmental change in VHF superiority.
Davidoff, Beaton, Done, & Booth, 1982	12 illiterate males, 12 male controls and 12 normal boys, aged 8 years. All right-handed.	Vertically oriented CVC nonsense syllables; consonant trigrams and three-letter words. Uni-	Recognition. Verbal report of letters in any order.	(R − L)/(R + L)	Overall RVF superiority for all stimuli for all three groups

Davidoff & Done, 1984	Expt. 1: 34 right-handed B & G aged 5.2 years, tested 4 times at 7-month intervals.	Vertically oriented three-letter strings (CCC's or words) arranged in homogeneous and mixed sets. Unilateral presentation.	Ss pressed one button if a letter of a word or CCC matched a letter presented at fixation, and another button if there were no match.	Proportion of errors for each VHF	Overall RVF superiority for CCC's at all testing sessions. RVF superiority for words at the 2nd, 3rd, and 4th testing sessions. Overall RVF superiority for mixed list of CCCs and words.
	Expt. 2: 25, 22, and 24 age-matched Ss acted as controls for each testing session in a cross-sectional study.	Same as Expt. 1	Same as Expt. 1	Same as Expt. 1	No visual field differences for trial blocks in which CCCs or words were presented alone, but RVF for blocks of trials in which both CCCs and words were mixed.
	Expt. 3: B & G aged 4 years, who could not yet name letters	3-letter words	Same as Expt. 1	Same as Expt. 1	LVF superiority for boys, no VHF difference for girls
Turkewitz & Ross–Kossak, 1984	72 right-handed 8-, 11-, & 13-year-old B & G	Photographs of female faces. Unilateral presentation.	Ss pointed to an array of four faces to indicate the face presented on a given trial.	Number of errors for each VHF	Overall LVF superiority. No developmental change in VHF superiority.
Miller, 1984	Expt. 1: 48 right-handed males & females aged 8.8, 11.9, & 22 years	Common four-letter words. Stimuli were presented singly or in pairs. Stimulus pairs were arranged vertically (unilateral presentation), horizontally (bilateral presentation), or diagonally (bilateral presentation).	Recognition. Verbal report. In two-element displays, only the item designated by a post-stimulus cue was to be reported.	Number of words correct for each VHF	LVF superiority for diagonal arrays for the 8-year-olds. RVF superiority for vertical arrays for 11-year-olds. RVF superiority for single words in 22-year-olds.
	Expt. 2: 36 right-handed males & females, aged 8.3, 10.8, & 19.1 years	Same as Expt. 1 except that words in positions not designated to be reported were replaced by 4-element repeating consonant strings (e.g., BBBB).	Same as Expt. 1	Same as Expt. 1	Overall RVF superiority. No developmental change in VHF superiority.
Saxby & Bryden, 1985	91 right-handed B & G aged 6–7, 9–10, & 13–14 years	Emotional: Male and female faces displaying different emotions. Ver-	Ss were required to judge whether pairs of sequentially presented	Lambda	LVF superiority for the emotional task. RVF superiority for the verbal task. No developmental

(continued)

Table 5-2 (*continued*)

Study	Subjects	Stimuli	Response	Score	Results
		bal: Upper and lower case letters. Unilateral presentation.	lateral and central stimuli were the same or different. Verbal report.		change in either RVF or LVF superiority.
Merola & Liederman, 1985	120 right-handed B & G, aged 10, 12, & 14 years	Two vertically arranged letter pairs were presented in each trial. Two letters were upright and two were inverted. Pairs of letters were presented unilaterally or bilaterally. For bilateral conditions letter pairs were presented on the horizontal in the top or bottom of the visual fields, or on a diagonal. Two interference conditions: (1) Separated: both letters in one letter pair were inverted. (2) Unseparated: one letter in each letter pair was inverted and one upright.	Ss were required to name a number that appeared at fixation, then to name as many of the presented letters as possible	Proportion of letters correctly named on a given trial R − L	Overall RVF superiority. No developmental change in VHF superiority. The "hemispheric independence" index, a measure of the advantage of distributing interfering stimuli across VHF's, was greater for 12- and 14-year-olds than for 10-year-olds.
Corballis, Macadie, Crotty, & Beale, 1985	10 right-handed B & G, aged 12.3 years. Control group for an LD study.	Upper-case letters F, G, & R in normal or backwards orientation. Letters rotated 60°, 120°, 180°, 240°, or 300° from upright. Unilateral presentation.	Recognition. Verbal report.	RT for stimuli presented in each VHF	No VHF differences

Abbreviations: B & G (boys and girls); CCC (consonant trigram); CV (consonant–vowel syllable); CVC (consonant–vowel–consonant word); EA (ear advantage); Expt. (experiment); G (grade); L (left); R (right); LD (learning-disabled); LE (left ear); RE (right ear); LEA (left-ear advantage); REA (right-ear advantage); LEM (left-ear monitoring); REM (right-ear monitoring); LH (left hand); RH (right hand); LVF (left visual half-field); RVF (right visual half-field); RT (reaction time); S (subject); SEL (socioeconomic level); VF or VHF (visual half-field).

Thus, although neither of these tasks yielded a significant LVF advantage, both showed an invariance of outcome across a wide age range.

The diversity of outcomes from studies of children's face perception is not surprising in light of the equally variable results from tachistoscopic studies of face perception in adults (see Bryden, 1982b). The asymmetry of performance is subject to the influence of numerous stimulus characteristics, such as exposure duration (Sergent, 1982), familiarity of the faces (Broman, 1978; Ross & Turkewitz, 1981), and number of dimensions on which the faces differ (Sergent, 1984). Furthermore, asymmetries have been defined in various ways—for example, in terms of reaction time, number of errors, and the minimum exposure duration necessary for a specified level of performance. As pointed out by Carey *et al.* (1980), "At every age task variables will influence the presence or absence of a right hemisphere advantage for faces as well as its absolute magnitude" (p. 266). The problem is compounded in developmental studies, for the relative importance of the various stimulus and task factors cannot be assumed to remain constant across different age levels.

Nonlinguistic stimuli other than faces have been presented to children's left and right half-fields, with mixed results. Some investigators have reported early asymmetries and the absence of age-related change. Young and Bion (1979), for example, found that dots were enumerated more quickly and more accurately if presented to the LVF than if presented to the RVF, and that this asymmetry was constant across the age range of 5 to 11 years. Although Young and Bion (1981) obtained the opposite asymmetry in a task requiring the naming of line drawings, this asymmetry also was established by the age of 5 years. Data reported by Witelson (1977c) suggest that 6- and 7-year-old boys match pairs of human figures more accurately when the figures are presented in the LVF than in the RVF.

Grant (1980, 1981) also reported an early-developing asymmetry, but in this case the asymmetry disappeared with increasing age. Grant's procedure entailed presenting colored squares to one VHF or the other and asking children to name the color they had seen. With children aged 5, 7, and 10 years, Grant (1980) found a curvilinear developmental pattern: The youngest children showed a significant LVF superiority; the middle group showed no asymmetry; and the eldest children showed a tendency toward LVF superiority, which was significant only for the girls. Longitudinal follow-up of 75 of the original 120 children confirmed this unusual developmental pattern (Grant, 1981). In explaining the pattern, Grant proposed that the color-naming task involves predominantly the right hemisphere but that, as children become increasingly familiar with colors, the task becomes "verbally biased." Subsequently, with the establishment of right-hemispheric language capacity, LVF superiority is reestablished.

Using a simple reaction time task in which the subject responds manually to flashes of light impinging on either the nasal or the temporal part of the retina, Jeeves (1972) found among right-handed boys an asymmetry favoring input to the right hemisphere. The results for right-handed boys between the ages of 9 and 12 years were similar to results obtained with right- and left-handed adults, but left-handed boys failed to show any asymmetry.

Other developmental patterns of VHF asymmetry have been reported, but there is little evidence that asymmetry increases with age. Lewandowski (1982) found no significant asymmetry in any of four age groups for the identification of slanted lines. Age-related laterality changes were found with another line-orientation task (Schaller & Dziadosz, 1976), but the changes are not readily ascribed to increasing degrees of cerebral lateralization. Preschoolers failed to show significant asymmetry; Grade 3 students showed significant RVF superiority; and most adults showed LVF superiority. This finding is reminiscent of a study by Braine (1968) in which Israeli children from Grades 3, 5, and 7, as well as university students, were administered a variety of tachistoscopic and nontachistoscopic tasks designed to detect asymmetries in the processing of predominantly nonverbal patterns and arrays. In general, the results suggested a right-biased "attentiveness" among children from Grades 3 and 5 and the opposite asymmetry among older children and adults.

STUDIES WITH VERBAL STIMULI

Presenting letters, digits, and words to children does not guarantee that verbal processing will occur. Tomlinson-Keasey and Kelly (1979), for instance, showed that the distinction between words and pictures is less important than other factors in determining perceptual asymmetry in a matching task. If linguistic stimuli can be detected or matched on the basis of physical identity (e.g., Broman, 1978; Reynolds & Jeeves, 1978a), then one cannot assume that the stimuli will be processed verbally. Similarly, the presentation of letters in unusual orientations (Corballis, Macadie, Crotty, & Beale, 1985) may necessitate nonverbal processing and thus make the task less linguistic than it otherwise might be. Clearly, young children who are unfamiliar with the alphabet cannot be expected to process letters verbally (Davidoff & Done, 1984). Under circumstances like these, failure to obtain a significant RVF advantage is more plausibly attributed to the nonverbal nature of the task than to the subjects' lack of language lateralization.

Because of its primacy, the 1953 study by Forgays provides a natural starting point for summarizing those VHF studies that involve linguistic stimuli. Forgays (1953) tested subjects at 12 educational levels on a task that required recognition of three- and four-letter words from the left or right VHF. Presentation was unilateral, with LVF and RVF trials mixed randomly. The results are illustrated in Figure 5-2. All three sources of variance in the education level × VHF analysis of variance turned out to be significant. There was an increase in overall performance with increasing educational level; RVF recognition exceeded LVF recognition; and the interaction reflected increasing asymmetry with increasing education level. There was no apparent difference between LVF and RVF performance for the youngest children, that is, for those in Grades 2 through 7. Cerebral dominance was not widely accepted as an explanation for VHF asymmetry at the time Forgays's study was conducted. Consequently, he attributed the age-related change in laterality to "selective retinal training coincident with the educational process through the conditions present in the reading of English text" (pp. 167–168).

Subsequent studies have not confirmed the developmental trend reported by Forgays (Ellis & Young, 1981; Garren, 1980; Marcel, Katz, & Smith, 1974; Marcel & Rajan, 1975; McKeever & Huling, 1970; Miller & Turner, 1973; Olson, 1973; Tomlinson-Keasey & Kelly, 1979; Tomlinson-Keasey, Kelly, & Burton, 1978; Turner & Miller, 1975). Olson (1973), using stimuli and procedures very similar to those used by Forgays, found a constant RVF superiority across the age range of 7 to 11 years (Grades 2–6). The only obvious difference between the respective procedures was Olson's inclusion of trials in which words were presented simultaneously in both VHFs. Both the unilateral and bilateral conditions, which were randomly interspersed, yielded significant RVF advantages.

Although the intermixing of unilateral and bilateral trials in the study by Olson (1973) might have contributed to the discrepancy between her results and those of Forgays (1953), studies with only unilaterally presented words also have yielded significant RVF advantages for children between the ages of 7 and 9 (Marcel, Katz, & Smith, 1974; Marcel & Rajan, 1975). McKeever and Huling (1970), using unilateral presentation of words, reported a marked RVF advantage for children in Grade 7, including a group of children whose average reading proficiency was below the Grade 4 level. Miller and Turner (1973), though failing to find a significant RVF superiority for unilaterally presented words among

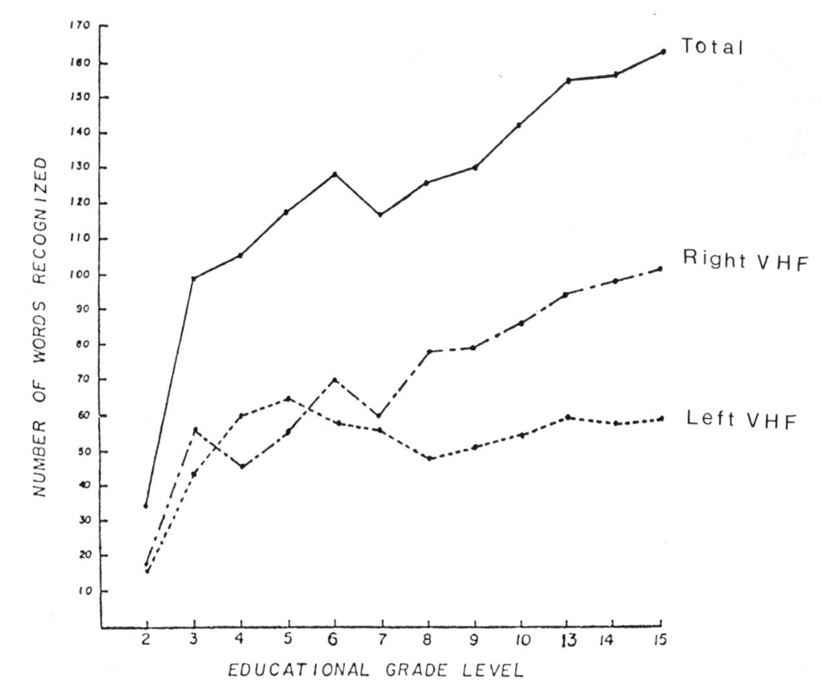

Figure 5-2. Mean number of three- and four-letter words recognized from the right and left visual half-fields as a function of grade level. Reprinted by permission from "The Development of Differential Word Recognition" by D. G. Forgays, 1953, *Journal of Experimental Psychology, 45,* p. 166. Copyright © 1953 by the American Psychological Association.

Grade 2 children, did find a significant effect among Grade 4 and Grade 6 children. Using a forced-choice response format, Turner and Miller (1975) obtained a RVF advantage for three-letter words in children from Grades 1 through 4. There was no evidence of an age-related increase in the asymmetry even when the children's scores were compared with those of university students.

In two studies involving same–different judgments of pictures and words presented in succession to the same VHF, only the youngest subjects (8-year-olds in one instance and 13-year-olds in the other) failed to show an RVF advantage for matched pairs of stimuli (Tomlinson-Keasey & Kelly, 1979; Tomlinson-Keasey, Kelly, & Burton, 1978). Subjects in all age groups, however, showed similar laterality patterns for unmatched stimulus pairs.

Even if one were to accept Forgays's (1953) evidence for late development of the RVF advantage for words, there is good reason to question his conclusion that the age-related change is dependent on training in the reading of English text. Carmon, Nachshon, and Starinsky (1976) found a significant RVF superiority among Israeli schoolchildren for both Hebrew words and Arabic numbers, even though the two kinds of material are scanned in opposite directions. Aaron and Handley (1975) found that a left-to-right scanning tendency increased in frequency after the age of 4 years in a sample of American children. Not only did the change occur prior to the beginning of systematic instruction in reading, but the left-to-right scanning tendency was not related to an enhanced RVF superiority for either verbal or nonverbal material in a tachistoscopic recognition task. Nonetheless, when the scanning required by the child's second language is opposite in direction to that required by the child's first language, VHF asymmetry for words in the second language may be affected, at least during the early stages of second-language acquisition (Silverberg, Bentin, Gaziel, Obler, & Albert, 1979).

When multiple letters are substituted for words as stimuli to be processed, the usual result is a significant RVF superiority that remains constant across the age range being sampled (Butler & Miller, 1979; Davidoff, Beaton, Done, & Booth, 1982; Davidoff & Done, 1984; Lewandowski, 1982; Merola & Liederman, 1985; Miller, 1971, 1973). Results from studies involving the presentation of single letters in the left or right VHF are somewhat more variable (Corballis *et al.,* 1985; Gross, Rothenberg, Schottenfeld, & Drake, 1978; Reynolds & Jeeves, 1978a; Saxby & Bryden, 1985); but the most common outcome, again, is a significant RVF advantage at all age levels.

Using a task that entailed detecting targets from sequentially presented letters that appeared in either the left or the right VHF, Reynolds and Jeeves (1978a) failed to find a significant RVF advantage in 7- and 8-year-olds, the youngest of their three age groups. It would be misleading, however, to cite this outcome as evidence that asymmetry increases with increasing age. First, the age × VHF interaction was not significant. Second, the average magnitude of the RVF advantage was somewhat greater for the younger children than for the two groups of older subjects. Apparently it was the relatively great variability of performance (expressed in reaction time), as well as the limited power of a statistical test based on only 12 subjects, that precluded finding a significant VHF effect for the 7- and 8-year-olds.

Miller (1971, 1973) found that children in Grades 1 and 2 (i.e., 6 to 8 years of age) are significantly more accurate in detecting a target letter when it appears among other letters in the RVF rather than the LVF. The asymmetry at this age level was at least as large as the similar asymmetry shown by older children and university students. These results are consistent with those from a longitudinal study by Davidoff and Done (1984) in which 34 children attempted to match a centrally presented letter to one of three letters presented in either the left or the right VHF. The children were tested four times, at approximately 7-month intervals, between the ages of 5 and 7 years. The investigators found little evidence of developmental change in the degree of VHF asymmetry. As a rule, the children maintained a consistent RVF superiority across four testing sessions. When administered to 4-year-olds with very limited knowledge of the alphabet, however, the same task did not yield a RVF advantage. Davidoff and Done concluded from their findings that "there is a left hemisphere involvement for letter matching present soon after knowledge of letter naming is achieved" (p. 317).

Single digits, presented unilaterally and alternated with digits presented on midline, have been shown to yield a RVF advantage in children (Yeni-Komshian, Isenberg, & Goldberg, 1975). Simultaneous bilateral presentation of digit arrays also yields a RVF advantage in children under some circumstances, but this laterality effect can be reversed if a nonverbal fixation-control stimulus is used in lieu of the customary fixation-control stimulus, that is, a centrally presented digit (Carter & Kinsbourne, 1979; Kershner, Thomae, & Callaway, 1977).

CONCLUSIONS

Tachistoscopic studies seem to be more susceptible than other kinds of laterality studies to the effects of methodological variables, most of which are poorly understood. These variables must be investigated and controlled before the method can be exploited effectively as a source of information about hemispheric specialization. In her foreword to a special issue of *Brain and Cognition* devoted to the methodology of VHF studies, Sergent (1986) warns that scientific "anarchy" may occur unless greater methodological rigor is brought to bear on tachistoscopic laterality studies.

The developmental literature, when considered in light of the ambiguities present in the adult literature, seems less chaotic than one might fear. Whereas it may not be possible to specify the precise circumstances that favor a reliable right or left VHF superiority in children, it seems clear that different categories of stimuli usually yield predictable asymmetries. Moreover, there is little evidence that the child's age has a major effect on the direction or magnitude of VHF asymmetries. Thus, even if one cannot predict the outcome associated with a given combination of stimulus and task factors, there is some basis for predicting that children will show an asymmetry similar to the asymmetry found with adults tested under similar conditions, and that the effect will be comparable for children of different ages. These conclusions are in accord with conclusions reached in previous reviews of VHF studies with children (Beaumont, 1982a; Witelson, 1977b; Young, 1982).

Tactile and Haptic Studies

Although the word "haptic" is a synonym for "tactile" (*Stedman's Medical Dictionary,* 1982), a distinction between the two terms is often made, such that "haptic" refers to active touch, or palpation, whereas "tactile" refers to passive stimulation of the cutaneous receptors (e.g., Witelson, 1977b). Thus, haptic tasks entail not only tactile stimulation but also motor activity and proprioceptive feedback. Most of the tasks to be discussed in this section are tests of *stereognosis,* the ability to recognize objects on the basis of active touch. Consequently, there is a major cognitive component to task performance, in addition to the sensory and motor components, and it is this cognitive component that has been the primary focus of attention. The studies are summarized in Table 5-3.

Haptic laterality resembles auditory laterality in certain respects. The rationale for asymmetries in both modalities is similar; that is, the crossed pathways from receptor organ to sensory cortex are thought to be functionally superior to the uncrossed pathways. Consequently, if one cerebral hemisphere is specialized for processing a particular kind of information, then relevant input from the side of the body opposite to the specialized hemisphere will be at an advantage relative to input from the ipsilateral side. In haptic as well as auditory tasks (see Henry, 1979, 1983), asymmetrical performance may be elicited by either unilateral (noncompetitive) or bilateral (competitive) stimulation. It appears, however, that haptic asymmetries are more readily elicited than auditory asymmetries in the absence of bilateral competition, perhaps because the superiority of the crossed pathways is more pronounced in the somatosensory system than in the auditory system (Sperry, Gazzaniga, & Bogen, 1969).

Three characteristics distinguish haptic methods from other methods for studying laterality. First, haptic techniques are particularly well suited for examining the processing of nonlinguistic stimuli, but poorly suited for examining linguistic processing, except perhaps in individuals who are blind. In contrast to the visual and auditory modalities, through which children normally receive their linguistic information, the tactile modality ordinarily is a source of only nonlinguistic input. Even though letter and word shapes have been used in haptic studies to induce linguistic processing, the salience of the linguistic aspect of these tasks is difficult to specify. If substantial spatial analysis is necessary before the stimulus can acquire linguistic significance for the subject, the processing may be primarily nonlinguistic in spite of the linguistic stimulus.

Table 5-3. Summary of Tactile and Haptic Studies

Study	Subjects	Stimuli	Response	Score	Results
Ghent, 1961	108 B & G, aged 5, 6, 7, 9 and 11 years	Graded series of nylon monofilaments applied to the ball of the thumb	Verbal report (presence/absence)	Tactual threshold for each hand (log force) as determined by the method of limits	Girls: At 5 years, dominant thumb was more sensitive; at 6–9 years nondominant thumb was more sensitive; no difference at 11 years. Boys: Overall increase in sensitivity with age. More sensitive with nondominant thumb at 11 years.
Witelson, 1974	47 right-handed boys, ranging in age from 6.4 to 14.3 years. Three age groups: 5.2, 10.2, and 13.1 years.	Nonsense shapes and letters. Both shapes and letters were presented simultaneously (dichhaptically).	Pointing to a visual display for forms and verbal identification for letters. Subjects used the left hand to point. A subgroup was tested again using the right hand to point. One to two weeks separated testing for letter and shape stimuli.	Percentage accuracy for each hand	Overall LH superiority for nonsense shapes. No developmental change in hand superiority. No hand difference for letters. When the nonsense shapes test was given after the letters test, the LH superiority disappeared. LH superiority was not present when the right hand indicated the Ss's choice.
Rudel, Denckla, & Spalten, 1974	80 right-handed B & G aged 7–8, 9–10, 11–12, and 13–14 years	Braille letters. Unilateral presentation.	Paired-associate learning of Braille letters and their verbal labels. Verbal report.	Number correct per hand	Overall RH superiority for girls and LH superiority for boys. RH superiority at age 7–8. LH superiority at age 13–14. The RH superiority was due primarily to the performance of the 7- to 8-year-old girls. The LH superiority was due to the performance of 13- to 14-year-old boys. Overall, for Ss except 7–8-year-olds, the LH performed better when it was tested after the RH than when it was tested first.
Witelson, 1976	200 right-handed B & G aged 6–7, 8–9, 10–11, 12–13 years	Nonsense shapes presented dichhaptically	Pointing to a visual display	Number correct per hand	Overall LH superiority for boys. No hand difference for girls. No developmental change in hand superiority.

Witelson, 1977a	156 right-handed boys aged 10.5 years (normal controls for LD group)	Pairs of meaningless shapes or pairs of letters. Dichhaptic presentation	Pointing response for shapes; naming of letters	Number of correct responses for each hand	Shapes: LH superiority Letters: No asymmetry
Witelson, 1977c	Study 1: 75 G & 100 B aged 6–7, 8–9, 10–11, & 12–14 years	Nonsense shapes. Dichhaptic presentation.	Pointing to a visual display	Number correct per hand	Only boys showed LH superiority for nonsense shapes. No developmental change in hand superiority for boys. Shapes presented to the LH were reported first more often than those presented to the RH for boys.
	Study 2: 27 G and 28 B aged 6–14 years	Pairs of letters. Dichhaptic presentation.	Free recall, verbal report	Number correct per hand	Boys showed RH superiority for letters. For girls there was no difference between LH and RH performance.
Rudel, Denckla, & Hirsch, 1977	120 right-handed males & females aged 7–8, 9–10, 11–12, 13–14, & 20–40 years	Pairs of Braille letters. Unilateral presentation.	Same/different judgments about two Braille letters. Verbal report	Frequencies and type (number, displacement, orientation) of errors for each hand.	LH superiority at ages 11–12 and 13–14. At ages 9–10 there was RH superiority.
LaBreche, Manning, Goble, & Markman, 1977	24 Ss, mean age 17.2 years Control group for a study of deaf children	Nonsense forms and letters. Dichhaptic presentation.	For nonsense forms Ss pointed to a visual array. For letters Ss wrote or finger–spelled their response.	Number correct per hand	Overall RH superiority for nonsense forms No hand differences for the letters task
Galin, Johnstone, Nakell, & Herron 1979	30 right-handed girls, aged 3 & 5 years	A fabric of specific texture was rubbed across the fingers of one hand. Either the identical fabric or a different fabric was subsequently rubbed across the fingers of the same or opposite hand.	Same/different judgment for fabric textures presented sequentially to the same or opposite hands. Verbal report.	Number of crossed and uncrossed matching errors	Total number of crossed (interhemispheric) errors decreased from ages 3 to 5. No hand difference.
Bakker & Van der Kleij, 1978	56 right-handed B & G aged 7.2 & 11.3 years	Mechanical stimulation of fingertips. Two fingers stimulated on each trial in medio-lateral or latero-medial direction (thumb excluded). Unilateral stimulation.	Identification of stimulated finger by pressing response knobs with nonstimulated hand (nonverbal condition) or by naming fingers according to numbers on a model (verbal condition).	Number of stimuli correctly localized at each hand	Overall RH superiority in verbal and nonverbal report conditions. No developmental change in hand superiority.

(continued)

Table 5-3 *(continued)*

Study	Subjects	Stimuli	Response	Score	Results
Cioffi & Kandel, 1979	112 B & G aged 7.5, 9.2, 10.8, & 12.5 years	(1) Nonsense shapes; (2) 2-letter words; (3) Consonant bigrams. Dichhaptic presentation.	Pointing to a visual display	Number correct per hand	Overall LH superiority for identification of nonsense shapes and RH superiority for identification of words. Boys identified more bigrams with the LH than did girls, but girls identified more bigrams with RH than did boys. No developmental change in hand superiority.
Flanery & Balling, 1979	64 right-handed males & females aged 7.2, 9.3, 11.3, & 23.8 years	Nonsense forms: (1) unilateral presentation, (2) dichhaptic presentation	Tactile matching. Same/different response made with hand signals	Number correct per hand	Correct responses: Overall LH superiority. No developmental change in hand superiority. Laterality coefficient: Absolute value of the laterality coefficient increased with age. The two older groups had more Ss showing LH superiority than the younger groups.
Affleck & Joyce, 1979	31 right-handed B & G, mean age 5 years	Nonsense shapes; dichhaptic presentation.	Pointing to a visual display	Number of correct responses for each hand.	LH superiority for boys, no difference for girls
Cranney & Ashton, 1980	20 right-handed B & G, aged 7 & 11.4 years Control group for a study with deaf children	Nonsense shapes. Dichhaptic presentation.	Pointing with the left hand to a visual display	Number correct per hand	No difference between RH and LH performance. No sex differences.
Klein and Rosenfield, 1980	30 B & G of heterogeneous handedness from G3. 13/15 boys and 11/13 girls showed RH preference; the rest were left-handed or of mixed handedness.	Nonsense forms and letters. Dichhaptic presentation.	Subjects used a "divining rod"–shaped double-handled pointer (held by both hands) to indicate their choices on a visual display.	Number correct per hand	Overall LH superiority for nonsense shapes. No hand difference for the letters task. No sex differences.
Posluszny & Barton, 1981	42 right-handed B & G aged 10 years. Subjects were preselected on the basis of scores on the Primary Mental Abilities	Nonsense shapes and 2-letter words. Dichhaptic presentation.	Words were reported verbally. Ss identified shapes from a visual display. No other information given	Number correct per hand Percentage correct Phi coefficient	No overall hand effects. Boys showed greater accuracy than girls on the shapes test. LH superiority for the high spatial/low verbal group for both types of stimuli

	test. Two groups: high spatial/low verbal; low spatial/high verbal.		regarding response mode for shapes task.	Percentage errors	High spatial/low verbal girls made more RH than LH errors on the words task; high spatial/low verbal boys made more RH than LH errors on the shapes task.
Yamamoto, 1980	42 B & G, aged 8.4, 10.5, & 12.6 years	Meaningful object forms (cow, tree, etc.). Unilateral presentation	Pointing to a visual display	Number of correct responses for each hand	LH superiority for 12-year-olds but no significant asymmetry for younger children
				RT for each hand	Age × Hand interaction, which reflects faster R than L RT for 8-year-olds and faster L than R RT for older children
				Laterality quotient $(L-R)/(L+R)$	Laterality quotient increased with age
Dawson, 1981	120 right-handed males & females in G1, G6, & university	Nonsense shapes. Dichhaptic presentation.	Verbal response. Ss reported the position number of shapes on a visual display that corresponded to the two palpated shapes.	Number correct per hand	Only males showed LH superiority for identifying nonsense shapes. No developmental change in hand advantage.
				Number of Ss showing a hand advantage	More males than females showed LH superiority; more females than males showed RH superiority.
Denes & Spinaci, 1981	80 right-handed B & G, aged 6, 8, 10 and 13 years	Nonsense shapes. Each shape was assigned a high or low association value. High-low association pairs were presented dichhaptically.	Pointing to a visual display	Number of identification errors	Overall LH superiority for nonsense shapes. Better performance for high association shapes than low association shapes. Decrease in errors over age. No sex effects.
Moreau & Milner, 1981	31 right-handed B & G, aged 5.4 years	Unilateral and bilateral stimulation of the L and R cheeks and hands. This included simultaneous stimulation of ipsilateral and contralateral face and hand sites.	Child indicated the site(s) touched by pointing	Omission errors (failure to identify a site touched)	Face test: Number of omissions greater for the R cheek than for the L cheek Hand test: No asymmetry of omission errors Face–hand test: Number of omissions greater on the R than on the L side
Etaugh & Levy, 1981	46 right-handed B & G, aged 4 and 5 years	Nonsense shapes Dichhaptic presentation	Pointing to a visual display	Number correct per hand	Overall LH superiority. No developmental change in hand superior-

(continued)

Table 5-3 *(continued)*

Study	Subjects	Stimuli	Response	Score	Results
					ity. No sex difference in hand superiority.
Vargha-Khadem, 1980	16 right-handed B & G from G7, G8, & G11 Control group for a study with deaf children	Pairs of abstract 3-letter nouns and nonsense shapes Dichhaptic presentation	Pointing to a visual display	Percentage accuracy for each hand	Overall RH superiority. The RH superiority was larger for the verbal stimuli than for the shapes.
Dalby & Gibson, 1981	15 right-handed boys, aged 9–12 years Control group for a study of LD boys	Steel rods, oriented from 18° to 162°, in steps of 18°, relative to the horizontal plane. Unilateral presentation.	Tactile matching. Ss palpated an array of 9 rods and selected the one with the same inclination as the rod previously felt with the same hand.	Number of correct trials per hand	Overall LH superiority
Hatta, Yamamoto, Kawabata, & Tsutui, 1981	48 right-handed B & G, aged 8.3, 10.5, & 12.4 years	Representational shapes (horse, cow, car). Unilateral presentation.	Pointing to a visual display with opposite hand	Percentage correct	The oldest group showed a LH superiority. No hand differences in the younger groups. Females showed greater accuracy with their RH. Males showed no hand differences.
Brizzolara, De Nobili, & Ferretti, 1982	16 B & G, aged 7.5 years, and 16 college students, aged 25 years. All Ss right-handed or ambidextrous	Wooden sticks, oriented from 9° to 171°, in steps of 18°, relative to the horizontal plane. Unilateral presentation.	Tactile matching. Ss palpated an array of 10 sticks and selected the one with the same inclination as the stick previously felt with the same hand.	Number correct per hand	Children: Overall LH superiority. Significant LH superiority for G but not B. Adults: Overall LH superiority. No sex difference.
Yamamoto & Hatta, 1982	32 right-handed B & G, aged 10.4–11.4 years	(1) Meaningful forms. Unilateral presentation.	Pointing with the opposite hand to a visual display	RT	Females showed RH superiority. Males showed no hand difference.
		(2) Two fingers of one hand were touched.	Pointing with the opposite hand to the fingers touched	Number correct per hand	Overall RH superiority
		(3) Children palpated digit shapes that were oriented up, down or 90° to the left or right.	Pointing with the opposite hand to a visual display	RT	Overall LH superiority

Cranney & Ashton, 1982	32 right-handed B & G aged 6.2 & 8.3 years Control group for a study of deaf children	Nonsense shapes. Unilateral presentation. Two shapes presented sequentially to the same hand or to opposite hands	Tactile matching. Same/different response made with hand signals	Number correct per hand	LH superiority for matching forms for the older age group. No sex differences
Gibson & Bryden, 1983	80 right-handed B & G, aged 8, 10, 12 and 14 years	Pairs of letters and pairs of nonsense shapes. Dichhaptic presentation.	Pointing to a visual array of shapes and letters. Poststimulus cueing indicated order of report.	Number of correct responses for each hand	LH superiority for nonsense shapes; no difference between hands in verbal condition. Overall greater accuracy with LH for children aged 8 and 12 years.
				Lambda	LH superiority for nonsense shapes. Stronger LH superiority for boys than girls.
Gibson & Bryden, 1984	20 right-handed B & G aged 11.0 years Control group for a study of deaf children	Letters and shapes. Dichhaptic presentation.	Pointing to a visual array of shapes and letters. Poststimulus cueing indicated order of report.	Number correct per hand	RH superiority for letters. LH more accurate for shapes than for letters. Males were more accurate with their LH, females with their RH.
				Lambda	Males showed overall LH superiority; females showed overall RH superiority.
Yamamoto, 1984	Expt. 1: 17 right-handed and 12 ambidextrous B & G, aged 5.3–6.2 years	Nonsense shapes. Unilateral presentation.	Tactile matching. Same/different response made verbally. Ss matched a comparison stimulus presented to the same hand.	Number correct per hand	LH superiority for males
	Expt. 2: Same as Expt. 1	Same as Expt. 1	Same as Expt. 1 except Ss matched a comparison stimulus presented to the contralateral hand.	Number correct per hand	No hand differences. Right-handed boys made fewer errors in the LH-to-RH condition than in the RH-to-LH condition.
Rose, 1984	72 right-handed B & G, aged 1.0, 2.0, & 3.4 years.	Pairs of three-dimensional stimuli	Children palpated objects and were subsequently shown the palpated object and a novel stimulus. Amount of time the child visually fixated the novel or familiar object was measured.	Ratio of fixation time for novel stimuli to total fixation time	LH superiority for the 2- and 3-year-olds but not for the 1-year-olds. 45%, 70%, & 75% of the 1-, 2-, and 3-year-olds showed LH superiority, respectively.

(continued)

Table 5-3 *(continued)*

Study	Subjects	Stimuli	Response	Score	Results
Rose, 1985	96 right-handed B & G, aged 2.0, 3.7, 4.5, & 5.6 years	Three-dimensional stimuli similar to those used by Rose, 1984, with the addition of harpsichord and flute music. Three conditions: music to right ear, left ear, and no music.	Children palpated objects and were subsequently shown the palpated object and a novel stimulus. Amount of time the child visually fixated the novel or familiar object was measured.	Ratio of fixation time for novel stimuli to total fixation time	Overall LH superiority. Ipsilateral musical input caused a decrement in LH performance for the 4- and 5-year-olds. For the 2- and 3-year-olds, contralateral input disrupted LH performance. Music interfered with RH performance across all ear × age groups.
Hassler & Birbaumer, 1986	120 B & G aged 9–14 years were tested 3 times with 1 year intervening each time. Divided into 3 groups on the basis of scores on Wing's Tests of Musical Intelligence. Group 1 consisted of children who had high scores and demonstrated an ability to compose or improvise; group 2 only had high scores; group 3 Ss were nonmusician controls. Handedness was mixed, with 101 right-handers and 19 left-handers.	Nonsense shapes. Dichaptic presentation.	Identification of shapes from a visual display. Verbal report.	Number correct per hand	Session 1: No overall hand difference. Right-handed boys in group 1 showed LH superiority. Session 2: No overall hand difference. Right-handed boys in group 2 showed LH superiority. Session 3: Right-handed boys showed nearly significant LH superiority.

Abbreviations: B & G (boys and girls); CCC (consonant trigram); CV (consonant–vowel syllable); CVC (consonant–vowel–consonant word); EA (ear advantage); Expt. (experiment); G (grade); L (left); R (right); LD (learning-disabled); LE (left ear); RE (right ear); LEA (left-ear advantage); REA (right-ear advantage); LEM (left-ear monitoring); REM (right-ear monitoring); LH (left hand); RH (right hand); LVF (left visual half-field); RVF (right visual half-field); RT (reaction time); S (subject); SEL (socioeconomic level); VF or VHF (visual half-field).

A second characteristic of haptic laterality is the existence of functional asymmetries at various distinct levels of analysis. If, as suggested by Rose (1984), the task of identifying an object through touch is determined by three mechanisms—tactual sensitivity, motor control, and information processing—then it is possible that each mechanism independently influences any observed difference between left- and right-hand performance. Right-handed adults show greater tactile sensitivity on the left hand than on the right (Semmes, Weinstein, Ghent, & Teuber, 1960; Weinstein & Sersen, 1961). This asymmetry, combined with unequal skill in moving the left and right hands, makes it difficult to attribute haptic asymmetries unequivocally to lateralized cognitive processing. A left-hand advantage for object recognition may be attributed either to right hemisphere processing or to an asymmetry of tactile sensitivity (or both). Failure to find a difference between the hands may be ascribed either to bilateral cognitive processing or to a right-hand advantage for palpation that nullifies the left-hand advantage associated with tactile sensitivity and right hemisphere processing.

Finally, the haptic literature is replete with studies showing that boys outperform girls, that boys show greater asymmetry, and that boys and girls show different developmental patterns. Reports of sex differences in children's laterality are not entirely lacking in the dichotic listening or VHF literature; but, on the whole, there is little reason to conclude that boys and girls differ in degree of laterality or in the age at which laterality is first manifested. In haptic studies, however, sex differences appear so frequently that it would be difficult to summarize the findings without considering separately the results for boys and for girls.

STUDIES OF TACTILE SENSITIVITY

Noting that the left hand of adults tends to be more sensitive to touch than the right hand, Ghent (1961) measured left- and right-hand sensory thresholds in children between the ages of 5 and 11 years in an attempt to specify the age at which the adult pattern of asymmetry first appears. Thresholds were established using the method of limits. Fine nylon monofilaments, graduated in caliber, were applied to the ball of the thumb in ascending and descending series; the children, who were blindfolded, indicated when they felt the stimulus. Because the results for boys did not resemble the results for girls, Ghent analyzed the data for each sex separately. For girls there was no overall change in threshold with increasing age, but there was a significant hand × age interaction such that 5-year-olds were significantly more sensitive in the dominant than in the nondominant hand, whereas girls between the ages of 6 and 9 showed a significant difference in the opposite direction. However, the eldest girls (the 11-year-olds) showed no asymmetry at all. The pattern for boys was very different. For boys there was significant bilateral improvement with age and a significant hand × age interaction that reflected lack of asymmetry until the age of 11 years, at which time the sensitivity of the nondominant hand exceeded that of the dominant hand.

If one overlooks the absence of asymmetry in 11-year-old girls, then the results support the conclusion that the adult pattern of tactile asymmetry develops by the age of 6 years in girls but not until sometime after the age of 9 in boys. Such a conclusion, however, is tenuous for at least two reasons. First, Ghent's findings, which are based on cross-sectional analyses, could easily have been distorted by sampling error, that is, by unrepresentative results in one or more cells of the design. Second, the findings pertain to dominant and nondominant hands rather than to right and left hands. Since left-handed children constituted 13% of the sample, the pooling of data from right- and left-handers may have obfuscated differences between the left and right hands in the right-handed children.

Additional evidence regarding asymmetry of children's tactile sensitivity is sparse, but two studies provide some information. Galin, Johnstone, Nakell, and Herron (1979) required 3- and 5-year-old girls to make same–different judgments after being touched twice on the hand with either two identical or two different fabrics. The same hand was touched twice on half of the trials (uncrossed condition), but both hands were touched sequentially on the other trials (crossed condition). Although the main point of this study was to show that young children have particular difficulty in the crossed condition—implying a deficiency of information transfer between hemispheres—the authors also tested for differences between left and right hands in the uncrossed condition and found no significant asymmetry. They did find, however, that in the crossed condition there were significantly fewer errors with a left–right order of stimulation than with a right–left order. If one assumes that memory for the first of the two fabrics is the performance-limiting aspect of the paradigm, then this latter finding would indicate a left-hand superiority in young girls.

Other sensitivity data are contained in a paper by Moreau and Milner (1981), who applied a double simultaneous stimulation test to 5-year-old children. In this procedure, the child is touched on the left hand, right hand, left cheek, or right cheek. Some trials entail touching only a single site, whereas other entail simultaneous touching of two sites. Data were analyzed separately for face, hand, and face–hand trials. No significant asymmetry for hands was found, but there were significantly fewer left-sided errors than right-sided errors for both the face and the face–hand trials. All of the face–hand trials involved double simultaneous stimulation, and the hand and face data were analyzed after single and double stimulation trials were combined. Consequently, these analyses do not reveal whether simple tactile sensitivity was asymmetrical or whether asymmetries were manifested only as asymmetrical "extinction" of one stimulus in the double stimulation condition. No significant sex differences were found.

In summary, there is insufficient evidence to permit any firm conclusions about the asymmetry of simple tactile sensitivity in children. When a difference is found, the left side of the body seems to be favored. The sex difference reported by Ghent (1961) has not been duplicated. Moreau and Milner's (1981) findings imply that tactile asymmetries may be found in young children of both sexes.

STUDIES WITH UNILATERAL STIMULATION

Of the studies involving information processing of greater complexity than detection, nearly half entail unilateral stimulation. These studies, though diverse in many respects, show some consistency of outcome when categorized according to the stimulus and task used. When finger localization—a process traditionally associated with the left hemisphere—is required, right-hand performance exceeds left-hand performance (Bakker & Van der Kleij, 1978; Yamamoto & Hatta, 1982). In this task the child is stimulated on two fingers in succession and then must identify the fingers stimulated and, in some instances, the order in which the fingers were stimulated. Right-hand superiority is found irrespective of whether the child responds by pointing to the stimulated fingers or by identifying the fingers verbally. Significant asymmetry has been reported in children as young as 7 years (Bakker & Van der Kleij, 1978), and there is no evidence of age or sex differences in laterality on this task.

Equally straightforward conclusions may be drawn with respect to a task traditionally associated with the right hemisphere—judgment of spatial orientation. Brizzolara, De Nobili, and Ferretti (1982) required adults and 7-year-old children to palpate a small stick with the tip of the index finger and then determine, by touch, which stick from a set of 10 has an orientation in space that matches the orientation of the test stick. The test stick and the set of 10 sticks were always felt with the same hand. A significant left-hand superiority was found for both groups, and there was no significant difference between groups in the magnitude of the asymmetry.

Whereas the results for these presumably well-lateralized tasks are encouraging, the data are sparse. Moreover, the results for other unilateral tasks are less straightforward. Not only are findings inconsistent from one study to the next, but the findings often are complicated by age and sex differences, and by age × sex interactions. A good example of such complications can be found in the literature on the recognition of Braille or Braille-like characters by sighted children.

In the first of two studies in which Braille letters were used, Rudel and her colleagues (Rudel, Denckla, & Spalten, 1974) taught 80 right-handed children between the ages of 7 and 14 years to read six Braille letters with the left hand and a different set of six letters with the right hand. Children responded by naming each letter. The main effect for hand was not significant, but there was a significant age × hand interaction such that the youngest group showed a right-hand superiority and the oldest group a left-hand superiority. When boys' and girls' data were analyzed separately, it was found that boys showed a significant left-hand superiority, whereas girls showed a significant right-hand superiority. This sex difference, however, was not constant across age groups: Only the oldest two groups of boys and the youngest two groups of girls showed a substantial degree of asymmetry.

In a subsequent study by Rudel, Denckla, and Hirsch (1977), the naming task was replaced by a discrimination task in which children and adults were required to determine whether two adjacent Braille letters were the same or different. This study did yield an overall left-hand superiority, but there was also a significant age × hand interaction. Performance of the left hand surpassed that of the right hand only in children above the age of 11 years. Even though Rudel *et al.* (1977) concluded that left-hand superiority is attained earlier in boys than in girls, sex differences in their data are not impressive. Clearly, the striking sex differences found in the earlier study were absent in the 1977 study.

In an experiment by Wagner (cited in Harris, 1978), right-handed university students and three groups of right-handed children accomplished a Braille-reading task similar to that used by Rudel *et al.* (1974). Unlike Rudel *et al.* (1974), Wagner found a significant left-hand advantage for this task. Although post hoc analyses suggested that asymmetrical performance may emerge earlier in males than in females, the primary analysis yielded neither a significant main effect for sex nor significant interactions involving subjects' sex.

The inconsistent results for Braille reading may be attributable to the inherent mixing of spatial and verbal components and a consequent tendency of subjects to approach the task with complex or divergent strategies. If so, haptic tests of object recognition (stereognosis) might yield more orderly results insofar as there is greater latitude for varying the stimuli along a verbal–nonverbal dimension. The findings, however, are not encouraging. Yamamoto and Hatta (1982), for example, reported a significant left-hand superiority in 10-year-old girls and boys when they attempted to identify digit-shaped stimuli, and a significant right-hand advantage in girls when they attempted to identify common objects. Boys showed no significant asymmetry in the identification of objects. One might have expected that if there were to be different outcomes for the two different stimulus categories, it would be the digits, presumably the more linguistic of the two kinds of stimuli, that would yield a right-hand superiority. In a study requiring same–different judgments of random shapes (Cranney & Ashton, 1982), performance asymmetries depended on the age of subjects. Eight-year-olds showed a significant left-hand advantage but neither 6-year-olds nor adults showed any significant asymmetry. No sex differences were found.

Other studies of haptic object recognition have yielded diverse and often contradictory results. Yamamoto (1984), using a sequential matching task, found a left-hand advantage for 5- and 6-year-old boys but not for girls. Another study, in which children responded by pointing to a visual display, yielded a significant left-hand advantage in 12-year-olds but not in 6- or 8-year-olds (Yamamoto, 1980). Sex differences were not reported. Hatta, Yamamoto, Kawabata, and Tsutui (1981) found a similar developmental pattern of hand differences in their study of 8-, 10-, and 12-year-olds, but those findings were qualified by a sex × hand interaction reflecting an overall right-hand superiority for girls and a lack of significant asymmetry for boys.

Some of the most promising results from studies of haptic asymmetry were reported by Rose (1984, 1985), who modified the object identification paradigm for use by very young children. An object is placed into the child's hand for 25 seconds and shielded from his or her view by the experimenter's hands. If the child fails to palpate the object spontaneously, the experimenter moves the object about in the child's hand. Following this haptic exploration, the child is shown the palpated object along with a novel object, and an experimenter times the duration of the child's visual fixation on each object.

In the 1984 study it was found that children at all age levels—1, 2, and 3 years—looked significantly longer at the novel stimulus than at the palpated stimulus. Moreover, among the two older groups, the effect was significantly greater on left-hand trials than on right-hand trials. No left-hand superiority was evident among 1-year-olds. There were no significant sex differences. In the subsequent study, Rose (1985) found a significant left-hand superiority in children between the ages of 2 and 5 years. The magnitude of this asymmetry did not change across the four age levels. Again, there were no sex differences. Thus, despite the conflicting findings from studies of object recognition in older children, Rose has obtained a reproducible left-hand advantage for tactile processing in preschool children of both sexes.

STUDIES WITH BILATERAL STIMULATION

The most popular paradigm for studying asymmetries of stereognosis is Witelson's (1974, 1976) dichhaptic task, which entails simultaneous palpation of objects by the left and right hands. The subject places both hands through openings in a box and uses the index and middle fingers of each hand to explore two different stimuli for a specified period, usually 10 seconds. At the end of this period, the subject responds by pointing to the palpated shapes on a visual display or, in the case of namable stimuli, by reporting the stimuli orally.

In Witelson's (1974) initial dichhaptic experiment, 47 right-handed boys between the ages of 6 and 14 years felt nonsense shapes and letters during two sessions that took place over a 2- to 3-week interval. This procedure yielded a significant material × hand interaction reflecting a left-hand advantage for shapes and a right-hand advantage for letters. Post hoc tests showed, however, that the left-hand superiority for shapes was significant only for boys who were tested first with shapes (i.e., before being tested with letters) and that the right-hand superiority for letters was not significant.

Witelson (1976) subsequently administered the dichhaptic shapes test to 100 right-handed girls and 100 right-handed boys between the ages of 6 and 13 years and found a significant left-hand superiority for boys but not for girls. Even the youngest boys showed a significant degree of left-hand superiority. Witelson's findings are illustrated in Figure 5-3.

If Witelson's (1974, 1976) primary findings are characterized in general terms as (1) left-hand superiority for dichhaptic shapes and (2) later onset of asymmetric performance

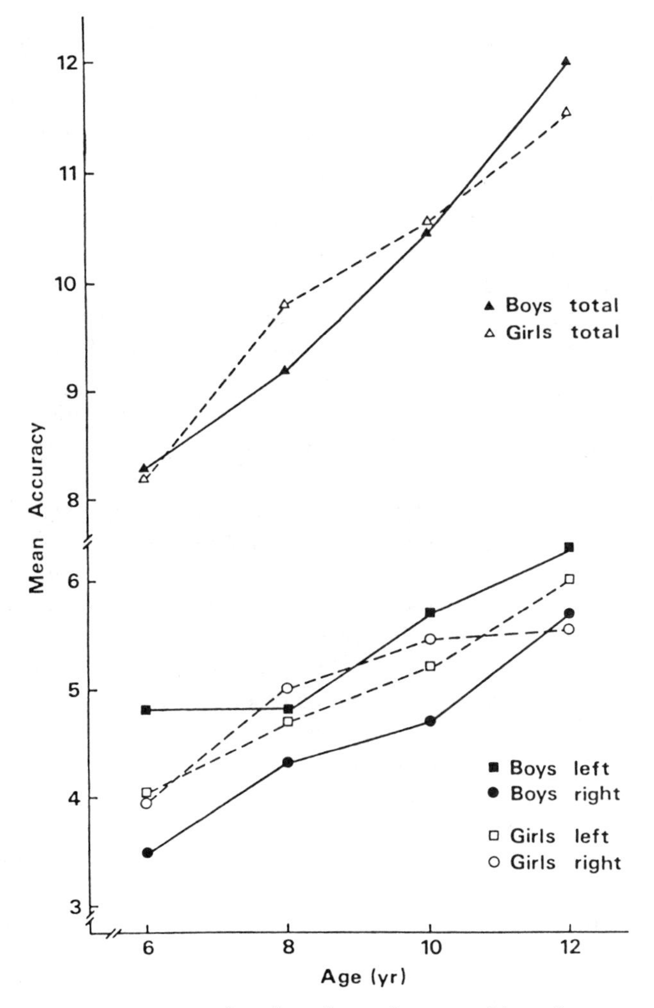

Figure 5-3. Mean accuracy scores, as a function of age, for recognition of nonsense shapes presented to the left and right hands on a dichhaptic stimulation test. Adapted by permission from "Sex and the Single Hemisphere: Right Hemisphere Specialization for Spatial Processing" by S. F. Witelson, 1976, *Science, 193,* p. 425.

in females than in males, then the former is much better supported than the latter by subsequent research. Although there are a few published failures to find a left-hand advantage for dichhaptically presented shapes (Cranney & Ashton, 1980; Hassler & Birbaumer, 1986; Vargha-Khadem, 1980), and one report of a significant right-hand advantage among adolescents (LaBreche, Manning, Goble, & Markman, 1977), the most common finding is that of an overall left-hand superiority that is invariant across subjects' age and sex (Cioffi & Kandel, 1979; Denes & Spinaci, 1981; Etaugh & Levy, 1981; Klein & Rosenfield, 1980; Posluzny & Barton, 1981). Even the lack of asymmetry reported by Vargha-Khadem (1980) is not too injurious to Witelson's claim insofar as there was a significant right-hand advantage for abstract three-letter nouns. In other words, the dissimilar outcomes for shapes and for words may be construed as being consistent with the assumption that the shapes task demands relatively more right-hemispheric resources. Of particular interest from a developmental perspective is Etaugh and Levy's (1981) report of a significant left-hand superiority in 4-year-old girls and boys.

Evidence that young girls and boys alike show left-hand superiority on the dichhaptic shapes test contradicts Witelson's claim about delayed lateralization of dichhaptic performance in girls. Other studies have yielded sex differences; but, even when sex differences are observed, they are seldom consistent across studies. For example, Affleck and Joyce (1979) found a significant left-hand superiority among boys but not girls at the age of 5 years, and Dawson (1981) found that males at each of three age levels from Grade 1 to university were more accurate than females with the left hand but not with the right. In contrast, Flanery and Balling (1979) failed to find a sex difference in any of three groups of children but found instead that adult males showed a stronger left-hand advantage than did adult females. Posluszny and Barton (1981) reported that 10-year-old boys outperformed 10-year-old girls on a shapes task (but not a dichhaptic words test) irrespective of the hand being tested. Thus, there was a sex difference in overall performance but not in laterality.

Gibson and Bryden (1983), recognizing the diversity of outcomes in the dichhaptic literature, speculated that some of the inconsistency might be attributable to the long (10-second) duration of stimulus presentation, as well as the lack of control over the order in which subjects report left- and right-hand stimuli. These characteristics presumably make the paradigm susceptible to influence by factors other than hemispheric specialization. In an attempt to minimize these influences, Gibson and Bryden (1983) shortened the presentation duration to 2 seconds and constrained the order in which left- and right-hand stimuli were to be reported. In applying this modified dichhaptic procedure to 80 right-handed children between the ages of 8 and 14 years, the authors obtained a significant left-hand advantage for shapes and no significant asymmetry for letters. There was a sex difference such that boys showed the greater left-hand advantage, but this difference applied equally to the verbal and nonverbal tasks. Moreover, degree of asymmetry varied as a nonmonotonic function of age. A significant asymmetry was found in 8- and 12-year-olds but not in 10- and 14-year-olds. At least some of the sex and age effects could be ascribed to the anomalous performance of 10-year-old girls, who tended to show a right-hand advantage irrespective of the stimulus material.

In a subsequent study (Gibson & Bryden, 1984), the same modified dichhaptic task was administered to 20 normal, right-handed 11-year-olds. In this study, the authors again obtained not only the expected hand × material interaction but also a significant hand × sex interaction that reflected greater left-hand superiority in males irrespective of the stimuli. Thus, the dichhaptic procedure as modified by Gibson and Bryden appears to yield a significant left-hand advantage for shapes, no significant hand difference for letters, and a sex difference such that males show a larger left-greater-than-right disparity for both shapes and letters. As Gibson and Bryden (1983) point out, a sex difference of this nature may reflect a peripheral factor such as differential sensitivity of the right hand, perhaps due to greater callosity in boys.

CONCLUSIONS

When the entire corpus of tactile laterality evidence—evidence concerning sensitivity as well as unimanual and dichhaptic perception—is considered, only a few conclusions seem to be warranted. The first and most fundamental of these is that asymmetries favoring the left side of the body occur frequently. One can only speculate as to whether many of these asymmetries reflect primarily sensory processes, in which case peripheral factors may underlie the asymmetry, or higher level perceptual and cognitive functions, in which case hemispheric specialization may be responsible for the asymmetrical performance.

A second important conclusion is that different laterality patterns are often obtained with verbal and with nonverbal stimuli. Even if the result is only that of asymmetrical performance with one category of material and symmetrical performance with another, a hand × material interaction shows that laterality is material-specific and thus unlikely to be entirely dependent on asymmetrical sensitivity.

Finally, it is clear from several studies, especially those of Rose (1984, 1985), that tactile asymmetries may be seen in young children of both sexes. When age or sex differences are found, it is often the youngest children or the females who do not show the expected left-hand advantage. Nonetheless, the sex and age differences reported thus far are too sporadic and too variable to nullify the evidence in favor of early asymmetry in both girls and boys.

Studies of Concurrent-Task Interference

Each of the three experimental paradigms discussed previously entails measuring an asymmetry of perception. Despite the proven usefulness of these paradigms, there are—in principle as well as in application—certain limitations in using perceptual (input) asymmetry as an index of hemispheric specialization. Some of these limitations may be avoided by using a laterality paradigm based on motor (output) performance.

One potential advantage of studying motor performance lies in the relatively overt nature of motor activity. Whereas perceptual asymmetries are often subject to covert influences such as attentional biases, scanning habits, and response biases, the various components of motor asymmetry usually are more easily observed. Finger tapping speed, for example, may be analyzed not only in terms of overall rate but also in terms of the velocity of upstroke and downstroke and the quickness with which the direction of movement can be reversed (see Peters, 1980). Other factors, such as fatigue effects and force modulation, are subject to measurement as well.

Motor tasks are also advantageous insofar as output processes are more distinctly lateralized than input processes (LeDoux, Wilson, & Gazzaniga, 1977; Searleman, 1977; Zaidel, 1978). Especially when the research question concerns the lateralization of language, the availability of a task based on speech output is useful. Even if motor tests of laterality should prove to be as problematic as perceptual tests, the motor tasks can nonetheless provide converging evidence of lateralized processing. In other words, it is not necessary that a motor task be superior to perceptual tasks, but only that it serve as an independent source of evidence.

Concurrent-task methods have a well-established history in human factors research and, more recently, in cognitive psychology (see Kahneman, 1973; Kinsbourne, 1981; Posner, 1982). The first application of concurrent-task methods to laterality research was an experiment by Kinsbourne and Cook (1971) in which 20 right-handed adults attempted to balance a dowel rod on their index finger while continuously reciting a sentence. Vocalization disrupted right-hand balancing but enhanced balancing with the left hand. This outcome was attributed to a combination of two effects: bilateral enhancement of manual performance due to distraction, and selective impairment of right-hand performance due to "hemisphere sharing," that is, to interference in the left hemisphere between speaking and right-hand balancing.

As additional data accumulated (e.g., Hicks, 1975) it became clear that speaking does not usually enhance the concurrent performance of either hand. Speaking usually disrupts concurrent manual performance but does so asymmetrically; that is, performance of the right hand is degraded more than that of the left. This asymmetrical pattern of interference generally occurs in right-handers but not in left-handers (Hicks, 1975; Lomas & Kimura, 1976; Sussman, 1982) and is found with an assortment of verbal tasks but seldom with nonverbal tasks (Dalby, 1980; Hellige & Longstreth, 1981; McFarland & Ashton, 1978a, 1978b, 1978c). Nonverbal tasks either interfere with the left hand more than with the right or else interfere about equally with both hands.

The data from adults, then, support Kinsbourne and Cook's (1971) initial impression that asymmetrical interference reflects a difference between intra- and interhemispheric sharing of capacity. The precise mechanism underlying the asymmetry, however, is a matter of considerable dispute. Kinsbourne and Hicks (1978) have suggested that the difference between intrahemispheric and interhemispheric interference illustrates a general principle of "functional cerebral distance." According to this view, there is a gradient of neural connectivity such that some pairs of brain loci are highly connected whereas others are relatively independent. Functional distance does not necessarily correspond to anatomical distance. Nevertheless, a particular site tends to be more highly interconnected with other loci in the same hemisphere than with corresponding (homologous) loci in the opposite hemisphere. Consequently, if two concurrent activities are inherently incompatible, the interference between them will be heightened when both are controlled by sites within the same cerebral hemisphere.

Friedman and Polson (1981) view the left and right hemispheres not as territories within a highly interconnected network, but as two discrete processing systems or "pools of resources." According to their model, neither the left nor the right hemisphere can be selectively activated, nor can the resources of one hemisphere be accessed by the other hemisphere. Asymmetrical interference in concurrent-task situations depends on the degree to which subjects draw on the resources of one hemisphere for the performance of both tasks. Another explanation for concurrent-task asymmetries was put forth by Lomas (1980; Lomas & Kimura, 1976), who argued that lateralized interference between speaking and manual activity depends on competition within the left hemisphere for a specific processing capacity—the capacity for controlling rapid, sequential repositioning of muscles in the absence of visual guidance.

Theoretical controversies notwithstanding, the concurrent-task method has been applied to normal children of different ages in an attempt to detect developmental changes in the pattern of left- and right-hand interference (see Table 5-4). For expository purposes these studies are dichotomized into those that entail motor–motor interference (usually interference between speaking and simultaneous manual activity) and those that entail cognitive–motor interference.

STUDIES OF MOTOR–MOTOR INTERFERENCE

Concurrent-task procedures have been readily adapted for children by simplifying both of the conjoined tasks. For example, young children can speak and perform a manual task simultaneously provided that the material to be recited consists of nursery rhymes, short word lists, or the like, and provided that the manual task involves repetitive tapping with the index finger. The vocal–manual interference paradigm, thus modified, has been used to address three main questions: Does speaking disrupt children's manual performance in the same asymmetrical manner as in adults? If so, what is the youngest age at which the asymmetry can be shown? Does the asymmetry of interference become greater with increasing age?

Answers to these questions have been remarkably consistent across studies. Kinsbourne and McMurray (1975), upon testing 48 kindergarten students, found that recitation of nursery rhymes and animal names slowed concurrent right-hand tapping more than left-hand tapping. Piazza (1977) duplicated this finding with right-handed 3-, 4-, and 5-year-olds. The magnitude of the asymmetry did not vary significantly across Piazza's three age groups. Moreover, the opposite pattern of interference was obtained when humming was substituted for reciting; that is, humming disrupted left-hand tapping more than it did right-hand tapping. Hiscock and Kinsbourne (1978) found a significant right-greater-than-left asymmetry of interference when children between the ages of 3 and 12 years performed concurrent recitation and finger tapping. Although there was a linear decline in overall interference with increasing age, the asymmetry remained constant across this broad age range. These findings are illustrated in Figure 5-4. Most other findings have been consistent with these early results (Dalby & Gibson, 1981; Hiscock, Antoniuk, Prisciak, & von Hessert, 1985; Hiscock & Kinsbourne, 1980b; Hiscock, Kinsbourne, Samuels, & Krause, 1987; Marcotte & LaBarba, 1985; Obrzut, Hynd, Obrzut, & Leitgeb, 1980; White & Kinsbourne, 1980; Willis & Hynd, 1987).

In these studies the expected asymmetry was found in the youngest children tested and, although overall interference usually diminished with increasing age, the degree of asymmetry did not change significantly. In only one instance did speaking fail to disrupt asymmetrically the manual performance of normal children (Hughes & Sussman, 1983), and this negative finding was based on a sample of only 12 children. There were three studies in which a significant age-related change in asymmetry was found, but the degree

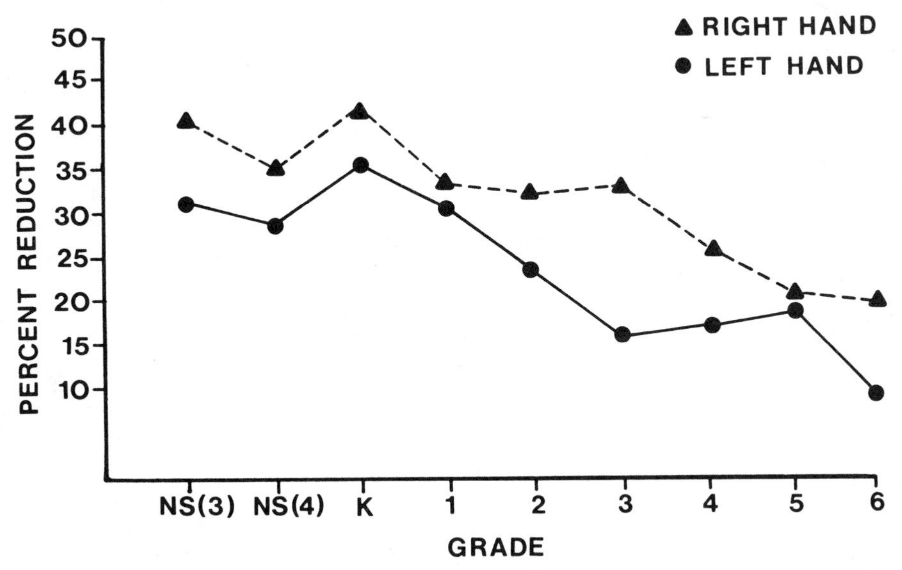

Figure 5-4. Mean reduction in right-hand and left-hand tapping rate, relative to the control conditions, when the concurrent task was recitation of a nursery rhyme. Reprinted by permission from "Ontogeny of Cerebral Dominance: Evidence from Time-Sharing Asymmetry in Children" by M. Hiscock and M. Kinsbourne, 1978, *Developmental Psychology, 14,* p. 324. Copyright © 1978 by the American Psychological Association.

Table 5-4. Summary of Concurrent-Task Studies

Study	Subjects	Manual Task	Concurrent Task	Results
McFarland & Ashton, 1975	16 right-handed B & G, aged 9, 10, 11, & 12 years	Pressing a button switch with one finger	Spatial task: Finding hidden figures Verbal task: Reading a section of a book Spatial–verbal control: Finding the missing letters from a spatially random alphabetic array	Two dependent measures: (1) mean intertap interval and (2) intertap variance (1) Mean intertap interval: Spatial task caused a decrement in LH performance, relative to no-activity control condition. Verbal task caused a decrement in RH performance, relative to no-activity control condition. (2) Intertap variance: Spatial task caused an increase in intertap variance for the LH. Verbal task caused an increase in intertap variance for the RH.
Kinsbourne & McMurray, 1975	48 B & G, aged 5.7 years (7 left-handers)	Speeded tapping of the index finger on a table top	Reciting a nursery rhyme Reciting four animal names	Both concurrent tasks caused a bilateral decrease in tapping rate. This effect was greater for the RH than for the LH.
Piazza, 1977	36 right-handed B & G, aged 3, 4, and 5 years	Speeded tapping of the index finger	Verbal: Reciting a familiar rhyme Nonverbal: Humming	RH tapping was slowed more than LH tapping by recitation. LH tapping was slowed more than RH tapping by humming. No developmental change in the asymmetry of interference
Cermak, Cermak, Drake, & Kenney, 1978	14 right-handed boys, aged 10.7 years Control group for a study of LD children	Speeded alternate tapping of a stylus on two metal plates	A dichotic listening task in which each S listened to 3 pairs of digit names and then immediately attempted to recall as many as possible. Tapping continued throughout both stimulus presentation and recall.	Both RH and LH tapping had no effect on subsequent recall from either RE or LE.
Hiscock & Kinsbourne, 1978	155 right-handed B & G, aged 3–12 years	Speeded tapping on a telegraph key using the index finger	Reciting a nursery rhyme Reciting 4 animal names	Both recitation tasks caused a greater decrement in RH tapping than in LH tapping. No developmental change in the asymmetry of interference, and the percentage of Ss showing asymmetric

				effects did not change across age levels.
Obrzut, Hynd, Obrzut, & Leitgeb, 1980	48 right-handed B & G, aged 8.0, 9.4, & 11.0 years Control group for a study of LD children	Speeded tapping on a telegraph key using the index finger	Reciting animal names	Recitation caused a greater decrement in RH than in LH tapping rate. No developmental change in the asymmetry of interference
White & Kinsbourne, 1980	105 right-handed B & G, aged 3.5–12.5 years	Speeded tapping on a metal key using the index finger	Verbal tasks: Reciting a nursery rhyme and as many animal names as possible Spatial task: Encoding nonsense shapes for subsequent recognition	For the verbal tasks the reduction in tapping rate in the dual-task condition was greater for the RH than the LH. 66% and 78% of the children showed this lateralized effect for the rhyme and animal naming tasks, respectively. For the rhyme task children produced more words during LH tapping than during RH tapping. For the spatial task the decrease in concurrent tapping rate was equivalent for the RH and LH. No developmental change in the asymmetry of interference
Hiscock & Kinsbourne, 1980b	155 right-handed B & G, aged 3–12 years. A subset of this sample (N = 115) was tested twice with 1 year intervening.	Speeded tapping on a telegraph key using the index finger	Reciting a nursery rhyme Reciting 4 animal names	(1) Cross-sectional findings: Recitation of the nursery rhyme caused a greater decrement in RH than LH tapping rate for boys but not for girls. Recitation of animal names caused a greater decrement in RH than LH tapping irrespective of sex. No developmental change in the asymmetry of interference (2) Longitudinal findings: No developmental change in the asymmetry of interference
Dalby & Gibson, 1981	15 boys aged 9–12 years Control group for a study of LD children	Alternate tapping of the first and second fingers on two adjacent keys on an electric typewriter	Verbal task: Reciting 4 animal names Spatial task: Solving problems from Ravens Progressive Matrices	Recitation caused a greater decrement in RH than in LH tapping rate. The spatial task caused a greater decrement in LH than in RH tapping rate.
Ashton & Beasley, 1982	20 right-handed B & G, aged 5–6 and 11–12 years Control group for a study	Speeded tapping, alternating between two buttons	Verbal task 1: Repeating a CV syllable. Verbal task 2: Repeating	RH tapping was slowed more than LH tapping with concurrent verbal tasks, but only for the 11–12 year-

(*continued*)

Table 5-4 *(continued)*

Study	Subjects	Manual Tasks	Concurrent Task	Results
	with deaf children		words ("dog-cat"). Nonverbal task: Finding hidden figures.	olds. Verbal task 2 produced greater interference than Verbal task 1. No asymmetric interference was produced by the nonverbal task.
Hiscock, 1982	86 right-handed B & G, aged 8.8, 9.9, & 11.1 years	Alternate tapping of two telegraph keys with the index finger. Task emphasis (emphasis on either the verbal or manual task) was manipulated within subjects.	Recitation of a tongue twister	Reciting the tongue twister caused a greater decrement in RH than in LH tapping rate. 85.5% of the children showed this asymmetry. The magnitude of asymmetry increased linearly with age.
Hughes & Sussman, 1983	12 right-handed children, aged 5.5 years. Control group for a study of language-disordered children	Speeded repetitive tapping on a metal disk	Verbal task 1: Describing a story or the events taking place in a set of pictures. Verbal task 2: Retelling a story using a set of picture cards as a visual aid. Nonverbal task: Making car noises	Both verbal tasks disrupted tapping more than the nonverbal task. Decrements in tapping rate during the verbal tasks were bilateral. During verbal task 1 the number of syllables produced during RH and LH tapping was equal. During verbal task 2 fewer syllables were produced during RH than LH tapping.
Marcotte & La-Barba, 1985	30 right-handed children aged 3–4, 5–6, & 13–14 years. Control group for a study of deaf children	Speeded tapping of a telegraph key with the index finger	Verbal task 1: Repeating a CV syllable. Verbal task 2: Reciting a list of animal names. Verbal task 3: Reciting a sentence	RH tapping was disrupted by all verbal tasks across all age groups. LH tapping was disrupted only for task 2 in the 3- to 4-year-old group. No developmental change in the asymmetry of interference
Hiscock, Kinsbourne, Samuels, & Krause, 1985	73 right-handed B & G, aged 6.7, 7.9, 8.8, & 10.0 years	Speeded tapping of a telegraph key with the index finger	Reciting a nursery rhyme	Dependent variables were percentage reduction in tapping rate relative to baseline and percentage change in variability (as measured by the coefficient of variation). Rate and variability were calculated using raw (unrestricted) data and data with intervals greater than 500 msec removed (restricted data). Rate: RH tapping was disrupted to a greater degree than LH tapping for both the restricted and unrestricted data.

Study	Subjects	Tapping task	Concurrent task	Results
				Variability: For the unrestricted data there was a greater increase in variability for the RH than for the LH for the youngest age group. When intervals greater than 500 msec were removed, there were no asymmetrical effects of talking on tapping across all grade levels. No developmental change in the asymmetry of interference
Hiscock, Antoniuk, Prisciak, & von Hessert, 1985	Expt. 1: 55 right-handed boys in G2–G5. Four groups: Younger good readers, younger poor readers, older good readers, older poor readers	Speeded tapping of a key with the index finger	Task 1: Reading a list of words aloud. Task 2: Reciting a tongue twister	Concurrent reading caused a greater RH than LH tapping rate decrement. This asymmetry was greater in poor readers. Concurrent reciting caused a greater decrement in RH than in LH tapping rate in both groups. No developmental change in the asymmetry of interference
	Expt. 2: 64 right-handed B & G in G2–G5	Same as Expt. 1	Spatial task: Encoding and recognizing the orientation of a line segment Verbal task: Silent reading	Encoding: No overall asymmetry of interference. Girls showed greater LH interference than did boys. Silent reading disrupted RH more than LH tapping. No developmental change in the asymmetry of interference
	Expt. 3: 64 right-handed children in G2–G5	Alternate tapping of two keys with the index finger	Spatial task: Same as Expt. 2 except that performance was self-paced to allow more than one trial of the line orientation task within each tapping trial	No overall asymmetry of interference. Girls showed no significant difference between LH and RH interference, but boys showed more RH than LH interference. For G2 children, performance on the line-orientation task was better with RH tapping than with LH tapping. No developmental change in the asymmetry of interference

Abbreviations: B & G (boys and girls); CCC (consonant trigram); CV (consonant–vowel syllable); CVC (consonant–vowel–consonant word); EA (ear advantage); Expt. (experiment); G (grade); L (left); R (right); LD (learning-disabled); LE (left ear); RE (right ear); LEA (left-ear advantage); REA (right-ear advantage); LEM (left-ear monitoring); REM (right-ear monitoring); LH (left hand); RH (right hand); LVF (left visual half-field); RVF (right visual half-field); RT (reaction time); S (subject); SEL (socioeconomic level); VF or VHF (visual half-field).

of asymmetry increased with age in two studies (Ashton & Beasley, 1982; Hiscock, 1982) and decreased in the other study (Hiscock, Kinsbourne, Samuels, & Krause, 1985). Consequently, there is no compelling reason to reject the conclusion that asymmetries of vocal–manual interference are invariant across the childhood years.

The evidence from studies of vocal–manual interference in children is not without problematic characteristics. The paradigm has been criticized because it tends to yield asymmetrical but bilateral interference effects in children rather than the largely unilateral effects often obtained with adults (Hughes & Sussman, 1983). In other words, speaking typically affects both left- and right-hand performance in children (even though the left hand is affected to a significantly lesser degree), whereas speaking tends to have a significant effect on adults' right-hand performance and little or no effect on their left-hand performance. The generality of this age difference, as well as its importance, are matters of dispute (cf. Kee, 1984; Sussman, 1984). Quite possibly the apparent difference between outcomes for children and for adults merely reflects differential capacity for performing the concurrent activities. When a pair of conjoined tasks is made sufficiently difficult for adults (e.g., Hicks, Provenzano, & Rybstein, 1975), the pattern of interference may resemble that usually found in children. Whatever the correct explanation, differences between adult and child interference patterns probably reflect factors other than speech lateralization (Sussman, 1984).

Another seeming anomaly is the unidirectionality of interference asymmetries. Speaking interferes asymmetrically with manual activity, but the manual activity has approximately the same effect on speaking irrespective of the hand used to perform the manual activity. Although this property of vocal–manual interference is not restricted to studies of children, it is better documented in studies of children than in studies of adults. Hiscock (1982) hypothesized that the absence of lateralized interference in the "opposite" direction (i.e., from manual activity to speaking) is attributable to subjects' tendency to protect their performance on the speech task. It was reasoned that, if there is little or no interference in that direction, then there can be little or no lateralization of interference. Data from Hiscock's (1982) study, however, failed to support the hypothesis. Even when task emphasis was altered so that children protected their tapping performance at the expense of speaking accuracy, the interfering effect of left-hand tapping on speaking was comparable to that of right-hand tapping. At present, the lack of reciprocal interference effects in the vocal–manual time-sharing paradigm remains enigmatic.

A third problem is the lack of a suitable nonverbal control task against which the unique effects of speaking can be identified. As noted previously, Piazza (1977) reported that humming interfered to a greater degree with concurrent left-hand performance than with right-hand performance. Although nonverbal vocalization, such as humming, might seem to be the ideal nonverbal counterpart to speaking, studies of adults consistently have failed to show that such tasks interfere more with left-hand performance than with right-hand performance (Kinsbourne & Hiscock, 1983a).

Without a suitable control for nonspecific effects, it is always possible that the asymmetry of interference between speaking and manual performance in right-handers is an artifact of the disparity between hands in the control condition. Left-hand performance, being relatively poor in the control condition, might be less susceptible than right-hand performance to further degradation in the concurrent-task condition. This possibility is supported by recent reports of reversed asymmetry of interference in left-handed adults (Orsini, Satz, Soper, & Light, 1985; Simon & Sussman, 1987). It has been suggested by Orsini *et al.* and by Simon and Sussman that the pattern of concurrent-task interference may be determined more by hand dominance than by speech lateralization.

Using a proportional rather than an absolute measure of change from single-task to dual-task performance often will eliminate range effects, making the measure of interference independent of performance in the control condition (Hiscock, 1982; Hiscock & Kinsbourne, 1978). The adequacy of this precaution can be assessed via regression analysis. An even more convincing argument against range artifacts is a crossover interaction such that right-hand performance exceeds left-hand performance in the single-task (control) condition, and left-hand performance exceeds right-hand performance in the dual-task condition (Kinsbourne & McMurray, 1975; Piazza, 1977). This outcome, though ruling out statistical artifacts, would not preclude the possibility that the opposite asymmetry of interference might be found in left-handers.

STUDIES OF COGNITIVE–MOTOR INTERFERENCE

The distinction between motor–motor interference and cognitive–motor interference is somewhat arbitrary. Recitation tasks have been classified as motor tasks even though there is a memory component; conversely, many of the cognitive tasks to be described in this section involve a substantial motor component. One of the most difficult tasks to classify is oral reading, which represents a complex combination of cognitive and motor activity. The so-called cognitive tasks, irrespective of motor involvement, extend the concurrent-task paradigm to various functions other than vocalization and thus greatly enhance the usefulness of the method for investigating children's hemispheric specialization.

In the first of the cognitive–motor studies, McFarland and Ashton (1975) required right-handed children to tap a button switch repetitively while performing each of three cognitive tasks: finding hidden figures, reading, and finding missing letters from an array. The three cognitive activities were defined as being spatial, verbal, and spatial–verbal, respectively. If one disregards the spatial–verbal condition and compares tapping in the other two dual-task conditions with tapping in a single-task control condition, then the results are straightforward. Performing the hidden-figures task reduced the speed and increased the variability of left-hand performance but had no significant effect on the right hand. Reading reduced the speed and increased the variability of right-hand performance but had no effect on the left hand. It appears that task-specific laterality was more pronounced in the youngest children (9-year-olds) than in the three older groups, but the small size of the sample limits one's ability to draw conclusions about the generality of this developmental pattern.

Results obtained by Dalby and Gibson (1981) support McFarland and Ashton's (1975) finding that performing a nonverbal task disrupts concurrent left-hand activity more than that of the right hand. More specifically, Dalby and Gibson (1981) found that solving problems from Raven's matrices test reduced left-hand tapping speed to a greater degree than right-hand tapping speed in 15 normal right-handed boys between the ages of 9 and 12 years. The verbal task, recitation of animal names, yielded the usual asymmetry; that is, the right-hand was slowed more than the left.

Even though other studies have not always shown left-greater-than-right interference for putatively nonverbal tasks, the interference pattern usually differs from that found when verbal tasks are performed. For example, White and Kinsbourne (1980), in their study of normal right-handed children between the ages of 3 and 12 years, found that encoding nonsense shapes generated only bilateral interference with concurrent finger tapping. In contrast, vocalization reduced right-hand tapping more than left-hand tapping. In two experiments described by Hiscock, Antoniuk, Prisciak, and von Hessert (1985), judging the orientation of line segments disrupted children's left- and right-hand finger tapping in comparable degrees. However, there was an unexpected sex difference underlying this result. In boys the interference was greater in the right hand than in the left, but girls showed a nonsignificant trend in the opposite direction. This sex difference was taken as evidence that factors such as strategy and skill level may influence the pattern of interference observed in concurrent-task studies involving cognitive activity. Strategy effects also seem to be implicated in the results of Willis and Hynd (1987), who found that interference patterns varied not only according to the modality of the cognitive task (i.e., auditory–vocal versus visual–motor) but also according to the demand for either successive or simultaneous processing.

The available concurrent-task evidence regarding the processing of faces is difficult to interpret. The two studies of face processing in adults, perhaps because the respective methods were dissimilar, yielded somewhat dissimilar results. McFarland and Ashton (1978c) found that performing a running memory-span task with faces as stimuli interfered to a greater degree with left-hand than with right-hand performance, but Bowers, Heilman, Satz, and Altman (1978) found that encoding faces slowed left- and right-hand performance by comparable amounts. The dissimilarity of these findings notwithstanding, both suggest that face encoding involves the right hemisphere to the extent that concurrent left-hand performance is disrupted at least as much as right-hand performance. In two studies of children, however, face encoding disrupted concurrent right-hand tapping more than left-hand tapping (Hiscock, Prisciak, & Antoniuk, 1983; Hiscock, *et al.*, 1987).

There are several possible explanations for the diversity of outcomes represented in this meager literature on face processing. Perhaps the different outcomes can be attributed to stimulus and task factors. More specifically, it has been suggested that face encoding takes place in the left hemisphere under certain conditions—for example when each face is studied for a lengthy duration or when the faces are difficult to discriminate (Sergent, 1982, 1984). Alternatively, there may be a true laterality difference between children and adults. Such a difference could stem from differential strategy for processing faces (Carey & Diamond, 1977; Carey *et al.*, 1980), or it could reflect an age-related difference in the cerebral representation of physiognomic information.

The concurrent-task paradigm provides a means for studying the lateralization of reading in a fairly naturalistic context. Hiscock, Antoniuk, Prisciak, and von Hessert (1985) reported that, irrespective of whether normal children read words aloud or silently, the reading slows simultaneous right-hand finger tapping more than left-hand tapping. The overall level of interference is much greater with oral reading than with silent reading, which indicates that motor–motor interference accounts for much of the disruptive effect of reading on concurrent finger tapping. However, the lower level of interference found in the silent reading condition—the interference that presumably is attributable to cognitive factors alone—is significantly lateralized.

Hiscock, Antoniuk, Prisciak, and von Hessert (1985) reported that relatively poor readers show significantly greater asymmetry of interference than do better readers. This finding was supported by Crossley and Hiscock (1987), who used regression analyses to show that reading achievement scores predict the amount of right-hand but not of left-hand interference in the concurrent-task situation. Lower reading scores were associated with greater interference from reading to right-hand finger tapping. These individual differences are consistent with the assumption that readers, irrespective of skill level, draw on resources of the left hemisphere for reading, but that the demand for resources is higher in less skilled readers, who consequently have fewer surplus resources to control simultaneous manual activity with the right hand.

Substituting cognitive tasks for speech tasks makes the matching of verbal and nonverbal tasks seem more plausible, but the goal of achieving a perfect match is probably unrealistic. Consider the study by Hiscock *et al.* (1987) in which children performed finger tapping while encoding numbers or faces for subsequent recognition. It was found that, even though numbers are more readily recognized than faces, the encoding of numbers is more disruptive of concurrent tapping. Apparently there is some characteristic of number encoding—perhaps rehearsal at a subvocal level—that is not present in face encoding, and this characteristic tends to disrupt concurrent finger tapping. Thus, even two tasks that appear to be very similar may involve components that are quite dissimilar and consequently may have quite dissimilar effects on concurrent manual performance. When there is no attempt to match the verbal and nonverbal tasks, any difference between tasks in the amount or pattern of interference generated may be attributable to factors other than hemispheric specialization, for example, floor or ceiling effects.

Another important issue in concurrent-task research is the selection of an appropriate criterion for assessing manual performance. As noted previously, Lomas and Kimura (1976) and Lomas (1980) argued that the manual task should require rapid repositioning of the hand in the absence of visual guidance. According to this argument, sequential tapping of different keys would be a more appropriate measure than would repetitive tapping of a single key. The evidence suggests otherwise, however, for several concurrent-task studies, especially those with children as subjects, have yielded highly asymmetric interference effects with repetitive tapping rate as the dependent variable.

Most investigators have measured manual performance in terms of tapping rate, but some have also examined the variability of tapping performance. Recently Kee, Morris, Bathurst, and Hellige (1986) reported that, in a task involving alternate tapping of two keys by adults, the expected asymmetry of interference materialized when tapping variability was analyzed, but not when tapping rate was analyzed. Under other circumstances, however, tapping rate appears to be the more sensitive index of lateralized interference (Hiscock, Kinsbourne, Samuels, & Krause, 1985). Moreover, there is some reason to believe that rate and variability reflect different mechanisms of intertask interference (Hiscock & Chipuer, 1986). If this issue is to be resolved, investigators must consider not only the kind of finger movement required (repetitive, alternating, or sequential tapping) but also the instructions given to subjects—that is, whether subjects are told to tap as rapidly as possible, to tap as regularly as possible, or to meet some other performance criterion.

CONCLUSIONS

When speaking is conjoined with finger tapping, right-handed children show a stronger interference effect on the right side than on the left. Asymmetric interference has been observed in 3-year-olds and, although the degree of overall interference tends to decrease with increasing age, the magnitude of the asymmetry usually remains constant. If speaking is replaced by a verbal activity without overt motor components, the overall disruption of manual activity usually is less marked, but the interference nevertheless tends to be lateralized. Various nonverbal tasks produce either the opposite asymmetry of interference or symmetric interference.

These findings from the concurrent-task paradigm parallel findings from dichotic listening studies with children. With both methods, an asymmetry is readily elicited using verbal material, but the opposite asymmetry is obtained only sporadically with nonverbal material. Both methods yield early asymmetries that do not appear to grow larger with increasing age. For both methods, the question of how to obtain the predicted asymmetry seems less salient than the question of how to interpret the asymmetries that occur quite regularly. As in the case of dichotic listening, correct interpretation of concurrent-task data depends on one's understanding of the underlying mechanisms. What is the performance-limiting factor that causes interference between two tasks? Why is interference often lateralized in only one direction, that is, in the nonmanual to manual direction? How does the concurrent-task performance of left-handers differ from the performance of right-handers, and what are the implications of that difference for understanding interference asymmetries in right-handers?

Depending on the answers to questions like these, the concurrent-task method may become an increasingly important source of information about children's hemispheric specialization. The method can provide information about the lateralization of speech output and can be used to study a variety of other phenomena. Its methodological and conceptual complexity, however, probably is sufficient to preclude rapid gains.

GENERAL PROBLEMS

In the preceding review of laterality studies with normal children, certain shortcomings were noted. These include lacunae and contradictions in the evidence as well as methodological problems inherent in each of the four paradigms chosen for examination. A comprehensive methodological critique of the four paradigms is not only beyond the scope of the present chapter but, indeed, beyond the scope of any work of manageable proportion. An entire issue of *Brain and Cognition* has been devoted to tachistoscopic methodology alone and even this treatment, according to the guest editor's own assessment, "is restricted in its scope and addresses only a small portion of the problems inherent in visual laterality studies" (Sergent, 1986, p. 130).

It would be misleading to claim that the methodological problems of child laterality studies are adequately explicated in the present chapter. There is, however, an advantage in surveying in one chapter the literature from several different paradigms. From this broader perspective one may more readily appreciate problems that stem not from the unique characteristics of one technique or modality, but from more general characteristics that are shared by different paradigms. Thus, without minimizing the importance of the more specific methodological problems, it is worthwhile to identify some of the broader problems in laterality research and, whenever possible, to propose some solutions to those problems.

The broad problems have been classified as (1) failure to acquire the necessary experimental control over laterality phenomena and (2) measurement problems. Each of these categories will be discussed in turn.

Inadequate Experimental Control

That behavioral asymmetry may be influenced by factors other than hemispheric specialization is hardly a novel idea. Recall that early investigators of tachistoscopic perception preferred to explain asymmetric performance in terms of habitual scanning habits (e.g., Forgays, 1953). Kinsbourne (1975) listed several attributes of the child and of the situation that might contribute to ear asymmetry or lack of asymmetry in a dichotic listening task—for example, the child's motivational level, the child's orientation toward the right or left side of space, and whether the stimulus material is construed as being verbal or nonverbal. Kinsbourne (1975) suggested that even "such ostensibly trivial matters as asymmetry of furnishings in the experimental room or as the experimenter standing to one side might bias the results in various directions" (p. 212).

Variables like these are of special interest within Kinsbourne's (1970) theoretical framework insofar as they relate to the relative activation of the left and right hemispheres and to the child's distribution of attention to the left and right ears. However, Bryden (1978, 1982a, 1982b) also has pointed out the importance of variables other than hemispheric specialization:

> In any measure of perceptual asymmetry, there is a certain amount of variability. Some of this variability is associated with hemispheric asymmetry, some with other factors—simply because we are dealing with an active, plotting, scheming organism. If we are to develop good measures of cerebral asymmetry using noninvasive techniques, we must attempt to maximize the variability associated with cerebral organization, and to minimize that associated with other factors. To do this, we must have a full and complete understanding of how subjects perform on the tasks we employ to measure laterality. (Bryden, 1982a, pp. 44–45)

Whether one views nonstructural factors as being intrinsic to the laterality phenomena under study (Kinsbourne, 1970) or as entirely extrinsic sources of variability (Bryden, 1982a), it is essential that these factors be examined carefully. Only by manipulating these variables within experiments will researchers be able to assess their contribution to performance asymmetries. Then, depending on the results of such experiments, investigators will be able to incorporate the nonstructural factors into more comprehensive models of laterality, or else to control these variables so that "pure" physiological asymmetries can be measured in isolation.

Some of the variables that influence laterality are undeniably extraneous, but the influence of those variables may be minimized through careful experimental design. For example, acquisition and fatigue effects may distort laterality estimates in any paradigm that entails measuring left- and right-sided performance sequentially. Such artifacts often can be minimized by counterbalancing the order in which the left and right sides are tested. Acoustic disparities between left- and right-ear channels in dichotic listening are sometimes difficult to eliminate, but the effects may be nullified by reversing the subject's earphones midway through the test.

The more interesting variables are factors such as processing strategies and attentional biases whose action may be inferred from certain between-group differences in laterality, as well as certain experimental outcomes that are not readily attributed to hemispheric specialization. Scanning habits associated with the reading of different languages may influence tachistoscopic laterality (cf. Carmon *et al.*, 1976; Mishkin & Forgays, 1952; Orbach, 1953; Silverberg *et al.*, 1979). Similarly, ear asymmetry has been reported to vary as a function of subjects' familiarity with the stimulus material. Experienced musicians show an REA on musical tasks that yield an LEA in the musically unskilled (Bever & Chariello, 1974; Johnson, 1977); speakers of the Thai language show an REA for intoned Thai words even though other subjects show an LEA (Van Lancker & Fromkin, 1977); and Morse Code instructors show an REA for Morse-like characters, whereas subjects unfamiliar with the code show an LEA (Papcun, Krashen, Terbeek, Remington, & Harshman, 1974). The same stimulus material may yield either an REA or an LEA depending on whether the material is presented in a verbal or nonverbal context (Spellacy & Blumstein, 1970).

Numerous investigators have discovered unexpected carry-over effects from one task to another, one hand to the other, one ear to the other, and so forth. Williams (1982) found that, in one instance, asymmetries of dichotic listening were related to habits of telephone usage: The magnitude of the REA was correlated ($r = .60$) with the strength of preference for holding the telephone receiver to the right ear. Kimura and Durnford (1974) reported a left VHF superiority for recognizing shapes only if the shape-recognition task was not preceded by a word-recognition task. When the word-recognition task was presented first, subjects showed a right VHF advantage for shapes. A similar phenomenon was observed by Witelson (1974) in her initial dichhaptic study; that is, children showed a left-hand superiority for recognizing shapes only if they had not previously accomplished the dichhaptic words task. This carry-over, or priming, effect was obtained in spite of a 10-day interval between the words and shapes tests. Unimanual haptic tasks often show an order effect such that the left hand, but not the right, benefits markedly from the prior experience of the other hand (Rudel *et al.*, 1974, 1977; Wagner, cited in Harris, 1980). Right-hand performance is similar regardless of which hand is tested first, but left-hand performance is improved substantially if the right hand has been tested previously.

Two other findings in the child literature illustrate vividly the biasing effect that seemingly incidental variables may have on the asymmetry of performance. Ironically, both of these biasing effects stem from attempts to increase the degree of control over the subject's attention. One of the findings concerns the fixation stimulus in the tachistoscopic paradigm; the other concerns focused attention in dichotic listening.

It has become practice in tachistoscopic studies to present a fixation stimulus at midline and to require the subject to report that stimulus before reporting stimuli from the lateral half-fields (Sperry, 1968). This procedure is designed to eliminate one source of variance, that is, eccentric fixation used by the subject as part of a strategy to maximize performance (McKeever & Huling, 1970). Usually a single digit is presented as the fixation-control stimulus at the same time that two other stimuli are presented, one in the left and one in the right VHF.

In their study of 5- and 6-year-old children, Kershner *et al.* (1977) found the expected right VHF superiority for digit triads when a central digit was used as the fixation-control stimulus, but the asymmetry was reversed when a shape (triangle, square, and asterisk) replaced the digit as the fixation-control stimulus. The crossover interaction between fixation stimulus and VHF, which was significant at $p < .0001$, is shown in Figure 5–5. This finding was confirmed by Carter and Kinsbourne (1979), who tested children between the ages of 5 and 12 years. Again, the laterality of children's performance was reversed when the category of the fixation-control stimulus was changed. Carter and Kinsbourne (1979) also reported a carry-over effect that was statistically significant for boys but not for girls. Boys who were tested initially with nonverbal fixation-control stimuli showed a reduced right VHF superiority during subsequent testing with verbal fixation-control stimuli, despite a 2- or 3-day interval between the two sessions. The fixation-control stimulus may influence adults' laterality under certain conditions (McKeever & van Eys, 1986), but the generality of the effect in studies of either adults or children is not known.

Identifying an important attentional factor in the auditory modality began with recognizing that free-report procedures for dichotic listening allow the child excessive freedom in allocating attention to one ear or the other (e.g., Bryden & Allard, 1978). Even though the REA of younger children tends to be no smaller than that of older children, the variability may be greater for the younger children, thus reducing the robustness of the ear effect in statistical tests (Kinsbourne & Hiscock, 1977). In an effort to reduce this variability, a series of studies was conducted in which the free-report procedure was replaced with a selective listening (focused-attention) task (Hiscock & Bergstrom, 1982; Hiscock & Chipuer, in preparation; Hiscock & Kinsbourne, 1977, 1980a; Hiscock, Kinsbourne, Caplan, & Swanson, 1979; Kinsbourne & Hiscock, 1977).

In some of the experiments, for the sake of administrative convenience, the child monitored one ear for a series of trials and then switched attention to the opposite ear. Half of the children within a sample listened first to the left ear, and half listened first to the

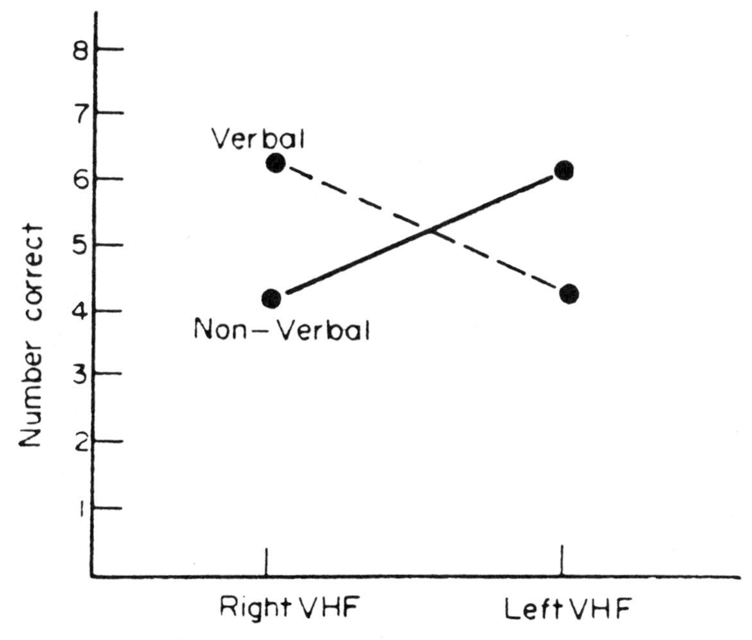

Figure 5-5. Mean number of digits recalled under verbal and nonverbal fixation conditions. Reprinted by permission from "Nonverbal Fixation Control in Young Children Induces a Left-Field Advantage in Digit Recall" by J. Kershner, R. Thomae, and R. Callaway, 1977, *Neuropsychologia, 15,* p. 572. Copyright © 1977 by Pergamon Journals Ltd.

right ear. It was soon discovered that the child was less successful in listening to the second ear than to the first ear. Consequently, as depicted in Figure 5-6, there was a significantly greater REA for those children who monitored the right ear first than for those who monitored the left ear first. Hiscock and Kinsbourne (1987), summing over four of these studies (Hiscock & Bergstrom, 1982; Hiscock & Chipuer, in preparation; Hiscock & Kinsbourne, 1980a; Hiscock *et al.*, 1979; $N = 277$ children), calculated that 88% of the children who monitored the right ear first showed an REA as compared with only 57% of the children who monitored the left ear first.

This order effect is not simply a transient switching difficulty or the product of fatigue, as it persists over a week-long interval (Hiscock & Bergstrom, 1982) and is absent when nondichotic stimuli are used (Hiscock & Chipuer, in preparation). Consequently, the effect has been termed a "priming bias." Studies with adults have established that this bias may be eliminated by substituting CV nonsense syllables for digit names (Hiscock & Stewart, 1984) or by using a signal detection test in lieu of free-report or selective listening procedures (Hiscock & Mackay, 1987). Apparently the bias is generated only when stimuli are readily localized in space and when multiple stimuli are to be reported.

These two effects—the fixation-control bias in VHF studies and the priming bias in dichotic listening—are but two examples of nonstructural (dynamic) factors that, under some circumstances, may exert a powerful influence on children's laterality. These factors can be readily manipulated within experiments; and, in the process of studying these factors, investigators may gain additional insight into mechanisms underlying perceptual asymmetries. Insofar as a factor is shown to be extraneous to hemispheric specialization, it can be controlled, thus permitting more precise measurement of remaining factors.

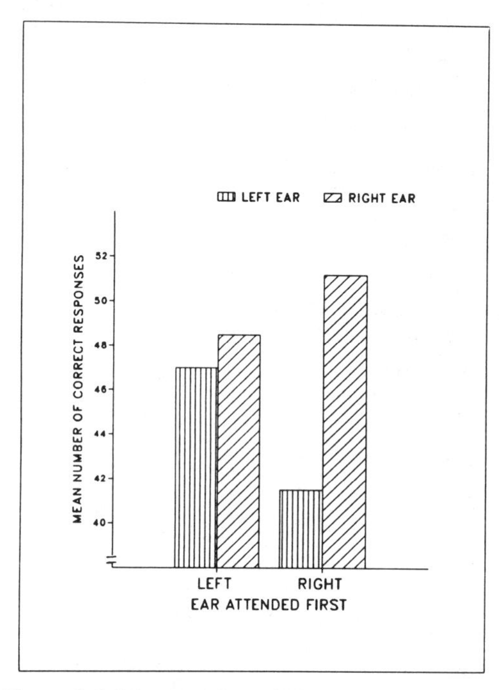

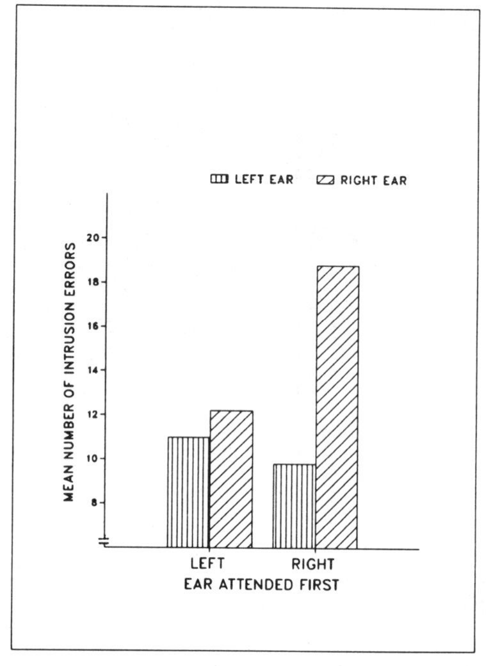

Figure 5-6. Mean number of digit names reported from the attended ear (left panel) and mean number of intrusion errors from the unattended ear (right panel) as a function of the order in which children monitored the left and right ears. Data from Hiscock and Kinsbourne (1980a).

Measurement Problems

It may seem surprising at first that there are significant difficulties involved in measuring behavioral asymmetries. The task seems almost trivial: Performance at one side of the body is to be compared with performance at the opposite side. For instance, the number of correct responses from the left VHF in a tachistoscopic task is to be compared with the number of correct responses from the right VHF. Under ideal circumstances, one would measure the difference between right- and left-sided performance over a number of trials and use that difference as an index of the individual's hemispheric specialization.

In actuality, the index obtained probably would not be strongly associated with the individual's hemispheric specialization as measured through invasive means (e.g., sodium amytal testing), or with an index obtained from another laterality task (e.g., dichotic listening). The index derived from the tachistoscopic task might bear only a weak relation to an index computed from subsequent performance on the identical task. Some of the reasons for the lack of association among different measures are described next. Whereas these measurement problems affect studies of adults as well as those of children, some are more pronounced in child studies, especially studies that encompass a wide age range.

RELIABILITY AND VALIDITY PROBLEMS

At least three problems lie within the domain of reliability and validity. One of these is limited retest reliability, or the difficulty of obtaining repeatable laterality measurements from an individual when the same test is used on different occasions. A second problem is limited concurrent validity, or the lack of an association between laterality measurements in different modalities or from different paradigms. Finally, there is the problem of predictive validity, or the limited power of laterality tests to predict hemispheric specialization as ascertained from more direct and definitive methods.

Perhaps the best way of describing these three intertwined problems is to begin with the problem of predictive validity, which Satz (1977) has termed the "inferential problem." Satz (1977) illustrated this problem using a hypothetical sample of 100 right-handers, 95% of whom have left-hemispheric speech representation, but only 70% of whom show an REA in dichotic listening. By Satz's calculation, the conditional probability of right-hemisphere speech, given an LEA in dichotic listening, is only .10. The investigator who concludes on the basis of a LEA that the individual has right-hemispheric speech will be incorrect 9 times out of 10.

This problem can be appreciated intuitively if one considers any population in which a specified outcome (e.g., right-hemispheric language representation) is very infrequent. Under such circumstances the validity of a predictive test must be very high if the test is to be useful because the investigator can achieve a high degree of predictive accuracy by simply betting against the rare outcome (e.g., by assuming that every right-hander has left-hemispheric speech representation). If 95% of the right-handed population has left-sided speech representation, then a laterality test would have to be almost perfectly valid if it is to improve the classification accuracy (95%) that can be achieved with only the knowledge that the subject is right-handed. The situation, however, may be quite different in studies of left-handers and certain clinically defined populations. The sparse data currently available from clinical samples provide limited support for the predictive validity of laterality measures within the respective populations (cf. Geffen & Caudrey, 1981; Kimura, 1961; Strauss, Gaddes, & Wada, 1987; Strauss & Wada, 1983; Warrington, 1981).

The inferential problem discussed here would constitute a major challenge for even the most valid and reliable of tests. The problem is compounded when tests are low in reliability and validity. The reliability of laterality scores depends on the task and the test–retest interval. Whereas children's scores may be moderately reliable within a testing session (Bakker, Van der Vlugt, & Claushuis, 1978) or over a short test–retest interval (Harper & Kraft, 1986; Hiscock & Kinsbourne, 1977), the reliability over a longer interval is often much poorer (Bakker *et al.*, 1979; Eling *et al.*, 1981; Hiscock, Chipuer, & Kinsbourne, 1986). Blumstein *et al.* (1975) have shown that, even when estimates of retest reliability fall in the .70 range, nearly one-third of subjects may reverse their laterality from the first to the second session. The reliability of right-minus-left scores (or of any other index derived from this difference) is limited by a high correlation between right and left scores. Unfortunately, in at least some laterality paradigms, right- and left-side scores tend to be highly correlated (e.g., Provins & Glencross, 1968).

Lack of reliability, in turn, limits concurrent validity, that is, correlations among laterality scores derived from different measures, whether within a modality or across modalities. As a rule, the correlations among laterality measures in children are unimpressive (e.g., Eling, 1983; Fennell, Bowers, & Satz, 1977; Hiscock *et al.*, 1986). For instance, Hiscock *et al.* (1986) obtained correlations no higher than .25 between dichotic listening asymmetry and asymmetry of the interference between speaking and finger tapping. Although there are factors other than low reliability (such as some of the nonstructural factors discussed previously) that might suppress the correlation between two laterality scores, it is clear from psychometric theory that concurrent validity cannot be high in the absence of an acceptable level of reliability (Nunnally, 1967).

LATERALITY INDICES

A measurement issue of special importance to developmental studies concerns the choice of an index for quantifying the degree of asymmetry. The most straightforward means of analyzing laterality data is to use raw scores for the right (R) and left (L) sides of the body (e.g., right and left VHF) as dependent variables in an analysis of variance. For the sake of convenience, one might calculate the difference between each individual's score for the right and for the left side—that is, $R-L$—and use that difference as the dependent variable. The effect for side (e.g., VHF) in the analysis of variance is eliminated when R and L scores are replaced by the $R-L$ difference, and the interactions between side and other design factors (e.g., the age × VHF interaction) also disappear. The main effect for each of the other factors (e.g., age), now acquires precisely the same F value as the interaction of that factor with side (e.g., age × VHF) in the analysis of raw scores. The analysis of raw scores and of difference scores thus lead to the same conclusion.

A major disadvantage of raw scores and difference scores—the one especially problematic in developmental studies—is that these scores are absolute measures of sidedness; that is, the range of values that they may assume depends on the subject's performance level. If a young child, for example, reports only 10 correct stimuli out of 100 in a dichotic listening task, then the greatest value that $R-L$ could assume would be 10. In contrast, an older child who reports 50 of the stimuli correctly could obtain a $R-L$ score of 50. Would the score of 50 reflect a degree of lateralization 5 times as great as that represented by the score of 10? Both scores are the highest scores possible for the respective performance levels. Consequently, a proportional index of laterality, such as $(R-L)/(R+L)$, would indicate that the degree of laterality is identical for both children.

The potential contradiction between absolute and relative laterality scores is illustrated in Figure 5-7, in which R and L scores are plotted against an abscissa of overall performance, that is, R and L values. The curves were generated by choosing values of R and L that would yield a constant value for $(R-L)/(R+L)$ across all levels of $R+L$. Thus despite an increase in the absolute degree of asymmetry with increasing overall performance, the proportional degree of asymmetry is constant.

The description of the scaling problem is not complete without mention of range restrictions at the upper limit of performance. As $R+L$ approaches its upper limit, the $R-L$ score will again be constrained. For example, in the case of the hypothetical dichotic listening test with a total of 100 stimuli, a child who reports 90 of the 100 stimuli correctly can achieve an $R-L$ score no greater than 10. Although this limitation is identical to that encountered by the child who reports only 10 stimuli correctly, there is a marked discrepancy in the possible range of proportional scores. The child with 10 correct responses could have an $(R-L)/(R+L)$ score as great as 1.00, but the child with 90 correct responses could have a score no greater than 0.11.

Authors who have concerned themselves with this problem of scaling have reacted in one of two ways. Some (Colbourn, 1978; Richardson, 1976) have argued that there is no satisfactory means of quantifying laterality and that, consequently, one must settle for nonparametric tests performed on rank-ordered scores. Other writers, however (e.g., Bryden & Sprott, 1981; Harshman & Krashen, 1972; Kuhn, 1973; Marshall, Caplan, & Holmes, 1975), have proposed mathematical transformations of raw scores that could be used to make laterality estimates comparable across various levels of performance. The degree to which different laterality indices actually achieve this objective is a matter of dispute (Birkett, 1977; Jones, 1983a, 1983b; Kinsbourne & Hiscock, 1983b; Levy, 1977; Marshall *et al.*, 1975; Sprott & Bryden, 1983). Moreover, Stone (1980) has shown that correlations between various laterality indices and total accuracy ($R+L$) have expected values that may deviate substantially from zero. Consequently, a correlation between a laterality score and $R+L$, or lack of a correlation, may be misleading.

With respect to this scaling problem, developmental research is a special case. Not

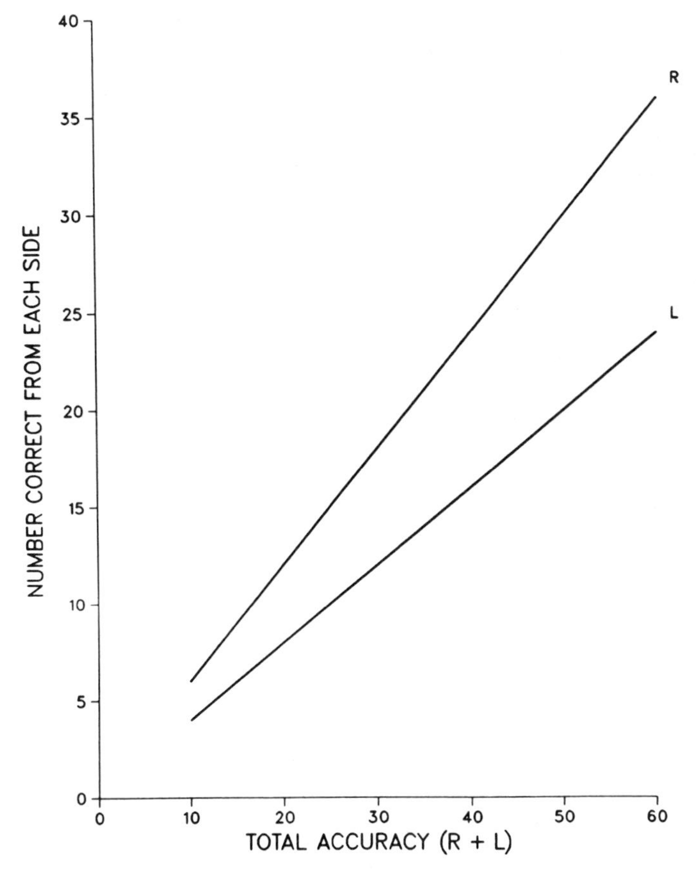

Figure 5-7. Mathematically derived plot of right-sided (R) and left-sided (L) accuracy as a function of total accuracy (R + L). Values were chosen so as to yield a constant laterality ratio [(R − L)/(R + L) = .20] acrosss the range of performance.

only do developmental studies often span a broad range of overall performance, but there is usually a high correlation between overall performance and age. Consequently, choosing a laterality index that will eliminate any correlation between laterality and overall performance will very likely constrain the correlation between laterality and age. Insofar as the purpose of the study is to examine age-related changes in laterality, the investigator may be begging the question by selecting a particular laterality index. Primarily for this reason, Jones (1983a) has argued in favor of using difference scores in laterality studies.

Alternatively, the developmental investigator might ascertain the manner in which different indices tend to bias the data across different levels of performance (see Figure 5-8) and then select two indices whose effects are opposite. If the outcome is the same regardless of the index chosen, then the results can be accepted with confidence. If not, then the results should be considered as indeterminate.

A similar approach may be taken, without using laterality indices, if the task can be scored for errors as well as correct responses. Hiscock and Kinsbourne (1980a), for example, found that the number of correct responses in a selective listening task increased between the ages of 3 and 12 years, and that the number of intrusions from the opposite ear decreased. The possible range of laterality, in terms of $R-L$ difference scores, thus increased with increasing age in the case of correct responses and decreased in the case of

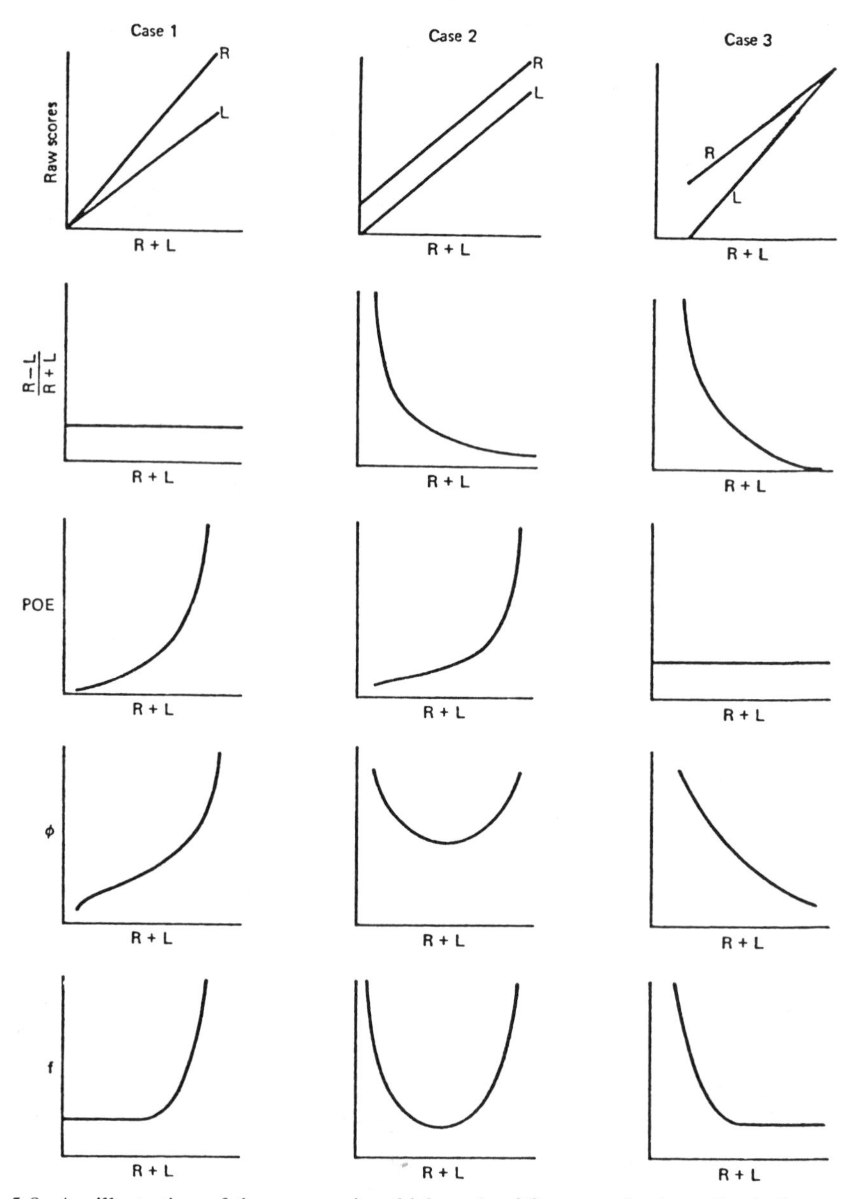

Figure 5-8. An illustration of the manner in which each of four popular laterality indices varies as a function of total performance (R + L). Considered separately are Case 1, in which the difference between right (R) and left (L) raw scores increases with increasing total performance; Case 2, in which the difference between R and L remains constant as total performance increases; and Case 3, in which the difference between R and L decreases as total performance increases. The laterality indices depicted are: (R − L)/(R + L) (e.g., Studdert-Kennedy & Shankweiler, 1970); percentage of error (POE) (Harshman & Krashen, 1972); the phi coefficient (Kuhn, 1973); and *f,* which is (R − L)/(R + L) for (R + L) < 50% and (R − L)/(T − (R + L)) for (R + L) > 50%, where T represents the maximum possible number of correct responses (Marshall, Caplan, & Holmes, 1975). Curves were generated with the following constraints: 60 trials, 2 responses per trial, mean R − L difference of 10. Reprinted by permission from "The Normal and Deviant Development of Functional Lateralization of the Brain" by M. Kinsbourne and M. Hiscock, 1983, in *Handbook of Child Psychology* (4th ed.), Vol. 2, *Infancy and Developmental Psychobiology,* edited by M. M. Haith and J. J. Campos, New York: Wiley. Copyright © 1983 by John Wiley and Sons, Inc.

intrusion errors. Separate analysis of variance for each dependent variable failed to yield a significant age-related change in degree of laterality. Insofar as similar results were obtained despite opposite scaling biases, the finding of developmental invariance in degree of laterality cannot be a statistical artifact. The same approach may be used with tasks that yield reaction times as well as correct-response scores. Reaction time will tend to decrease with increasing age, whereas the number of correct responses will tend to increase (e.g., Eling *et al.*, 1981). A bias introduced by applying a laterality index to one dependent variable will be reversed when the same laterality index is applied to the other dependent variable.

POST HOC ANALYSES

In many of the studies reviewed in this chapter, the phenomena of primary interest were manifested as age × side, sex × side, or age × sex × side interactions in analysis of variance. Regardless of whether these interactions were statistically significant, investigators often performed post hoc tests to determine whether the side effect (e.g., REA) was significant at each age level or within each age–sex cell. Occasionally the failure to find a significant difference at one grade level or within one age–sex cell would lead to suggestions of a previously undiscovered developmental process. Ingram (1975), for example, apparently failed to find a significant age × sex × ear interaction but did discover, by a posteriori *t*-tests, that 4-year-old girls failed to show a significant REA. The REA was significant for 4-year-old boys and for both girls and boys at ages 3 and 5 years. Citing a similar anomaly in two other sets of data, Ingram (1975) speculated that the findings may reflect "periods of cerebral reorganization such that left hemisphere mechanisms are temporarily pre-empted by functions other than speech" (p. 104). The anomaly, however, failed to materialize in subsequent studies (e.g., Hiscock & Kinsbourne, 1977, 1980a).

Apart from the dubious legitimacy of post hoc tests in the absence of a significant interaction, there are issues of statistical power and sampling error. The magnitude of behavioral asymmetries is often modest, and the variability across subjects is often great. By using sufficiently large samples in the analysis of variance, the statistical power necessary to detect the weak effects can be obtained. If, however, those samples are decomposed into several age–sex cells, the number of subjects per cell usually will be quite small. When *t*-tests or analyses of variance are performed on a cell-by-cell basis, the power of the tests is limited, sometimes leading to results that do not reach the $p = .05$ level of significance, that is, Type II errors. Test performed on data from the youngest children are particularly susceptible insofar as the variability of these data tends to be especially great (see Kinsbourne & Hiscock, 1977). On the other hand, a large number of *t*-tests or *F*-tests may lead to spurious postive results, that is, Type I errors.

Although these problems may be ameliorated by using more appropriate post hoc tests such as the Newman-Keuls test, a better alternative in many cases is trend analysis, which can be used to decompose an age × side or age × sex × side interaction into linear, quadratic, and higher order trends. A significant age linear trend × side interaction, for example, would indicate a linear increase (or decrease) with age in the magnitude of asymmetry. A significant quadratic component would indicate a substantial deviation from linearity, which could reflect a true developmental pattern or perhaps a floor or ceiling effect. Whereas multiple comparisons are based on pairs of data points, trend analyses are based on the overall pattern of results across the different age levels. Whereas multiple comparisons often lead to overinterpretation of idiosyncrasies in the data, trend analyses guide the investigator toward specific conclusions regarding linear and nonlinear developmental changes.

DIRECTIONS FOR FUTURE RESEARCH

If knowledge of laterality in children is to be advanced significantly beyond the present level of understanding, investigators must strive to do more than just collect more data. Although there is no obvious solution for the major problems in laterality research, a higher level of understanding might nonetheless be attained if certain objectives are met.

One of these objectives is to improve the reliability of laterality tests. A useful first step is the development of tasks in which scores for the left and right sides of the body are not highly correlated. In accomplishing this, researchers would be removing one of the major limitations on reliability. Reliability would also increase insofar as investigators are able to identify and control those nonstructural factors that influence laterality, such as attentional bias and strategy.

A second objective is the assessment and ultimate improvement of validity. For this purpose, criteria must be defined with sufficient precision as to enable the comparison of paradigms. One possible criterion is the proportion of right-handed children who show the expected asymmetry in a particular test. On an ideal laterality task, nearly 100% of right-handed children would show the expected asymmetry. Another potentially useful criterion is the task's power to differentiate right- and left-handers. The ideal laterality task would yield the expected asymmetry in right-handers significantly more often than in left-handers. This criterion, when combined with the first, will help to ensure that asymmetrical performance in right-handers is attributable to hemispheric specialization and not to some biasing factor. A third criterion is the power of the laterality task to predict hemispheric specialization as ascertained by Wada test, positron emission tomography (PET scanning), event-related brain potentials, and the like. As more powerful techniques for measuring brain physiology become available, and especially as such techniques become available for use with normal children, the usefulness of this approach for validating laterality measures becomes much greater.

During the first 25 years of laterality research, it has been customary for investigators to report findings based on an arbitrary set of experimental parameters. For example, one may find a REA in children for natural-speech words, presented in sets of 3 pairs per trial, at 60 dB(A), and with a presentation rate of 2 pairs per second. But does one find the same ear asymmetry when the presentation rate is decreased to 1 pair per second? Is an REA of comparable magnitude obtained for single pairs of words? Does degradation of the stimuli alter the ear advantage? Only rarely in developmental studies have investigators varied attributes of the stimulus or task in a parametric fashion. Yet, it is clear that factors such as perceptual difficulty, memory load, and response demands may affect laterality. In the future, it will be increasingly important for researchers to ascertain the generality of their findings across various stimulus and task parameters. Sampling is a concept that should apply not only to the selection of subjects from a population of children, but also to the selection of experimental parameters from a multidimensional parametric space. Parametric studies should help to resolve some of the apparent contradictions that abound in the laterality studies currently available.

Finally, one would expect that, as laterality research progresses, there will be less emphasis on the presence or absence of laterality per se and more emphasis on the mechanisms underlying performance. As noted previously, trends in this direction can already be detected. Even if investigators continue to regard the asymmetry itself as the phenomenon of primary interest, they should be cognizant of associated phenomena that may have developmental importance. Dichotic listening, for example, can be used to obtain information not only about ear asymmetry but also about the development of the ability to allocate and switch attention (Geffen & Sexton, 1978; Geffen & Wale, 1979; Sexton & Geffen, 1979) and about children's strategies for processing multiple stimuli (Witelson & Rabinovitch, 1971). The tachistoscopic method can provide information about developmental change in children's ability to process conflicting inputs simultaneously (Merola & Liederman, 1985). The concurrent-task method is particularly well adapted for providing insight into developmental changes in children's capacity to process different kinds of information (Hiscock *et al.*, 1987).

Regardless of whether laterality research ultimately can be justified in terms of the knowledge it yields about the development of hemispheric specialization for various processes, laterality methods, because they address behavioral questions, can provide valuable insight into the development of the processes themselves.

ACKNOWLEDGMENT

Preparation of this chapter was supported in part by a grant from the Medical Research Council of Canada. The author is grateful to Matthew Decter and Roxanne Inch for their invaluable help.

REFERENCES

Aaron, P. G., & Handley, A. C. (1975). Directional scanning and cerebral asymmetries in processing visual stimuli. *Perceptual and Motor Skills, 40,* 719–725.

Affleck, G., & Joyce, P. (1979). Sex differences in the association of cerebral hemispheric specialization of spatial function with conservation task performance. *Journal of Genetic Psychology, 134,* 271–280.

Ashton, R., & Beasley, M. (1982). Cerebral laterality in deaf and hearing children. *Developmental Psychology, 18,* 294–300.

Bakker, D. J. (1973). Hemispheric specialization and states in the learning-to-read process. *Bulletin of the Orton Society, 23,* 15–27.

Bakker, D. J., Hoefkens, M., & Van der Vlugt, H. (1979). Hemispheric specialization in children as reflected in the longitudinal development of ear asymmetry. *Cortex, 15,* 619–625.

Bakker, D. J., & Van der Kleij, P. C. M. (1978). Development of lateral asymmetry in the perception of sequentially touched fingers. *Acta Psychologica, 42,* 357–365.

Bakker, D. J., Van der Vlugt, H., & Claushuis, M. (1978). The reliability of dichotic ear asymmetry in normal children. *Neuropsychologia, 16,* 753–757.

Barroso, F. (1976). Hemispheric asymmetry of function in children. In R. W. Rieber (Ed.), *The neuropsychology of language*. New York: Plenum.

Basser, L. S. (1962). Hemiplegia of early onset and the faculty of speech with special reference to the effects of hemispherectomy. *Brain, 85,* 427–460.

Beaumont, J. G. (1982a). Developmental aspects. In J. G. Beaumont (Ed.), *Divided visual field studies of cerebral organisation* (pp. 113–128). London: Academic Press.

Beaumont, J. G. (Ed.) (1982b). *Divided visual field studies of cerebral organisation.* London: Academic Press.

Berlin, C. I., Hughes, L. F., Lowe-Bell, S. S., & Berlin, H. L. (1973). Dichotic right ear advantage in children 5 to 13. *Cortex, 9,* 394–402.

Best, C. T., Hoffman, H., & Glanville, B. B. (1982). Development of infant ear asymmetries for speech and music. *Perception and Psychophysics, 31,* 75–85.

Bever, T. G. (1971). The nature of cerebral dominance in speech behavior of the child and adult. In R. Huxley & E. Ingram (Eds.), *Language acquisition: Models and methods* (pp. 231–261). London: Academic Press.

Bever, T. G., & Chariello, R. J. (1974). Cerebral dominance in musicians and non-musicians. *Science, 185,* 537–539.

Birkett, P. (1977). Measures of laterality and theories of hemispheric process. *Neuropsychologia, 15,* 693–696.

Bissell, J. C., & Clark, F. (1984). Dichotic listening performance in normal children and adults. *American Journal of Occupational Therapy, 38,* 176–183.

Blumstein, S., Goodglass, H., & Tartter, V. (1975). The reliability of ear advantage in dichotic listening. *Brain and Language, 2,* 226–236.

Borowy, T., & Goebel, R. (1976). Cerebral lateralization of speech: The effects of age, sex, race, and socioeconomic class. *Neuropsychologia, 14,* 363–370.

Bowers, D., Heilman, K. M., Satz, P., & Altman, A. (1978). Simultaneous performance on verbal, nonverbal and motor tasks by right-handed adults. *Cortex, 14,* 540–556.

Bradshaw, J. L., Nettleton, N. C., & Taylor, M. J. (1981). The use of laterally presented words in research into cerebral asymmetry: Is directional scanning likely to be a source of artifact? *Brain and Language, 14,* 1–14.

Braine, L. G. (1968). Asymmetries of pattern perception observed in Israelis. *Neuropsychologia, 6,* 73–88.

Brizzolara, D., De Nobili, G. L., & Ferretti, G. (1982). Tactile discrimination of direction of lines in relation to hemispheric specialization. *Perceptual and Motor Skills, 54,* 655–660.

Broman, M. (1978). Reaction-time differences between the left and right hemispheres for face and letter discrimination in children and adults. *Cortex, 14,* 578–591.

Bryden, M. P. (1970). Laterality effects in dichotic listening: Relations with handedness and reading ability in children. *Neuropsychologia, 8,* 443–450.

Bryden, M. P. (1978). Strategy effects in the assessment of hemispheric asymmetry. In G. Underwood (Ed.), *Strategies of information processing* (pp. 117–149). London: Academic Press.

Bryden, M. P. (1982a). The behavioral assessment of lateral asymmetry: Problems, pitfalls, and partial solution. In R. N. Malatesha & L. C. Hartlage (Eds.), *Neuropsychology and cognition* (Vol. 2, pp. 44–54). The Hague: Martinus Nijhoff.

Bryden, M. P. (1982b). *Laterality: Functional asymmetry in the intact brain.* New York: Academic Press.

Bryden, M. P. (1983). *Studies of functional asymmetry in the intact brain.* Paper presented at the meeting of the Canadian Psychological Association, Winnipeg, Manitoba.

Bryden, M. P., & Allard, F. A. (1978). Dichotic listening and the development of linguistic processes. In M. Kinsbourne (Ed.), *Asymmetrical function of the brain* (pp. 392–404). New York: Cambridge University Press.

Bryden, M. P., & Allard, F. A. (1981). Do auditory perceptual asymmetries develop? *Cortex, 17,* 313–318.

Bryden, M. P., Munhall, K., & Allard, F. (1983). Attentional biases and the right-ear effect in dichotic listening. *Brain and Language, 18,* 236–248.

Bryden, M. P., & Sprott, D. A. (1981). Statistical determination of degree of laterality. *Neuropsychologia, 19,* 571–581.

Bryson, S., Mononen, L. J., & Yu, L. (1980). Procedural constraints on the measurement of laterality in young children. *Neuropsychologia, 18,* 243–246.

Butler, D. C., & Miller, L. K. (1979). Role of approximation to English and letter array length in the development of visual laterality. *Developmental Psychology, 15,* 522–529.

Caplan, B., & Kinsbourne, M. (1981). Cerebral lateralization, preferred cognitive mode, and reading ability in normal children. *Brain and Language, 14,* 349–370.

Carey, S., & Diamond, R. (1977). From piecemeal to configurational representation of faces. *Science, 195,* 312–314.

Carey, S., Diamond, R., & Woods, B. (1980). Development of face recognition—A maturational component? *Developmental Psychology, 16,* 257–269.

Carmon, A., Nachshon, I., & Starinsky, R. (1976). Developmental aspects of visual hemifield differences in perception of verbal material. *Brain and Language, 3,* 463–469.

Carter, R. L., Hohenegger, M. K., & Satz, P. (1982). Aphasia and speech organization in children. *Science, 218,* 797–799.

Carter, G. L., & Kinsbourne, M. (1979). The ontogeny of right lateralization of spatial mental set. *Developmental Psychology, 15,* 241–245.

Cermak, S. A., Cermak, L. S., Drake, C., & Kenney, R. (1978). The effect of concurrent manual activity on the dichotic listening performance of boys with learning disabilities. *American Journal of Occupational Therapy, 32,* 493–499.

Cioffi, J., & Kandel, G. L. (1979). Laterality of stereognostic accuracy of children for words, shapes, and bigrams: A sex difference for bigrams. *Science, 204,* 1432–1434.

Colbourn, C. J. (1978). Can laterality be measured? *Neuropsychologia, 16,* 283–289.

Corballis, M. C., Macadie, L., Crotty, A., & Beale, I. L. (1985). The naming of disoriented letters by normal and reading-disabled children. *Journal of Child Psychology and Psychiatry, 26,* 929–938.

Corballis, M. C., & Morgan, M. J. (1978). On the biological basis of human laterality: I. Evidence for a maturational left–right gradient. *Behavioral and Brain Sciences, 2,* 261–336.

Cranney, J., & Ashton, R. (1980). Witelson's dichhaptic task as a measure of hemispheric asymmetry in deaf and hearing populations. *Neuropsychologia, 18,* 95–98.

Cranney, J., & Ashton, R. (1982). Tactile spatial ability: Lateralized performance of deaf and hearing age groups. *Journal of Experimental Child Psychology, 34,* 123–134.

Crossley, M., & Hiscock, M. (1987). Concurrent-task interference indicates asymmetric resource allocation in children's reading. *Developmental Neuropsychology, 3–4,* 207–225.

Dalby, J. T. (1980). Hemispheric timesharing: Verbal and spatial loading with concurrent unimanual activity. *Cortex, 16,* 567–573.

Dalby, J. T., & Gibson, D. *(1981).* Functional cerebral lateralization in subtypes of disabled readers. *Brain and Language, 14,* 34–48.

Davidoff, J. B., Beaton, A. A., Done, D. J., & Booth, H. (1982). Information extraction from brief verbal displays: Half-field and serial position effects for children, normal and illiterate adults. *British Journal of Psychology, 73,* 29–39.

Davidoff, J. B., & Done, D. J. (1984). A longitudinal study of the development of visual field advantage for letter matching. *Neuropsychologia, 22,* 311–318.

Davidoff, J. B., Done, J., & Scully, J. (1981). What does the lateral ear advantage relate to? *Brain and Language, 12,* 332–346.

Dawson, G. D. (1981). Sex differences in dichhaptic processing. *Perceptual and Motor Skills, 53,* 935–944.

Denes, G., & Spinaci, M. P. (1981). Influence of association value in recognition of random shapes under dichhaptic presentation. *Cortex, 17,* 597–602.

Dorman, M. F., & Geffner, D. S. (1974). Hemispheric specialization for speech perception in six-year-old black and white children from low and middle socio-economic classes. *Cortex, 10,* 171–176.

Eling, P. (1983). Comparing different measures of laterality: Do they relate to a single mechanism? *Journal of Clinical Neuropsychology, 5,* 135–147.

Eling, P., Marshall, J. C., & Van Galen, G. (1981). The development of language lateralization as measured by dichotic listening. *Neuropsychologia, 19,* 767–773.

Ellis, A. W., & Young, A. W. (1981). Visual hemifield asymmetry for naming concrete nouns and verbs in children between seven and eleven years of age. *Cortex, 17,* 617–624.

Entus, A. K. (1977). Hemispheric asymmetry in processing of dichotically presented speech and nonspeech stimuli by infants. In S. J. Segalowitz & F. A. Gruber (Eds.), *Language development and neurological theory* (pp. 63–73). New York: Academic Press.

Etaugh, C., & Levy, R. B. (1981). Hemispheric specialization for tactile–spatial processing in preschool children. *Perceptual and Motor Skills, 53,* 621–622.

Fennell, E. B., Bowers, D., & Satz, P. (1977). Within-modal and cross-modal reliabilities of two laterality tests. *Brain and Language, 4,* 63–69.

Fennell, E. B., Satz, P., & Morris, R. (1983). The development of handedness and dichotic ear listening asymmetries in relation to school achievement: A longitudinal study. *Journal of Experimental Child Psychology, 35,* 248–262.

Flanery, R. C., & Balling, J. D. (1979). Developmental changes in hemispheric specialization for tactile spatial ability. *Developmental Psychology, 15,* 364–372.

Forgays, D. G. (1953). The development of differential word recognition. *Journal of Experimental Psychology, 45,* 165–168.

Friedman, A., & Polson, M. C. (1981). Hemispheres as independent resource systems: Limited capacity processing and cerebral specialization. *Journal of Experimental Psychology: Human Perception and Performance, 7,* 1031–1058.

Galin, D., Johnstone, J., Nakell, L., & Herron, J. (1979). Development of the capacity for tactile information transfer between hemispheres in normal children. *Science, 204,* 1330–1332.

Garren, R. B. (1980). Hemispheric laterality differences among four levels of reading achievement. *Perceptual and Motor Skills, 50,* 119–123.

Gates, A., & Bradshaw, J. L. (1977). The role of cerebral hemispheres in music. *Brain and Language, 4,* 403–431.

Geffen, G. (1976). Development of hemispheric specialization for speech perception. *Cortex, 12,* 337–346.

Geffen, G. (1978). The development of the right ear advantage in dichotic listening with focused attention. *Cortex, 14,* 169–177.

Geffen, G., & Caudrey, D. (1981). Reliability and validity of the dichotic monitoring test for language laterality. *Neuropsychologia, 19,* 413–423.

Geffen, G., & Sexton, M. A. (1978). The development of auditory strategies of attention. *Developmental Psychology, 14,* 11–17.

Geffen, G., & Wale, J. (1979). Development of selective listening and hemispheric asymmetry. *Developmental Psychology, 15,* 138–146.

Geffner, D. S., & Dorman, M. F. (1976). Hemispheric specialization for speech perception in four-year-old children from low and middle socio-economic classes. *Cortex, 12,* 71–73.

Geffner, D. S., & Hochberg, I. (1971). Ear laterality performance of children from low and middle socioeconomic levels on a verbal dichotic listening task. *Cortex, 8,* 193–203.

Ghent, L. (1961). Developmental changes in tactual thresholds on dominant and nondominant sides. *Journal of Comparative and Physiological Psychology, 54,* 670–673.

Gibson, C., & Bryden, M. P. (1983). Dichhaptic recognition of shapes and letters in children. *Canadian Journal of Psychology, 37,* 132–143.

Gibson, C. J., & Bryden, M. P. (1984). Cerebral laterality in deaf and hearing children. *Brain and Language, 23,* 1–12.

Gilbert, J. H. V., & Climan, I. (1974). Dichotic studies in 2–3 year olds: A preliminary report. In *Speech communication seminar Stockholm* (Vol. 2). Uppsala: Almqvist & Wiksell.

Glanville, B. B., Best, C. T., & Levenson, R. (1977). A cardiac measure of cerebral asymmetries in infant auditory perception. *Developmental Psychology, 13,* 55–59.

Goodglass, H. (1973). Developmental comparisons of vowels and consonants in dichotic listening. *Journal of Speech and Hearing Research, 16,* 744–756.

Gordon, D. P. (1983). The influence of sex on the development of lateralization of speech. *Neuropsychologia, 21,* 139–146.

Grant, D. W. (1980). Visual asymmetry on a color-naming task: A developmental perspective. *Perceptual and Motor Skills, 50,* 475–480.

Grant, D. W. (1981). Visual asymmetry on a color-naming task: A longitudinal study with primary school children. *Child Development, 52,* 370–372.

Gross, K., Rothenberg, S., Schottenfeld, S., & Drake, C. (1978). Duration thresholds for letter identification in left and right visual fields for normal and reading-disabled children. *Neuropsychologia, 16,* 709–715.

Hardyck, C. (1983). Seeing each other's points of view: Visual perceptual lateralization. In J. B. Hellige (Ed.), *Cerebral hemisphere asymmetry: Method, theory and application* (pp. 219–254). New York: Praeger.

Hardyck, C. (1986). Cerebral asymmetries and experimental parameters: Real differences and imaginary variations? *Brain and Cognition, 5,* 223–239.

Harper, L. V., & Kraft, R. H. (1986). Lateralization of receptive language in preschoolers: Test–retest reliability in a dichotic listening task. *Developmental Psychology, 22,* 553–556.

Harris, L. J. (1978). Sex differences in spatial ability: Possible environmental, genetic and neurological factors. In M. Kinsbourne (Ed.), *Asymmetrical function of the brain* (pp. 405–522). Cambridge: Cambridge University Press.

Harris, L. J. (1980). Which hand is the "eye" of the blind?—A new look at an old question. In J. Herron (Ed.), *Neuropsychology of left-handedness* (pp. 303–329). New York: Academic Press.

Harshman, R., & Krashen, S. (1972). An "unbiased" procedure for comparing degree of lateralization of dichotically presented stimuli. *UCLA Working Papers in Phonetics, 23,* 3–12.

Hassler, M., & Birbaumer, N. (1986). Witelson's dichhaptic stimulation test and children with different levels of musical talent. *Neuropsychologia, 24,* 435–440.

Hatta, T., Yamamoto, M., Kawabata, Y., & Tsutui, K. (1981). Development of hemisphere specialization for tactile recognition in normal children. *Cortex, 17,* 611–616.

Hécaen, H. (1976). Acquired aphasia in children and the ontogenesis of hemispheric functional specialization. *Brain and Language, 3,* 114–134.

Hellige, J. B., & Longstreth, L. E. (1981). Effects of concurrent hemisphere-specific activity on unimanual tapping rate. *Neuropsychologia, 19,* 395–406.

Henry, R. G. J. (1979). Monaural studies eliciting an hemispheric asymmetry: A bibliography. *Perceptual and Motor Skills, 48,* 335–338.

Henry, R. G. J. (1983). Monaural studies eliciting an hemispheric asymmetry, a bibliography: II. *Perceptual and Motor Skills, 56,* 915–918.

Hicks, R. E. (1975). Intrahemispheric response competition between vocal and unimanual performance in normal adult human males. *Journal of Comparative and Physiological Psychology, 89,* 50–60.

Hicks, R. E., Provenzano, F. J., & Rybstein, E. D. (1975). Generalized and lateralized effects of concurrent verbal rehearsal upon performance of sequential movements of the fingers by the left and right hands. *Acta Psychologica, 39,* 119–130.

Hiscock, M. (1982). Verbal–manual time sharing in children as a function of task priority. *Brain and Cognition, 1,* 119–131.

Hiscock, M., Antoniuk, D., Prisciak, K., & von Hessert, D. (1985). Generalized and lateralized interference between concurrent tasks performed by children: Effects of age, sex, and skill. *Developmental Psychology, 1,* 29–48.

Hiscock, M., & Bergstrom, K. J. (1982). The lengthy persistence of priming effects in dichotic listening. *Neuropsychologia, 20,* 43–53.

Hiscock, M., & Chipuer, H. (1986). Concurrent performance of rhythmically compatible or incompatible vocal and manual tasks: Evidence for two sources of interference in verbal–manual timesharing. *Neuropsychologia, 24,* 691–698.

Hiscock, M., & Chipuer, H. (in preparation). *Persistence of laterally biased attention in children's selective listening for dichotic and monaural stimuli.*

Hiscock, M., Chipuer, H., & Kinsbourne, M. (1986). *Task specificity of children's laterality.* Paper presented at the meeting of the International Neuropsychological Society, Denver, Colorado.

Hiscock, M., & Kinsbourne, M. (1977). Selective listening asymmetry in preschool children. *Developmental Psychology, 13,* 217–224.

Hiscock, M., & Kinsbourne, M. (1978). Ontogeny of cerebral dominance: Evidence from time-sharing asymmetry in children. *Developmental Psychology, 14,* 321–329.

Hiscock, M., & Kinsbourne, M. (1980a). Asymmetries of selective listening and attention switching in children. *Developmental Psychology, 16,* 70–82.

Hiscock, M., & Kinsbourne, M. (1980b). Asymmetry of verbal–manual time sharing in children: A follow-up study. *Neuropsychologia, 18,* 151–162.

Hiscock, M., & Kinsbourne, M. (1987). Specialization of the cerebral hemispheres: Implications for learning. *Journal of Learning Disabilities, 20,* 130–143.

Hiscock, M., Kinsbourne, M., Caplan, B., & Swanson, J. M. (1979). Auditory attention in hyperactive children: Effects of stimulant medication on dichotic listening performance. *Journal of Abnormal Psychology, 88,* 27–32.

Hiscock, M., Kinsbourne, M., Samuels, M., & Krause, A. E. (1985). Effects of speaking upon the rate and variability of concurrent finger tapping in children. *Journal of Experimental Child Psychology, 40,* 486–500.

Hiscock, M., Kinsbourne, M., Samuels, M., & Krause, A. E. (1987). Dual task performance in children: Generalized and lateralized effects of memory encoding upon the rate and variability of concurrent finger tapping. *Brain and Cognition, 6,* 24–40.

Hiscock, M., & Mackay, M. (1987). A signal detection procedure eliminates priming biases in dichotic listening. *Neuropsychologia, 25,* 507–517.

Hiscock, M., Prisciak, K., & Antoniuk, D. (1983). *Laterality of dual-task interference in children: Effects of task, age, and academic skill.* Paper presented at the meeting of the International Neuropsychological Society, Mexico City.

Hiscock, M., & Stewart, C. (1984). The effect of asymmetrically focused attention upon subsequent ear differences in dichotic listening. *Neuropsychologia, 22,* 337–351.

Hughes, M., & Sussman, H. M. (1983). An assessment of cerebral dominance in language-disordered children via a time-sharing paradigm. *Brain and Language, 19,* 48–64.

Hynd, G. W., & Obrzut, J. E. (1977). Effects of grade level and sex on the magnitude of the dichotic ear advantage. *Neuropsychologia, 15,* 689–692.

Hynd, G. W., Obrzut, J. E., Weed, W., & Hynd, C. R. (1979). Development of cerebral dominance: Dichotic listening asymmetry in normal and learning-disabled children. *Journal of Experimental Child Psychology, 28,* 445–454.

Inglis, J., & Sykes, D. H. (1967). Some sources of variation in dichotic listening performance in children. *Journal of Experimental Child Psychology, 5,* 480–488.

Ingram, D. (1975). Cerebral speech lateralization in young children. *Neuropsychologia, 13,* 103–105.

Jeeves, M. A. (1972). Hemisphere differences in response rates to visual stimuli in children. *Psychonomic Science, 27,* 201–203.

Johnson, P. R. (1977). Dichotically stimulated ear differences in musicians and nonmusicians. *Cortex, 13,* 385–389.

Jones, B. (1979). Sex and visual field effects on accuracy and decision making when subjects classify male and female faces. *Cortex, 15,* 551–560.

Jones, B. (1980). Sex and handedness as factors in visual-field organization for a categorization task. *Journal of Experimental Psychology: Human Perception and Performance, 6,* 494–500.

Jones, B. (1983a). Measuring degree of cerebral lateralization in children as a function of age. *Developmental Psychology, 19,* 237–242.

Jones, B. (1983b). Some problems with Bryden and Sprott's "Statistical determination of degree of lateralization." *Neuropsychologia, 21,* 295–298.

Jones, B., & Anuza, T. (1982). Sex differences in cerebral lateralization in 3- and 4-year old children. *Neuropsychologia, 20,* 347–350.

Kahneman, D. (1973). *Attention and effort.* Englewood Cliffs, NJ: Prentice-Hall.
Kamptner, L., Kraft, R. H., & Harper, L. V. (1984). Lateral specialization and social–verbal development in preschool children. *Brain and Cognition, 3,* 42–50.
Kee, D. W. (1984). Comments on Hughes and Sussman's time-sharing study of cerebral laterality in language-disordered and normal children. *Brain and Language, 22,* 354–356.
Kee, D. W., Morris, K., Bathurst, K., & Hellige, J. E. (1986). Lateralized interference in finger tapping: Comparisons of rate and variability measures under speed and consistency tapping instructions. *Brain and Cognition, 5,* 268–279.
Kershner, J. R., Thomae, R., & Callaway, R. (1977). Nonverbal fixation control in young children induces a left-field advantage in digit recall. *Neuropsychologia, 15,* 569–576.
Kimura, D. (1961). Cerebral dominance and the perception of verbal stimuli. *Canadian Journal of Psychology, 15,* 166–171.
Kimura, D. (1963). Speech lateralization in young children as determined by an auditory test. *Journal of Comparative and Physiological Psychology, 56,* 899–902.
Kimura, D. (1967). Functional asymmetry of the brain in dichotic listening. *Cortex, 3,* 163–175.
Kimura, D., & Durnford, M. (1974). Normal studies on the function of the right hemisphere in vision. In S. J. Dimond & J. G. Beaumont (Eds.), *Hemisphere function in the human brain* (pp. 25–47). London: Paul Elek.
Kinsbourne, M. (1970). The cerebral basis of lateral asymmetries in attention. In A. F. Sanders (Ed.), *Attention and performance III* (pp. 193–201). Amsterdam: North-Holland.
Kinsbourne, M. (1975). Cerebral dominance, learning, and cognition. In H. R. Myklebust (Ed.), *Progress in learning disabilities* (Vol. 3, pp. 201–218). New York: Grune & Stratton.
Kinsbourne, M. (1981). Single channel theory. In D. H. Holding (Ed.), *Human skills* (pp. 65–89). Chichester, Sussex: Wiley.
Kinsbourne, M., & Cook, J. (1971). Generalized and lateralized effects of concurrent verbalization on a unimanual skill. *The Quarterly Journal of Experimental Psychology, 23,* 341–345.
Kinsbourne, M., & Hicks, R. E. (1978). Functional cerebral space: A model for overflow, transfer and interference effects in human performance: A tutorial review. In J. Requin (Ed.), *Attention and performance VII* (pp. 345–362). Hillsdale, NJ: Erlbaum.
Kinsbourne, M., & Hiscock, M. (1977). Does cerebral dominance develop? In S. J. Segalowitz & F. A. Gruber (Eds.), *Language development and neurological theory* (pp. 171–191). New York: Academic Press.
Kinsbourne, M., & Hiscock, M. (1983a). Asymmetries of dual-task performance. In J. B. Hellige (Ed.), *Cerebral hemisphere asymmetry: Method, theory, and application* (pp. 255–334). New York: Praeger.
Kinsbourne, M., & Hiscock, M. (1983b). The normal and deviant development of functional lateralization of the brain. In M. M. Haith & J. J. Campos (Eds.), *Handbook of child psychology* (4th ed.): *Vol. 2. Infancy and developmental psychobiology* (pp. 157–280). New York: Wiley.
Kinsbourne, M., & McMurray, J. (1975). The effect of cerebral dominance on time sharing between speaking and tapping by preschool children. *Child Development, 46,* 240–242.
Klein, S. P., & Rosenfield, W. D. (1980). The hemispheric specialization for linguistic and non-linguistic tactile stimuli in third grade children. *Cortex, 16,* 205–212.
Knox, C., & Kimura, D. (1970). Cerebral processing of nonverbal sounds in boys and girls. *Neuropsychologia, 8,* 227–237.
Kraft, R. H. (1981). The relationship between right-handed children's assessed and familial handedness and lateral specialization. *Neuropsychologia, 19,* 697–705.
Kraft, R. H. (1982). The relationship of ear specialization to degree of task difficulty, sex and lateral preference. *Perceptual and Motor Skills, 54,* 703–714.
Kraft, R. H. (1984). Lateral specialization and verbal/spatial ability in preschool children: Age, sex and familial handedness differences. *Neuropsychologia, 22,* 319–335.
Krashen, S. D. (1973). Lateralization, language learning, and the critical period: Some new evidence. *Language Learning, 23,* 63–74.
Kuhn, G. M. (1973). The phi coefficient as an index of ear differences in dichotic listening. *Cortex, 9,* 450–456.
LaBreche, T. M., Manning, A. A., Goble, W., & Markman, R. (1977). Hemispheric specialization for linguistic and nonlinguistic tactual perception in a congenitally deaf population. *Cortex, 13,* 184–194.
Larsen, S. (1984). Developmental changes in the pattern of ear asymmetry as revealed by a dichotic listening task. *Cortex, 20,* 5–17.
Larsen, S., & Hakonsen, K. (1983). Absence of ear asymmetry in blind children on a dichotic listening task compared to sighted controls. *Brain and Language, 18,* 192–198.

LeDoux, J. E., Wilson, D. H., & Gazzaniga, M. S. (1977). Manipulo-spatial aspects of cerebral lateralization: Clues to the origin of lateralization. *Neuropsychologia, 15,* 743–750.

Lenneberg, E. H. (1967). *Biological foundations of language.* New York: Wiley.

Levy, J. (1977). The correlation of the phi function of the difference score with performance and its relevance to laterality experiments. *Cortex, 13,* 458–464.

Levy, J., & Reid, M. (1978). Variations in cerebral organization as a function of handedness, hand posture in writing and sex. *Journal of Experimental Psychology: General, 107,* 119–144.

Lewandowski, L. (1982). Hemispheric asymmetries in children. *Perceptual and Motor Skills, 54,* 1011–1019.

Lokker, R., & Morais, J. (1985). Ear differences in children at two years of age. *Neuropsychologia, 23,* 127–129.

Lomas, J. (1980). Competition within the left hemisphere between speaking and unimanual tasks performed without visual guidance. *Neuropsychologia, 18,* 141–150.

Lomas, J., & Kimura, D. (1976). Intrahemispheric interaction between speaking and sequential manual activity. *Neuropsychologia, 14,* 23–33.

Mackay, M., & Hiscock, M. (1986). Attentional shifting in dichotic listening: A signal detection analysis [Abstract]. *Canadian Psychology, 27,* 368.

Marcel, T., Katz, L., & Smith, M. (1974). Laterality and reading proficiency. *Neuropsychologia, 12,* 131–139.

Marcel, T., & Rajan, P. (1975). Lateral specialization for recognition of words and faces in good and poor readers. *Neuropsychologia, 13,* 489–497.

Marcotte, A. C., & LaBarba, R. C. (1985). Cerebral lateralization for speech in deaf and normal children. *Brain and Language, 26,* 244–258.

Marshall, J. C., Caplan, D., & Holmes, J. M. (1975). The measure of laterality. *Neuropsychologia, 13,* 315–321.

Marzi, C. A. (1986). Transfer of visual information after unilateral input to the brain. *Brain and Cognition, 5,* 163–173.

McFarland, K., & Ashton, R. (1975). A developmental study of the influence of cognitive activity on an ongoing manual task. *Acta Psychologia, 39,* 447–456.

McFarland, K., & Ashton, R. (1978a). The influence of brain lateralization of function on a manual skill. *Cortex, 14,* 102–111.

McFarland, K., & Ashton, R. (1978b). The influence of concurrent task difficulty on manual performance. *Neuropsychologia, 16,* 735–741.

McFarland, K., & Ashton, R. (1978c). The lateralized effects of concurrent cognitive and motor performance. *Perception and Psychophysics, 23,* 344–349.

McFie, J. (1952). Cerebral dominance in cases of reading disability. *Journal of Neurological and Neurosurgical Psychiatry, 15,* 194–199.

McKeever, W. F., & Huling, M. D. (1970). Lateral dominance in tachistoscopic word recognition of children at two levels of ability. *Quarterly Journal of Experimental Psychology, 22,* 600–604.

McKeever, W. F., & Van Eys, P. (1986). Evidence that fixation digits can contribute to visual field asymmetries in lateralized tachistoscopic tasks. *Brain and Cognition, 5,* 443–451.

Merola, J. L., & Liederman, J. (1985). Developmental changes in hemispheric independence. *Child Development, 56,* 1184–1194.

Messina, T. M. F., & Fogliani, A. M. (1981). Children's reaction times to verbal and nonverbal tachistoscopic stimuli exposed to the left and right visual hemifields. *Perceptual and Motor Skills, 52,* 459–462.

Miller, L. K. (1971). Developmental differences in the field of view during tachistoscopic presentation. *Child Development, 42,* 1543–1551.

Miller, L. K. (1973). Developmental differences in the field of view during covert and overt search. *Child Development, 44,* 247–252.

Miller, L. K. (1981). Perceptual independence of the hemifields in children and adults. *Journal of Experimental Child Psychology, 32,* 298–312.

Miller, L. K. (1984). Sources of visual field interference in children and adults. *Journal of Experimental Child Psychology, 37,* 141–157.

Miller, L. K., & Turner, S. (1973). Development of hemifield differences in word recognition. *Journal of Educational Psychology, 65,* 172–176.

Mirabile, P. J., Porter, R. J., Jr., Hughes, L. F., & Berlin, C. I. (1978). Dichotic lag effect in children 7 to 15. *Developmental Psychology, 14,* 277–285.

Mishkin, M., & Forgays, D. G. (1952). Word recognition as a function of retinal locus. *Journal of Experimental Psychology, 43,* 43–48.

Moreau, T., & Milner, P. (1981). Lateral differences in the detection of touched body parts in young children. *Developmental Psychology, 17,* 351–356.

Morris, R., Bakker, D., Satz, P., & Van der Vlugt, H. (1984). Dichotic listening ear asymmetry: Patterns of longitudinal development. *Brain and Language, 22,* 49–66.

Moscovitch, M. (1977). The development of lateralization of language functions and its relation to cognitive and linguistic development: A review and some theoretical speculations. In S. J. Segalowitz & F. A. Gruber (Eds.), *Language development and neurological theory* (pp. 193–211). New York: Academic Press.

Nagafuchi, M. (1970). Development of dichotic and monaural hearing abilities in young children. *Acta Otolaryngologica, 69,* 409–414.

Nunnally, J. C. (1967). *Psychometric theory.* New York: McGraw-Hill.

Obrzut, J. E., Boliek, C. A., & Obrzut, A. (1986). The effect of stimulus type and directed attention on dichotic listening with children. *Journal of Experimental Child Psychology, 41,* 198–209.

Obrzut, J. E., Hynd, G. W., Obrzut, A., & Leitgeb, J. L. (1980). Timesharing and dichotic listening asymmetries in normal and learning-disabled children. *Brain and Language, 11,* 181–194.

Obrzut, J. E., Hynd, G. W., Obrzut, A., & Pirozzolo, F. J. (1981). Effect of directed attention on cerebral asymmetries in normal and learning-disabled children. *Developmental Psychology, 17,* 118–125.

Obrzut, J. E., Obrzut, A., Bryden, M. P., & Bartels, S. G. (1985). Information processing and speech lateralization in learning-disabled children. *Brain and Language, 25,* 87–101.

Olson, M. E. (1973). Laterality differences in tachistoscopic word recognition in normal and delayed readers in elementary school. *Neuropsychologia, 11,* 343–350.

Orbach, J. (1953). Retinal locus as a factor in the recognition of visually perceived words. *American Journal of Psychology, 65,* 555–562.

Orsini, D. L., Satz, P., Soper, H. V., & Light, R. K. (1985). The role of familial sinistrality in cerebral organization. *Neuropsychologia, 23,* 223–232.

Orton, S. T. (1937). *Reading, writing and speech problems in children.* New York: Norton.

Papcun, G., Krashen, S. D., Terbeek, D., Remington, R., & Harshman, R. (1974). Is the left hemisphere specialized for speech language and/or something else? *Journal of the Acoustical Society of America, 55,* 319–327.

Peters, M. (1980). Why the preferred hand taps more quickly than the non-preferred hand: Three experiments on handedness. *Canadian Journal of Psychology, 34,* 62–71.

Piazza, D. M. (1977). Cerebral lateralization in young children as measured by dichotic listening and finger tapping tasks. *Neuropsychologia, 15,* 417–425.

Porter, R. J., Jr., & Berlin, C. I. (1975). On interpreting developmental changes in the dichotic right-ear advantage. *Brain and Language, 2,* 186–200.

Posluszny, R., & Barton, K. (1981). Dichhaptic task performance as a function of ability pattern, sex, and hand preference. *Perceptual and Motor Skills, 53,* 435–438.

Posner, M. I. (1982). Cumulative development of attentional theory. *American Psychologist, 37,* 168–179.

Provins, K. A., & Glencross, D. J. (1968). Handwriting, typewriting and handedness. *Quarterly Journal of Experimental Psychology, 20,* 282–289.

Reynolds, D. McQ., & Jeeves, M. A. (1978a). A developmental study of hemisphere specialization for alphabetic stimuli. *Cortex, 14,* 259–267.

Reynolds, D. McQ., & Jeeves, M. A. (1978b). A developmental study of hemisphere specialization for recognition of faces in normal subjects. *Cortex, 14,* 511–520.

Richardson, J. T. E. (1976). How to measure laterality. *Neuropsychologia, 14,* 135–136.

Rose, S. A. (1984). Developmental changes in hemispheric specialization for tactual processing in very young children: Evidence from cross-modal transfer. *Developmental Psychology, 20,* 568–574.

Rose, S. A. (1985). Influence of concurrent auditory input on tactual processing in very young children: Developmental changes. *Developmental Psychology, 21,* 168–175.

Ross, P., & Turkewitz, G. (1981). Individual differences in cerebral asymmetries for facial recognition. *Cortex, 17,* 199–213.

Rudel, R. G., Denckla, M. B., & Hirsch, S. (1977). The development of left-hand superiority for discriminating Braille configurations. *Neurology, 27,* 160–164.

Rudel, R. G., Denckla, M. B., & Spalten, E. (1974). The functional asymmetry of Braille letter learning in normal, sighted children. *Neurology, 24,* 733–738.

Satz, P. (1976). Cerebral dominance and reading disability: An old problem revisited. In R. M. Knights & D. J. Bakker (Eds.), *The neuropsychology of learning disorders* (pp. 273–294). Baltimore, MD: University Park Press.

Satz, P. (1977). Laterality tests: An inferential problem. *Cortex, 13,* 208–212.

Satz, P., Bakker, D. J., Teunissen, J., Goebel, R., & Van der Vlugt, H. (1975). Developmental parameters of the ear asymmetry: A multivariate approach. *Brain and Language, 2,* 171–185.

Satz, P., Rardin, D., & Ross, J. (1971). An evaluation of a theory of specific developmental dyslexia. *Child Development, 42,* 2009–2021.

Satz, P., & Sparrow, S. (1970). Specific developmental dyslexia: A theoretical formulation. In D. J. Bakker & P. Satz (Eds.), *Specific reading disability: Advances in theory and method* (pp. 17–39). Rotterdam: Rotterdam University Press.

Saxby, L., & Bryden, M. P. (1984). Left-ear superiority in children for processing auditory emotional material. *Developmental Psychology, 20,* 72–80.

Saxby, L., & Bryden, M. P. (1985). Left visual-field advantage in children for processing visual emotional stimuli. *Developmental Psychology, 21,* 253–261.

Schaller, M. J., & Dziadosz, G. M. (1976). Developmental changes in foveal tachistoscopic recognition between prereading and reading children. *Developmental Psychology, 12,* 321–327.

Schulman-Galambos, C. (1977). Dichotic listening performance in elementary and college students. *Neuropsychologia, 15,* 577–584.

Searleman, A. (1977). A review of right hemisphere linguistic capabilities. *Psychological Bulletin, 84,* 503–528.

Segalowitz, S. J., & Gruber, F. A. (1977). *Language development and neurological theory.* New York: Academic Press.

Semmes, J., Weinstein, S., Ghent, L., & Teuber, H-L. (1960). *Somatosensory changes after penetrating brain wounds in man.* Cambridge, MA: Harvard University Press.

Sergent, J. (1982). Basic determinants in visual-field effects with special reference to the Hannay *et al.* (1981) study. *Brain and Language, 16,* 158–164.

Sergent, J. (1984). Processing of visually presented vowels in the cerebral hemispheres. *Brain and Language, 21,* 136–146.

Sergent, J. (1986). Prolegomena to the use of the tachistoscope in neuropsychological research. *Brain and Cognition, 5,* 127–130.

Sexton, M. A., & Geffen, G. (1979). Development of three strategies of attention in dichotic monitoring. *Developmental Psychology, 15,* 299–310.

Silverberg, R., Bentin, S., Gaziel, T., Obler, L. K., & Albert, M. L. (1979). Shift of visual field preference for English words in native Hebrew speakers. *Brain and Language, 8,* 184–190.

Simon, T. J., & Sussman, H. M. (1987). The dual task paradigm: Speech dominance or manual dominance? *Neuropsychologia, 25,* 559–570.

Sommers, R. K., & Taylor, M. L. (1972). Cerebral speech dominance in language-disordered and normal children. *Cortex, 8,* 224–232.

Spellacy, F. J., & Blumstein, S. (1970). The influence of language set on ear preference in phoneme recognition. *Cortex, 6,* 430–439.

Sperry, R. W. (1968). Hemispheric disconnection and unity in conscious awareness. *American Psychologist, 23,* 723–733.

Sperry, R. (1982). Some effects of disconnecting the cerebral hemispheres. *Science, 217,* 1223–1226.

Sperry, R. W., Gazzaniga, M. S., & Bogen, J. E. (1969). Interhemispheric relationships: The neocortical commissures; syndromes of hemisphere disconnection. In P. J. Vinken & G. W. Bruyn (Eds.), *Handbook of clinical neurology* (Vol. 4, pp. 273–290). Amsterdam: North-Holland.

Sprott, D. A., & Bryden, M. P. (1983). Some problems with "Some problems with Bryden and Sprott's 'Statistical determination of degree of lateralization.' " *Neuropsychologia, 21,* 299–300.

Stedman's Medical Dictionary (24th ed.). (1982). Baltimore and London: Williams and Wilkins.

Stone, M. A. (1980). Measures of laterality and spurious correlation. *Neuropsychologia, 18,* 339–345.

Strauss, E., Gaddes, W. H., & Wada, J. (1987). Performance on a free-recall dichotic listening task and cerebral speech dominance determined by the carotid amytal test. *Neuropsychologia, 25,* 747–754.

Strauss, E., & Wada, J. (1983). Lateral preferences and cerebral speech dominance. *Cortex, 19,* 165–177.

Studdert-Kennedy, M., & Shankweiler, D. P. (1970). Hemispheric specialization for speech perception. *Journal of the Acoustical Society of America, 48,* 579–594.

Sussman, H. M. (1982). Contrastive patterns of intra-hemispheric interference to verbal and spatial concurrent tasks in right-handed, left-handed and stuttering populations. *Neuropsychologia, 20,* 675–684.

Sussman, H. M. (1984). A reply to Kee's comments on Hughes and Sussman's time-sharing study of cerebral laterality in language-disordered and normal children. *Brain and Language, 22,* 357–358.

Tomlinson-Keasey, C., & Kelly, R. R. (1979). A task analysis of hemispheric functioning. *Neuropsychologia, 17,* 345–351.

Tomlinson-Keasey, C., Kelly, R. R., & Burton, J. K. (1978). Hemispheric changes in information processing during development. *Developmental Psychology, 14,* 214–223.

Turkewitz, G., & Ross-Kossak, P. (1984). Multiple modes of right-hemisphere information processing: Age and sex differences in facial recognition. *Developmental Psychology, 20,* 95–103.

Turner, S., & Miller, L. K. (1975). Some boundary conditions for laterality effects in children. *Developmental Psychology, 11,* 342–352.

Van Duyne, H. J., Gargiulo, R. M., & Gonter, M. A. (1984). The effect of word presentation rate on monaural and dichotic ear-asymmetry in school age children. *International Journal of Clinical Neuropsychology, 6,* 175–183.

Van Lancker, D., & Fromkin, V. A. (1977). Hemispheric specialization of pitch and "tone": Evidence from Thai. *Journal of Phonetics, 1,* 101–109.

Vargha-Khadem, F. (1980). Hemispheric specialization for the processing of tactual stimuli in congenitally deaf and hearing children. *Cortex, 16,* 277–286.

Vargha-Khadem, F., & Corballis, M. C. (1979). Cerebral asymmetry in infants. *Brain and Language, 8,* 1–9.

Waber, D. P. (1977). Sex differences in mental abilities, hemispheric lateralization, and rate of physical growth at adolescence. *Developmental Psychology, 13,* 29–38.

Warrington, E. (1981). *The significance of laterality effects.* Paper presented at the annual meeting of the International Neuropsychological Society, Atlanta, Georgia.

Weinstein, S., & Sersen, E. A. (1961). Tactual sensitivity as a function of handedness and laterality. *Journal of Comparative and Physiological Psychology, 54,* 665–669.

Wexler, B. E., & Halwes, T. (1983). Increasing the power of dichotic methods: The fused rhymed words test. *Neuropsychologia, 21,* 59–66.

Whitaker, H. A., & Ojemann, G. (1977). Lateralization of higher cortical functions: A critique. In S. J. Dimond & D. A. Blizard (Eds.), *Evolution and lateralization of the brain. Annals of the New York Academy of Sciences, 299,* 459–473.

White, M. J. (1969). Laterality differences in perception: A review. *Psychological Bulletin, 72,* 387–405.

White, M. J. (1972). Hemispheric asymmetries in tachistoscopic information-processing. *British Journal of Psychology, 63,* 497–508.

White, N., & Kinsbourne, M. (1980). Does speech output control lateralize over time? Evidence from verbal–manual time-sharing tasks. *Brain and Language, 10,* 215–223.

Williams, S. (1982). Dichotic lateral asymmetry: The effects of grammatical structure and telephone usage. *Neuropsychologia, 20,* 457–464.

Willis, W. G., & Hynd, G. W. (1987). Lateralized interference effects: Evidence for a processing style by modality interaction. *Brain and Cognition, 6,* 112–126.

Witelson, S. F. (1974). Hemispheric specialization for linguistic and nonlinguistic tactual perception using a dichotomous stimulation technique. *Cortex, 10,* 3–17.

Witelson, S. F. (1976). Sex and the single hemisphere: Right hemisphere specialization for spatial processing. *Science, 193,* 425–427.

Witelson, S. F. (1977a). Developmental dyslexia: Two right hemispheres and none left. *Science, 195,* 309–311.

Witelson, S. F. (1977b). Early hemispheric specialization and interhemispheric plasticity: An empirical and theoretical review. In S. J. Segalowitz & F. A. Gruber (Eds.), *Language development and neurological theory* (pp. 213–287). New York: Academic Press.

Witelson, S. F. (1977c). Neural and cognitive correlates of developmental dyslexia: Age and sex differences. In C. Shagass, S. Gershon, & A. J. Friedhoff (Eds.), *Psychopathology and brain dysfunction* (pp. 15–49). New York: Raven Press.

Witelson, S. F., & Rabinovich, M. S. (1971). Children's recall strategies in dichotic listening. *Journal of Experimental Child Psychology, 12,* 106–113.

Woods, B. T., & Teuber, H-L. (1978). Changing patterns of childhood aphasia. *Annals of Neurology, 32,* 239–246.

Yamamoto, M. (1980). Developmental changes for hemispheric specialization of tactile recognition by normal children. *Perceptual and Motor Skills, 51,* 325–326.

Yamamoto, M. (1984). Intra- and inter-hemispheric tactile identification matching in young children. *Japanese Psychological Research, 26,* 120–124.

Yamamoto, M., & Hatta, T. (1982). Sex, task difference, and hemispheric differences in somatosensory function of normal children. *Psychologia, 25,* 115–120.

Yeni-Komshian, G. H., Isenberg, D., & Goldberg, H. (1975). Cerebral dominance and reading disability: Left visual field deficit in poor readers. *Neuropsychologia, 13,* 83–94.

Yeni-Komshian, G. H., & Paul-Brown, D. (1982). Perception of temporally competing speech stimuli in preschool children. *Brain and Language, 17,* 166–179.

Young, A. W. (1982). Asymmetry of cerebral hemispheric function during development. In J. W. T. Dickerson & H. McGurk (Eds.), *Brain and behavioural development* (pp. 168–202). Glasgow: Blackie.

Young, A. W., & Bion, P. J. (1979). Hemispheric laterality effects in the enumeration of visually presented collections of dots by children. *Neuropsychologia, 17,* 99–102.

Young, A. W., & Bion, P. J. (1980). Absence of any developmental trend in right hemisphere superiority for face recognition. *Cortex, 16,* 213–221.

Young, A. W., & Bion, P. J. (1981). Identification and storage of line drawings presented to the left and right cerebral hemispheres of adults and children. *Cortex, 17,* 459–464.

Young, A. W., & Ellis, H. D. (1976). An experimental investigation of developmental differences in ability to recognise faces presented to the left and right cerebral hemispheres. *Neuropsychologia, 14,* 495–498.

Zaidel, E. (1978). Auditory language comprehension in the right hemisphere following cerebral commissurotomy and hemispherectomy: A comparison with child language and aphasia. In A. Carramazza & E. B. Zurif (Eds.), *Language acquisition and language breakdown: Parallels and divergencies* (pp. 229–275). Baltimore, MD: Johns Hopkins University Press.

Zaidel, E. (1983). Disconnection syndrome as a model for laterality effects in the normal brain. In J. B. Hellige (Ed.), *Cerebral hemisphere asymmetry: Method, theory and application* (pp. 95–151). New York: Praeger.

6

Electrophysiological Indices of the Early Development of Lateralization for Language and Cognition, and Their Implications for Predicting Later Development

DENNIS L. MOLFESE
JACQUELINE C. BETZ
Southern Illinois University at Carbondale

A number of advances in the study of the electrophysiological correlates related to the development of lateralization have been noted since the first serious study in 1972 (Molfese, 1972). Prior to that time, the general belief had been that the two hemispheres of the brain were equally capable of supporting language functions and that any signs of lateralization of function would not appear until sometime between 2 and 3 years of age (Lenneberg, 1967, p. 67). The electrophysiological research investigating hemisphere differences and their development has gone through a steady progression in development itself. Our belief is that this work can be broken down into four distinct research periods or stages. In the first stage of this work, between 1972 and 1976, researchers first concentrated their efforts on determining whether this methodological tool could be used to investigate functional lateralized differences between the hemispheres in young infants prior to the onset of language and speech development (Molfese, 1972; 1973; Molfese, Freeman, & Palermo, 1975; Molfese, Nunez, Seibert, & Ramaniah, 1976). Once it was ascertained that evoked potential and EEG procedures could detect differences in hemispheric responding in early infancy, the next stage involved a series of studies investigating the stimulus characteristics that evoked such lateralized responses. It was hoped that by identifying the specific stimulus characteristics that triggered such lateralized responses, one could begin to unravel the underlying mechanisms that subserved these lateralized functions (Molfese & Molfese, 1979a, 1979b, 1980). Given the general belief that early signs of lateralization could be used to identify children at risk for developmental disorders (Orton, 1937), the next logical stage for this research approach was to use these electrophysiological procedures to determine whether such evidence of early lateralized processes could be used to predict later language development (Molfese & Molfese, 1985, 1988; Molfese & Searock, 1986). Finally, the current stage of research finds researchers pressing the electrophysiological procedures even further in hopes of studying the emergence of early word meanings and their underlying concepts (Molfese *et al.* 1985).

This chapter will review the investigations of early lateralization through these four research stages. First, however, a general introduction concerning evoked potential procedures is provided for readers who may not be readily familiar with the technique.

ELECTROPHYSIOLOGICAL PROCEDURES

To those unfamiliar with the characteristics of an evoked potential recorded from the scalp, it may appear at first glance to be only a squiggly wave running across a piece of paper or a computer screen. In fact, the evoked potential is a synchronized portion of the ongoing EEG pattern. Basically, such evoked potential waveforms are thought to reflect changes in brain activity over time as reflected by changes in the amplitude or height of the wave at different points in its time course. What distinguishes the evoked potential from the more traditional EEG measure is that the event-related potential (ERP) is a portion of the ongoing EEG activity of the brain that is time-locked to the onset of some event in the infant's environment. The ongoing EEG activity reflects a wide range of neural activity related to the myriad of neural and body self-regulating systems as well as the various sensory and cognitive functions ongoing in the brain at that time. The ERP, on the other hand, because of this time-locked feature, has been shown more likely to reflect both general and specific aspects of the evoking stimulus and the infant or young child's perceptions and decisions regarding the stimulus. It is this time-locking feature that enables researchers to pinpoint, with some degree of certainty, portions of the electrical response that occurred while the child's attention was focused on a discrete event.

The ERP recording procedure involves a number of steps. First, the infant's head is measured and positions are marked to indicate where electrodes are to be placed. Next, these positions are cleaned with a pumice paste to lower skin impedances, thereby assuring that the electrodes will be able to detect a better signal. The pumice paste is then cleaned off and a small amount of electrode-conducting paste is rubbed onto the scalp. Small disk-shaped electrodes are then filled with the electrode cream and placed on the infant's scalp at these prepared positions. The electrodes are connected via wires to amplifiers that amplify the ERP by 20,000 to 100,000 times. These amplifiers also contain filters that keep out some of the system and biological noise that the investigator does not want to study. The output from these amplifiers is connected in turn to a computer, which collects the ERPs from each electrode for each stimulus presented. Once all the electrodes are in place and connected to the amplifiers and the computer, the stimuli can be presented to the infant while it is in a reasonably quiet state.

The ERP detected at the scalp, of course, is not by any means an exact and completely stable pattern reflecting only those discrete neural events directly related to the evoking stimulus, the task, or the subject's state. Clearly, it is in part only a by-product of the brain's bioelectrical response to such an event, which begins at levels well below that of the cortex as the stimulus information is transformed by the sensory systems and progresses through the brain stem, into the midbrain, and on upward into the higher centers of the brain. Moreover, such signals that originate within the brain must travel through a variety of tissues of different densities, conductivity, and composition (e.g., neurons, glial cells, fiber tracts, cerebral spinal fluid, bone, muscle) before they reach the recording electrode placed on the scalp of an infant. Consequently, the final version of the ERP recorded at the scalp is a composite of a variety of complex factors, some of which relate directly to the stimulus situation and some of which do not. Because of this moment-by-moment variability in the ERP, which results from moment-by-moment changes in the physiology of the infant, in most cases researchers have resorted to a system of collecting a number of ERPs to a stimulus within a single recording session, summing these responses, and then calculating an averaged evoked response. It is reasoned that this averaged response is more likely to have buried within it the repetitive activity that reflects the processing of the stimulus from one time to the next. The non-stimulus-related activity that is not time-locked to the onset of the stimulus would be expected to average out or be minimized in the averaged waveform of the ERP. Subsequent analyses of the ERP are then conducted on the averaged waveforms. These analysis approaches have a range of options, including amplitude and latency measures, area measures, discriminant function procedures, and other multivariate approaches including principal-components analysis.

The ERP procedure has a number of strengths, including its ability to employ identical procedures with all participants, regardless of age, so that direct comparisons can be made between infants and adults in terms of discrimination abilities. Although the waveshapes of the ERP's will change from infancy to adulthood, one can assess whether the brain responses at these different ages discriminate reliably between different stimulus, subject, and task characteristics. Moreover, the ERP procedures can be used to obtain response information from subjects who either have difficulty in responding in a normal fashion (as in the case of individuals with brain damage) or who cannot respond because of language or maturity factors (as with young infants and children). They also provide information concerning both between-hemisphere differences as well as within-hemisphere differences. Finally, the procedure provides time-related information. It can reveal the onset of one stimulus relative to another and provide information about the different points in time when such information is detected.

On the other hand, the reader should also keep in mind is that the ERP procedure is *not* some infallible technique that will magically answer all of our most probing neuropsychological questions. Like all other neuropsychological procedures, it is a technique with its advantages and disadvantages, its strengths and weaknesses. Our bias is that the ERP technique is strongest when coupled with other procedures in an experimental situation based firmly on an established research literature, but where the procedure can address questions in part beyond the limits of more traditional techniques. At the same time, one major area of weakness results from the lack of experienced investigators with competencies in language and cognitive development. It is difficult for an area to advance, a tool to be developed, or rapid progress to be made with so few involved. This chapter, however, is not the appropriate forum for an in-depth treatise on these issues (see Molfese, 1983).

STAGE 1: EVIDENCE FOR FUNCTIONAL LATERALITY FOR SPEECH PERCEPTION IN YOUNG INFANTS

The first evidence of functional lateralization in early infancy can be traced to a 1972 dissertation. Investigators at that time generally held to the equipotentiality model of Lenneberg and others, although there had been no direct test of this model. Lenneberg, on the basis of Basser's (1962) data, had argued that the two hemispheres remained unspecialized for language until sometime during language development, between 2 and 3 years of age. Basser had reviewed 102 cases involving infants and young children with hemiplegia of early onset. Hemispherectomies were performed in 35 of these cases either before productive language skills could be observed or after such skills had emerged. Although his paper reviews a number of the 102 cases, the 35 hemispherectomy cases are most relevant to Lenneberg's argument. There were 17 cases of left hemispherectomy and 18 cases of right hemispherectomy carried out between 20 months and 31 *years* of age. These cases were further divided into two distinct groups: Group 1, composed of 25 cases (12 left and 13 right hemispherectomies) who suffered the lesion *before* speech onset, and Group 2, which consisted of 10 cases (5 left and 5 right hemispherectomies) who experienced the lesion *after* speech onset. In examining the postoperative data to evaluate the impact of the hemispherectomy on speech abilities, Basser reported that for Group 1, 10 left and 10 right hemispherectomized children displayed *no* change in language skills. However, an examination of the postoperative group who underwent surgery *after* speech onset showed some speech loss for a time after surgery. Consequently, from Basser's data it appeared that speech skills were disturbed primarily if the surgery was carried out on individuals who had developed speech prior to the lesion. Importantly, however, no differences were noted between children as a function of side of hemispherectomy. Three left and three right hemispherectomized children responded similarly in Group 2. Basser's data, then, would suggest that the hemispheres are equipotential for speech both *before* and *after* speech onset! Curiously, both Basser and Lenneberg used the data from Group 1 to support an equipotential model prior to speech onset, while ignoring the data from Group 2.

At any rate, the argument that language development and lateralization would emerge simultaneously seemed a very cogent one at the time. Given that many language skills emerge sometime after 18 months of age, it seemed reasonable, given the relationship thought to exist between lateralization and language, that lateralization of these skills should also occur during this time. However, a now classic paper by Eimas, Siqueland, Jusczyk, and Vigorito (1971) indicated that young infants, even prior to 4 months of age, possessed some ability to discriminate between speech sounds in a manner similar to that long noted in adults. Using a nonnutritive sucking procedure, Eimas *et al.* were able to demonstrate that these young infants could discriminate between voiced and voiceless consonant sounds. Molfese speculated that if such young infants were able to discriminate between speech sounds in a manner similar to adults, then they might in fact possess some early language-related skills. If, indeed, there was some relationship between language and laterality onset, then the presence of such early language perception skills might signal the presence of early lateralization for such skills. Given that such skills would be expected to increase with further language development, Molfese speculated that the lateralization of these skills would also increase as the infant developed. To this end, Molfese designed and executed an evoked-potential study designed to assess changes in hemisphere differences from early in infancy into the childhood and adult years (Molfese, 1972, 1973).

A series of speech and nonspeech sounds were presented aurally through a speaker positioned over the listener's head. Auditory event-related potentials were recorded in response to each sound from the left and right temporal regions (T3 and T4 of the Ten–Twenty International Electrode System; Jasper, 1958) of 10 infants between 1 week and 10 months of age (mean age = 5.8 months), 11 children between 4 and 11 years of age (mean age = 6.0 years), and 10 adults from 23 to 29 years of age (mean age = 25.9 years). The speech stimuli consisted of the consonant–vowel syllables *ba* and *dae* and the monosyllabic words *boy* and *dog*. The nonspeech materials consisted of a piano chord and a burst of white noise. Measures of differences in the amplitudes of the auditory evoked responses between the largest positive peak and the largest negative peak within a response indicated that hemispheric differences did in fact exist in these infants. In general, the magnitude of the left-hemisphere auditory ERP was greater than that for the right hemisphere in response to the speech stimuli for 27 of the 31 individuals tested. This relationship, however, was reversed for the nonspeech materials. In the latter case, the amplitudes of the right-hemisphere auditory evoked responses (AERs) were greater than the left when evoked by the piano chord (for 30 of 31 subjects) and noise (for 29 of 31 subjects). Since the proportion of subjects of each age level showing lateralized patterns of responding did not change, the data were interpreted to indicate that lateralized responses were as prevalent in the infant group as in the adult group. Hemisphere differences clearly were present in young infants, long before the period predicted by Lenneberg. However, as noted by Molfese *et al.* (1975), the magnitude of such hemispheric differences decreased with age. This finding made these early results even more puzzling because they contradicted the long-held belief that hemispheric differences would increase during early development.

A subsequent study by Molfese, Nunez, Seibert, and Ramaniah (1976) also noted hemispheric effects with young infants. In this case they presented five different sounds to a group of 14 newborn infants less than 2 days of age. The stimuli included a consonant–vowel syllable, [gae], a vowel, [ae], two multiple formant nonspeech sounds with formant frequencies that matched the mean frequency of each of the speech stimuli, but which were 1 Hz in width, and a 500-Hz tone. Analyses of the AERs, which included a principal-components procedure followed by an analysis of variance, indicated that a late-occurring portion of neonates' brain responses (which peaked 880 msec following stimulus onset) discriminated sounds that contained a rapid initial frequency transition from those that did not. This response occurred for both speech and nonspeech sounds. A second portion of the auditory ERP reflected hemispheric differences that were most marked 624 msec following stimulus onset. Finally, the AERs of the male infants differed from those recorded from the female infants in the region approximately 600 msec following stimulus onset.

Other laboratories also noted evidence of early lateralized responses to speech sounds. Barnet, de Sotillo, and Campos (1974) recorded AERs from anterior parietal scalp locations (C3 and C4) of normal and malnourished infants between 5 and 12 months of age (mean age = 8 months) while clicks and the infants' names were presented. Only the normal infants showed a clear-cut lateralized pattern of responding. Eleven of 16 infants produced larger left-hemisphere than right-hemisphere responses to the speech stimuli, whereas three infants generated larger right-hemisphere responses. No differences were noted for two infants. Larger right-hemisphere responses were noted across all these infants for the click sounds.

Davis and Wada (1977) used a somewhat different procedure to analyze the auditory and visual evoked responses than was used by Molfese or Barnet. They recorded evoked responses from 16 infants from 2 to 11 weeks of age. However, instead of speech sounds or names, they used an auditory stimulus consisting of 0.1-ms click presented 40 times through earphones placed on the infants's chest approximately 4 inches from the ears. The visual stimulus employed consisted of a 10-μs flash presented via a photostimulator located approximately 30 inches from the infant's face. Scalp potentials were recorded from the left and right temporal (T3 and T4) and occipital (O1 and O2) scalp locations with activity referred to linked ear references. The waveforms were analyzed using two different analysis procedures: coherence and power spectra analysis. The coherence procedure provided information concerning the degree of similarity in the form of the waves. Davis and Wada noted that the form of the waveforms evoked by the auditory stimuli were more similar within the left than in the right hemisphere. No hemispheric differences, however, occurred in response to the visual stimuli. The second analysis procedure, power spectra analysis, which measured the amount of different frequencies in the waveforms, also noted lateralized responses. Frequencies elicited by the visual stimulus in the 3- to 9-Hz range were greater for the right occipital than the right temporal site, while no differences were noted within the left hemisphere. This effect was reversed for the auditory click stimulus, with greater power noted for the left temporal than for the occipital site, while no differences were noted between the right temporal and occipital sites. Interestingly, the results of the Davis and Wada paper were among the first to point out differences occurring within hemispheres as well as between hemispheres. Such an effect marked a substantial departure from previous infant and adult work, which simply focused on between-hemisphere differences.

Investigators using other electrophysiological procedures successfully noted early hemispheric differences. Gardiner, Schulman, and Walter (1973) and Gardiner and Walter

(1977) reported hemispheric differences for EEG power distributions in four infants 6 months of age when the infants listened to continuous segments of speech and music. The EEG patterns were recorded over four locations on the scalp above each hemisphere (and referred to linked mastoids). Continuous plots of the laterality ratio versus time were recorded for each pair of symmetrical locations and then calculated from stimulus onset to offset. The parietal and temporal locations yielded hemispheric differences, with the largest changes occurring in the posterior temporal–parietal areas. For all infants, the power spectrum between 3 and 5 Hz decreased over the left-hemisphere leads during the speech condition, whereas a similar decrease was noted over the right hemisphere leads during the music condition.

Early hemispheric differences were also noted when visual stimuli were presented (Crowell, Jones, Kapuniai, & Nakagawa, 1973; Crowell, Kapuniai, & Garbanati, 1979). Crowell *et al.* (1973) found evidence of differential hemispheric driving in the right hemisphere of newborn infants in response to presentations of rhythmic visual stimuli. Crowell *et al.* placed electrodes over the left (O1) and right occipital (O2) areas of 97 full-term infants. Repetitive light flashes were presented at 3 per second for 4 seconds. The EEG patterns were recorded during stimulation and later tested for evidence of photic driving—an increase in the EEG spectral frequency to the same frequency as the repetitive stimulus. Photic driving was found in 36 infants (37% of the total group tested). Of this latter group, 18 infants showed unilateral driving, with 16 showing right-hemisphere driving and two infants showing driving in the left hemisphere. Since adults in a similar situation show bilateral driving, the presence of a unilateral response in nearly 20% of the infants tested was thought to indicate the presence of early functional hemispheric differences, perhaps in the form of a more developed right-hemisphere occipital area.

Subsequently Crowell and his associates, who tested 217 infants at several ages, replicated these earlier findings and further noted that the lateralized differences appeared to decrease with age (Crowell, Kapuniai, & Garbanati, 1979). At 2 days of age, 12% of the infants showed bilateral driving, but at 30 days of age, 48% of the infants showed this pattern. Such results may be comparable to that reported by Molfese (as noted earlier), as concerns the decrease in hemispheric differences with age and could reflect changes in the manner in which the two hemispheres communicate with each other as the various commissures interconnecting them mature.

Finally, an investigation by Shucard, Shucard, Cummings, and Campos (1981) noted that female infants responded with greater left-hemisphere amplitude responses to tones used as "probe stimuli" during verbal and nonverbal stimulus presentations, whereas males produced larger right-hemisphere responses under these conditions. Eight male and 8 female infants between the ages of 10 weeks, 6 days and 13 weeks, 2 days were tested. Shucard *et al.* argued on the basis of these findings that hemisphere activation and subsequent differences in hemispheric responding are "more dependent on the sex of the infant than on the type of stimulus the infant is receiving" (p. 99).

Although the studies reviewed so far (and outlined in Table 6-1) indicate consistent findings of differential hemispheric responding to a variety of auditory and visual stimuli, it continued to remain unclear at that time how to interpret these findings. Did the two hemispheres discriminate between the speech and nonspeech materials on the basis of very discrete features, or did they respond at a more general level to collections of features? Or did the two hemispheres, early in development, simply respond to everything differently, perhaps as a function of the sex of the infant, as Shucard *et al.* argued? It was out of this early beginning that the next set of investigations into early hemispheric specialization developed.

Table 6-1. Studies in Which Researchers Have Identified Hemispheric Differences in Human Infants Using Electrophysiological Procedures

Study	Subjects/ages	Stimuli
Molfese, 1972	10 infants aged 7 days–10 mo.	2 syllables
Molfese, Freeman, & Palermo, 1975		2 words Piano chord Noise burst
Crowell, Jones, Kapuniai, & Nakagawa, 1973	97 neonates	Light flashes
Gardiner, Schulman, & Walter, 1973	4 normal infants aged 6 mo.	Speech and nonspeech segments
Barnet, de Sotillo, & Campos, 1974	16 normal infants and 16 malnourished infants, aged 5–12 mo.	Infants' own names
Molfese, Nunez, Seibert, & Ramaniah, 1976	Full-term neonates $n = 14$	Speech and nonspeech consonant and vowel 500-Hz tone
Davis & Wada, 1977	16 infants aged 2–11 wk.	Clicks, light flashes
Gardiner & Walter, 1977	4 infants aged 6 mo.	Speech and nonspeech segments
Molfese & Molfese, 1979a	Neonates, $n = 16$	PLACE contrasts
	Young infants, $n = 16$, aged 2–5 mo	VOT contrasts
Molfese & Molfese, 1979	Neonates, $n = 16$	VOT contrasts
Crowell, Kapuniai, & Garbanati, 1979	217 infants aged 2–30 days	Light flashes
Molfese & Molfese, 1980	11 preterm infants aged 35.8 wks GA	PLACE contrasts
Molfese & Molfese, 1985	Neonates, $n = 16$	PLACE contrasts

STAGE 2: THE SEARCH FOR EARLY HEMISPHERIC SPECIFICITY

Prior to this time, the studies in the initial period just described seemed designed primarily to demonstrate the presence of early hemispheric differences rather than to investigate the nature of such differences. Little was known about the cortical mechanisms responsible for such differences or about the acoustic features that might evoke such differences. This lack of information was due in part to the use of relatively gross stimulus features or experimental designs that simply intended to discern if speech versus nonspeech materials would elicit lateralized hemispheric responding in these young infants. For example, in the case of Molfese *et al.* (1975), although effects were indeed noted between the speech and nonspeech materials, the stimuli varied along many other dimensions as well. These materials differed in numbers of formants, formant bandwidths, overall frequency ranges, and the presence or absence of rapid frequency transitions, to note just a few of the confounding factors. Consequently, although such hemispheric differences appeared to change depending on the stimulus class (speech versus nonspeech), the specific stimulus characteristics that distinguished the two classes of stimuli could not be readily identified. Clearly, the next step needed in this process was one in which stimulus, task, and subject variables such as sex could be more systematically manipulated and evaluated.

In many respects, the study by Molfese *et al.* (1976) set the tone for this next period of research. They had noted that the AERs discriminated between different acoustic cues. Although no interactions were found in that study between hemisphere responding and specific stimulus features, there were several nonsignificant trends that hinted at such effects. With improved stimulus controls and a more elaborate analysis procedure, Molfese and his colleagues undertook a series of studies to determine whether the infant's electrophysiological responses to speech cues (Molfese & Molfese, 1979a, 1979b, 1980) were comparable to that noted for older children and adults (Molfese, 1978a, 1978b, 1980a, 1980b; Molfese & Hess, 1978; Molfese & Schmidt, 1983; Molfese, 1984) and, furthermore, whether such responses were in fact lateralized early in development.

Molfese and his colleagues concentrated their work during this period on two speech cues that had received a great deal of attention from researchers using behavioral techniques over the previous 20 years, *voice onset time* (VOT) and *place of articulation* (PLACE). This work is outlined in Table 6-2.

Voice Onset Time

Previous researchers had identified VOT, the temporal relationship between laryngeal pulsing and the onset of consonant release, as an important cue for the perceived distinction between voiced and voiceless forms of stop consonants such as *b* and *p* (Liberman, Cooper, Shankweiler, & Studdert-Kennedy, 1967). Adult listeners appear to discriminate a variety of speech sounds by the phonetic labels attached to them. Adults can readily discriminate between consonants from different phonetic categories, such as [ba] and [pa], while they perform at only chance levels when attempting to discriminate between two different [ba] sounds that differ acoustically to the same extent as the [ba]–[pa] difference (Lisker & Abramson, 1970). This pattern of discrimination for *between–phonetic category contrasts* while chance levels of discrimination are noted for *within-category contrasts* is referred to as "categorical perception." Studies with infant (Eimas *et al.*, 1971; Eilers, Gavin, & Wilson, 1980), children (Streeter, 1976), and adult listeners (Lisker & Abramson, 1970) have demonstrated categorical perception and discrimination for a wide range of contrasts, such as voicing (*ba, pa; ga, ka*) and place of articulation (*ba, da, ga*).

The classic work by Eimas *et al.* (1971) investigating early categorical perception in young infants, when viewed against a backdrop of reports that language perception skills were lateralized (Kimura, 1961; Shankweiler & Studdert-Kennedy, 1967; Studdert-Kennedy & Shankweiler, 1970), provided one obvious approach to studying early lateralization for specific language-related cues. Clearly, if infants possessed such skills, one would expect that these skills should be lateralized to one hemisphere, generally the left, while the other hemisphere (the right) would not show such abilities. Molfese (1978b), in a follow-up to work by Dorman (1974), attempted to determine whether categorical discrimination of VOT could be assessed using ERP procedures and, if present, whether such discriminations were confined to one hemisphere.

Before the work could begin with young infants, Molfese first had to determine whether such effects occurred for adults. To this end, Molfese (1978b) recorded ERPs from the left and right temporal regions of 16 adults during a phoneme identification task. The adults were presented with randomly ordered sequences of synthesized bilabial stop consonants with VOT values of +0 ms, +20 ms, +40 ms, and +60 ms. In the +0 ms case, the onset of consonant release and vocal fold vibration would occur simultaneously, whereas in the +60-ms condition the onset of laryngeal pulsing was delayed for 60 ms after consonant release. The ERPs were recorded in response to each sound; then, after a brief delay, the adults pressed a series of keys to identify the sound they had heard. Two regions of the ERP (one component centered around 135 ms and the second occurring between 300 and 500 ms following stimulus onset) did change systematically as a function of the sound's phonetic category—a categorical discrimination effect. Stop consonant sounds with VOT values of +0 and +20 ms (sounds identified as *ba*) were discriminated from those with VOT values of +40 and +60 ms (sounds identified as *pa*). However, the ERPs did not discriminate between the sounds from the same category. There were no differences in the waveforms between the +0 and +20 ms sounds or between the +40 and +60 ms sounds. Electrophysiological studies employing similar stimuli with a variety of different populations have replicated this finding (Molfese & Hess, 1978; Molfese & Molfese, 1979b; Molfese, 1980a; Molfese & Molfese, 1988). Surprisingly, however, in all these studies at least one region of the ERP in which this categorical discrimination effect was noted across the different age groups occurred over the *right* temporal region.

Similar effects were noted with 4-year-old children in a study involving the velar stop consonants *k, g*. Molfese and Hess (1978) recorded AERs from the left and right temporal scalp regions of 12 preschool-age children (mean age = 4 years, 5 months) in response to randomly ordered series of synthesized consonant–vowel syllables in which the initial consonant varied in VOT from +0 ms, to +20 ms, to +40 ms, to +60 ms. Upon analysis of the AERs, they, like Molfese (1978b), also found a categorical discrimination effect whereby one late-occurring portion of the waveform (peak latency = 444 ms) changed systematically in response to consonants from different phonetic categories but did not respond differentially to consonants from within the same phonetic category. As in the case of Molfese (1978b), this effect occurred over the right hemisphere. Unlike the adult study by Molfese, however, they found a second portion of the auditory ERP that occurred earlier in the waveform, before this right-hemisphere effect, and which was detected by electrodes placed over *both* hemispheres. This earlier auditory ERP component also discriminated the voiced from the voiceless consonants in a categorical manner (peak latencies = 198 and 342 ms). Similar results have recently been reported by Molfese and Molfese (1988) with 3-year-old children.

This work was later extended to include newborn and older infants (Molfese & Molfese, 1979b). In the work with newborn infants, they presented the four consonant–vowel syllables used by Molfese (1978b) to 16 infants between 2 and 5 months of age (mean = 3 months, 25 days). AERs were again recorded from the left and right temporal locations. Analyses revealed that one portion or component of the auditory ERP, recorded from over the right hemisphere approximately 920 ms following stimulus onset, discriminated between the different speech sounds in a categorical manner. As in the case of Molfese and Hess, they also noted a second portion of the auditory ERP that was present over both hemispheres and that also discriminated between the consonant sounds categorically. The major portion of this component occurred 528 ms following stimulus onset. These results, then, paralleled the findings of Molfese and Hess in noting two portions of the auditory ERP that discriminated between the speech sounds categorically. These included a bilateral component that occurred first in the waveform, followed by a right-hemisphere lateralized component that occurred later in time and also discriminated between the sounds categorically. A final portion of the ERP waveform was found to differ between the two hemispheres across all the different stimuli.

A second experiment described by Molfese and Molfese (1979b) failed to note any such bilateral or right-hemisphere lateralized effects with 16 newborn infants under 48 hours of age on the basis of group analyses. However, a recent study by Kurtzberg (personal communication) employing a different evoked-potential test procedure suggests that at least some young infants may be able to discriminate between voiced and voiceless consonant sounds.

One discrepancy between the adult study of Molfese (1978b) and the studies with children (Molfese & Hess, 1978; Molfese & Molfese, 1988) and infants (Molfese & Molfese, 1979b) concerns the absence of a bilateral effect with the adult population studied by Molfese. At first it was speculated that such a bilateral effect might drop out with further maturation and development. However, a more recent study with adults (Molfese, 1980a), suggests that the bilateral effect remains in adults but that the area in which this effect can be noted is more restricted. The difference, then, between the two age groups could be due to the shrinking size of the electrical fields over which the effect can be detected. As individuals age, the scalp potentials become more and more differentiated, with more differences in electrical activity being noted between even closely adjacent electrode sites.

Molfese (1980a) conducted a second study with adults to determine whether the laterality effects noted for the VOT stimuli were elicited by only speech stimuli or whether similar electrophysiological effects could be noted for both speech and nonspeech sounds. Such a comparison would allow conclusions to be reached regarding similarities in mechanisms that might subserve the perception of materials with similar temporal delays (+0, +20, +40, +60 ms). If the right hemisphere and bilateral categorical effects occurred for nonspeech stimuli containing comparable temporal delays, it would be clear that such effects would be due to the temporal nature of the cues rather than to their ''speech'' quality. Molfese used four ''tone onset time'' (TOT) stimuli (from Pisoni, 1977). Each TOT stimulus was 230 ms in duration and consisted of two tones. The TOT stimuli differed from each other in the onset of the lower frequency tone (500 Hz) relative to the higher frequency tone (1,500 Hz). The lower tone began at the same time as the upper tone for the O-ms TOT stimulus; the lower tone lagged behind the upper tone by 20 ms for the +20-ms TOT stimulus. This delay increased to 40 ms and 60 ms, respectively, for the +40- and +60-ms TOT stimuli. Both tones ended simultaneously. AERs were recorded from 16 adults. Analyses indicated that one region of the auditory ERP centered around 330 ms and common to electrodes placed over the temporal, central, and parietal regions of the right hemisphere categorically discriminated the +0- and +20-ms TOT sounds from the +40- and +60-ms sounds. No comparable changes were noted over the left hemisphere at this latency. However, bilateral responses were noted earlier in time from the left and right parietal regions 145 ms following stimulus onset and over the central areas at 210 ms. Interestingly, these bilateral effects were detected by electrodes placed over regions that were not sampled in the original Molfese (1978b) study. Thus, the lack of bilateral effects in the original study appears to result from the use of a more restricted sampling of electrical activity. Consequently, as in the case of the infant and child studies, processing of the temporal cue appeared to involve both bilateral responses which occurred earlier in time, followed by later right-hemisphere lateralized responses. The work by Molfese and Molfese (1988) with 3-year-old children, employed both the VOT stimuli used by Molfese and Hess and the TOT stimuli of Molfese (1980a). They found that both stimulus sets produced identical right-hemisphere responses. It appears, then, that these changes noted in the ERP are indeed the result of responses to temporal delays rather than to some general ''speech'' quality per se.

Although the right-hemisphere discrimination of the VOT cue seems paradoxical in light of arguments that language processes are carried out primarily by the left hemisphere, two developments may address this concern. First, even clinical studies of VOT suggest that VOT may be discriminated, if not exclusively, then at least in part, by the right hemisphere (for a review of this literature, see Molfese, Molfese, & Parsons, 1983). For example, Miceli, Caltagirone, Gainotti, and Payer-Rigo (1978), using a nondichotic pair presentation task, noted that the left-brain-damaged aphasic group made fewest errors with stimuli differing in voicing but not in place of articulation. Blumstein, Baker, and Good-

Table 6-2. Studies in Which Researchers Have Identified Hemispheric Differences in Human Infants Related to Place of Articulation and Voice Onset Time (VOT) Discrimination Using Electrophysiological Procedures

Study	Subjects/ages	Stimuli	Sites	Results
		Consonant place of articulation discrimination		
Molfese & Molfese, 1980	Preterm infants, $n = 11$	*bae, gae* Phonetic and nonphonetic transitions	T3, T4	No PLACE effects
Molfese & Molfese, 1979a	Full-term infants, $n = 16$	*bae, gae* Speech and nonspeech formants	T3, T4	LH: 192 ms Bilateral: 630 ms
Molfese & Molfese, 1985	Full-term infants, $n = 16$	*ba, da, ga* *bi, di, gi* *bu, du, gu*	T3, T4	LH: 168 ms Bilateral: 664 ms
		Categorical VOT discrimination		
Molfese & Molfese, 1979a	Full-term infants, $n = 16$	*ba* to *pa* 0-, 20-, 40-, 60-ms	T3, T4	No VOT effects
Molfese & Molfese, 1979b	Young infants, $n = 16$, aged 2–5 mo	*ba* to *pa* 0-, 20-, 40-, 60-ms	T3, T4	RH: 920 ms Bilateral: 528 ms

glass (1977) also noted fewer errors for voicing contrasts than for place contrasts with left-hemisphere-damaged Wernicke aphasics. Finally, Perecman and Kellar (1981), based on their own findings that left-hemisphere-damaged patients continue to match sounds on the basis of voicing but not place, speculated that voicing could be processed by either hemisphere but that the PLACE cue was more likely to be processed by only the left hemisphere. Second, the eletrophysiological studies of Molfese and his colleagues point to several regions of the brain that appear responsive to voicing contrasts.

Three general findings have emerged from this series of VOT/TOT studies. First, the discrimination of the temporal delay cue common to voiced and voiceless stop consonants can be detected by electrophysiological measures—specifically, the ERPs recorded from electrodes placed on the scalp over the hemispheres. Second, from at least 2 months of age, if not before, the infant's brain appears capable of discriminating voiced from voiceless stop consonants in a categorical manner. Third, categorical discrimination across different ages appears to be carried out first by bilaterally represented mechanisms within both hemispheres and then, somewhat later in time, by right-hemisphere lateralized mechanisms.

Place of Articulation

Several studies with infants and adults were also undertaken during this period to identify the correlates of acoustic and phonetic cues that are important to the perception of consonant place of articulation information (Molfese, 1978a, 1980b, 1984; Molfese, Buhrke, & Wang, 1985; Molfese, Linnville, Wetzel, & Leicht, 1985; Molfese & Schmidt, 1983; Molfese & Molfese, 1979a, 1980, 1985). As in the case of the VOT temporal cue, these studies of the PLACE cue, which monitored electrical activity from multiple electrode regions, identified both lateralized and bilateral hemisphere responses that discriminated between the different consonant sounds. Furthermore, such discriminations were present from birth. There were some important differences, however, both in the development of ERP responses to the PLACE cue and in the character of the lateralized responses, which distinguished the perception of this cue from that for VOT. These differences are noted next.

ADULTS

In the first study in this series, Molfese (1978a) attempted to isolate the neuroelectrical correlates of the second formant transition, the cue to which listeners attend in order to discriminate between different consonant sounds. In this study, he presented a series of consonant–vowel syllables in which the stop consonants varied in place of articulation, formant structure, and phonemic transition quality characteristics. Changes in the place cue signaled either the consonant *b* or *g*. The formant structure variable referred to a set of nonspeech sounds that contained formants composed of sine waves 1 Hz in bandwidth, whereas a set of speech sounds contained formants with speech like bandwidths of 60, 90, and 120 Hz for formants 1 through 3. The phonetic transition quality cue referred to two stimulus properties in which one stimulus set contained formant transitions that normally characterize human speech patterns and the second set contained an unusual pattern not found in the initial consonant position in human speech patterns. Auditory ERP responses were recorded from the left and right temporal regions of 10 adults in response to randomly ordered series of consonant–vowel syllables that varied in consonant place of articulation, bandwidth, and phonetic transition quality. Two regions of the auditory ERP that peaked at 70 and 300 ms following stimulus onset discriminated consonant phonetic transition quality and place of articulation only over the left-hemisphere temporal electrode site. As in the case of Molfese (1978b), who also used only a single left-hemisphere temporal site, no bilateral place discrimination was noted. Similar left hemisphere PLACE discrimination effects have since been noted by Molfese (1980b), Molfese and Schmidt (1983), and Molfese (1984), with the exception that, with the inclusion of auditory ERP data collected from more electrode recording sites over each hemisphere, consistent discrimination of the place cues were noted for both hemispheres (bilateral effects).

Several general findings from these adult studies should be noted at this time. In the case of the adult studies reviewed to this point, when multiple electrode sites are employed, bilateral stimulus discrimination effects are noted. Furthermore, these bilateral effects invariably occur early in the waveform and prior to the onset of the lateralized PLACE discrimination responses. This temporal relationship between bilateral and lateralized effects also can be noted with the VOT discrimination studies. Finally, in addition to stimulus related hemisphere effects, portions of the AERs are found to vary between hemispheres that are unrelated to stimulus, task, or subject features. Apparently, during the discrimination process both hemispheres initially discriminate between the PLACE and VOT stimuli at the same time, somewhere approximately 100 ms following stimulus onset. Shortly afterwards, at approximately 300 ms following stimulus onset, the left hemisphere discriminates between differences in the PLACE cue, while the right hemisphere at approximately 400 ms will discriminate the VOT or temporal offset cue. Finally, throughout this time and afterwards, there are brief periods of activity during which time the two hemispheres are doing quite different things, which may be unrelated to the discrimination of the stimuli that are then being perceived.

INFANTS

In a replication/extension of this PLACE discrimination work with newborn and preterm infants, Molfese and Molfese (1979a, 1980) noted a similar pattern of lateralized and bilateral responses. Unlike those findings for VOT, PLACE discrimination was clearly present from birth. In this study, AERs were recorded from the left and right temporal regions (T3 and T4) of 16 full-term newborn human infants within 2 days of birth. These data were recorded while the infants were presented series of consonant–vowel syllables that differed in the second formant transition (F2, which signaled the place of articulation information), and formant bandwidth. As with adults, one auditory ERP component that appeared only over the left-hemisphere recording site discriminated between the two consonant sounds when they contained normal speech formant characteristics (peak latency = 168ms). A second region of the auditory ERP varied systematically over both hemispheres and also discriminated between the two speechlike consonant sounds (peak latency = 630 ms). Finally, the AERs differed between hemispheres at approximately 288 ms following stimulus onset. This hemisphere difference occurred across all stimuli.

In a replication and extension of this work, Molfese and Molfese (1985) presented a series of consonant–vowel syllables that varied in PLACE and formant structure. Two different consonant sounds *(b, g)* combined with three different vowel sounds were presented with speech or nonspeech formant structures. AERs were again recorded from the left and right temporal regions (T3, T4). As in the case of Molfese and Molfese (1979a), analyses identified two regions of the auditory ERP that discriminated the PLACE difference. One region, with a peak latency of 168 ms, was detected only over the left-hemisphere site as discriminating between the two different consonant sounds; a second region, with a peak latency of 664 ms, discriminated this PLACE difference and was detected by electrodes placed over both hemispheres. Interestingly, the lateralized effect noted for these infants for the PLACE cue occurred *before* that for the bilateral effect, a finding opposite to that noted for adults studied under similar circumstances. However, the reversal of the temporal relationship between the bilateral and lateralized responses appears to be a legitimate one, given that virtually identical results were found by Molfese and Molfese (1985) and Molfese and Molfese (1979a) with different populations of infants and somewhat different stimulus sets that contained the PLACE variable. This temporal pattern of initial lateralized responses followed by bilateral responses is opposite to that noted previously for both VOT and PLACE cues for adults as well as that found for infants exposed to changes in the VOT/temporal cue. Clearly, such differences in the ERP effects suggest that different mechanisms subserve the perception and discrimination of the different speech related cues.

The relationship between the lateralized and bilateral responses are not clear at this time. It does appear, however, that the bilateral response may develop after the lateralized one, both ontogenetically and phylogenetically. For example, Molfese and Molfese (1980) noted only the presence of left-hemisphere lateralized responses in 11 preterm infants born on average 35.9 weeks postconception. Stimuli identical to those employed in Molfese (1978a) with adults were presented to these infants while AERs were recorded from the left- (T3) and right-hemisphere (T4) temporal regions. As found with the full-term infants (Molfese & Molfese, 1979a), a portion of the auditory ERP recorded from over the left hemisphere discriminated between speech stimuli containing different consonant transition cues. An additional left-hemisphere component differentiated only between the nonphonetic consonants, a finding similar to that reported by Molfese (1978a) with adults, with the exception that adults were sensitive to both phonetic and nonphonetic contrasts. Another auditory ERP component responded differently to speech versus nonspeech formant structures. Finally, hemisphere differences in the AERs that were not stimulus related could be noted across a large portion of the waveforms between 200 ms and 704 ms.

Two separate studies with rhesus monkeys, one in which PLACE perception was studied (Molfese, Laughlin, Morse, Linnville, Wetzel, & Erwin, 1986), and one in which VOT was studied (Morse, Molfese, Laughlin, Linnville, & Wetzel, 1987), found left and right lateralized categorical discrimination responses, respectively, but no bilateral responses were noted. A recent VOT discrimination study with two breeds of dogs, collies and beagles, also noted a right-hemisphere lateralized categorical discrimination response but no bilateral one (Adams, Moltese, & Betz, 1987). Given the absence of the bilateral response in nonhuman primates and other mammals, it may be possible that it is the bilateral response that discriminates humans from other organisms in the perception of speech cues—not, as has usually been argued, the lateralized mechanisms.

On the basis of the electrophysiological data collected during this period, it appears that hemispheric differences in young infants, as well as in adults, are multidimensional. First, at some point during the auditory ERP to virtually all stimuli tested to date using this procedure, the two hemispheres, in both infants and adults, respond differently to all stimuli. This general hemispheric effect seems most pronounced in the preterm infants, with many different regions varying between the two hemispheres (Molfese & Molfese, 1980), but is also present in newborn and 1-year-old infants (Molfese & Searock, 1986), preschool-age children (Molfese & Hess, 1978; Molfese & Molfese, 1988), and adults (Molfese, 1978a, 1978b, 1980a, 1984; Molfese & Schmidt, 1983). Second, different regions of the auditory ERP elicited by the different auditory stimuli appear to be lateralized differently, depending on the evoking stimuli. The temporal cue, VOT, elicits a right-hemisphere response, while the PLACE cue elicits a left-hemisphere response. Third, the different lateralized responses for specific speech cues such as VOT and PLACE may appear at different points in development. The PLACE response seems clearly to be in place at birth, although no such effects have been noted extensively for the cue VOT.

STAGE 3: ELECTROPHYSIOLOGICAL INDICES OF EARLY LATERALIZED PROCESSES AS A MEANS TO PREDICT FUTURE LANGUAGE DEVELOPMENT

Researchers such as Orton and Lenneberg have long argued that the presence of lateralization of language functions is an indicator of language development and, more generally, of cognitive development. Although a number of different arguments and theories have been posited regarding the relationship between lateralization and language development, most arguments may be reduced to the premise that if lateralization develops normally, language development will also develop normally. However, exactly what must be lateralized in order to ensure such normal development? Are hemisphere differences per se the appropriate measure that should be used to predict long-term development? Or are the lateralized discriminations of some aspect of the infant or child's environment better predictors of later development? Given the current findings regarding the early identification of a variety of types of hemisphere differences in young infants, it appeared to some investigators that the question of the role of lateralization in language development could at last be more directly tested (Molfese & Molfese, 1985, Molfese & Searock, 1986).

Molfese and Molfese (1985, 1986) attempted to establish the predictive validity of a variety of factors in predicting long-term outcomes in language development from measures taken shortly after birth and during the first years of life. A variety of measures were used, including demographic variables, behavioral scales, and AERs. The specific issue under study concerned whether general hemisphere differences per se or specific lateralized discrimination abilities would best identify children with underdeveloped language skills.

Sixteen infants were studied longitudinally from birth through their 3rd birthday. During this time information was collected on factors such as gender, birth weight, length, gestational age, scores on the Obstetric Complications Scale (Littman & Parmalee, 1978), the Brazelton Neonatal Assessment Scale (Als, Tronick, Lester, & Brazelton, 1977), the Bayley Scales of Infant Development (Bayley, 1969), the Peabody Picture Vocabulary Test (Dunn, 1965), and the McCarthy Scales of Children's Abilities (McCarthy, 1972), as well as parental ages, incomes, educational levels, and occupations. In addition, AERs were recorded from the left and right temporal areas (T3 and T4), at birth and again at 6-month intervals through the child's 3rd birthday in response to the synthetic speech stimuli employed by Molfese (1980b) and Molfese and Schmidt (1983). These stimuli were chosen because they had been found to produce reliable general hemispheric difference effects as well as bilateral and lateralized discrimination effects. In addition, eight other stimulus tokens were added to the auditory ERP test battery in order to facilitate tests of generalizability across the different PLACE and vowel contrasts. Such stimuli appeared, then, to be ideally suited for determining whether general hemispheric differences per se or specific lateralized discrimination abilities were the best predictors of later language skills.

Analyses of the auditory ERP data did in fact indicate that electrophysiological measures recorded at birth could identify children who performed better or worse on language tasks 3 years later. Moreover, the best predictor of later development was the presence of a lateralized speech sound discrimination ability. The newborn infants in which left-hemisphere-generated AERs reliably discriminated between the different consonant sounds at birth were more likely to develop better language skills 3 years later. Children who performed poorer at 3 years of age failed to make such discriminations as newborn infants.

At certain electrode sites (hemispheres), and under certain stimulus conditions, one component of the auditory ERP that occurred between 88 and 240 ms reliably discriminated between children who scored above 50 (the High MCVP group) on the McCarthy Scales of Children's Abilities and those who scored lower (the Low MCVP group). Only the AERs recorded from over the left hemisphere of the High MCVP group systematically discriminated between the different consonant speech sounds. The right-hemisphere responses of this group, on the other hand, discriminated between the different nonspeech stimuli. However, the Low MCVP group displayed no such lateralized discrimination for either the speech or the nonspeech sounds. A second portion of the auditory ERP with a late peak latency of 664 ms also discriminated between the High and Low MCVP groups. Unlike the earlier peak, however, this component occurred over both hemispheres and consequently reflected bilateral activity. This second component did not behave in exactly the same manner as the first. It was able to discriminate between speech and nonspeech stimuli. In addition, its ability to discriminate between consonant sounds depended on which vowel followed the consonant. In other words, this auditory ERP component was much more context sensitive. A third segment of the auditory ERP (peak latency = 450 ms) that only varied across hemispheres failed to discriminate between the two different groups. Thus, it appears that hemispheric differences per se were not sufficient to discriminate at birth between infants who 3 years later would develop better or poorer language skills. Furthermore, given that the auditory ERP components that discriminated between the two groups were sensitive to certain speech and nonspeech contrasts but not to others, it appears that the AERs reflect the organism's sensitivity to specific language-related cues rather than the overall readiness of the brain to respond to any general stimulus in its environment.

A stepwise multiple regression model of these data was developed using the Peabody and McCarthy scores as the dependent variables and the AER components obtained at birth that best discriminated the different consonant sounds as the independent variables. This model accounted for 78% of the total variance in predicting McCarthy scores from the brain responses, whereas 69% of the variance was accounted for in predicting Peabody scores (Molfese & Molfese, 1986). Clearly, there appears to be a strong relationship between early ERP discrimination of speech-related stimuli and later language skills.

A subsequent study by Molfese and Searock (1986) noted that this relationship between early ERP activity and later language skills continues to exist at 1 year of age. AERs were recorded from 16 infants within 2 weeks of their first birthday. A series of three vowel sounds with speech formant structure and three nonspeech tokens containing 1-Hz-wide formants that matched the mean frequencies of the speech sounds were presented to these infants, and their auditory ERPs were recorded in response to each sound. Two regions of the ERPs, one centered between 300 and 400 ms, and another centered around 200 ms following stimulus onset, discriminated between the 1-year-old infants who 2 years later would perform better or worse on the McCarthy language tasks. Infants who were able to discriminate between more vowel sounds performed better on the language tasks at 3 years of age.

One interpretation of these results is that early discrimination abilities may relate directly to later language development. The children who performed better on language tasks at age 3 not only discriminated between consonant sounds alone and consonant sounds in combination with different vowel sounds, but also discriminated between different speech sounds and between different nonspeech sounds. Such a pattern of responding could suggest that the more linguistically advanced children were at an advantage in the language development process because their nervous systems could make finer discriminations along a variety of different dimensions. Perhaps the earlier an infant can discriminate between speech sounds in its environment, the more likely that infant will be able to use such information to discriminate sound differences. This is clearly an important process in that it will play a major role in the child's learning to discriminate between words with different meanings and to produce these words as his or her language develops.

These results concerning the long-term prediction of later language skills from brain wave activity recorded at birth are still very new. It is clear that more extensive testing with a larger and more heterogeneous population is needed to determine whether such results will continue to be found under more elaborate and extensive test procedures. Such a project is now underway at a number of laboratories. Should these results be confirmed, a number of clear benefits will be derived.

STAGE 4: LATERALIZATION AND EARLY WORD ACQUISITION

The research described so far has indicated that there are clear indicators of lateralization from the earliest points in infancy and that such lateralized responses are multidimensional and complex. Clearly, some speech discrimination abilities seem to be lateralized from birth, while others are not. In addition, other patterns of hemispheric differences are noted that do not appear to be related to the stimulus or subject variables under investigation. In this latter case it appears that one hemisphere is simply responding differently than the other hemisphere to all stimuli.

Another point that is supported by the previously described research is that hemispheric differences appear to be related to later language development providing that the lateralized hemispheric response is one that discriminates specific stimulus features. More general hemispheric differences that occur regardless of the evoking stimulus do not appear to predict later development with any accuracy.

The current research carries us into one more region of study concerning hemispheric differences. Given that we now know that hemispheric differences are present from birth and that such differences do in fact relate to later development, one possible next step would be to identify more specifically the relationships between such early forms of lateralization and the early emerging language systems.

The emergence of language in the human child presumes several important perceptual abilities: the comprehension of human speech sounds, and the learning that patterns of speech sounds are linked in an arbitrary way to objects in the infant's environment as "names." As noted earlier, researchers investigating human speech perception have found that infants in the first few months of life discriminate between a variety of human speech sounds in a manner similar to that of adult listeners. In fact, comparable research with nonhuman primates (Molfese *et al.*, 1986; Morse, Molfese, Laughlin, Linnville, & Wetzel, 1987) and other mammals (Adams *et al.*, 1987) has indicated that these speech perceptual abilities are not unique to humans. Yet little is known about the infant's beginning comprehension of "names" for objects. Although a few investigators have catalogued the words first comprehended by infants, beginning around 8 months of age, the process whereby the infant learns that particular speech sound patterns are arbitrarily associated with specific referents have largely gone unstudied.

The present series of investigations was designed to study the development of the comprehension of "names." Perhaps one reason that so little is known about this learning process is that the early stages of word recognition are not easy to demonstrate using standard behavioral procedures.

ERP procedures had been successfully used to discriminate between words that were known and words that were not known to a group of sixteen 16-month-old children (Molfese, *et al.* 1985). In that study, a series of words identified by parents and independent observers as understood by the child were presented to him or her while the AERs were recorded. These children also listened to groups of words that both parents and observers believed that the children did not understand. Analyses of the brain responses recorded from over the left side of the head indicated that frontal, temporal, and parietal areas of the left hemisphere discriminated reliably between words that were known and words that were unknown to the children. Although such results suggest that AERs can discriminate differences in words' meanings in young children, it is possible that these effects were due instead to differences in familiarity. The brain responses to known words might have differed from those elicited by the unknown words simply because the known words were phonetically more familiar to the child. To address this issue, a second study was conducted (Wetzel & Molfese, 1986).

This study attempted to determine whether familiarity with speech stimuli would produce brain responses similar to those found for the word materials. In this procedure, eleven 14-month-old infants first listened to a nonsense CVCV over a 2-day period. Parents were asked to have their child play with a Frisbee for three times on each of the 2 days designated for training, with 15 minutes being allowed for each of the six play sessions. Six of the children heard "toto" during the familiarization process, while five children heard "gigi." This procedure was used to decrease the likelihood that any experimental effects might be due to acoustic differences between the stimuli instead of due to differences in amount of previous exposure to the different stimuli. On the third day, AERs were recorded to this now familiar CVCV and to a novel CVCV. Electrodes were placed over the left and right sides of the head at the following locations: T3 and T4, midway between the external meatus of the left ear and Fz (FL); midway between the right external meatus and Fz (FR); midway between the left external meatus and Pz (PL); over the right side of the head midway between the right ear's external meatus and Pz (PR). These electrode placements were over the left frontal, temporal, and parietal areas of the brain and the corresponding areas of the right hemisphere. If the latencies and scalp distributions of the brain responses found in this study were identical to those found in the known–unknown word study, it was felt that the familiarity hypothesis could not be rejected. In fact, however, results indicated that only the brain responses recorded over both the left- and right-hemisphere frontal areas discriminated between the familiar and nonfamiliar CVCVs. In addition, the major peak in the AER that discriminated these differences occurred at 360 ms, not at the 630 ms previously found for the known–unknown word distinction. Consequently, it appears that the earlier ERP findings noted in the above first experiment did indeed reflect meaning differences and not differences in familiarity.

Given that these ERP procedures appear suited to the study of early word meanings and their differences in young infants, the next step is to attempt to investigate in a more detailed fashion the nature of those word differences. Can such ERP procedures be used to study the development of specific word meanings in young infants? It is to this question that our lab has now turned.

ACKNOWLEDGMENTS

Support for this work was provided by the National Science Foundation (BNS8004429, BNS8210846), the National Institutes of Health (R01 HD17860), and the Office of Research Development and Administration (2-10947), Southern Illinois University at Carbondale.

REFERENCES

Adams, C. A., Molfese, D. L., & Betz, J. C. (1987). Electrophysiological correlates of categorical speech perception for voicing contrasts in dogs. *Developmental Neuropsychology, 3,* 175–189.

Als, H., Tronick, E., Lester, B., & Brazelton, T. (1977). The Brazelton Neonatal Behavioral Assessment Scale (BNAS). *Journal of Abnormal Child Psychology, 5,* 215–231.

Barnet, A., de Sotillo, M., & Campos, M. (1974). *EEG sensory evoked potentials in early infancy malnutrition.* Paper presented at the meeting of the Society for Neurosciences, St. Louis, MO.

Basser, L. S. (1962). Hemiplegia of early onset and the faculty of speech with special reference to the effects of hemispherectomy. *Brain, 85,* 427–460.

Bayley, N. (1969). *Bayley Scales of Infant Development: Birth to two years.* New York: Psychological Corporation.

Blumstein, S., Baker, E., & Goodglass, H. (1977). Phonological factors in auditory comprehension in aphasia. *Neuropsychologia, 15,* 19–30.

Crowell, D. H., Jones, R. H., Kapuniai, L. E., & Nakagawa, J. K. (1973). Unilateral cortical activity in newborn humans: An early index of cerebral dominance? *Science, 180,* 205–208.

Crowell, D. H., Kapuniai, L. E., & Garbanati, J. A. (1979). Hemispheric differences in human infant rhythmic responses to photic stimulation. In J. E. Desmedt (Ed.), *Cerebral evoked potentials in man.* Basel: Karger.

Davis, A. E. & Wada, J. A. (1977). Hemispheric asymmetries in human infants: Spectral analysis of flash and click evoked potentials. *Brain and Language, 4,* 23–31.

Dorman, M. (1974). Auditory evoked potential correlates of speech sound discrimination. *Perception and Psychophysics, 15,* 215–220.

Dunn, L. (1965). *Peabody Picture Vocabulary Test.* Circle Pines, MN: American Guidance Service.

Eilers, R., Gavin, W., & Wilson, W. (1980). Linguistic experience and phonemic perception in infancy: A cross-linguistic study. *Child Development, 50,* 14–18.

Eimas, P. D., Siqueland, E., Jusczyk, P., & Vigorito, J. (1971). Speech perception in infants. *Science* (Washington, DC), *171,* 303–306.

Gardiner, M. F., & Walter, D. O. (1977). Evidence of hemispheric specialization from infant EEG. In S. Harnad,

R. Doty, L. Goldstein, J. Jaynes, & G. Krauthamer, (Eds.), *Lateralization in the nervous system* (pp. 481–500). New York: Academic Press.

Gardiner, M. F., Schulman, C., & Walter, D. O. (1973). Facilitative EEG asymmetries in infants and adults. In *Cerebral Dominance: BIS Conference Report No. 34*, pp. 37–40.

Jasper, H. H. (1958). The ten–twenty electrode system of the International Federation of Societies for Electroencephalography: Appendix to report of the committee on methods of clinical examination in electroencephalography. *Journal of Electroencephalography and Clinical Neurophysiology, 10*, 371–375.

Kimura, D. (1961). Cerebral dominance and the perception of verbal stimuli. *Canadian Journal of Psychology, 15*, 166–171.

Lenneberg, E. (1967). *Biological foundations of language*. New York: Wiley.

Liberman, A. M., Cooper, F. S., Shankweiler, D., & Studdert-Kennedy, M. (1967). Perception of the speech code. *Psychological Review, 74*, 431–461.

Lisker, L., & Abramson, A. S. (1970). The voicing dimension: Some experiments in comparative phonetics. In *Proceedings of the 6th International Congress of Phonetic Sciences* (pp. 563–567). Prague: Academia.

Littman, B., & Parmalee, A. H. (1978). Medical correlates of infant behavior. *Pediatrics 61*, 470–474.

McCarthy, D. (1972). *Manual for the McCarthy Scales of Children's Abilities*. New York: Psychological Corporation.

Miceli, G., Caltagirone, C., Gianotti, G., & Payer-Rigo, P. (1978). Discrimination of voice versus place contrasts in aphasia. *Brain and Language, 6*, 47–51.

Molfese, D. L. (1972). *Cerebral asymmetry in infants, children and adults: Auditory evoked responses to speech and music stimuli*. Unpublished doctoral dissertation, Pennsylvania State University.

Molfese, D. L. (1973). Cerebral asymmetry in infants, children and adults: Auditory evoked responses to speech and noise stimuli. *Dissertation Abstracts International*, 34(3-B), 1298.

Molfese, D. L. (1978a). Left and right hemisphere involvement in speech perception: Electrophysiological correlates. *Perceptual Psychophysiology, 23*, 237–243.

Molfese, D. L. (1978b). Neuroelectrical correlates of categorical speech perception in adults. *Brain and Language, 5*, 25–35.

Molfese, D. L. (1980a). Hemispheric specialization for temporal information: Implications for the perception of voicing cues during speech perception. *Brain and Language, 11*, 285–299.

Molfese, D. L. (1980b). The phoneme and the engram: Electrophysiological evidence for the acoustic invariant in stop consonants. *Brain and Language, 9*, 372–376.

Molfese, D. L. (1983). Event related potentials and language processes. In A. W. K. Gaillard & W. Ritter (Eds.), *Tutorials in ERP research: Endogenous components* (pp. 345–368). The Hague: North Holland.

Molfese, D. L. (1984). Left hemispheric sensitivity to consonant sounds not displayed by the right hemisphere: Electrophysiological correlates. *Brain and Language, 22*, 109–127.

Molfese, D. L., Buhke, R. A., & Wang, S. (1985). The right hemisphere and temporal processing of consonant transition durations: Electrophysiological correlates. *Brain and Language, 26*, 49–62.

Molfese, D. L., Freeman, R. B., & Palermo, D. S. (1975). The ontogeny of brain lateralization for speech & nonspeech stimuli. *Brain and Language, 2*, 356–368.

Molfese, D. L., & Hess, T. M. (1978). Speech perception in nursery school age children: Sex and hemisphere differences. *Journal of Experimental Child Psychology, 26*, 71–84.

Molfese, D. L., Laughlin, N. K., Morse, P. A., Linnville, S. E., Wetzel, W. F., & Erwin, R. J. (1986). Neuroelectrical correlates of categorical perception for place of articulation in normal and lead-treated rhesus monkeys. *Journal of Clinical and Experimental Neuropsychology 8(6)*, 680–696.

Molfese, D. L., & Molfese, V. J. (1979a). Hemisphere and stimulus differences as reflected in the cortical responses of newborn infants to speech stimuli. *Developmental Psychology, 15(5)*, 505–511.

Molfese, D. L., & Molfese, V. J. (1979b). Infant speech perception: Learned or innate. In H. A. Whitaker & H. Whitaker (Eds.), *Advances in Neurolinguistics* (Vol. 4, pp. 225–238). New York: Academic Press.

Molfese, D. L., & Molfese, V. J. (1980). Cortical response of preterm infants to phonetic and nonphonetic speech stimuli. *Developmental Psychology, 16(6)*, 574–581.

Molfese, D. L., & Molfese, V. J. (1985). Electrophyiological indices of auditory discrimination in newborn infants: The bases for predicting later language development? *Infant Behavior and Development, 8*, 197–211.

Molfese, D. L., & Molfese, V. J. (1986). Psychophysical indices of early cognitive processes and their relationship to language. In J. E. Obrzut & G. W. Hynd (Eds.), *Child neuropsychology: Vol. 1. Theory and research* (pp. 95–116). New York: Academic Press.

Molfese, D. L., & Molfese, V. J. (1988). Right hemisphere responses from preschool children to temporal cues contained in speech and nonspeech materials: Electrophysiological correlates. *Brain and Language, 33*, 245–249.

Molfese, D. L., Nunez, V., Seibert, S. M., & Ramaniah, N. V. (1976). Cerebral asymmetry: Changes in factors affecting its development. *Annals of the New York Academy of Sciences, 280,* 821–833.

Molfese, D. L., & Schmidt, A. (1983). An auditory evoked potential study of consonant perception in different vowel environments. *Brain and Language, 18,* 57–70.

Molfese, D. L., & Searock, K. (1986). The use of auditory evoked responses at one year of age to predict language skills at 3 years. *Australian Journal of Communication Disorders, 14,* 35–46.

Molfese, D. L., Wetzel, W. F., Linnville, S. Imbasciate, C., Leicht, D., Courtney, C., Baldwin, K., & Adams, C. (1985). *Word recognition in 16-month-old infants: Electrophysiological indices.* Paper presentation at the 57th Midwestern Psychological Association Meeting, May 2, 1985.

Molfese, V. J., & Molfese, D. L. (1985). Predicting a child's preschool language performance from perinatal variables. In R. Dillon & R. R. Schmeck (Eds.), *Individual differences in cognition* (Vol. 2, pp. 95–117). New York: Academic Press.

Molfese, V. J., Molfese, D. L., & Parsons, C. (1983). Hemisphere involvement in phonological perception. In S. Segalowitz (Ed.), *Language functions and brain organization* (pp. 29–49). New York: Academic Press.

Morse, P. A., Molfese, D. L., Laughlin, N. K., Linnville, S. & Wetzel, F. (1987). Categorical perception for voicing contrasts in normal and lead-treated rhesus monkeys: electrophysiological indices. *Brain and Language, 30,* 63–80.

Orton, S. (1937). *Reading, writing and speech problems in children.* New York: Horton.

Perecman, E., & Kellar, L. (1981). The effect of voice and place among aphasic, nonaphasic right-damaged and normal subjects on a metalinguistic task. *Brain and Language, 12,* 213–223.

Pisoni, D. B. (1977). Identification and discrimination of the relative onset time of two component tones: Implications for voicing perception in stops. *Journal of the Acoustical Society of America, 61,* 1352–1361.

Shucard, J. L., Shucard, D. W., Cummings, K. R., & Campos, J. J. (1981). Auditory evoked potentials and sex related differences in brain development. *Brain and Language, 13,* 91–102.

Shankweiler, M., & Studdert-Kennedy, D. (1967). Identification of consonants and vowels presented to left and right ears. *Quarterly Journal of Experimental Psychology, 14,* 69–63.

Studdert-Kennedy, M., & Shankweiler, D. (1970). Hemisphere specialization for speech perception. *Journal of the Acoustical Society of America, 48,* 579–594.

Streeter, L. A. (1976). Language perception of two-month-old infants shows effects of both innate mechanisms and experience. *Nature, 259,* 39–41.

Wetzel, W. F., & Molfese, D. L. (1986). *Electrophysiological correlates of familiar versus unfamiliar material in 14-month-old infants.* Poster presentation at the 58th Midwestern Psychological Association Meeting, May 9, 1986.

7

Cerebral Asymmetry and Emotion: Developmental and Individual Differences

RICHARD J. DAVIDSON
University of Wisconsin–Madison

NATHAN A. FOX
University of Maryland, College Park

Although the role of the two cerebral hemispheres in cognition has been extensively studied over the past 20 years, comparatively little has been written on hemispheric function and emotion. Even less is known about the role of the development of cortical function in the ontogeny of emotional behavior. There are undoubtedly many reasons that this is so. Probably the most important and least explicit is the prevailing bias against the view that the cortex has anything to do with emotion. Traditionally, the cortex is viewed as the seat of human higher cognitive functions. If any role in emotion is ascribed to the cortex, it is an inhibitory one, with cortical regions functioning to suppress subcortical limbic activity. More will be said later about this bias, which has crept into contemporary theorizing on the role of the two hemispheres in emotion.

A second reason for the relative lack of attention to emotion in studies of cerebral asymmetries is the lack of sufficient recognition of the importance of introhemispheric specificity. Differences in functional specialization exist in different cortical regions along the rostral–caudal plane. Many of the asymmetries associated with language and other cognitive functions are mediated by posterior cortical areas (e.g., parietal and posterior temporal regions). Recent findings in both normals (e.g., Davidson, 1984a) and brain-damaged subjects (e.g., Robinson, Kubos, Starr, Reo, & Price, 1984) indicate that asymmetries related to the actual generation of emotion are localized in the anterior cortical regions. To tap asymmetries in these regions, methods other than standard behavioral paradigms involving dichotic listening and divided visual field presentations are required.

Over the past 15 years, a growing body of literature has developed on cerebral asymmetries associated with emotion (see Davidson, 1984a; Silberman & Weingartner, 1986; and Tucker, 1981, for reviews). Some controversy exists about the interpretation of the available evidence. In the first section of this chapter, we briefly summarize adult data on asymmetry and emotion and review the various interpretations that have been offered to explain these findings. We will show several of the current interpretive schemes to be seriously deficient and will highlight those that offer the most promise. We will emphasize individual differences in hemispheric activation and their relation to affective behavior, and we will present studies in adults that indicate that the two cerebral hemispheres are differentially lateralized for the experience of certain positive and negative emotions. We use the adult literature to provide a context in which to examine the evidence on the development of emotion and its relation to cerebral asymmetry. The profound changes in emotional behavior that occur naturally over the first 2 years of life offer an ideal "model system" to study lateralization related to emotion. Moreover, individual differences in basic parameters of affect have been noted in very young infants (e.g., Goldsmith *et al.*, 1987). We will stress the relation between individual differences in activation asymmetries and affective responsiveness during the first year of life.

LATERALIZATION OF EMOTIONAL FUNCTIONS: CORE NEUROPSYCHOLOGICAL EVIDENCE

The data on the lateralization of emotional functions come from several different sources. Perhaps the earliest references to asymmetries of this nature come from reports of the affective consequences of brain damage. Alford (1933) and Goldstein (1939) were among the first to note a high incidence of negative affect and "catastrophic" reactions among patients with unilateral left-hemisphere damage. A very different form of emotional reaction has been observed following unilateral damage to the opposite hemisphere. In patients with right-hemisphere damage, indifference or euphoria has been noted to predominate as a consequence of the brain injury (for early reports, see, e.g., Denny-Brown, Meyer, & Horenstein, 1952; Hecaen, Ajuriaguerra, & Massonet, 1951). Gainotti (1969, 1972), who systematically compared patients with unilateral right- and left-sided lesions on emotional behavior, found that left-hemisphere lesions produced more frequent displays of the catastrophic reaction, whereas patients with right-hemisphere lesions showed a higher incidence of joking, indifference, and anosognosia. In a retrospective study of cases of pathological laughter and crying, Sackeim and associates (Sackeim *et al.*, 1982) found that left-sided lesions were more frequently associated with crying, whereas right-sided lesions were more often accompanied by laughter. In none of these studies was the location of the lesion within the hemisphere considered in the analyses.

An important series of recent studies has begun to evaluate systematically the effects of lesion location on affective behavior. Robinson and his colleagues, in a number of elegant studies, have found that the proximity of a left-hemisphere lesion to the frontal pole (assessed by CT scan) is correlated with the severity of depressive symptomatology (Robinson & Benson, 1981; Robinson & Szetela, 1981; Robinson *et al.*, 1984). The closer the lesion to the frontal pole, the more severe the depression. Among patients with left hemisphere lesions, Robinson *et al.* (1984) have reported a −.54 correlation between distance of the lesion from the frontal pole and severity of depressive symptomatology (based on a composite of several different indices). Out of the group of 30 patients who were studied by Robinson *et al.* (1984), 8 met research diagnostic criteria for major depressive disorder. Among these 8 patients, 6 had left anterior lesions.

The association of frontal lobe damage with affective disturbance is not surprising in light of the unique anatomical situation of this brain region. The frontal lobes have extensive anatomical reciprocity with various limbic structures directly implicated in the control of emotion (Nauta, 1964, 1971). A variety of neuropsychological evidence links damage of particular frontal lobe areas to deficits in affective regulation (e.g., Akert, 1964; Luria, 1966, 1973; Pribram, 1973). In recent research, frontal lobe lesions have been found to impair both voluntary and spontaneous facial expressions (Kolb & Milner, 1981a, 1981b). For these and other reasons, the cortical region most likely to participate in the generation of emotional processes is the frontal region. As noted later, brain electrical activity recorded from this region is more consistently related to emotional behavior than is activity from other cortical regions that have been sampled.

Several other lines of research with clinical populations support the differential lateralization of positive and negative affect. These include studies on the effects on mood of unilateral injections of sodium amytal, lateralized dysfunctions in patients with affective disorders, and the differential effects of left- versus right-sided electroconvulsive therapy. These data have been extensively reviewed (e.g., Davidson, 1984a) and will not be considered here. In general, the evidence from these other sources has been consistent with the findings from the brain damage data.

In normal subjects, a variety of procedures have been employed to make inferences about underlying hemispheric asymmetries associated with emotion. The large body of literature that has been generated on the perception of emotional information indicates that the right hemisphere, particularly the parietal region, plays an essential role in this process (see reviews by Bryden, 1982; Etcoff, 1986). Moreover, some workers have suggested that the right-hemisphere superiority in the perception of emotional information is independent of the more general superiority of this hemisphere in visuospatial tasks (e.g., Etcoff, 1986). Unfortunately, the superiority of the right hemisphere on tasks requiring the perception of emotional information has been interpreted by some to reflect an overall advantage of this hemisphere in the "processing" of emotion. As will be underscored, the posterior regions of the hemispheres actively participate in perceptual tasks, whereas the anterior regions have been implicated in tasks involving the generation of behavior such as emotional expression. It is in the anterior regions, *when emotion is recruited,* that differential asymmetries as a function of affective valence have been observed.

One of the most effective methods for examining asymmetries in hemispheric activation during the generation of emotion is to record the EEG in response to stimuli that elicit affect and assess asymmetries in activation as a function of the nature of the emotion that is elicited. This strategy has been used extensively in adult (e.g., Bennett, Davidson, & Saron, 1981; Davidson, Schaffer, & Saron, 1985; Davidson, Schwartz, Saron, Bennett, & Goleman, 1979) and infant (Davidson & Fox, 1982; Fox & Davidson, 1986, 1987, 1988) studies. In most of the studies to be described, asymmetries in the frontal and parietal scalp regions were compared in response to stimuli that were designed to elicit a range of different positive and negative emotions. On the basis of the brain damage literature described earlier, it was hypothesized that greater relative left frontal activation would accompany epochs of positive affect compared with epochs of negative affect, and vice versa. One additional important prediction was that parietal asymmetry would not differentiate between positive and negative affect.

EEG STUDIES OF STIMULUS-ELICITED AFFECT IN ADULT AND INFANT POPULATIONS

In the EEG studies to be described below the major dependent variable has been power in the alpha (8–13 Hz) band for experiments with adults and power in the lower frequencies (1–12 Hz) for the infant studies. Decreases in power in these frequency bands have been interpreted to reflect increased activation (Lindsley & Wicke, 1974; Shagass, 1972). Asymmetries in activation between the hemispheres have been examined by comparing the power values derived from homologous electrode locations (for a detailed review of the methodological issues involved in EEG studies of cerebral asymmetry, see Davidson, in press).

In one of the first studies designed to evaluate anterior and posterior EEG asymmetries associated with differential affective responding, Davidson *et al.* (1979) exposed 16 right-handed subjects to videotaped segments of popular television programs that were judged to vary in affective content. While viewing the videotapes, subjects were instructed to rate continuously the degree to which they experienced positive versus negative affect by pressing up and down on a pressure-sensitive gauge. The output of this pressure transducer was digitized to provide a quantitative measure of affective self-report.

EEG was recorded from the left and right frontal (F3 and F4) and parietal (P3 and P4) regions referred to common vertex (Cz). Activity in the alpha band was extracted from the EEG, integrated, and digitized. The electro-oculogram (EOG) was also recorded and epochs confounded by eye movement artifact were eliminated. To obtain an independent measure of the subjects' affective response to the video stimuli, two channels of facial EMG were also recorded—from the zygomatic (which tenses during smiling) and frontalis (associated with tension and frowning) regions. EMG data were also integrated and digitized.

To test the major hypotheses, the 30-second epoch *each subject* judged to be most positive was compared with the one rated as most negative. This information was derived from the pressure transducer data. The positive and negative epochs deviated from the central neutral position by comparable amounts. The positive and negative epochs were first compared on an alpha laterality ratio score ($R - L/R + L$ alpha power). Higher numbers on this score indicate greater relative left-sided activation. Davidson and colleagues found significantly greater relative left frontal activation during the epochs subjects judged as most positive than during those they judged as most negative. Parietal asymmetry did not discriminate between conditions. Analysis of the separate alpha power from the right and left frontal sites indicated that the difference between conditions was a function of changes in both hemispheres. The positive epochs were associated with less left frontal and more right frontal α compared with the negative epochs.

To confirm independently that the epochs that subjects self-rated as positive and negative produced expressive changes consistent with these emotional shifts, the integrated EMG recorded from the zygomatic and frontalis muscle regions was examined. Positive segments elicited reliably more zygomatic and less frontalis activity than did negative segments. Several other studies in adults using a variety of different affect elicitors were performed and confirmed the basic effect described here (e.g., Bennett, Davidson, & Saron, 1981; Davidson *et al.*, 1985).

Research with human infants confirms the presence of hemispheric lateralization for the expression of emotion during the first year of life (Davidson & Fox, 1982; Fox & Davidson, 1986, 1987). Davidson and Fox (1982) tested 10-month-old infants in two studies examining EEG during the presentation of emotion-eliciting stimuli. Ten-month-olds were chosen for these initial developmental studies because most investigators agree that by this age, infants display facial signs of all the primary emotions (Campos, Barrett, Lamb, Goldsmith, & Stenberg, 1983). In these two studies a videotape of an actress laughing and crying (order was counterbalanced across subjects) was presented to the infants. The findings from the two studies were virtually identical, and the effects were independently significant for each experiment. Parietal asymmetry did not discriminate between the happy and sad segments. Similar to the adult findings, the frontal asymmetry score did discriminate between conditions, with greater relative left-sided activation elicited in response to the happy segments compared with the sad segments (see Table 7-1). When the separate contributions of the left and right frontal regions were examined, it was the left hemisphere that changed more than the right between conditions. The left hemisphere was more active during happy compared to sad video segments. Across both studies, 20 of the 24 infants showed equal or greater relative left frontal activation during happy versus sad epochs. These findings were the first to demonstrate that the frontal asymmetry for positive

Table 7-1. Mean (Standard Deviation) Frontal Laterality Ratio Score (F4 − F3/F4 + F3 1–12 Hz Activity) by Condition for the Two Studies Described

		Condition	
Study	N	Happy	Sad
1	10	.021 (.051)	−.001 (.032)
2	14	.073 (.100)	.032 (.115)

Source: Davidson and Fox (1982).

Note: Higher numbers indicate greater relative left-sided activation.

versus negative affect that was found in adults is present in infants in the first year of life.

In a subsequent study, Fox and Davidson (1987) recorded EEG from 35 10-month-old infants during a stranger approach/mother approach/maternal separation sequence. Infant facial and vocal behavior was videotaped during the experiment. From inspection of the videotapes, it was clear that there were two general behavioral patterns that occurred in response to maternal separation. Of the 14 infants for whom there was artifact-free EEG during this condition, 6 cried at maternal separation, while the remainder did not cry. The EEG data were examined as a function of the two different patterns of behavioral response during separation. Infant EEG for criers and noncriers in the condition just before the separation (mother reaching toward the infant, following an approach sequence) was compared to EEG during the separation condition. Results of the analyses revealed that infants who cried showed a complete reversal in their pattern of frontal activation between the mother-reach and maternal-separation conditions. In response to mother reach, these subjects showed left-sided activation, whereas in response to maternal separation the criers exhibited right frontal activation. The noncriers showed no difference in left frontal activation between conditions. Interestingly, compared with the mother-reach condition, in response to maternal separation the noncriers showed a pronounced inhibition of right frontal activation (an increase in power). Seven of the 9 subjects (3 of 4 criers and 4 of 5 noncriers) displayed these changes in frontal asymmetry between the mother-reach and maternal-separation conditions.

The finding of differences in frontal EEG asymmetry that distinguish between infants who differed in their response to maternal separation is consistent with the notion that changes in frontal EEG are related to the expression of different positive and negative emotions (Davidson, 1984a, 1984b; Fox & Davidson, 1984). The infants who cried in response to maternal separation showed an increase in relative right frontal activation in this condition compared with the preceding condition, but those infants who did not cry in response to this stressor showed a decrease in activation of the right frontal region. Coding of infant facial behavior during the separation condition revealed that infants that protested separation exhibited expressions of anger, distress and sadness, whereas those not crying exhibited expressions of interest. This pattern of emotional expressiveness during the separation condition is similar to that reported by Izard and colleagues (Shiller, Izard, & Hembree, 1986). The decreased activation of the right frontal region in the noncriers may reflect an active inhibition in this cortical area. The degree to which infants exhibited this inhibition may be associated with individual differences in the maturation of certain brain regions associated with the ability to regulate emotional expression.

Table 7-2. Means and Standard Deviations for Log Power in the 3- to 6-Hz Band Separately for the Left and Right Frontal and Parietal Regions, by Condition

		Frontal		Parietal	
		Left	Right	Left	Right
Water	M	.35	−.14	1.42	1.23
	S.D.	1.42	1.55	.96	1.01
Sugar	M	.44	.70	1.06	1.38
	S.D.	1.12	1.00	.93	.82
Citric	M	.33	.34	1.42	1.39
	S.D.	1.59	1.47	1.00	.78

Source: Fox and Davidson (1986).

Although these data on 10-month-olds suggest that the frontal asymmetry is ''hard-wired,'' it is certainly possible that a considerable amount of learning relevant to emotion and its motor sequelae occurs during the first 10 months. In an attempt to extend the finding of frontal asymmetry differences between positive and negative affect back even earlier, Fox and Davidson (1986) performed a study with newborns. To elicit approach and withdrawal reactions, they exposed infants to different tastes presented via pipette on the tongue. To acclimate subjects to the procedure, distilled water was presented first followed by a sucrose solution and then by citric acid. Infants' facial behavior was videotaped while EEG was recorded from the left and right frontal and parietal scalp regions according to the methods described earlier. Analysis of the videotapes indicated that facial signs of disgust were present in equal amounts in response to the initial introduction of water and in response to citric acid. EEG in response to the water condition revealed right-hemisphere activation (reductions in right-hemisphere power in the 3- to 6-Hz and 6- to 12-Hz bands) in both regions compared with the other two conditions. The sucrose condition produced greater relative left-sided activation in both regions compared with the water condition (See Table 7-2).

The findings from this study generally support the view that asymmetry of hemispheric activation in response to affective stimuli is present at birth. Although the water condition had originally been presented as a neutral condition, which was predicted to fall in between the two taste conditions, it was found unexpectedly that the greatest difference in EEG asymmetry was between the water and sucrose conditions. The facial data indicate that the water condition was associated with the display of expressions of disgust. Perhaps this was a function of the water always being the first stimulus condition. The procedure of introducing a pipette into the infants' mouth may, in itself, possess certain aversive qualities. Although this analysis may explain the finding of right-sided activation for the water condition, it does not explain the lack of a right-sided effect for the citric acid condition, during which facial signs of disgust were also present. It may be that electrocortical manifestations of emotion habituate prior to behavioral signs in infants of this age, but the current evidence does not permit us to offer any more definitive explanation.

One other unexpected finding from this study was that the right-sided activation in response to the water condition was found at both frontal and parietal scalp locations. It might be that the differentiated activation of different functional regions of the cortex does not emerge until later in the first year of life. Recent findings using measures of regional brain metabolism in human infants are consistent with this suggestion (Chugani & Phelps, 1986).

FRONTAL ASYMMETRY AND EXPRESSION OF FACIAL SIGNS OF EMOTION

Although the adult and infant studies described here demonstrate a relation between frontal EEG asymmetry and the subjective experience of emotion or behavioral changes reflecting emotion, they do not precisely specify the essential continuum along which the frontal region is lateralized for emotion. Specifically, it is unclear whether differences in frontal asymmetry reflect hedonic tone or are more specifically associated with particular discrete emotions. Do different positive and negative emotions share the property of being associated with the same general pattern of frontal activation asymmetry? If so, this would provide some support for a dimensional conception of emotion. If, on the other hand, different emotions are associated with unique signatures of brain activity, support would be given to a discrete conceptualization of emotion. Following Kinsbourne (1978), Davidson (Davidson, 1984; Davidson *et al.*, 1979; Reuter-Lorenz & Davidson, 1981) proposed that the frontal asymmetry that was observed in the EEG was a reflection of a basic asymmetry for the control of approach versus withdrawal behavior. It was argued that these behavioral systems require very different motor programming and that the motor specialization of the left hemisphere is uniquely suited for the control of approach, while that of the right hemisphere is appropriate for the control of withdrawal (see Davidson, 1984a, 1984b; Davidson *et al.*, 1979; and Reuter-Lorenz & Davidson, 1981). Fox and Davidson (1984) expanded this argument to include a developmental perspective. On the basis of this scheme, positive emotions that are accompanied by approach should be associated with left frontal activation, whereas negative emotions accompanied by withdrawal should be associated with right frontal activation. Certainly, not all negative emotions are regularly associated with withdrawal. For example, sadness may not elicit withdrawal, and anger is sometimes associated with approach where the angered individual wishes to strike out at the object or person responsible for frustrating a sought-after goal. The emotions of disgust and fear would be those most likely associated with right frontal activation because of their association with withdrawal behavior.

To explore differences in EEG asymmetry during emotions associated with approach and withdrawal in adults, Davidson, Ekman, Saron, and Friesen (1988) exposed subjects to films designed to elicit primarily happiness and disgust while brain activity was monitored (from the left and right frontal and parietal scalp regions) and the subjects' facial behavior was unobtrusively videotaped. In this experiment, the facial expressions were used to specify epochs during which particular discrete emotions were present. EEG during the period coincident with the display of expressions of happiness and disgust was then examined. The videotaped records were coded off line using Ekman and Friesen's (1984) Emotion Facial Action Coding System (EMFACS) for the presence of discrete facial expressions of emotion. Onset and offset times for facial expressions of happiness and disgust were determined, and artifact-free EEG during these periods was extracted for analysis. The results from this experiment support the hypothesis that discrete emotions associated with approach and withdrawal are differentially lateralized to the left and right frontal regions, respectively. During facial expressions of disgust, there was significantly more relative right frontal activation than during facial signs of happiness. No differences in parietal asymmetry were observed between emotions. As a control procedure, EEG was extracted from the entire positive and negative film periods, irrespective of the presence or absence of facial behavior. No differences were found in EEG asymmetry at either frontal or parietal sites between periods extracted from the positive versus the negative film. In other words, the use of facial signs of emotion to flag epochs during which affect was

Table 7-3. Number of Infants Displaying Smiles with and without Orbicularis Oculi Activity in Response to the Stranger- and Mother-Approach Conditions

	With orbicularis	Without orbicularis
Stranger approach	5	15
Mother approach	21	6

Source: Fox and Davidson (1988).

Note: Difference in the incidence of the two types of smiling between the two conditions is significant ($p = .005$ by Fisher's Exact Test).

experienced was quite fruitful in revealing those periods during which the EEG reflected differences as a function of emotion.

Similar questions were also investigated in 10-month-old infants (Fox & Davidson, 1988). Facial behaviors were coded from a sample of 35 10-month-old infants who were presented with the stranger and mother approach sequences.

The periods of artifact-free EEG that coincided with the presence of the discrete emotions of joy, sadness, and anger were extracted. The strategy for examining brain activity during the presence of discrete facial signs of emotion was dictated by the frequency of occurrence of different expressions that were coincident with artifact-free EEG. Facial signs of joy, sadness, and anger occurred with sufficient frequency to permit analysis.

Infants were observed to exhibit smiles to both stranger and mother during the two different approaches. Examination of the EMFACS data revealed, however, that during the stranger approach infants displayed significantly more instances of smiles without orbicularis compared to the mother-approach condition (see Table 7-3). Smiles in the absence of orbicularis activity are expressions that involve only the action of the zygomatic major muscle, whereas the other form of smiling is comprised of actions of both the zygomatic major and orbicularis oculi muscles, an observation made originally by Darwin (1872) and more recently confirmed by Ekman (Ekman & Friesen, 1982). Examination of the EEG during the periods of these two different types of smiles revealed that frontal asymmetry discriminated between them. During the expression of ''orbicularis smiles,'' infants exhibited greater relative left frontal activation than during the expression of smiles without orbicularis activity. During the latter periods, infants displayed right frontal activation. Parietal EEG did not discriminate between these conditions. Interestingly, infants were more likely to exhibit gaze aversion following a smile without orbicularis activity than following the other form of smiling. Gaze aversion, particularly to an approaching unfamiliar person, has been interpreted as a sign of withdrawal. Thus, smiles without orbicularis activity, considered by some to be unfelt and exhibited during approach of a stranger, may be viewed as an initial component of withdrawal to a mildly stressful unfamiliar event. This response was associated with right frontal activation. Approach of the mother, a positive event, was accompanied by genuine expressions of happiness and left frontal activation. The pattern of differential cerebral activation during specific emotion expressions thus seems to be evident as early as 10 months of age. Those expressions of emotion associated with approach elicited relative left frontal activation, whereas those associated with withdrawal elicited relative right frontal activation.

The analyses of EEG during facial signs of sadness and anger indicated that the presence of these expressions in conjunction with crying was associated with greater relative right frontal activation than was the display of these same expressions in the absence of crying. Again, parietal EEG did not discriminate between epochs during which crying was present or absent.

INDIVIDUAL DIFFERENCES IN FRONTAL ACTIVATION ASYMMETRY: RELATION TO AFFECTIVE STYLE IN ADULTS AND INFANTS

Pronounced differences among individuals are typical in both EEG and behavioral measures of asymmetry. Levy (1983) has suggested that the diversity among dextrals in the magnitude and direction of asymmetries on behavioral measures of "cerebral lateralization" may reflect true variations in "patterns of asymmetric hemispheric arousal that were superimposed on a relatively invariant pattern of hemispheric specialization" (p. 476). Levy underscores the inconsistency between the percentage of subjects who would be expected to show lateralization of verbal processing to the left hemisphere and the percentage who actually show right-field advantages for verbal material on dichotic and divided visual field tasks. She argues that this discrepancy is a function of individual differences in asymmetrical hemispheric arousal and infers the magnitude of such differences on the basis of behavioral asymmetries. Levy and her colleagues (Levy, Heller, Banich, & Burton, 1983) have reported a number of robust relations between individual differences in "hemispheric arousal" and performance on a variety of tasks that presumably differentially require the activation of the two hemispheres.

Recordings of EEG asymmetries provide a more direct method for inferring individual differences in hemispheric activation. A number of workers have demonstrated that individual differences in EEG asymmetry are reliable over a 1- to 3-week period (Amochaev & Salamy, 1979; Ehrlichman & Wiener, 1979). Several investigators have reported that individual differences in resting EEG activation asymmetry recorded from the posterior scalp regions are related to performance differences on verbal and spatial cognitive tasks (e.g., Davidson, Taylor, & Saron, 1979; Furst, 1976; Glass & Butler, 1977). For example, Davidson, Taylor, and Saron (1979) found that greater right parietal activation during rest was associated with better performance on a face recognition task. Measures of frontal EEG asymmetry from the same points in time were uncorrelated with cognitive performance.

Since our studies on emotion indicated that frontal asymmetries were related to the valence of affective responding, it was of interest to determine whether individual differences in affective style were related to variations in resting frontal activation asymmetry. In a first attempt to explore this issue, Davidson and colleagues (Schaffer, Davidson, & Saron, 1983) selected subjects on the basis of extreme scores on the Beck Depression Inventory. Depressed and nondepressed subjects were compared on resting eyes-closed frontal and parietal activation asymmetry (based on measures of alpha power) recorded before and after a series of experimental tasks that lasted approximately 2 hours. Frontal asymmetry discriminated between the depressed and nondepressed groups. The major group difference was that there was less left frontal activation among the depressed than among the nondepressed subjects. Parietal asymmetry recorded from the same points in time failed to discriminate between groups. These findings underscore the specificity of frontal asymmetry for affect and indicate that individual differences on this measure are related to affective style.

In more recent work with adults, Tomarken and Davidson (1988) have found that individual differences in resting frontal and anterior temporal asymmetry predict the intensity of response to emotional films in two separate studies using different film clips. For example, in a sample of 22 normal right-handed female subjects, greater relative right frontal activation during rest was significantly correlated with increased intensity of fear in response to films designed to elicit negative affect. This pattern was present in response to each of the two negative films that were presented. Parietal asymmetry from the same points in time was unrelated to subject's rating of emotional intensity. In addition to assessing self-reported emotion following each of the film clips, subjects' emotional experience following each resting baseline was also examined in order to determine whether resting asymmetries are related to spontaneous emotion during the baseline periods themselves. It was found that resting activation asymmetry was unrelated to emotion reported during the baseline period. Thus, the subjects who showed right frontal activation during this time were not simply in a dysphoric mood when they arrived for the experiment. Subjects with extreme right versus left frontal activation were not discriminable on any emotion scale from the baseline rating period.

Davidson and Fox (1988) have recently explored the relation between resting frontal asymmetries and affective behavior in infants. Resting EEG was recorded from the left and right frontal and parietal scalp regions for a 30-second period from 19 normal 10-month-old infants (all born to two right-handed parents). The mother was present in the room during the baseline measurement. Following this period, two standardized approach sequences were presented. The first involved a stranger approaching the infant (with mother present), and the second consisted of the mother approaching. Following the mother approach sequence, the mother was instructed to turn around and leave the room. The duration of this period was 60 seconds unless the infant was judged by the experimenter to be extremely upset, at which time the trial was terminated by having the mother reenter the subject room and comfort her baby. The infant was videotaped during all periods of the experiment.

In response to the maternal separation period, we coded the presence or absence of sustained crying. Of the 14 infants with usable EEG during the baseline period, 7 were coded as criers and 7 as noncriers during this period. We then examined the EEG during the baseline period to determine whether the criers could be discriminated from the noncriers. Asymmetries in the frontal and parietal region in the 6- to 8-Hz frequency band were compared between criers and noncriers. This frequency band was chosen because the majority of power in the infant EEG occurs between these frequencies and it has been used in our previous research with infants of this age (Fox & Davidson, 1987). We found a reliable difference between criers and noncriers in frontal asymmetry. The criers displayed significantly more relative right-sided frontal activation during rest than did the noncriers. No differences in parietal asymmetry were obtained between these groups. Of the 7 infants who cried in this situation, only one did not show absolute right frontal activation during the baseline period. Figure 7-1 presents the frontal and parietal baseline data separately by hemisphere for the criers and noncriers.

The facial behavior of the infants during the baseline period was coded in order to ascertain whether subjects who subsequently cried in response to maternal separation were simply in a more dysphoric mood when they first arrived for the experiment. In that case, the frontal asymmetry differences in the baseline period would be interpreted differently. This is the same question we asked of our adult data. There we examined whether resting frontal asymmetries were related to subjects' self-reported emotional experiences during the same resting period. Since data of this type are obviously unavailable for infants, we used facial behavior as an index of emotional reactivity. Table 7-4 presents the data on the duration of different emotion expressions coded during the baseline period for the infants who subsequently went on to cry and for those who did not cry in response to maternal separation. As can be seen from this table, there were no differences in the incidence of any of the emotion expressions coded during baseline between criers and noncriers.

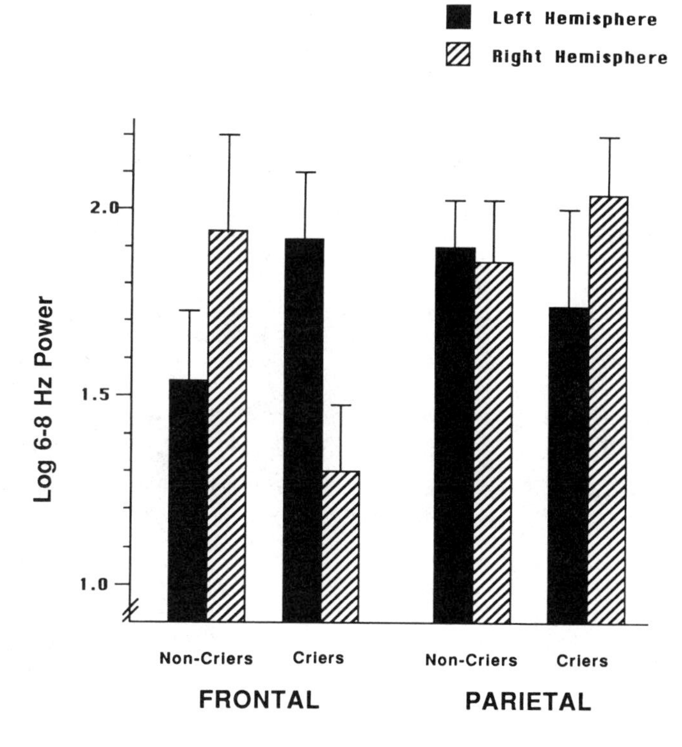

Figure 7-1. Mean log 6–8-Hz power for the resting baseline period in the left and right frontal and parietal regions for criers and noncriers. Decreases in 6–8-Hz power are indicative of increases in activation. Error bars are standard errors of the mean. Reprinted with permission from "Frontal Brain Asymmetry Predicts Infants' Response to Maternal Separation" by R. J. Davidson and N. A. Fox, 1988, paper submitted for publication.

Table 7-4. Mean Duration in Seconds of Facial Affect for Criers ($N=6$) and Noncriers ($N=7$) during the Baseline Period

		Criers	Noncriers
Interest	Mean	9.5	11.3
	S.D.	8.6	7.8
No expression	Mean	17.0	15.1
	S.D.	8.2	8.9
Joy/surprise	Mean	2.4	3.2
	S.D.	2.9	3.2
Negative affect	Mean	0.5	1.4
	S.D.	0.9	1.3

Source: Davidson and Fox (1987).

Note: The no-expression category represents the mean number of seconds during which no facial signs of emotion were present. The negative-affect category represents the mean number of seconds during which facial signs of any of the negative emotions (anger, fear, distress, sadness, disgust) were expressed.

Table 7-5. Summary of the Studies Conducted by the Authors Described in This Chapter

Citation	Subjects	Conditions	Measures	Results
		Task effects		
Davidson *et al.*, 1979	16 adults	Self-rated positive and negative epochs	P3, P4, F3, F4 alpha	Neg. cond.—right fron. activ. pos. cond.—left fron. activ. No parietal diff.
Davidson & Fox, 1982	24 10-month-old infants	Videotape of actress portraying happiness and sadness	P3, P4, F3, F4 1–12 Hz activity	Happy epoch—more left fron. activ. compared with sad epoch. No parietal diff.
Fox & Davidson, 1986	33 full-term infants 2–3 days old	Distilled water, sucrose, and citric acid solutions	P3, P4, F3, F4 3–6 Hz power	Sucrose—more facial signs of interest and left-sided activ. Water—facial sign of disgust and right-sided activ.
Davidson *et al.*, 1987	22 adults	Facial signs of happiness and disgust	P3, P4, F3, F4 alph power	Disgust—greater right fron. activ. compared with happy. No parietal diff.
Fox & Davidson, 1987b	35 10-month-old infants	Smiles with and without orbicularis	P3, P4, F3, F4 3–12 Hz power	Orbicularis smile—left fron. activ. Non-orbicularis smile—right fron. activ.; No parietal diff.
		Individual differences		
Schaffer *et al.*, 1983	6 depressed 9 nondepressed	Eyes closed baseline	P3, P4, F3, F4 alpha	Depressed Ss—less left fron. activ. compared with nondepressed. No parietal diff.
Tomarken & Davidson, 1988	22 adults	Eyes open baseline; negative film clips	P3, P4, F3, F4 alpha power	Right fron. activ. correlated with greater self-reported fear; Parietal asymmetry uncorr.
Davidson & Fox, 1988	19 10-month-old infants	Eyes open baseline; maternal separation	P3, P4, F3, F4 5–9 Hz power	Ss who cried to materal separation—greater right fron. activ. during baseline. No parietal diff.
Fox & Davidson, 1987a	35 10-month-old infants	Mother approach; maternal separation	P3, P4, F3, F4 3–5 Hz power	Criers—left fron. activ. during mother reach and right fron. activ. during separation. Noncriers—less right fron. activ. during separation versus mother reach. No parietal diff.

Note: Fron. = frontal; activ. = activation; diff. = difference; neg. = negative; pos. = positive; cond. = condition; uncorr. = uncorrelated. The first half of the table presents the studies examining task effects. The second half summarizes the studies on individual differences. Subjects in all adult studies were right-handed, and those in all infant studies were born to two right-handed parents.

WHAT DO FRONTAL ACTIVATION ASYMMETRIES REFLECT?

The data reviewed in this chapter (see Table 7-5 for a summary) indicate that differences in frontal activation asymmetry are observed in response to stimuli that elicit certain positive and negative emotional reactions. The data also indicate that right frontal activation might occur during resting baseline conditions when neither self-report nor facial behavior indicates that negative emotion is present. In these circumstances, relative right-sided resting frontal activation was found to predict the intensity of the subsequent response to negative affective elicitors. Thus, the combination of available evidence indicates that under certain circumstances, right frontal activation is associated with concurrent negative affect, but in other circumstances it is not. This pattern of findings leads to the proposal that right frontal activation marks a vulnerability to experience certain negative emotions. In this situation, the threshold for the elicitation of negative affect might be lower. Given a moderately intense negative stimulus, we would predict that those subjects with baseline right frontal activation would respond more intensely than would subjects displaying left frontal activation. A weak negative stimulus should be capable of eliciting negative affect only among those who are relatively vulnerable. Subjects with strong left frontal activation may represent an "invulnerable" group who require an extremely intense elicitor to trigger negative affect.

Precisely why subjects with right frontal activation should be more vulnerable to the experience of negative affect is not currently known. It may be that such subjects appraise situations differently than do those not so affected. It may be that appraisal is the same in both types of subjects and that it is the magnitude of the response that differs. Subjects with strong right frontal activation may appraise a situation as only mildly stressful, yet not be capable of regulating their extreme response. For example, in response to the negative films (Tomarken & Davidson, 1988), a subject might report that she knew the stimulus was a film and there was nothing objective to be scared of, yet she couldn't keep herself from experiencing a very strong reaction. Still another possibility is that subjects with both left- and right-sided resting frontal activation appraise the situation similarly and respond with similar intensity. In this model, what distinguishes the subjects is the availability of coping responses among those with left frontal activation. These subjects may be capable of quickly terminating their reaction, whereas subjects with right frontal activation may lack the requisite coping skills to minimize the duration of the negative affective response.

Choosing the best model among these alternatives to explain the meaning of individual differences in resting frontal activation asymmetry necessitates research specifically designed to answer this question. Such investigation will require accurate measures of appraisal and coping processes as well as the duration and intensity of the emotional reaction in question. The complexity in the interpretation of individual differences in resting frontal activation asymmetries underscores the relevance of basic emotion theory to studies on psychophysiological responses to emotional stimuli. It is clear that emotion is a multicomponential set of phenomena which can only be unraveled by careful attention to its differentiated nature. This requires a detailed examination of relations between physiological changes and specific emotion sub-components.

SUMMARY AND CONCLUSIONS

In this chapter, we reviewed selected findings on the lateralization of emotion in adults and infants. At the outset, we emphasized the importance of the distinction between *perception* and *production* of emotion. We suggested that overall right-hemisphere superiority (across valence) is present for the perception of emotion, but that once emotion is recruited, differential lateralization of certain positive and negative emotions is found. This differential lateralization is most prominently observed in recordings of brain electrical activity from the frontal region. We proposed that the fundamental continuum along which the anterior regions of the hemispheres are lateralized for emotion is approach and withdrawal, and we presented evidence for the presence of this asymmetry in young infants. In two studies, one with adults and one with infant subjects where EEG was extracted during facial signs of emotion, facial signs of emotions associated with withdrawal were associated with right frontal activation compared with facial signs of emotions associated with approach.

Pronounced individual differences are present in resting measures of EEG activation asymmetries. A series of findings was presented in both adults and infants that indicate that these EEG differences among subjects are related to differences in emotional style or reactivity. In adults, subjects scoring high on the Beck Depression Inventory have decreased left frontal activation during rest compared with nondepressed controls (Schaffer *et al.*, 1983). And greater right frontal activation during rest was correlated with increased intensity of self-reported fear in response to films designed to elicit negative affect (Davidson & Tomarken, 1987). Finally, among 10-month-old infants, those with resting right frontal activation were more likely to cry in response to brief maternal separation than were subjects showing left frontal activation during rest (Davidson & Fox, 1987). In the latter two studies, measures of affect during the baseline periods themselves were unrelated to resting frontal activation asymmetries.

The findings reported in this chapter provide the basis for the assertion that right frontal activation is a contributory cause to the experience of certain forms of negative affect. The presence of right frontal activation during rest was said to represent a vulnerability for the experience of negative affect. Precisely what the frontal asymmetry represents will require additional research wherein the subcomponents of emotion are systematically disentangled and related to EEG measures. Appraisal and coping are two subcomponents that may be related to the frontal asymmetries we have reported. It is clear that future research in this area must combine the sophistication that is now available in both behavioral studies of emotion and cerebral psychophysiology.

ACKNOWLEDGMENTS

The research described in this chapter was supported in part by grants from NIMH (MH#40747) and the Graduate School of the University of Wisconsin to RJD, NSF grant #BNS-8317229 to NAF and RJD and NICHD grant HD#17899 to NAF.

REFERENCES

Akert, K. (1964). Comparative anatomy of the frontal cortex and thalamocortical connections. In J. M. Warren & K. Akert (Eds.), *The frontal granular cortex and behavior* (pp. 372–396). New York: McGraw-Hill.

Alford, L. B. (1933). Localization of consciousness and emotion. *American Journal of Psychiatry, 12,* 789–799.

Amochaev, A., & Salamy, A. (1979). Stability of EEG laterality effects. *Psychophysiology, 16,* 242–246.

Bennett, J., Davidson, R. J., & Saron, C. (1981). Patterns of self-rating in response to verbally elicited affective imagery: Relation to frontal vs. parietal EEG asymmetry. *Psychophysiology, 18,* 158.

Bryden, M. P. (1982). *Laterality: Functional asymmetry in the intact brain.* New York: Academic Press.

Campos, J. J., Barrett, K. C., Lamb, M. E., Goldsmith, H. H., & Stenberg, C. (1983). Socioemotional development. In M. M. Haith & J. J. Campos (Eds.), *Handbook of child psychology: Vol. II. Infancy and developmental psychobiology* (pp. 783–915). New York: Wiley.

Chugani, H. T., & Phelps, M. E. (1986). Maturational changes in cerebral function in infants determined by 18FDG positron emission tomography. *Science, 231,* 840–843.

Darwin, C. (1872/1976). *The expression of emotion in man and animals.* Chicago: University of Chicago Press.

Davidson, R. J. (1984a). Affect, cognition and hemispheric specialization. In C. E. Izard, J. Kagan, & R. Zajonc (Eds.), *Emotion, cognition and behavior* (pp. 320–365). New York: Cambridge University Press.

Davidson, R. J. (1984b). Hemispheric asymmetry and emotion. In K. Scherer & P. Ekman (Eds.), *Approaches to emotion* (pp. 39–57). Hillsdale, NJ: Erlbaum.

Davidson, R. J. (in press). EEG measures of cerebral asymmetry: Conceptual and methodological issues. *International Journal of Neuroscience.*

Davidson, R. J., Ekman, P., Saron, C., & Friesen, W. (1988). *EEG asymmetry during facial expressions of happiness and disgust.* Manuscript in preparation.

Davidson, R. J., & Fox, N. A. (1982). Asymmetrical brain activity discriminates between positive versus negative affective stimuli in human infants. *Science, 218,* 1235–1237.

Davidson, R. J., & Fox, N. A. (1988). *Frontal brain asymmetry predicts infants' response to maternal separation.* Paper submitted for publication.

Davidson, R. J., Schaffer, C. E., & Saron, C. (1985). Effects of lateralized stimulus presentations on the self-report of emotion and EEG asymmetry in depressed and non-depressed subjects. *Psychophysiology, 22,* 353–364.

Davidson, R. J., Schwartz, G. E., Saron, C., Bennett, J., & Goleman, D. J. (1979). Frontal versus parietal EEG asymmetry during positive and negative affect. *Psychophysiology, 16,* 202–203.

Davidson, R. J., Taylor, N., & Saron, C. (1979). Hemisphericity and styles of information processing: Individual differences in EEG asymmetry and their relationship to cognitive performance. *Psychophysiology, 16,* 197.

Denny-Brown, D., Meyer, S. T., & Horenstein, S. (1952). The significance of perceptual rivalry resulting from parietal lesion. *Brain, 5,* 433–471.

Ehrlichman, H., & Wiener, M. S. (1979). Consistency of task-related EEG asymmetries. *Psychophysiology, 16,* 247–252.

Ekman, P., & Friesen, W. V. (1982). Felt, false and miserable smiles. *Journal of Nonverbal Behavior, 6,* 238–252.

Ekman, P., & Friesen, W. V. (1984). *EMFACS coding manual.* Unpublished manuscript, University of California, San Francisco.

Etcoff, N. L. (1986). The neuropsychology of emotional expression. In G. Goldstein & R. E. Tarter (Eds.), *Advances in clinical neuropsychology* (Vol. 3, pp. 127–179). New York: Plenum.

Fox, N. A., & Davidson, R. J. (1984). Hemispheric substrates of affect: A developmental model. In N. A. Fox & R. J. Davidson (Eds.), *The psychobiology of affective development* (pp. 353–381). Hillsdale, NJ: Erlbaum Associates.

Fox, N. A., & Davidson, R. J. (1986). Taste-elicited changes in facial signs of emotion and the asymmetry of brain electrical activity in human newborns. *Neuropsychologia, 24,* 417–422.

Fox, N. A., & Davidson, R. J. (1987). Electroencephalogram asymmetry in response to the approach of a stranger and maternal separation in 10-month-old infants. *Developmental Psychology, 23,* 233–240.

Fox, N. A., & Davidson, R. J. (1988). Patterns of brain electrical activity during facial signs of emotion in 10-month-old infants. *Developmental Psychology, 24,* 230–236.

Furst, C. J. (1976). EEG asymmetry and visuospatial performance. *Nature, 260,* 254–255.

Gainotti, G. (1969). Reactions ''Catotrophiques'' et manifestations d'indifference au cours des atteintes cerebrais. *Neuropsychologia, 7,* 195–204.

Gainotti, G. (1972). Emotional behavior and hemispheric side of lesion. *Cortex, 8,* 41–55.

Glass, A., & Butler, S. R. (1977). Alpha EEG asymmetry and speed of left hemisphere thinking. *Neuroscience Letters, 4,* 231–235.

Goldsmith, H. H., Buss, A. H., Plomin, R., Rothbard, M. K., Thomas, A., Chess, S., Hinde, R. A., & McCall, R. B. (1987). Roundtable: What is temperament? Four approaches. *Child Development, 58,* 505–529.

Goldstein, K. (1939). *The organism.* New York: Academic Book Publishers.

Hecaen, H., Ajuriaguerra, J. D., & Massonet, J. (1951). Les troubles visu, constructifs par lesions parieto-occipitales droctes. Roles des perturbations resticularies. *L'Encephale, 1,* 122–179.

Kinsbourne, M. (1978). Biological determinants of functional bisymmetry and asymmetry. In M. Kinsbourne, (Ed.), *Asymmetrical function of the brain* (pp. 3–13). New York: Cambridge University Press.

Kolb, B., & Milner, B. (1981a). Performance of complex arm and facial movements after focal brain lesions. *Neuropsychologia, 17,* 491–503.

Kolb, B., & Milner, B. (1981b). Observations on spontaneous facial expression after focal cerebral excisions and after intracarotid injection of sodium amytal. *Neuropsychologia, 19,* 505–514.

Levy, J. (1983). Individual differences in cerebral hemisphere asymmetry: Theoretical issues and experimental considerations. In J. B. Hellige (Ed.), *Cerebral hemisphere asymmetry: Method, theory and application* (pp. 465–497). New York: Praeger.

Levy, J., Heller, W., Banich, M. T., & Burton, L. A. (1983). Are variations among right-handed individuals in perceptual asymmetries caused by characteristic arousal differences between the hemispheres? *Journal of Experimental Psychology: Human Perception and Performance, 9,* 329–359.

Lindsley, D. B., & Wicke, J. D. (1974). The electroencephalogram: Autonomous electrical activity in man and animals. In R. F. Thompson & M. M. Patterson (Eds.), *Bioelectric recording techniques: B. Electroen-*

cephalography and human brain potentials. New York: Academic Press.
Luria, A. R. (1966). *Higher cortical functions in man*. New York: Basic Books.
Luria, A. R. (1973). *The working brain*. New York: Basic Books.
Nauta, W. J. H. (1964). Some efferent connections of the prefrontal cortex in the monkey. In J. M. Warren & K. Akert (Eds.), *The frontal granular cortex and behavior* (pp. 397–409). New York: McGraw-Hill.
Nauta, W. J. H. (1971). The problem of the frontal lobe: A reinterpretation. *Journal of Psychiatric Research, 8,* 167–187.
Pribram, K. H. (1973). The primate frontal cortex—Executive of the brain. In K. H. Pribram & A. R. Luria (Eds.), *Psychophysiology of the frontal lobes* (pp. 293–314). New York: Academic Press.
Reuter-Lorenz, P., & Davidson, R. J. (1981). Differential contributions of the two cerebral hemispheres to the perception of happy and sad faces. *Neuropsychologia, 19,* 609–613.
Robinson, R. G., & Benson, D. F. (1981). Depression in aphasic patients: Frequency, severity and clinical–pathological correlations. *Brain and Language, 14,* 282–291.
Robinson, R. G., & Szetela, B. (1981). Mood change following left hemispheric brain injury. *Annals of Neurology, 9,* 447–453.
Robinson, R. G., Kubos, K. L., Starr, L. B., Reo, K., & Price, T. R. (1984). Mood disorders in stroke patients: Importance of location of lesion. *Brain, 107,* 81–93.
Sackeim, H. A., Weiman, A. L., Gur, R. C., Greenburgh, M., Hungerbuhler, J. P., & Geschwind, N. (1982). Pathological laughing and crying: Functional brain asymmetry in the experience of positive and negative emotions. *Archives of Neurology, 39,* 210–218.
Schaffer, C. E., Davidson, R. J., & Saron, C. (1983). Frontal and parietal EEG asymmetries in depressed and non-depressed subjects. *Biological Psychiatry, 18,* 753–762.
Shagass, C. (1972). Electrical activity of the brain. In N. S. Greenfield & R. H. Sternbach (Eds.), *Handbook of psychophysiology* (pp. 263–328). New York: Holt, Rinehart and Winston.
Shiller, V. M., Izard, C. E., & Hembree, E. A. (1986). Patterns of emotional expression during separation in the strange situation. *Developmental Psychology, 22,* 378–383.
Silberman, E. K., & Weingartner, H. (1986). Hemispheric lateralization of functions related to emotion. *Brain and Cognition, 5,* 322–353.
Tomarken, A. J., & Davidson, A. J. (1988). Resting anterior EEG asymmetry predicts affective response to emotional films. Manuscript in preparation.
Tucker, D. M. (1981). Lateral brain function, emotion and conceptualization. *Psychological Bulletin, 89,* 19–46.

8

Right-Brain Training: Some Reflections on the Application of Research on Cerebral Hemispheric Specialization to Education

LAUREN JULIUS HARRIS
Michigan State University

Most scientists and educators agree that the application of scientific research on human behavior to the solution of educational and other social problems is a worthy and appropriate goal. They also surely will agree that any such enterprise poses formidable problems. The scientific research itself should be sufficiently advanced so that some application can be reasonably contemplated; the nature and scope of the educational problem must be understood; persons taking responsibility for the application must understand both the scientific data and the educational problem; the practical and theoretical limits of the application must be ascertained and respected; and, perhaps above all, polemicism and excessive zeal must be curbed so as to discourage the all-too-human appetite for fads and quick fixes. In this chapter I discuss these issues as they pertain to applications of scientific research that, in recent years, has become of keen interest to educators—namely, research on the functions of the left and right hemispheres of the cerebral cortex.

TEACHING THE LEFT BRAIN: THE OLD ORTHODOXY

Application of research on hemispheric specialization to problems in education is hardly new. Indeed, possibilities began to be suggested practically on the heels of the first reports of lateral specialization in the 1860s by the French physician and anthropologist Paul Broca (1861, 1863; Broca, 1865). For an account of one early-20th-century educational movement, see Harris (1980, 1985a, 1985b). Because so much of the early research on lateral specialization focused on the linguistic capacities of the left hemisphere, educational application was largely geared to the analysis and treatment of deficits in language and related skills. One well-known formulation was that of the American neurologist and psychiatrist Samuel T. Orton (1928, 1937). Let us briefly recall this work before we consider applications of lateralization research in our own day.

Following Broca's first clinical reports on the role of the anterior part of the left hemisphere for speech (1861, 1863), further clinical evidence suggested that the left hemisphere was the seat not only of speech but of a host of other linguistic and intellectual skills as well, including the comprehension of speech (Wernicke, 1874) and the capacities to read and write (e.g., Dejerine, 1891). Given the importance of these capacities for normal cognition, the left hemisphere began to assume the status of the dominant or master hemisphere, superior in every important way to its dextral counterpart. In time, the concept of cerebral dominance came to be understood and used in an absolute sense, with the left hemisphere regarded as the dominant or major hemisphere for all cognitive domains, and the right hemisphere as nondominant or minor, at most a weak, mute, less talented version of the left hemisphere.

It was in this context that Orton's theory and the applications that grew out of it were developed. Orton (1928, 1937) noted that children who had profound difficulties in reading and writing (but who otherwise seemed to be intellectually normal) showed frequent and prolonged confusions in recalling the directional orientation of letters and words. Many of these children were what Orton called "motor intergrades"; that is, they showed incomplete or mixed lateral motor dominance, expressed as inconsistent hand preference or as a disjunction of hand preference from foot or eye preference. To explain this combination of symptoms, Orton made two assumptions: First, the cerebral hemisphere dominant for visual language skills recorded letters and words in the correct (veridical) orientation, whereas the other, nondominant hemisphere recorded them in reversed orientation; second, the incomplete, or mixed, motor dominance in the motor-intergrade child reflected incomplete, or mixed, cerebral dominance. This assumption carried with it a further implication—that lateral specialization was itself a maturational phenomenon and normally increased with age. Orton, therefore, proposed that the motor-intergrade child's directional confusion in reading and writing arose from the lack of unilateral dominance of the visual language area of the brain.

From his analysis, Orton developed a complex, multisensory program for remediation that included—but only as a relatively minor feature—measures to correct the child's motoric inconsistencies. For example, if a child who wrote (badly) with his right hand showed clear signs that his left hand was naturally dominant (as indexed by other motor tests), Orton suggested a trial period of change to left-hand use to see whether some of the child's writing problems might be alleviated (see Orton, 1937, Chapter 3).

Orton's remedial programs were experimental and highly individualized. He emphatically rejected any "simplified and universally applicable formula" (1937, p. 143) as is evident in his cautious and undogmatic proposals for changing a child's writing hand. Unfortunately, many others have been avid for formula, the result too often being the promotion of rigid, simpleminded programs. Perhaps the most notorious example is that of Doman and Delacato and their collaborators under the auspices of the "Institutes for the Achievement of Human Potential" (Delacato, 1959, 1966; Doman, Spitz, Zucman, Delacato, & Doman, 1960). Convinced that the presumably missing unilateral hemisphere dominance in the disabled reader could be directly established by dominance training of hand, foot, eye, as well as ear (a possibility that Orton himself rejected on theoretical grounds; 1937, p. 174), they have made this training part of a radical therapeutic program (the so-called patterning method) in which they promise to cure everything from reading, writing, and other language problems to neuromuscular disorders and mental subnormality. The program not only restricts use of the subordinate limb and eye; it also bans music from the child's environment on the assumption that any nonlinguistic activity will disrupt the progress of cerebral dominance training (see Delacato, 1966, p. 27).

CURRENT DEVELOPMENTS IN RESEARCH ON LATERAL SPECIALIZATION

In Orton's day, the scientific analysis of lateral specialization was still quite limited. Since then, especially in the last two decades, and most especially in the years since the first Brock conference in 1975 (Segalowitz & Gruber, 1977), research on lateral specialization has grown substantially. The result has been the corroboration and amplification, as well as the correction, of certain earlier views.

In the correction department, I think it fair to say that Orton's (1937) application of lateralization principles to reading disability has been found wanting. As Zangwill (1960, p. 14) pointed out more than a quarter-century ago, the notion that one-half of the brain records patterns correctly, the other half incorrectly, was "decidedly speculative" and has found little acceptance among neuropsychologists. This verdict has not changed today. Likewise, after much research, there is no indication that mixed or incomplete *motor* dominance is related simply or directly either to cerebral dominance or to reading disability and other language problems (Naylor, 1980; Young & Ellis, 1981). This is not to say that developmental disorders of language are unrelated to anomalies of lateralization or that Orton was incorrect in some of his other characterization of disabled readers (for discussion, see Corballis, 1983, Chapter 8; Geschwind, 1982; and Harris & Carlson, Chapter 12, this volume).

There also is no evidence for the Doman-Delacato view that unilateral cerebral dominance for language functions can be enhanced by direct training of the contralateral limb (a view that, as I said, Orton himself rejected). Therefore, even if there were a simple, direct relationship between mixed cerebral dominance and language disabilities, attempts to remediate such problems through motor training would lack scientific foundation (see discussion in Kinsbourne & Hiscock, 1978).[1]

There have been many developments, too—both amplification and correction—in our understanding of the general principles of lateral specialization. This progress has been greatly assisted through new studies of clinical populations, including commissurotomy patients and patients with unilateral cortical lesions; through the use of new methods of assessing lateral functional specialization in neurologically normal individuals, including dichotic listening, recognition of briefly (tachistoscopically) exposed visual stimuli, dichaptic perception, and conjugate gaze deviation; and with the aid of both old and new methods of monitoring real-time cerebral activity (e.g., electroencephalography and regional cerebral blood flow).

One major result of contemporary research has been to provide a more careful specification of the kinds of component skills underlying left-hemisphere specialization for language. These include analyzing consonant sounds, processing rapidly changing acoustic events (a defining feature of consonants), dealing with grammatical categories, and classifying objects into standard linguistically defined categories (see review in Best, Chapter 1, this volume).

Another major result has been a dramatic change in our understanding of the functions of the right hemisphere. Only a few decades ago, the right hemisphere was still widely thought to be an inferior organ, largely lacking any special functions of its own. Today we know that it plays a special and, in many instances, leading role in the mediation of a variety of cognitive tasks. These tasks perhaps are best described as requiring the detection, processing, recognition, and memory of information that does not lend itself to linguistic description or analysis. In fact, Broca's contemporaries, the English neurologist John Hughlings Jackson, 1915, and *passim,* and the French-American neurologist Charles E. Brown-Séquard (1877) anticipated several of these new developments, although their views were not generally heeded at the time; see Benton (1972) and Harrington (1985). Examples include the encoding of certain components of musical structure (Gates & Bradshaw, 1977), face recognition and the interpretation of facial expression (Bryden & Ley, 1983), visualization in the third dimension, and appreciation of spatial relationships (Benton, 1985;

Harris, 1980b). The right hemisphere, though largely lacking the capacity to support speech, appears to provide an adequate substrate for more restricted aspects of linguistic processing, including the comprehension of spoken words (Gainotti, Caltagirone, Miceli, & Masullo, 1981; Searleman, 1977). New research also has confirmed and elaborated the earlier view (Jackson, 1874/1915) that the right hemisphere plays a leading role in analyzing the prosodic, as distinct from the semantic or syntactic, features of language (Ross, 1981).

All these new developments pertain to research on what are referred to conventionally as cognitive abilities. In recent years, neuropsychologists also have begun to study cerebral specialization for the perception, experience, and expression of affect and emotional state, functions once largely relegated to subcortical areas (see Chapter 3 by Denenberg and Chapter 7 by Davidson & Fox, this volume; see also reviews in Heilman & Satz, 1983). Although there is agreement as to the fact of the cortex's role, there are disagreements about the nature of lateral specialization with respect to the valence of the emotion. Some studies suggest that the right hemisphere plays the leading role in the mediation of negative emotions, the left hemisphere in the mediation of positive emotions (see reviews by Bruyer, 1980; Campbell, 1982; Sackeim *et al.*, 1982); other research points in precisely the reverse direction (e.g., Levy, Heller, Banich, & Burton, 1983; Tucker, Stenslie, Roth, & Shearer, 1981); and still other research suggests that the right hemisphere takes the lead in the mediation of all emotional states, whether positive or negative (e.g., Bryden & Ley, 1983; Carlson & Harris, 1986; Moscovitch & Olds, 1982; Schwartz, Davidson, & Maer, 1975). It is beyond the scope of this chapter to attempt to explain and reconcile these disparate views, except to note that studies differ in such potentially important factors as subject populations, dependent measures (perception versus expression), and even—and perhaps most crucially—precise definitions of "positive" and "negative" (see review in Tucker, 1981).

In light of this new, more comprehensive view of lateral specialization, we have had to change our notion of the concept of "cerebral dominance" and to give up the old terms "major" and "minor" hemispheres. If we say "cerebral dominance" today, we do not mean it in the old sense. Rather, we must add, "Dominant for what?"

In addition to studies further charting the respective functions of the cerebral hemispheres, the decade since the first Brock conference has also seen progress in our understanding of several other major issues pertaining to lateralization. One prominent area of work has been on individual differences. Much of this work has focused on the differences between right-handers and left-handers in the organization of language. From Broca's day until the 1940s, it was widely supposed that in left-handers, the right hemisphere rather than the left is the speech-dominant side. The new research shows, however, that in the majority of left-handers, perhaps two-thirds or more, the left hemisphere is the dominant side for speech, just as it is in nearly all right-handers (Hecaen & Ajuriaguerra, 1964; Hecaen & Sauguet, 1971; Satz, 1980). (For an analysis of Broca's own position and of further developments through the 1940s, see Harris, 1988.)

New research also has fostered a better appreciation of the possibility of individual differences within ostensibly homogeneous groups, such as right-handers. For instance, ordinary right-handed adults may differ in their characteristic patterns of hemispheric arousal, with some persons showing more phasic left-hemispheric arousal, others more right-hemispheric arousal. In one study (Levy *et al.*, 1983), the individual differences were suggested on the basis of reliable differences in patterns of performance in the perception of chimeric faces in a free-viewing task. Other measures also have been used, most prominently conjugate gaze deviation. Where the usual finding (Kinsbourne, 1972; Kocel, Galin, Ornstein, & Merrin, 1972) is that the eyes tend to move rightward for questions requiring predominantly verbal analysis (thus indicating relatively greater left-hemispheric arousal), leftward for questions requiring the analysis of spatial relations (greater right-hemispheric arousal), there are individual differences in the strength of the effect, such that, under certain test conditions, some individuals preferentially move their eyes to the right, irrespective of problem type, whereas others show preferential movement to the left (e.g., Gur, Gur, & Harris, 1975). Some neuropsychologists have adopted the term "hemisphericity" in reference to this possible dimension of individual differences. There also have been attempts to determine whether the individual patterns of performance on these tests are associated with such variables as college major or occupation, on the view that, say, left hemisphericity would be over-represented among individuals whose academic disciplines or occupations ostensibly draw heavily on linguistic–logical skills (e.g., lawyers), whereas right hemisphericity would be overrepresented among those whose work seems to require a relatively greater measure of spatial–artistic ability (e.g., artists). The results to date are, at best, inconclusive. Some findings are consistent with the model (e.g., Arndt & Berger, 1978; Dabbs, 1980), but the differences are small and often difficult to replicate. It would seem that, whatever their line of work or cognitive style, people generally are not definable in such typologically simple terms as "left-" or "right-brained" (see review in Beaumont, Young, & McManus, 1984).

Finally, in contrast to just 10 years ago, we have a vastly improved understanding of the developmental nature of lateral specialization. Through the 1960s, a widely accepted theory (implicit, as I have suggested, in Orton's model) was that lateral specialization is progressive, increasing with age from either no or limited specialization in infancy to full specialization by adolescence or adulthood (Lenneberg, 1967). The evidence today indicates instead that the cerebral hemispheres are structurally and functionally different even in early infancy and that, notwithstanding the many neurological and neurobehavioral changes that take place over time, the extent of lateral specialization itself does not appear to change (see Chapters 1 by Best, 2 by Witelson & Kigar, 4 by Turkewitz, 5 by Hiscock, 6 by Molfese & Betz, and 12 by Harris & Carlson, this volume; see also Kinsbourne & Hiscock, 1978, 1983, and reports in Young, Segalowitz, Corter, & Trehub, 1983).

TEACHING THE RIGHT BRAIN

Even as the new scientific developments have revealed the errors in certain earlier educational applications, new applications have been inspired. Of all the scientific developments to come to light in the last decade, however, what has most captured educators' fancy pertains not to language and the left hemisphere, nor to any of the other issues reviewed here. It is, instead, the disclosures of the talents of the right side of the brain. Whereas earlier research on the language functions of the left hemisphere drew educators' attention to the left hemisphere and to disabilities in such basic language skills as reading and writing, the more recent revelations of the cognitive capacities of the right hemisphere have inspired concern among educators for nonlinguistic (or at least not obviously linguistic) skills. Entire disciplines, such as music, art, and mathematics, have been assimilated into this category, along with more specific cognitive capacities ranging from visualization and imagination to creativity and intuition. The new research on cortical specialization for emotion also has been noted, but the only view to become well known is that the right hemisphere is specialized for emotion and affect in general.

In the new reports on right-hemisphere specialization, many educators, therefore, have extracted a new educational message: Where, in their estimation, individuals show deficient interest or skill in music, art, visualization, creativity, empathy, and all other presumptively nonlogical, nonlinguistic abilities, the reason must be either overdevelopment of (and over-reliance on) the left hemisphere, or underdevelopment of the right. From this conviction has emerged an educational movement favoring the training of the right brain that is far stronger than the older movement for training the left. This right-brain movement began in the early 1970s and grew so swiftly that, by 1977, the psychologist Daniel Goleman, then the associate editor of *Psychology Today,* called it the "fad of the year" and asked, "Is our romance with the right side of the brain too hot not to cool down?" (Goleman, 1977, p. 89). Goleman thought not, noting that "As with all such fads, excitement over the two-minded brain may soon peak" (p. 89).

Goleman was wrong. Today, more than a decade later, there are no signs of any letup. Numerous—even numberless—benefits are claimed from stimulating the right brain; special mental exercises are advocated; conventional education (the old orthodoxy), with its emphasis on reading, writing, and other "analytic" skills, is denounced as "left-brained," and its failings are contrasted with the virtues of the new right-brain psychology. Finally, all this is propagated, with missionary zeal, through the news media, public conferences and workshops, education journals, popular science magazines like *Brain–Mind Bulletin* and *Science Digest,* and an ever-expanding stream of pop psychology and self-help books such as *The Right Brain* (Blakeslee, 1980), *Drawing on the Right Side of the Brain* (Edwards, 1979) *The Aquarian Conspiracy* (Ferguson, 1980), *The Psychology of Consciousness* (Ornstein, 1972), and *Whole-Brain Thinking* (Wonder & Donovan, 1984). Indeed, the right-brain gospel has penetrated so deeply into the public consciousness that it has become a preoccupation not only of the general public but of our favorite comic book characters as well. The characters in "Peanuts," "Frank and Ernest," and other American comic strips speak often—and amusingly—on the subject. There is, in short, a mania in the land—or, to use Marcel Kinsbourne's apt term, a "dichotomania."

The "Sorry Results" of Left-Brain Education

The statements of the right-brain advocates play on a variety of related themes. From the beginning, the major theme seems to be that conventional education, by focusing on left-hemisphere training, has led to a functional deterioration of the right hemisphere and, consequently, of right-hemisphere skills. A professor of music education, in an article in the *Music Educators Journal,* puts it this way: Conventional education has developed the left hemisphere "to the detriment of the 'whole' person" and tends "to minimize and even atrophy right-hemisphere thinking, which is responsible for music processing of stimulus input" (Regelski, 1977, p. 44).

A similar point is made in an article in *Today's Education* by the principal of the University Elementary School of the Graduate School of Education at the University of California, Los Angeles: "The [scientific] findings . . . powerfully suggest that schools have been beaming most of their instruction through a left-brained input (reading and listening) and output (talking and writing) system, thereby handicapping all learners" (Hunter, 1976, pp. 46–47). This principal's views were quoted extensively in the *New York Times* in a story on "The Brain's Division of Labor" (Landsmann, 1978).

A professor of mathematics and science education agrees. Writing in *Arithmetic Teacher,* he says: "Our society emphasizes and rewards left-hemisphere activities. This is particularly true of our schools. A premium is placed on being able to put ideas into words, to state them explicitly, and to operate with rules'' (Wheatley, 1977, p. 38). According to still another advocate, ''by only stimulating left brain processes, a competitive antagonistic relationship with the right brain may result because of the overdevelopment of left brain skills'' (Rubenzer, 1982, p. 10). This antagonistic relationship, he goes on to say, is intensified as the child progresses through school—a phenomenon ''amply supported by the fact that a student's measured creativity (right-brain function) actually decreases'' over the schooling period (p. 10). This particular writer is the state coordinator of gifted education for the New Mexico State Department of Education, and these and similar declarations appear in a document, ''Educating the Other Half: Implications of Left/Right Brain Research'' (Rubenzer, 1982), published by the ERIC Clearinghouse on Handicapped and Gifted Children under the auspices of the Council for Exceptional Children. ERIC documents are regarded as authoritative and are widely distributed to school systems throughout the United States.

What especially worries these critics is that the left-brain approach is followed even for supposedly right-brain disciplines. Thus, the professor of mathematics and science education quoted earlier notes that ''the mathematics curriculum in most schools provides little encouragement of right-hemisphere thought'' (Wheatley, 1977, p. 38); another mathematics teacher asserts that ''the climate militates against it'' (Loviglio, 1981, p. 12).

Significantly, even some language teachers, members of what we might call the left-brain establishment, have added their voices to the call. Writing in an official publication of the Phi Delta Kappa Educational Foundation, a university professor of education is joined by a member of the (American) National Council of Teachers of English to decry the school's role as ''a primary conveyor of the linear/sequential mode of consciousness and its functions'' (Grady & Luecke, 1978, p. 13). A high school English teacher, in an article in the *Journal of Creative Behavior,* concludes that there is ''little need to be concerned about the left-brain abilities of most individuals. The traditional schooling experience provides more than adequate practice in developing the power of the already dominant left hemisphere'' (Myers, 1982, p. 205).

The result of this traditional schooling is said to be a kind of left-brain dominance, or hegemony. According to an article in *The Gifted Child Quarterly,* ''this leaves only a few functions such as spatial and artistic forms to the right'' (Beckman, 1977, p. 155).

Rewards of Right-Brain Education

For these critics of the educational curriculum, the left hemisphere is not only alive and well in the public schools, but the once-favored program for establishing left-hemispheric dominance has been all *too* successful. The promised remedy is educational courses and mental exercises that stimulate greater use of the right brain, or ''hemispheric balance in the curriculum'' (Grady & Luecke, 1978, p. 18).

The rewards will be bountiful. Mathematical skill will improve—''problem solving will be enhanced by greater use of the right hemisphere'' (Wheatley, 1977, p. 38). Education in engineering, said to be dominated by left-brained analytical approaches, will be transformed (Williamson & Hudspeth, 1982). Art will blossom: ''A new way of seeing will be developed by tapping the special functions of the right hemisphere'' (Edwards, 1979, p. vii); and because art is the key to ''unlocking the illusive qualities of the right hemisphere,'' it might provide the means for society itself to ''become a bit more balanced'' (''Leonardo Was a Southpaw,'' 1977, p. 23). Creativity, that most cherished of American commodities, also will be enhanced: ''Since creativity . . . might be further developed in the right hemisphere, a new major thrust in education, which might educate the whole brain of the child, could evolve out of current efforts to stimulate early right hemisphere functioning'' (Beckman, 1977, p. 115; see also Hermann, 1981). At the very least, encouraging right-brain processes will mean that the ''reduction in creative thinking abilities can be effectively counteracted. . . .'' (Rubenzer, 1982, p. 10).

Even language (or conventionally left-hemisphere) skills will be improved. A university professor of English and creative arts, sensing the change in climate and evidently not wanting to be left behind, offers advice in a book entitled *Writing the Natural Way: Using Right-Brain Techniques to Release Your Expressive Powers* (Rico, 1983).

One educator, quoted in *Education Digest,* even forsees a new scientific rationale for ''outdoor education.'' The reason is that the ''mystique'' of the outdoors, which ''many outdoor educators insist . . . makes for effective learning and development of the whole child . . . achieves its ultimate impact on an individual in experiences which are probably sensed and interpreted in the right hemisphere'' (Staley, 1980, p. 46).

Mental health will improve, too. For example, the reported rise in the suicide rate among 10- to 13-year-old schoolchildren convinced Rubenzer of the need for more ''affective education (a right-brain function) within the schools.'' (1982, p. 16). In fact, whole systems of psychotherapy have been developed on the basis of certain extrapolations from the laterality literature. The scientifically most pretentious of these is known as Neurolinguistic Programming, or NLP (Bandler & Grinder, 1979). NLP began in 1975 and has quickly achieved cult status.

The promised reward of the new right-brain regime extend even beyond education, creativity, and mental health. The beneficiaries will also include businessmen and managers. Indeed, they were among the first to take notice. In 1976, a professor in the Faculty of Management at McGill University made the following stunning declaration in the *Harvard Business Review: ''The important policy processes of managing an organization rely to a considerable extent on the faculties identified with the brain's right hemisphere. Effective managers seem to revel in ambiguity; in complex, mysterious system with relatively little order''* (Mintzberg, 1976, p. 53; emphasis in original). Remarkably, this unflattering picture of the effective manager inspired many letters of agreement, although one chief executive officer modestly suggested that it is possible to ''overemphasize the predominance of intuition among managers'' and that ''too much creativity and intuition without enough homework will get a large, old, technically stable company in trouble fast'' (Fishwick, 1976, p. 170).

How to Teach (or Reach) the Right Brain

To accomplish their many goals, advocates of right-brain education are, as I have said, proposing—and promoting—educational or therapeutic programs that supposedly will directly strengthen the right hemisphere or will provide a means of gaining direct access to it.

One general recommendation is simply that we listen to music and look at art. In the schoolroom, Brandwein (1977) urges teachers to help students ''seek multiple evidence and to process it both discretely and holistically,'' to honor intuition as a complementary function of intelligence, to avoid ''narrowness of categorization,'' to give children ''more waiting time for responses,'' and to be more tolerant of children's wrong answers and of their excursions into dreams and fantasy. He also recommends ''show and tell'' as ''a perfect example of an activity that stimulates both sides of the brain'' (p. 56).

Where books are concerned, right-brain advocates encourage the augmenting of the "left-brain material"—the words and sentences—with drawings, graphs, and other "right-brain" illustrations. Grady and Luecke (1978) also call for the greater use of television, which, as another writer (a high school principal) pointed out, "is primarily a right-brained input system augmented by the temporal (left-brained) input of speech" (Hunter, 1976, p. 48). Grady and Luecke (1978) lament the fact that "in most classrooms, however, not only is television ignored, but all right hemispheric visual stimuli are often absent" (p. 18).

Grady and Luecke (1978) also suggest adding "learning experiences outside the traditional school curriculum," including "meditation in its many forms: TM, yoga, Sufi, biofeedback, biorhythms, and hypnosis" (p. 16).

> People are flocking to these classes for the personal fulfillment claimed for a "wonder weekend" of meditation. These popular, holistic, and metaphoric experiences and others like them suggest that many people are right hemisphere illiterates in need of training and are seeking this training outside of school. Perhaps schools should recognize that such a deficit exists in their curricula and make the needed changes. (Grady & Luecke, 1978, pp. 17–18)

Rubenzer (1982) agrees. His ERIC document includes a list of no fewer than 36 specific activities "to stimulate integrated right-brain processes," including biofeedback (e.g., having students raise finger temperatures), progressive relaxation, eidetic imagery training, mirror drawing, "transmodal exercises" (e.g., imagining the colors of certain musical tones), mime and charades, photography, "guided fantasy," and so on. He even recommends the temporary use of the nondominant hand or foot to perform everyday functions.

For managers in the workplace, Prince (1978) suggests yet another practice:

> One day a week, make it a rule that no one in the office or plant can use the word no. (The right hemisphere has no equivalent of no.) If something is not acceptable, the person must deal with it by saying, "yes, if . . ."; Give a 30 second explanation of something, and ask to guess what you're getting at. (Prince, 1978, p. 59)

The new approach is now being incorporated into computer software. According to a recent review ("Whole Brain Education: Software to Develop Both Halves of Johnny's Brain," 1985), computers can help develop the right-brained approach to thinking by means of software programs that rotate patterns, create shapes, and display colors and sound. The reviewer notes that "the very logical and highly technological computer may in fact be an important tool for teaching rather illogical, intuitive, and creative skills" (p. 130). The review ends with a listing of "good whole brain [software] packages," including one called "Whole Brain Spelling."

Betty Edwards, the author of *Drawing on the Right Side of the Brain* (1979), proposes still other exercises, all designed to "release creative potential and tap into the special drawing abilities of the right half of the brain" (quotation from back cover). One exercise is to copy a fairly detailed pencil drawing by Picasso of Igor Stravinsky seated in a chair. Edwards asserts that when we view this or any drawing in our usual way, that is, in upright orientation, this encourages what she calls a left-brain, or L-mode, approach. The reason is that when the picture is upright, we see it as a meaningful and therefore nameable (left-brain) form, with the usual features such as hands, ears, and so on. To put the student into the more appropriate right-hemisphere, or R-mode, state, Edwards recommends making the drawing indecipherable (that is, not nameable) by inverting it. The result, in Edwards's experience, is a vast improvement in drawing skill: "Presumably, the left hemisphere, confused and blocked by the unfamiliar image and unable to symbolize as usual, turned off, and the job passed over to the right hemisphere" (Edwards, 1979, p. 55).

Several other promoters of right-brain education recommend exercises that involve eye movements. These programs are being advertised under different names and by different people and seem to be targeted at somewhat different audiences. The version mentioned earlier, Neurolinguistic Programming, also casts the widest net, aiming at virtually all individuals interested in "personal improvement" (Dilts, 1983a, 1983b). Another version, being marketed under a program called "The Neuropsychology of Achievement," seems to be directed more at business managers, personnel directors, and the like (S. Devore, described in Trubo, 1982), as is a program offered through an "Applied Creative Thinking Workshop" (Hermann, 1981).

According to a publicity release for the "achievement" program (Trubo, 1982), there are "nine specific eye positions which arouse the nervous system and allow a person to fine-tune and tap into the images he has already created." Thus, the right-handed person who wishes to activate visual memory can do so most effectively with his eyes in the upper-left position; for auditory memory, laterally left. The lateral eye movements are said to arouse cortical (hemispheric) structures, thereby providing us access to higher cognitive processes. The author contends that simply by combining the lateral eye movements with downward movements, limbic system structures can be accessed as well, thereby facilitating access to noncognitive processes. Which noncognitive processes depends on which lateral direction: "Emotions and feelings can best be tapped with the eyes in a lower left position," whereas "body motions are accessed when the eyes are shifted lower right . . ." (Trubo, 1982).

As a last example, the promoter of something called "whole-brain learning" promises "brain–mind expansion" through the use of "megasubliminal" tape-recordings. Unlike "mere motivation tapes," these are "7 leveled or tracked—3 hearable by left brain and 4 unhearable by right brain—bypassing your resistance to positive change." The tapes cost $195 and are advertised regularly in the *New York Times* ("Whole or ½ Brain?," 1986). Readers also are invited to pay $1,400 to attend seminars in order to become "certified in accelerated teaching and learning."

Individual Differences: "Left-Brained" and "Right-Brained" Individuals

At the same time as our culture and our educational institutions are supposedly making most people overwhelmingly left-brained, the advocates of "hemispheric balance" also have become aware of—and deeply impressed by—the neuropsychological research on individual differences ("hemisphericity"). But to them, the implications of this research are simple and straightforward: Whereas the majority of individuals are "left-brained" (and not just the lawyers, writers, and accountants), a minority are "right-brained"; that is, somehow certain people have not only managed to escape the social–cultural–neurological hegemony of the left hemisphere, but have come to depend on their right hemispheres as much as the majority depend on their left. Some advocates of right-brain education have relied on neuropsychological tests such as the EEG or dichotic listening to identify these individuals, using the lateral direction and magnitude of difference in performance as the index of "hemisphericity." Others have made the diagnosis on the basis of the patterns of strengths and weaknesses on certain psychologial tests. For example, Bogen, DeZare, TenHouten, and Marsh (1972) compared the ratio of performance on the Street Gestalt Completion Test (on the assumption that it required predominantly right-hemisphere strategies) with the performance on the Similarities Subtest of the Wechsler Adult Intelligence Scale (on the assumption that it required predominantly left-hemisphere strategies), where high ratios were assumed to reflect more right-hemisphere thinking, low ratios more left-hemisphere thinking.

Other advocates of right-brain education are using mere self-report as the measure of hemispheric dominance. For example, the educational psychologist E. P. Torrance and his colleagues (Torrance, Reynolds, Riegel, & Ball, 1977) have devised a ''Style of Thinking'' questionnaire on which respondents can rate themselves on 36 different items, each with three alternatives, one said to signify ''left-hemisphere specialization,'' another signifying ''right-brain'' specialization,'' and the third indicating an ''integrative style.'' Examples of alternatives signifying a ''left-hemisphere specialization'' include ''not good at remembering faces'' and ''inhibited in expression of feelings and emotions''; the ''right-brain'' alternatives are ''not good at remembering names'' and ''able to express feelings and emotions freely.'' Alternatives signifying an ''integrated'' or ''balanced'' brain style are ''equally good at remembering names and faces'' and ''controlled in expression of feelings and emotions.'' Some of the other items ask for self-ratings of inventiveness, psychic ability, creativity, and preference for multiple-choice versus open-ended tests. This particular test was developed as a *research* instrument for the study of learning style and creativity, but the authors invited their readers to use the instrument ''either for research or guidance purposes'' (Torrance *et al.*, 1977, p. 563). It therefore may be in use in ordinary classrooms as a means of identifying ''left-'' and ''right-brained'' schoolchildren.

Such questionnaires have become popular in magazine and newspaper stories about lateral specialization, so that ordinary citizens also can ascertain their cerebral strengths and weaknesses. These tests are much like the ''personality'' tests that have long been a staple of the popular press. One questionnaire (''Left–Right Brain Role Is Studied'' *Chicago Tribune,* April 22, 1984) invited its readers to ''Test yourself. Are you right-brained or left-brained?'' This questionnaire consisted of 21 different items similar to those mentioned earlier. The authors were identified as two professors of education at Brigham Young University.

Who are the ''right-brained'' individuals revealed by these tests? A disproportionately large number have been reported to be members of certain ethnic and racial minorities. In perhaps the first such report (Bogen *et al.*, 1972), Hopi Indians, urban blacks, and rural and urban whites were compared on the Street Gestalt/Similarities ratio, mentioned earlier. The Hopis had the highest ratio, urban black women next, followed by urban black men, rural whites, and urban whites, leading the investigators to conclude that Hopi Indians and blacks were relatively more right-hemispheric in their thinking than were whites.

Another study, using EEG as a measure, found that when bilingual Hopi children listened to a story in Hopi, they showed relatively less alpha activity (signifying relatively greater activation) recorded over the right hemisphere than when they listened to a story in English (Rogers, TenHouton, Kaplan, & Gardiner, 1977).

A third study consisted of a demonstration by educational psychologists that right-handed American Navajo college students showed a *left*-ear (or right-hemisphere) advantage for identification of dichotically presented consonant–vowel syllables such as ''pa,'' ''ba,'' and ''ga,'' whereas right-handed ''Anglo,'' Caucasian students showed the more usual right-ear (left-hemisphere) advantage (Scott, Hynd, Hunt, & Weed, 1979). Similar differences were later reported between Navajo Indian and Anglo children (Hynd & Scott, 1980).

The authors of these reports explained these differences as manifestations of the roles of language and culture. The Hopi language was said to be more involved with the perceptual field, so that speech was linked immediately with its context, in contrast to English, which separates the user from the perceptual field (Rogers *et al.*, 1977). Likewise, the Navajo culture and the Navajo language (said to be more literal and concrete than English) made the Navajo's *thought* itself more ''apperceptive,'' more in tune with the spatial environment—hence, more ''right-hemispheric'' (Scott *et al.*, 1979).

All the reports cited here were published in professional neuropsychological journals. Recently, however, similar claims about the right-brained Indian have appeared in journals directly aimed at professional educators who work with Indian people (McShane, 1980; Ross, 1982).

Given the new atmosphere of right-brain advocacy, one might think that Native Americans, blacks, and other supposedly ''right-hemisphere-dominant'' individuals would be held up as examples of the benefits of right-brain thinking, as models to be admired and emulated by the left-brained majority. Sometimes they are. More often, however, they are presented as problems for our usual left-brain educational system—round right-hemispheric pegs who do not fit in our square left-hemispheric holes. This view is expressed by the professor of science–mathematics education quoted earlier:

> Students who do not find school very relevant could well be right-brain oriented. To them, the many left-brain tasks just do not make sense. There is also evidence that the urban poor tend to be right-hemisphere oriented, while middle-class persons are more left-hemisphere oriented. If this is true, it would explain why many urban poor do not succeed in our schools and why they claim irrelevancy of many of the tasks asked of them in school. (Wheatley, 1977, p. 38)

Similarly, the professors of education who assessed ''brainedness'' with questions about skill at remembering names or faces concluded that the ''many right-brained children'' do poorly because they are taught by ''left-oriented teachers using left-oriented materials'' and because they are being evaluated by ''left-oriented measures'' (''Left–Right Brain Role Is Studied,'' 1984).

The solution proposed by some critics is to adjust the educational programs by playing to these children's already well-developed right hemispheres. One method is the increased use of ''right-brained'' television, whereby ''the whole world is able to receive information without the complex left-brained processing that reading demands'' (Hunter, 1976, p. 48).

> Therefore, predominantly right-brained individuals can take their proper place in the sun. . . . Information about the Arab–Israeli conflict, for example, is no longer privileged communication for left-brained individuals who read about it; right-brained individuals can find out about the conflict through the primarily visual medium of television. (Hunter, 1976, p. 48)

The right-brain advocates see the question of individual differences simply in terms of left brain and right brain and make their diagnoses accordingly on the basis of the direction and strength of laterality scores. Practitioners of Neurolinguistic Programming also use laterality measures but have devised a somewhat different typology of individuality. According to the originators of NLP (Bandler & Grinder, 1979), the major individual difference is in the modality of the representational system, some people being predominantly auditory, some visual, and some tactual. Like the left-brain, right-brain typology, the key to the representational system is the direction of eye movements, only now the diagnosis depends on a combination of horizontal and vertical movements, with the visual mode represented by upward movements, the auditory by horizontal movements, and the kinesthetic (along with smell and taste) with downward movements—but to the right only. To be successful, the therapist must identify each style and adjust the therapy accordingly.

EVALUATION

These are only a few examples of the activities of the new right-brain movement. As I said earlier, more than a decade after the movement began, interest, rather than tapering off, is accelerating in pace. Given these developments, we would expect members of the scientific community to be paying serious attention to the right-brain advocates and to be speaking out about how neuropsychological research is being applied. Some have done so. Practically at the beginning of the movement, David Galin, in an address in 1974 to the American Association for the Advancement of Science, warned against "dichotomania" and noted that "the specialization of the two halves of the brain is being offered as everybody's favorite pair of polar opposites: obsessive–hysteric, rational–mystical," and so on (quoted in Goleman, 1977, p. 149). Similar warnings have come from Corballis (1980), Kinsbourne (1982), Levy (1985), and the educational psychologists Hardyck and Haapenen (1979). So far, however, there has not been a thorough analysis of the specific educational claims or any of the other applications. In my own previous attempts, I mostly tried an oblique attack by recalling the rise and fall of an earlier and now forgotten movement having certain parallels to the current day (Harris, 1978, 1985a, 1985b).

What can be said, then, about the call for "hemispheric balance" in the school, the workplace, and even life itself? And what of the mental exercises being proposed to bring this about? Could the right-brain advocates be right? After all, since we know much more about the nature of cerebral specialization today than in Orton's time, or even 10 years ago, should not the translation of this knowledge into practice have a better chance of being successful? Maybe so, but, for all the reasons outlined at the beginning of this chapter, the results, so far, seem to me to have been—to put it bluntly—a waste of time and, in some hands, a scandalous misuse of science. Let us look at these reasons more closely.

Misunderstanding and Misrepresentation of Neuropsychological Evidence

The most general problem is that—with certain important exceptions to be mentioned later—the champions of right-brain education fundamentally misunderstand and misrepresent the basic neuropsychological evidence. It is not hard to see why, since almost none of them have formal scientific training in neuropsychology. Instead, virtually all of their information about lateral specialization has come from their own professional journals (in education, music, management, and so on); from magazines, newspaper "science" reports, and popular books like those I quoted from earlier; and from lectures and workshops by people usually hardly more knowledgeable than their audiences. To make matters worse, all these "authorities" regularly lean on one another for documentation of their arguments. Thus Goodspeed (1983), the investment counselor, cites Mintzburg (1976), the management professor; the educators Grady and Luecke (1978) cite Ornstein (1976) and Samples (1976); the engineers Williamson and Hudspeth (1982) cite Blakeslee (1980), Edwards (1979), and

Ferguson (1980); and so forth. Where the primary literature itself is mentioned, it is typically through secondary or even tertiary citations, or else it is given equal weight with the popular accounts, as Rubenzer (1982) does throughout his ERIC document.

As is typical of all such accounts, gross generalizations are the norm; subtleties, complexities, inconsistencies, and nonreplicable findings are passed over; and frequently even the clearest, best substantiated principles are misconstrued. The result has all the depth of a cartoon. Indeed, an installment of the comic strip "Frank and Ernest" will serve the point. One character, reading his newspaper, says to the other: "This science column says that the left half of the brain is dominant in right-handed people, and the right half is dominant in left-handed people. And that's why left-handed people are the only ones in their right minds." The first statement misrepresents the relationship between handedness and cerebral organization, as well as the nature of dominance itself, but it very likely *is* just what the cartoonist himself read in a "science column" in the daily newspaper.

The result of this public miseducation has been the establishment and proliferation within the right-brain movement of several fundamental errors about the nature of lateral specialization. All are evident in one form or another in the excerpts quoted from earlier.

MISTAKEN CHARACTERIZATION OF COGNITIVE SKILLS

One of the more pervasive of these errors is to characterize highly complex, multidimensional cognitive processes as simple and unidimensional, and thereby to suppose that they can be localized *in toto* in either the left brain or the right. Language, reading, and writing thus are made the *exclusive* province of the left hemisphere, just as artistic ability, emotion, intuition, and other not obviously linguistic capacities are made the exclusive province of the right hemisphere. But there is no evidence that only one hemisphere is involved in *any* cognitive activity or task. Even during language tasks, which unquestionably depend more on the left hemisphere, both hemispheres are involved, as we know from studies of regional cerebral blood flow during mental activity. During a language task, blood flow is greater to the left hemisphere, but it increases on the right side as well, and this is true even for speech—the dimension of language that appears to be the most clearly lateralized (Lassen, Ingvar, & Skinhøj, 1978).

If both cerebral hemispheres are involved even in well-lateralized left-hemispheric tasks, the evidence indicates that even more joint involvement for so-called right-brain skills. Consider artistic ability. It is understandably comforting for art educators to suppose that artistry is a unique property of the right brain and that stimulating the right brain should enhance the ability to draw (Edwards, 1979). The neuropsychological evidence, however, indicates that both hemispheres contribute, although in different ways, the left hemisphere being more involved in the identification of details and internal elements, the right hemisphere in the analysis of location, orientation, and dimensionality. Thus, drawings made by patients with unilateral left or right parietal injuries both show impairments, but generally of different kinds, which means that we cannot say that the drawings made by the right-parietal patients are necessarily worse in some absolute sense (see Warrington, 1969). Nor can "musical ability" be localized in one hemisphere or the other. It depends, among other things, on the particular components of music involved (and, by implication, on the cognitive processes underlying musical ability). For example, in tests of music perception, rhythm tends to be left-lateralized, pitch and tonality right-lateralized (Borchgrevink, 1982). And, as with drawing, none of these relationships are absolute; they depend on the individual's strategy and skill as well as the familiarity of the type of material employed (see Gates & Bradshaw, 1977).

As for "creativity," the original basis for supposing that the right cerebral hemisphere plays the dominant role evidently was inspired by reports from the neuropsychological literature that "visual imagery" is mediated by the right hemisphere, and from largely anecdotal reports that "visual imagery" plays an important role in the thinking and problem solving of "creative scientists" (e.g., Hadamard, 1954; Kruger, 1976; West, 1976). An early experimental study of conjugate gaze deviation has also proved to be influential. In a small sample of mathematics professors and graduate students, those who more often looked left while reflecting were rated as using more imagery, were more artistically diverse, and, for the professors only, were rated (by graduate students) as being more creative than were those who looked right (Harnad, 1972).

These are interesting findings but very thin strands on which to build an educational program for enhancing "creativity," especially given the awesome difficulties in defining and measuring creativity. These difficulties are only exacerbated by the fact that "creativity" is one of those vague words whose frequency of use lies in inverse proportion to the carefulness of use. Ours, after all, is a democratic age, a time when, on a television variety show, the violinist Itzhak Perlman might be followed by a performing dog, the juxtaposition perhaps suggesting that the dog is no less talented than the man. Even when "creativity" is defined with some rigor, there is no evidence that it is the predominant, let alone the exclusive, responsibility of the right hemisphere of the brain. Rather, the nature of the task itself is crucial, and both cerebral hemispheres are involved (Torrance & Mourad, 1979; for an excellent critique, see Katz, 1979).

MISUNDERSTANDING OF THE NATURE OF INDIVIDUAL DIFFERENCES IN COGNITIVE SKILLS

From supposing that highly complex (and still ill-defined) cognitive processes are exclusively under the control of one cerebral hemisphere or the other, it is easy to slip into a further misunderstanding—that people who are relatively weak in one kind of cognitive skill must make inadequate use of the side of their brain that is the presumptive site of that skill. This is the only way I can understand the astonishing claim, by the mathematics professor quoted earlier, that some individuals "have such dominance of one hemisphere that the other hemisphere is rarely activated" (Wheatley, 1977, p. 38).

Does anyone have such dominance of one hemisphere that "the other hemisphere is rarely activated"? The closest candidate, perhaps, would be someone with lateralized (usually right posterior parietal) brain injury who shows the symptom of hemi-neglect (neglect of the hemi-space contralateral to the lesion) even to the point of failing to recognize his own limbs on that side (Critchley, 1969; Denny-Brown & Banker, 1952; Heilman, Watson, & Valenstein, 1985). Levy (1977) has speculated that in patients with this disorder, the injured side is insufficiently aroused and activated, and it is this hypoarousal and activation that leads to a loss of the dynamic balance between the hemispheres and thereby to hemi-neglect. Of course, most people are not brain-injured, and the "inattention" or neglect that some normal persons show to music, art, and other nonlinguistic domains is hardly to be equated with the hemi-neglect syndrome of the brain-injured patient.

If we can safely reject the claim that in some neurologically normal individuals, one hemisphere is so dominant that the other hemisphere is rarely activated, can we also reject the weaker and thus perhaps more reasonable claim that individuals relatively poor in one kind of skill make inadequate use of the cerebral hemisphere that is the presumptive site of that skill? As so stated, I think we must reject this claim, on the basis of the evidence available. To say this, however, is not to say that there are no differences in thinking style between highly musical or creative or mathematically gifted persons and persons less gifted (there undoubtedly are) or that such differences might not prove to be relatable *in some way* to individual differences in complex patterns of hemispheric organization or characteristic patterns of, say, phasic activation during the performance of certain mental tasks. My impression is that they will be relatable eventually. As mentioned earlier, there already is evidence suggesting that ordinary right-handed adults show individual differences in characteristic patterns of hemispheric arousal (Levy *et al.,* 1983). But this is still a long way from saying that the psychological differences, whatever they may be, between creative and less creative persons, or between lawyers and artists, or accountants and mechanics, are reducible to simple differences in such dimensions of neural activity. As I said earlier, the neuropsychological evidence itself cannot be accommodated to any such simple view.

All such considerations should make us extremely cautious about reports, like those cited earlier, that certain ethnic, racial, or social-class groups are more or less right- or left-hemisphere "dominant" than others. In fact, virtually all of these reports have been shown to be inadequate in one way or another. For instance, the early report by Bogen *et al.* (1972), which concluded that Hopi Indians and blacks were relatively more right hemispheric in their thinking than were whites, was criticized by Zook and Dwyer (1976) on the grounds that the only appreciable differences between the groups were on the Verbal Similarities Test and not on the Street Gestalt test (the "right-hemisphere" test). The critics suggested that the results therefore were merely a reflection of culture-based differences in performance on verbal IQ tests.

As for the comparisons of Navajos and Anglos on dichotic listening tests, the earlier conclusion that the Navajo has greater right-hemisphere dominance for language (Hynd & Scott, 1980; Scott *et al.,* 1979) has been challenged. McKeever (1981) found instead that both the direction and the magnitude of language laterality scores were identical in Anglo and Navajo subjects, both for a task different from the one used originally (McKeever, 1981) and for essentially the same task (McKeever & Hunt, 1984). McKeever and Hunt (1984) concluded that "right-handed Navajos are, like other right-handers, strongly left hemisphere superior for auditory receptive language processes. . . . There thus remains, to our knowledge, no convincing evidence that any neurologically normal right-handed population possesses reversed hemispheric specialization of language function" (p. 541). The vast majority of neuropsychologists will, I think, concur with this conclusion.[2]

VIEW OF CEREBRAL HEMISPHERES AS ISOLATED AND NONINTERACTING

Whatever else the pop psychology accounts get wrong about lateral specialization, several of them do point out correctly that the hemispheres are joined together by the corpus callosum and that this organ provides for communication between the hemispheres. Nevertheless, in saying this, they also manage to convey still another mistaken idea—that in some, perhaps many, individuals the cerebral hemispheres work more or less in functional isolation from each another. Recall in this connection the questionnaire that scores the answer, "equally good at remembering names and faces," as meaning that "both sides of the brain are interactive." Is the implication that respondents who are rated as either "right-brained" or "left-brained" have *non*interactive brains?

This particular misunderstanding about interhemispheric communication appears to have its roots in overgeneralizations from certain of the more dramatic effects of commissurotomy to individuals with intact commissures. Commissurotomy patients, under certain circumstances, do show remarkable disconnection effects reflecting the functional isolation of the cerebral hemispheres. Normal persons, however, are not split brains. And even adults whose cerebral hemispheres have been separated by commissurotomy have numerous strategies and means for engaging both hemispheres in problem solving and mentation. That is why the demonstration of lateralized functioning even in these individuals usually requires the application of rigidly controlled experimental procedures. If this is true in split brains, it would be true *a fortiori* in normal persons.

Does the Right Hemisphere Need Exercise?

The aforementioned remarks also begin to show what is mistaken in the notion that the right hemisphere is a sort of endangered species that needs special exercise and encouragement to survive. I would say, instead, that the right hemisphere gets plenty of exercise. The best evidence, as already mentioned, is that the cerebral hemispheres are inherently specialized for their respective functions, work normally from the outset, and receive ample opportunities to do what they are genetically programmed to do merely in the course of normal everyday living in an environment that is open to all of our senses every day of our lives. This is no less true in the school environment, even in the so-called left-brained classroom where the emphasis is heavily on reading, writing, talking, and listening. To assert that all such instruction is "beaming . . . through a left-brained input . . . and output, thereby handicapping all learners" (Hunter, 1976, p. 46) is to liken normal schoolchildren to split-brain patients under rigidly controlled experimental procedures of lateralized stimulus presentation. The normal school environment has been characterized in a variety of ways, both positive and negative. This description, surely, is not one of the more felicitous. And even though the study of music is inadequately supported by our educational institutions, the result does not seem to be a lack of interest in music by the average adolescent. (Those earphones embracing every teenage head surely are not piping in "left-hemispheric" news and literary debates!)

Effectiveness of Suggested Right-Brain Exercises

Earlier we recalled how the proposed link between disabilities in reading and other language skills and incomplete dominance of the left hemisphere had inspired a theory of remediation through direct motor training and other supposed left-hemisphere exercises. We also noted criticisms both of the "evidence" for the "therapy" and of the premise behind it. The question is: Are the exercises called for today by advocates of right-hemisphere training any more likely to be successful, even if we were to accept the doubtful premise that the right hemisphere needs special exercise in the first place? Let us consider some of the proposals more closely.

The general recommendation that we listen to music, look at art, and make greater use of drawings and other nonverbal illustrations seems hardly controversial in itself except in its justification—that is, that because such activities are not explicitly verbal or sequential and, by implication, not left-hemispheric, they must be explicitly and exclusively right-hemispheric. As for Brandwein's (1977) suggestions that teachers give children "more waiting time for responses," use "show and tell," and "seek multiple evidence" and process it "both discretely and holistically," one imagines that they would inspire yawns from most experienced primary-grade teachers once they see past the pretentious neuropsychological terminology.

No less than Brandwein's (1977) vague and banal suggestions, the more specific and focused exercises likewise are based on misunderstandings and overgeneralizations of the neuropsychological literature. Consider the proposal from the neurolinguistic programmers and other promoters of eye movement exercises that we can activate and gain access to images presumably stored in different parts of the brain merely by fixing our gaze in a certain direction along the vertical and horizontal axes. The authors of one version of this program claim support from "university research and our own experience to prove that the eye movements work" (S. Devore, quoted in Trubo, 1982, unpaginated).

To begin with, we can ignore any of the claims pertaining to the relationship between the vertical dimension and the limbic system, for example, that eye movements down and to the left result from greater arousal of right limbic structures. This is pure fancy, inspired, one can only suppose, by the authors' learning that the limbic system lies "below" the cerebral cortex. The question of the relationship between *lateral* gaze deviation and question type, however, is another matter. As already mentioned, there is evidence from studies of conjugate gaze deviation that the eyes tend to move in a direction contralateral to the side of presumptive greater hemispheric activation during mental problem solving. The popularizers, however, drastically exaggerate the strength and reliability of the relationship, whereas the evidence reveals something rather more evanscent, probably for both methodological and conceptual reasons (e.g., Berg & Harris, 1980; Ehrlichman & Weinberger, 1979). But suppose the relationship were strong and highly reliable. Could we then accept the claim that the phenomenon can be exploited to enhance cognitive performance? That is, if performing a verbal memory problem results in greater phasic activation of the left hemisphere, thereby driving the eyes to the right, then does merely looking to the right (or the left) *itself* raise the arousal level of the opposite hemisphere, thereby assisting in the retrieval of either verbal memories (with right-looking) or nonverbal memories (with left-looking)? This question, in fact, is the subject of a growing body of research. In one of the first such studies (Hines & Martindale, 1974), left-looking, induced by having the subjects (presumably college students) wear goggles with tape on the right half of each lens, resulted in enhanced performance on the Remote Associates Test (Mednick & Mednick, 1967), on a test of "creativity," and on two subtests of the Culture Fair Intelligence Test (Cattell & Cattell, 1959), a nonverbal test. The difference was statistically reliable but very small, no comparable effect was found on performance on a different "creativity" test or on verbal tests with *right*-looking, and the effect was confined to males. The results of a number of subsequent studies have been mixed as well; but, generally speaking, inducing visual fixation to the right has been associated with enhanced verbal performance (e.g., Gross, Franko, & Lewin, 1978; Lempert & Kinsbourne, 1982; Walker, Wade, & Waldman, 1982), and fixation to the left has been associated with enhanced performance on spatial tasks (Gross *et al.,* 1978; LaTorre & LaTorre, 1981; Walker *et al.,* 1982). Recently the effect has even been demonstrated for performance on an "emotional" as distinct from a cognitive task. The investigator, accepting the still-contested view that positive emotions are related to left-hemisphere activity and negative emotions to right-hemisphere activity, demonstrated an association between direction of visual fixation and performance on a test designed to reflect optimism about future life events. The subjects—a small number of American college students—scored higher on "optimism" in the eyes-right than the eyes-left condition. The conclusion was that the rightward orientation had induced a positive mood, thereby affecting the personal judgment (Drake, 1984). The effect, however, was weak, in one experiment being significant for only one of seven individual life events ("Having a happy life"), in a second experiment for only one of five life events ("Traveling to Europe").

The results of these new experiments thus are mixed but provocative. Certainly they point to new directions for further and more refined scientific study, but they seem far too weak to have any practical uses at this time. As far as I know, none of these new findings have trickled down to the popular science literature. If and when they do, I fear there will be the usual wild extrapolations. One can imagine the "optimism" study inspiring a new mental health exercise wherein everyone from schoolchildren to business executives is told to sit with eyes right in order to activate the "positive" left hemisphere and to promote good feeling and optimism. Imagine, too, the dilemma for those who believe that the left hemisphere is already overexercised, but that the alternative—arousing the right hemisphere by moving the eyes to the left—would engender *negative* feelings.

Consider as an alternative "hemispheric access" strategy Edwards's (1979) proposal that by inverting the picture we wish to copy, we can suppress the "interference" of the left hemisphere, and in this way gain access to the right hemisphere and dramatically improve our drawing skill. Whether this particular exercise will yield the results claimed remains to be seen. The students' copies reproduced in Edwards's book are impressive, but we are not told whether they are representative. (A reasonably careful test of college students, carried out by a group of my undergraduate students, failed to show any remotely similar differences in overall quality between the Picasso drawing when copied in the inverted orientation versus the upright orientation.) Even supposing, however, that the exercise works, it might not be for the reasons proposed by Edwards. For example, her own characterization of the process of copying an inverted picture suggests that the picture, no longer easily recognizable as a gestalt or whole, is now copied in a more feature-by-feature (i.e., line-by-line) manner. The practical effect may be for the individual to break the picture into many smaller parts and to work on each part by itself until the entire picture is completed. (When I tried the exercise, the effect was like painting with the paint-by-number books of my childhood.) Thus, to the extent that inverting the picture affects the way it is copied, it may be to promote a strategy closer to the information-processing style associated with the left, not the right, hemisphere. The fact that body parts are less likely to be recognized and named may be less consequential. This new characterization of the task is consistent, furthermore, with research on visual field differences on face-recognition tasks. Upright faces generally are more likely to be recognized when tachistoscopically projected to the left visual half-field (right hemisphere), but inverted faces are better recognized in the right visual half-field (left hemisphere), possibly because the subject, no longer able to discern facial expression, now must rely on a more analytic, feature-by-feature strategy (see Leehy, Carey, Diamond, & Cahn, 1978; Levine, 1985). (Many other factors also must be considered, since procedural conditions can crucially determine which hemifield advantage is obtained in any given experiment with faces or any other stimulus; see Sergent & Bindra, 1981.)

A Streak of Antiliteracy in the New Movement

Aside from its misrepresentation of the neuropsychological evidence, its tendentious analysis of the school environment, and its aggressive promotion of various neuropsychological nostrums, there is something else that troubles me about the "right-brain" movement. It is one thing to attempt to balance the supposed overemphasis on "left-brain thinking" by trying out this or that sort of exercise, by pressing for support for music and the arts, or by advocating intuition and creativity. It is another thing altogether for the critics to attack what they call "left-brain education" in order to promote an educational philosophy and practice that celebrates or at least seeks to excuse anti-intellectualism, illiteracy, and irrationality. This attitude pervades much of the literature on right-brain education. For examples, recall the argument that an outdoor (right-brain) education will provide "a world as a classroom that is whole and unfragmented by content disciplines such as math, science

. . . with no artificial boundaries . . . as might be found in textbooks and curriculum guides'' (Staley, 1980, p. 47), or the statement by the high school English teacher that ''there is little need to be concerned about the left-brain abilities of most individuals'' (Myers, 1982, p. 205). It is hard to credit the complacency in this teacher's remark. If he was reflecting on his own students' competence in reading and writing, either his students are highly atypical or he has badly misjudged them. Ours is hardly a golden age of clear reasoning and precise use of language. Finally, recall the school principal who, speaking on behalf of all ''right-brained'' individuals, endorsed the use of television, which will let ''the whole world . . . receive information without the complex left-brained processing that reading demands'' (Hunter, 1976, p. 48). Television perhaps could be a valuable adjunct to education, although evidence to date is not especially promising. It is, however, a poor substitute for reading, whose positive contribution is unquestioned.

In sum, the right-brain enthusiasts are urging us, as one of them has put it, to cease our worship of rationality and to ''get in touch'' with our right hemispheres (M. Ferguson, 1980). A critic had the right name for this sort of talk—''blatant hucksterism'' (Jones, 1980, p. 847).

CONCLUSIONS

I hope no one will take my remarks to mean that music and the visual and plastic arts have no proper place in education; that intuition, imagination, and visualization should not be encouraged and honored as valuable parts of thinking and problem solving; that hands-on experiences (field trips and the like) are of no educational value; that instructional methods should not be sensitive to children's different interests and learning styles, levels of skill, and rates of development; or that diagrams and drawings are not necessary supplements or even, under appropriate circumstances, alternatives to the written word. All of these unquestionably are important and worthy goals and practices, which we should vigorously pursue. We can even agree with Rudolph Arnheim (1969, p. 3) that, beyond kindergarten, ''the senses lose educational status,'' and the schoolchild is too often fitted into the verbal world of schoolteachers who are generally unaware of the significance of nonverbal components of thought. We also are rightly concerned when, even in an engineering school, a course in ''visual thinking'' is regarded as an aberration rather than ''as a discipline that should be incorporated into an engineer's repertoire of skills'' (see E. S. Ferguson, 1977, for an enlightening analysis of the role of nonverbal thought in technology); and we can justly call our education incomplete if we can read and write our native language but not the universal symbols of musical notation, or if we have studied and been moved in mind and heart by Lord Byron's *Don Juan* or Shakespeare's *Othello* while remaining deaf to Mozart's *Don Giovanni* and Verdi's *Otello*. But we do not make the case any more convincingly for any of these goals through portentous announcements about ''right-hemisphere deterioration'' or ''hemispheric unbalance.'' Rather, we shall have to justify these goals on the same grounds as have been articulated by educators and humanists long before anyone ever heard about the cerebral hemispheres. Educators who are displeased with the educational curriculum should present the case for change on its own merits and not seek to win scientific respectability for their arguments by dressing them in neuropsychological jargon. Likewise, educators who are unhappy with the way certain already well-established disciplines—such as mathematics or reading—are taught should work for change. But they should not justify their recommendations (and rationalize their failures) through simple-minded dichotomies about left- and right-brain specialization, learning styles, and the nature of the academic disciplines. Then, of course, they must show that the new ways truly improve on the old. In education, "innovation" is a cheap and common commodity. Hard support, however, is both rare and dear. (See, for example, Guthrie, 1978, and other essays in Benton & Pearl, 1978.)

As for the snake oil salesmen peddling their expensive wares to schools, to business and industry, and to the insatiable consumers of mental health "quick fixes," I doubt that anything that anyone could say to them would make any difference. Their motivation looks like pure greed, and they evidently are being well rewarded by school administrators, corporate officers, and private citizens who have more dollars than sense.

The Scientist's Responsibilities

Finally, in all these matters, neuropsychologists themselves are not entirely blameless, for in some respects we have been participants, albeit usually unwitting participants, in the promotion of this fad. Our support has taken several forms. First, it is not just the educators and other nonscientists who have sounded the alarm bells about the evils of left-brain education. Some prominent scientists have as well and, in fact, were among the first to do so. I said earlier that, with certain important exceptions, the champions of right-brain education fundamentally misunderstand the basic neuropsychological evidence. The scientist-advocates of right-brain education are the exceptions to whom I was referring. That is, I am hardly suggesting that *they* misunderstand the scientific evidence, but I do think that in their sincere desire to reach out beyond the scientific community to the general public, they have oversimplified both the evidence and the educational issues. Unquestionably, the most prominent figure has been Roger W. Sperry. In 1973, in a chapter for a scholarly book, he wrote that "our educational system, as well as science in general, tends to neglect the nonverbal form of intellect." This is a modest statement with which many scientists and scholars might well agree. Sperry went on, however, to reduce this assessment to stark neurological terms: "What it comes down to is that modern society discriminates against the right hemisphere."

A year later, Sperry presented the same analysis to an audience of engineers (1974) and then the following year (1975) to the readers of a mass-circulation lay magazine, *Saturday Review*. There he wrote:

> . . . that our educational system and modern society generally (with its very heavy emphasis on communication and on early training in the three Rs) discriminates against one whole half of the brain. I refer, of course, to the non-verbal, non-mathematical minor hemisphere, which, we find, has its own perceptual, mechanical, and spatial mode of apprehension and reasoning. In our present school system, the attention given to the minor hemisphere of the brain is minimal compared with the training lavished on the left, or major, hemisphere. (p. 33)

This passage was quoted in an essay on the brain in a special issue of *Mosaic*, a publication of the National Science Foundation ("A Window to the Brain," 1976, p. 19).

Perhaps inspired by Sperry's example, other scientists made similar suggestions and assertions, this time in educational journals and newsletters. For example, Galin, notwithstanding his own earlier warning against "dichotomania," wrote in the journal *Child Education:* "It appears that our schools have been tutoring only the left half of the brain" (1976, p. 17). Another asserted, in the *UCLA Educator*, that society has put too much emphasis on left-hemisphere skills, and that an elementary school program restricted to the three R's "will educate mainly one hemisphere" (Bogen, 1975, p. 11). Still another wrote, in the leading education journal, *Instructor,* "If we agree that most present-day curriculums stimulate primarily the left brain, then we recognize the need for content, method, and materials that will utilize the right brain in an equally vigorous manner'' (Ornstein, 1977, p. 56). Nor has this disposition for overstatement been confined to questions about education. In a book addressed to the lay public, a prominent neuropsychologist extrapolates from research on the behavior of split-brain patients to expound on a remarkable variety of other matters, ranging from the factors leading to the formation of religious beliefs to the reasons that social welfare systems fail (Gazzaniga, 1986).

Two scientists have also let their names be used in public endorsement of one of the most prominent of the ''right-brain'' self-help books. Sophisticated readers may be suspicious when the author of *The Aquarian Conspiracy* (Ferguson, 1980) praises *The Tao Jones Averages: A Guide to Whole-Brained Investing* (Goodspeed, 1983) as ''A fresh perspective in intuitive investing'' (quoted on back cover). Suspicion may be allayed, however, when Sperry, speaking of Edwards's (1979) book on drawing, says that ''her application of the brain research findings to drawing conforms well with the available evidence . . .'' (quoted on back cover), and when a distinguished cognitive psychologist calls it ''a marvelously fresh approach to drawing . . .'' (J. Bruner, quoted on back cover). Would the sentiments have been as charitable had Edwards made the same strong claims in an article submitted for publication in a scientific or scholarly journal?

We neuropsychologists also may help, however unwittingly, to promote the dichotomania that we criticize in others when we describe neuropsychological phenomena with certain shorthand phrases in place of more complex and refined statements. An example is the common use of the term ''left-brain skills'' to refer to reading, writing, and analytical problem solving or the tendency to speak informally and jocularly of, say, lawyers and athletes as ''left-brain types'' and ''right-brain types,'' respectively. We know this is caricature, not characterization, but the distinction may be lost on our students or even on those of our psychologist colleagues who are unfamiliar with the neuropsychological literature.

Furthermore, however much *we* understand that the cerebral hemispheres work mutually and interactively, we promote a different view whenever, in referring, say, to a typically modest visual field advantage on a tachistoscopic recognition test, we conclude that the contralateral hemisphere was necessarily the site of the requisite information processing of the stimulus input. Given the experimental method, we can be sure only that the input was lateralized and that the stimulus, therefore, had been projected first to one hemisphere. In the case of split-brain patients, of course, we are on surer ground, although even here, as noted earlier, we cannot be totally confident that only one hemisphere is involved.

Finally, we risk misleading not only ourselves but the general public as well by the terms we use to describe the basic phenomena of lateral cerebral specialization. In our technical shorthand, we commonly say that one or the other hemisphere ''saw'' or ''heard'' something, ''thought about'' or ''solved'' a problem, or ''painted,'' ''wrote,'' or ''spoke.'' This sort of language engenders the peculiar fiction that hemispheres are beings, homunculi, capable not only of problem solving and a host of actions in the external environment, but even of personhood, and since persons can be taught, it is a small logical step to the conclusion that hemispheres can be taught as well. But neither individual hemispheres nor, indeed, whole brains solve problems, nor do they see, hear, remember, feel, paint or speak. These are instances of what the philosopher Gilbert Ryle (1949) called ''category-mistakes.'' *People,* not cerebral hemispheres, do these things. As Robinson has said, in reference to the way certain scientists were speaking of the cerebral hemispheres after commissurotomy:

The plain fact is that hemispheres are not predicated of failures, confusions, contradictions, percepts, judgments. Need we remind ourselves again that a wedding invitation filed in the middle drawer does not confer an invitation on the drawer? We have every right to describe [postcommissurotomy] Smith as feeling restored after a walk in the garden and a spinach souffle but, short of humor, we would not discuss hemispheres, minor or major, this way. (1976, p. 77)

Robinson later remarked that his suggestions for restraint in this sort of characterization were "greeted with gracious indifference" (1982, p. 908). Still, one must keep on trying.

What all these examples tell me is that even the most sophisticated scientists can be swept up in the enthusiasm for dichotomization. As Corballis (1980) has said, there must be something about the left–right dimension that lends itself to this sort of overstatement. Perhaps, he suggests, it is part of the universal appeal of all dualities. But if even we in the field are so disposed, we can hardly expect cool restraint in people lacking scientific training and eager for solutions to pressing social problems. All the more reason for us to be careful how we talk about our work, lest we help to promote the very mistakes and misunderstandings that we rightfully deplore in others.

Finally, I trust that no one will take my remarks to mean that I object *in principle* to pressing for advances in educational practice, mental health, or business and industry through the application of scientific evidence about the nervous system and about cerebral specialization in particular. I do not object; my concern is only with the kind of (in my estimation) unwarranted application documented here.

What *should* neuropsychologists tell educators and the general public about the brain and about lateral specialization? In our academic lectures and public speeches, we should present the basic research in appropriate detail and with the qualifications and cautions always necessary in a developing science, and we should speak out vigorously against the misuse of our work. What, then, should we say are the *valid* ways to apply our research to educational and other societal problems? Perhaps some day, as Zaidel (1985, p. 312) has suggested, we shall have learned, say, to tailor learning environments to individual cognitive–cerebral organization and to improve individual performance on specific tasks through controlled shifts in cerebral balance. But, as he goes on to say, we have not yet reached that point. Today, then, I think our only honest statement would be like the one made by Hardyck and Haapenen in 1979: Research on lateral specialization as yet provides "no scientific basis . . . for any reorganization of curricular, teaching, or testing programs within contemporary educational practice" (p. 219). The public should be wary of anyone making promises to the contrary.

ACKNOWLEDGMENTS

Preparation of this chapter was supported in part by a grant from the Michigan State University Foundation.

NOTES

1. Medical and behavioral scientists have responsibly and effectively analyzed all the health claims made by the Doman-Delacato group and have shown them to be spurious (see Cohen, Birch, & Taft, 1970; Robbins & Glass, 1968; and the statements by the American Academy for Cerebral Palsy, 1968, and the American Academy

of Pediatrics, 1968). Nevertheless, some of the promoters of this scheme, prominently Doman, are still on the scene today. According to Reynolds (1984, p. 234), some school districts in the United States continue to employ Doman-Delacato programs "as the primary model for exceptional children within their jurisdiction" (see also Reynolds, 1981).

2. The reasons for the disparities between these two groups of studies are still unclear. The crucial difference may be that McKeever's Navajo subjects were assimilated into Anglo culture (all had been recruited from the local college), whereas Scott and Hynd's Navajo subjects were unassimilated. Scott and Hynd's results thus might indicate that their subjects did not treat the dichotic sounds as linguistic stimuli. If so, then the more revealing way of assessing their side of language dominance would have been to use minimal speech contrasts in Navajo rather than in English. Had that been done, my guess is that the results would be very similar to McKeever's, that is, a right-ear (left-hemisphere) advantage. (For an incisive review of the literature on the "right-brained Indian," see Chrisjohn and Peters, 1986.)

REFERENCES

"A window to the brain." (1976). *Mosaic, 7*(2), 14–19. Washington, DC: National Science Foundation.

American Academy for Cerebral Palsy (and other organizations). (1968). The Doman-Delacato treatment of neurologically handicapped children. *Developmental Medicine and Child Neurology, 10,* 243–246.

American Academy of Pediatrics. (1968). The Doman-Delacato treatment of neurologically handicapped children. *Journal of Pediatrics, 72,* 750.

Arndt, S., & Berger, D. (1978). Cognitive mode and asymmetry in cerebral functioning. *Cortex, 14,* 78–86.

Arnheim, R. (1969). *Visual thinking.* Berkeley: University of California Press.

Bandler, R., & Grinder, J. (1979). *Frogs into princes: Neuro-linguistic Programming.* Moab, UT: Real People Press.

Beaumont, J. G., Young, A. W., & McManus, I. C. (1984). Hemisphericity: A critical review. *Cognitive Neuropsychology, 1,* 191–212.

Beckman, L. (1977). The use of the Block Design sub test as an identifying instrument for spatial children. *The Gifted Child Quarterly, 21,* 113–116.

Benton, A. L. (1972). The "minor" hemisphere. *Journal of the History of Medicine and Allied Sciences, 27,* 5–14.

Benton, A. L. (1985). Visuoperceptive, visuospatial, and visuoconstructive disorders. In K. M. Heilman & E. Valenstein (Eds.), *Clinical neuropsychology* (2nd ed.) (pp. 151–185). New York: Oxford University Press.

Benton, A. L., & Pearl, D. (Eds.). (1978). *Dyslexia: An appraisal of current knowledge.* New York: Oxford University Press.

Berg, M. R., & Harris, L. J. (1980). The effects of experimenter location and subject anxiety on cerebral activation as measured by lateral eye movements. *Neuropsychologia, 18,* 89–93.

Blakeslee, T. R. (1980). *The right brain: A new understanding of the unconscious mind and its creative powers.* Garden City, NY: Anchor Press/Doubleday.

Bogen, J. E. (1975). The other side of the brain: VII. Some educational aspects of hemispheric specialization. *UCLA Educator, 17,* 24–32.

Bogen, J. E., DeZare, R., TenHouten, W. D., & Marsh, J. F. (1972). The other side of the brain: IV. The A/P ratio. *Bulletin of the Los Angeles Neurological Societies, 37,* 49–61.

Borchgrevink, H. M. (1982). Prosody and musical rhythm are controlled by the speech hemisphere. In M. Clyne (Ed.), *Music, mind, and brain: The neuropsychology of music* (pp. 151–157). New York and London: Plenum.

Brandwein, P. (1977). The duality of the brain: A symposium in print with Paul Brandwein and Robert Ornstein. *Instructor, 58,* 56–58.

Broca, P. (1861). Remarques sur le siège de la faculté du langage articulé, suiviés d'une observation d'aphemie (perte de la parole). *Bulletins de la Société Anatomique, 6,* 330–357.

Broca, P. (1863). Localisation des fonctions cérébrales. Siège du langage articulé. *Bulletins de la Société d'Anthropologie, 4,* 200–203.

Broca, P. (1865). Sur le siège de la faculté du langage articulé. *Bulletins de la Société d'Anthropologie de Paris, 6,* 377–393.

Brown-Séquard, C. E. (1877). Dual character of the brain: The Toner Lectures (Lecture II). *Smithsonian Miscellaneous Collections* (pp. 1–21). Washington, DC: Smithsonian Institution.

Bruyer, R. (1980). Implication différentielle des hémisphères cérébraux dans les conduites émotionelles. *Acta Psychiatrica Belgica, 80,* 266–284.
Bryden, M. P., & Ley, R. G. (1983). Right-hemisphere involvement in the perception and expression of emotion in normal humans. In K. M. Heilman & P. Satz (Eds.), *Neuropsychology of human emotion* (pp. 6–44). New York: Guilford.
Campbell, R. (1982). The lateralization of emotion: A critical review. *International Journal of Psychology, 17,* 211–229.
Carlson, D. F., & Harris, L. J. (1986). Perception of happiness and sadness in free-viewing of chimeric faces. Paper presented at the Fourteenth Annual Meeting of the International Neuropsychological Society, February 4–8, Denver Colorado.
Cattell, R. B., & Cattell, A. K. S. (1959). *Handbook for the Culture Fair Intelligence Test.* Champaign, IL: Institute for Personality and Ability Testing.
Chrisjohn, R. D., & Peters, M. (1986). The pernicious myth of the right-brained Indian. *Canadian Journal of Indian Education, 13,* 62–71.
Cohen, H. J., Birch, H. G., & Taft, L. T. (1970). Some considerations for evaluating the Doman-Delacato "patterning" method. *Pediatrics, 45,* 302–314.
Corballis, M. C. (1980). Laterality and myth. *American Psychologist, 35,* 284–295.
Corballis, M. C. (1983). *Human laterality.* New York: Academic Press.
Critchley, M. (1969). *The parietal lobes.* New York: Hafner Press.
Dabbs, J. (1980). Left–right differences in cerebral blood flow and cognition. *Psychophysiology, 17,* 548–551.
Dejerine, J. (1891). Sur un cas de cecité verbale avec agraphie suivi d'autopsie. *Memoires de la Société de Biologie, 3,* 197–201.
Delacato, C. H. (1959). *The treatment and prevention of reading problems.* Springfield, IL: Thomas.
Delacato, C. H. (1966). *Neurological organization and reading.* Springfield, IL: Thomas.
Denny-Brown, D., & Banker, B. (1952). The significance of perceptual rivalry resulting from parietal lesions. *Brain, 75,* 433–471.
Dilts, R. (1983a). *Applications of Neuro-linguistic Programming.* Cupertino, CA: Meta Publications.
Dilts, R. (1983b). *Roots of Neuro-linguistic Programming.* Cupertino, CA: Meta Publications.
Doman, R. J., Spitz, E. B., Zucman, I., Delacato, C. H., & Doman, G. (1960). Children with severe brain injuries: Neurological organization in terms of mobility. *Journal of the American Medical Association, 174,* 257–262.
Drake, R. (1984). Lateral asymmetry of personal optimism. *Journal of Research in Personality, 18,* 497–507.
Edwards, B. (1979). *Drawing on the right side of the brain: A course in enhancing creativity and artistic confidence.* Los Angeles: Tarcher.
Ehrlichman, H., & Weinberger, A. (1979). Lateral eye movements and hemipsheric asymmetry: A critical review. *Psychological Bulletin, 85,* 1080–1101.
Ferguson, E. S. (1977). The mind's eye: Non-verbal thought in technology. *Science, 197,* 827–836.
Ferguson, M. (1980). *The aquarian conspiracy: Personal and social transformation in the 1980s.* Los Angeles: Tarcher.
Fishwick, J. P. (1976). Letter to Editor. *Harvard Business Review, 54,* 170.
Gainotti, G., Caltagirone, C., Miceli, G., & Masullo, C. (1981). Selective semantic–lexical impairment of language comprehension in right brain-damaged patients. *Brain and Language, 13,* 201–211.
Galin, D. (1976). Educating both halves of the brain. *Childhood Education, 53,* 17–20.
Gates, A., & Bradshaw, J. L. (1977). Music perception and cerebral asymmetries. *Cortex, 13,* 390–401.
Gazzaniga, M. S. (1986). *The social brain: Discovering the networks of the mind.* New York: Basic Books.
Geschwind, N. (1982). Why Orton was right. *Annals of Dyslexia, 32,* 13–30.
Goleman, D. (1977). Split-brain psychology: Fad of the year. *Psychology Today, 11,* 88–90, 149–150.
Goodspeed, B. W. (1983). *The Tao Jones Averages: A guide to whole-brained investing.* New York: E. P. Dutton.
Grady, M. P., & Luecke, E. A. (1978). *Education and the brain (Fastback 108).* Bloomington, IN: Phi Delta Kappa Educational Foundation.
Grinder, J., & Bandler, R. (1976). *The structure of magic II: A book about communication and change.* Palo Alto, CA: Science and Behavior Books.
Gross, Y., Franko, R., & Lewin, I. (1978). Effects of voluntary eye movements on hemispheric activity and choice of cognitive mode. *Neuropsychologia, 16,* 653–657.
Gur, R., Gur, R., & Harris, L. J. (1975). Cerebral activation, as measured by subjects' lateral eye movements, is influenced by experimenter location. *Neuropsychologia, 13,* 35–44.
Guthrie, J. T. (1978). Principles of instruction: A critique of Johnson's "Remedial approaches to dyslexia." In

A. L. Benton & D. Pearl (Eds.), *Dyslexia: An appraisal of current knowledge* (pp. 423–432). New York: Oxford University Press.

Hadamard, J. (1954). *An essay on the psychology of invention in the mathematical fields.* New York: Dover.

Hardyck, C. & Haapanen, R. (1979). Educating both halves of the brain: Educational breakthrough or neuromythology? *Journal of School Psychology, 17,* 219–230.

Harnad, S. R. (1972). Creativity, lateral saccades, and the nondominant hemisphere. *Perceptual and Motor Skills, 34,* 653–654.

Harrington, A. (1985). Nineteenth-century ideas on hemisphere differences and "duality of mind" (target article with commentaries). *The Behavioral and Brain Sciences, 8,* 617–659.

Harris, L. J. (1979). *Two-brain education: Historical perspective on a contemporary fad.* Paper presented at the Annual Meetings of the International Neuropsychological Society, February 1, New York, N.Y.

Harris, L. J. (1980a). Left-handedness: Early theories, facts, and fancies. In J. Herron (Ed.), *Neuropsychology of left-handedness* (pp. 3–78). New York: Academic Press.

Harris, L. J. (1980b). Which hand is the "eye" of the blind?—A new look at an old question. In J. Herron (Ed.), *Neuropsychology of left-handedness* (pp. 303–329). New York: Academic Press.

Harris, L. J. (1985a). Teaching the right brain: Historical perspective on a contemporary educational fad. In C. T. Best (Ed.), *Hemispheric function and collaboration in the child* (pp. 231–274). Orlando, FL: Academic Press.

Harris, L. J. (1985b). The Ambidextral Culture Society and the "duality of mind." *The Behavioral and Brain Sciences, 8,* 639–640.

Harris, L. J. (1988). *Broca on the relationship between handedness and cerebral speech dominance: Have Broca's views been misconstrued?* If so, by whom, when, and why? Paper presented at the 11th Annual European Meetings of the International Neuropsychological Society, July 5–7, Lahti, Finland.

Hecaen, H., & Ajuriaguerra, J. de (1964). *Left-handedness: Manual superiority and cerebral dominance.* New York and London: Grune and Stratton.

Hecaen, H., & Sauguet, J. (1971). Cerebral dominance in left-handed subjects. *Cortex, 7,* 19–48.

Heilman, K. M., & Satz, P. (Eds.). (1983). *Neuropsychology of human emotion.* New York: Guilford Press.

Heilman, K. M., Watson, R. T., & Valenstein, E. (1985). Neglect and related disorders. In K. M. Heilman & E. Valenstein (Eds.), *Clinical neuropsychology* (2nd ed.) (pp. 243–293). New York: Oxford University Press.

Hermann, N. (1981). The creative brain. *Training and Development Journal, 35,* 11–16.

Hines, D., & Martindale, C. (1974). Induced lateral eye-movements and creative and intellectual performance. *Perceptual and Motor Skills, 39,* 153–154.

Hunter, M. (1976). Right-brained kids in left-brained schools. *Today's Education, 65,* 45–48.

Hynd, G. W., & Scott, S. A. (1980). Propositional and appositional modes of thought and differential cerebral speech in Navajo Indian and Anglo children. *Child Development,* 51, 909–911.

Intuitive skills for future managers. (1983). *Bulletin of Management.* The Bureau of National Affairs, Inc. September 1, No. 1744, pp. 2, 7.

Jackson, J. H. (1915). On the nature of the duality of the brain. *Brain, 38,* 80–103. (Reprinted from *Medical Press and Circular,* 1874, *1,* 19–25, 41–49, 63–70.)

Jones, E. (1980). Review of Marilyn Ferguson, *The aquarian conspiracy: Personal and social transformation in the 1980s* (Los Angeles: Tarcher). *Contemporary Psychology, 25,* 846–847.

Katz, A. N. (1979). Creativity and the cerebral hemispheres [Letter]. *American Psychologist, 34,* 279–280.

Kinsbourne, M. (1972). Eye and head turning indicates cerebral lateralization. *Science, 176,* 539–541.

Kinsbourne, M. (1982). Hemispheric specialization and the growth of human understanding. *American Psychologist, 37,* 411–420.

Kinsbourne, M., & Hiscock, M. (1978). Cerebral lateralization and cognitive development. In J. S. Chall & A. F. Mirsky (Eds.), *Education and the brain: The seventy-seventh yearbook of the National Society for the Study of Education* (pp. 169–222). Chicago: University of Chicago Press.

Kinsbourne, M., & Hiscock, M. (1983). The normal and deviant development of functional lateralization of the brain. In P. H. Mussen (Ed.), *Infancy and developmental psychobiology: Vol. 2. Handbook of child psychology* (4th ed.) (pp. 222–280). New York: Wiley.

Kocel, K., Galin, D., Ornstein, R., & Merrin, E. (1972). Lateral eye movement and cognitive mode. *Psychonomic Science, 27,* 223–224.

Kruger, T. H. (1976). *Visual imagery in problem solving and scientific creativity.* Derby, CT: Seal Press.

Landsmann, L. (1978). The brain's division of labor. *New York Times,* April 30, Spring Survey of Education, Section 12, p. 24.

Lassen, N. A., Ingvar, D. H., & Skinhøj, E. (1978). Brain function and blood flow. *Scientific American, 239,* 62–71.

La Torre, R. A., & La Torre, A. M. (1981). Effect of lateral eye fixation on cognitive processes. *Perceptual and Motor Skills, 52,* 487–490.

Leehy, S., Carey, S., Diamond, R., & Cahn, A. (1978). Upright and inverted faces: The right hemisphere knows the difference. *Cortex, 14,* 411–419.

Left–right brain role is studied. (1984). *Chicago Tribune,* April 22, Section 6, p. 3.

Lempert, H., & Kinsbourne, M. (1982). Effect of laterality of orientation on verbal memory. *Neuropsychologia, 20,* 211–214.

Lenneberg, W. H. (1967). *Biological foundations of language.* New York: Wiley.

Leonardo was a southpaw. (1977). *Art News, 76,* 22–23.

Levine, S. C. (1985). Developmental changes in right-hemisphere involvement in face recognition. In C. T. Best (Ed.), *Hemispheric function and collaboration in the child* (pp. 157–191). Orlando, FL: Academic Press.

Levy, J. (1977). Hemi-inattention after commisurotomy. In E. A. Weinstein & R. P. Friedland (Eds.), *Hemi-inattention and hemispheric specialization* (pp. 83–92). New York: Raven Press.

Levy, J. (1985). Right brain, left brain: Fact and fiction. *Psychology Today,* May, pp. 38–44.

Levy, J., Heller, W., Banich, M. T., & Burton, L. A. (1983). Art variations among right-handed individuals in perceptual asymmetries cased by characteristic arousal differences between hemispheres? *Journal of Experimental Psychology: Human Perception and Performance, 9,* 329–359.

Loviglio, L. (1981). Mathematics and the brain: A tale of two hemispheres. *The Massachusetts Teacher, 60*(5), 8–12.

McKeever, W. F. (1981). Evidence against the hypothesis of right hemisphere language dominance in the Native American Navajo. *Neuropsychologia, 19,* 595–598.

McKeever, W. F., & Hunt, L. J. (1984). Failure to replicate the Scott *et al.* finding of reversed ear dominance in the native American Navajo. *Neuropsychologia, 22,* 539–541.

McShane, D. (1980). A review of the scores of American Indian children on the Wechsler Intelligence Scales. *White Cloud Journal, 1,* 3–10.

Mednick, S. A., & Mednick, M. T. (1967). *Remote Associates Test: Examiners' manual.* Boston: Houghton Mifflin.

Mintzberg, H. (1976). Planning on the left side and managing on the right. *Harvard Business Review, 54,* 49–58.

Moscovitch, M., & Olds, J. (1982). Asymmetries in spontaneous facial expression and their possible relation to hemispheric specialization. *Neuropsychologia, 20,* 71–81.

Myers, J. T. (1982). Hemisphericity research: An overview with some implications for problem solving. *Journal of Creative Behavior, 16,* 197–211.

Naylor, H. (1980). Reading disability and lateral asymmetry: An information-processing analysis. *Psychological Bulletin, 87,* 531–545.

Ornstein, R. E. (1972). *The psychology of consciousness.* San Francisco: Freeman.

Ornstein, R. E. (1977). The duality of the mind: A symposium in print with Paul Brandwein and Robert Ornstein. *Instructor, 58,* 54–56.

Orton, S. T. (1928). A physiological theory of reading disability and stuttering in children. *New England Journal of Medicine, 199,* 1046–1052.

Orton, S. T. (1937). *Reading, writing, and speech problems in children.* New York: Norton.

Prince, G. (1978). Putting the other half of the brain to work. *Training: The Magazine of Human Resource Development, 15,* 57–61.

Regelski, T. A. (1977). Music education and the human brain. *Education Digest, 4*(3), 44–47 (condensed from *Music Educators Journal,* 1977, *63,* 30–38).

Reynolds, C. R. (1981). The neuropsychological basis of intelligence. In G. W. Hynd & J. E. Obrzut (Eds.), *Neuropsychological assessment and the school age child: Issues and procedures* (pp. 87–124). New York: Grune and Stratton.

Reynolds, C. R. (1984). Hemisphericity and neuropsychological approaches in education: Evidence for an aptitude X treatment interaction—and a caution. In M. K. Raina (Ed.), *Education of the left and the right: Implications of hemispheric specialization* (pp. 223–239). Atlantic Highlands, NJ: Humanities Press.

Rico, G. L. (1983). *Writing the natural way: Using right-brain techniques to release your expressive power.* Los Angeles: J. P. Tarcher.

Robbins, M. P., & Glass, G. V. (1968). The Doman-Delacato rationale: A critical analysis. In J. Hellmuth (Ed.), *Educational Therapy* (Vol. 2, pp. 321–377). Seattle, WA: Special Child Publications.

Robinson, D. N. (1976). What sort of persons are hemispheres? Another look at "split-brain" man. *British Journal of Philosophy of Science, 27,* 73–78.

Robinson, D. N. (1982). Cerebral plurality and the unity of self. *American Psychologist, 37,* 904–910.

Rogers, L., TenHouten, W., Kaplan, C., & Gardiner, M. (1977). Hemispheric specialization of language: An EEG study of bilingual Hopi Indian children. *International Journal of Neuroscience, 8,* 1–6.

Ross, A. C. (1982). Brain hemispheric functions and the Native American. *Journal of American Indian Education,* May, 2–5.

Ross, E. D. (1981). The aprosodias: Functional–anatomic organization of the affective components of language in the right hemisphere. *Archives of Neurology, 38,* 561–569.

Rubenzer, R. L. (1982). Educating the other half: Implications of left/right brain research. A publication of ERIC Clearinghouse on Handicapped and Gifted Children. Report #ISBN-0-86586-141-2. Reston, VA: Council for Exceptional Children, Publication #264.

Ryle, G. (1949). *The concept of mind.* London: Hutchinson House.

Sackeim, H. A., Greenberg, M. S., Weiman, A. L., Gur, R. C., Hungerbuhler, J. P., & Geschwind, N. (1982). Hemispheric asymmetry in the expression of positive and negative emotions: Neurologic evidence. *Archives of Neurology, 39,* 210–218.

Samples, B. (1976). *The metaphoric mind.* Reading, MA: Addison-Wesley.

Satz, P. (1980). Incidence of aphasia in left-handers: A test of some hypothetical models of cerebral speech organization. In J. Herron (Ed.), *Neuropsychology of left-handedness* (pp. 189–198). New York: Academic Press.

Schwartz, G. E., Davidson, R. J., & Maer, F. (1975). Right hemisphere lateralization for emotion in the human brain: Interactions with cognition. *Science, 190,* 286–288.

Scott, S., Hynd, G., Hunt, L., & Weed, W. (1979). Cerebral speech lateralization in the native American Navajo. *Neuropsychologia, 17,* 89–92.

Searleman, A. (1977). A review of right hemisphere capabilities. *Psychological Bulletin, 84,* 503–528.

Segalowitz, S. J., & Gruber, F. A. (Eds.). (1977). *Language development and neurological theory.* New York: Academic Press.

Sergent, J., & Bindra, D. (1981). Differential hemispheric processing of faces: Methodological considerations and reinterpretations. *Psychological Bulletin, 89,* 541–555.

Sperry, R. W. (1973). Lateral specialization of cerebral function in the surgically separated hemispheres. In F. J. McGuigan & R. A. Schoonover (Eds.), *The psychobiology of thinking* (pp. 209–229). New York: Academic Press.

Sperry, R. W. (1974). Messages from the laboratory. *Engineering Sciences, 37,* 29–32.

Sperry, R. W. (1975). Left brain, right brain. *Saturday Review,* August 9, 30–33.

Staley, F. A. (1980). Hemispheric brain research and outdoor education. *Education Digest, 46,* 46–49.

Torrance, E. P., & Mourad, S. (1979). Role of hemisphericity in performance on selected measures of creativity. *Gifted Child Quarterly, 23,* 44–45.

Torrance, E. P., Reynolds, C. R., Riegel, T., & Ball, O. (1977). Your style of learning and thinking, Forms A and B: Preliminary norms, abbreviated notes, scoring keys, and selected references. *Gifted Child Quarterly, 21,* 563–573.

Trubo, R. (1982). How to tap your brain's success circuits. *Success, The Magazine for Achievers,* March (reprint, unpaginated).

Tucker, D. M. (1981). Lateral brain function, emotion, and conceptualization. *Psychological Bulletin, 89,* 19–46.

Tucker, D. M., Stenslie, C. E., Roth, R. S., & Shearer, S. L. (1981). Right frontal lobe activation and right hemisphere performance: Decrement during a depressed mood. *Archives of General Psychiatry, 38,* 169–174.

Walker, E., Wade, S., & Waldman, I. (1982). The effect of lateral visual fixation on response latency to verbal and spatial questions. *Brain and Cognition, 1,* 399–404.

Warrington, E. K. (1969). Constructional apraxia. In P. J. Vinken & G. W. Bruyn (Eds.), *Handbook of clinical neurology* (Vol. 4, pp. 67–83). Amsterdam: North Holland.

Wernicke, C. (1874). *Der aphasische Symptomencomplex.* Breslau: Cohen & Weigert.

West, S. A. (1976). Creativity, altered states of awareness, and artificial intelligence. *Journal of Altered States of consciousness, 2,* 219–230.

Wheatley, G. G. (1977). The brain hemispheres' role in problem solving. *Arithmetic Teacher, 25,* 36–39.

Whole brain education: Software to develop both halves of Johnny's brain (1985). *Computer Buyer's Guide and Handbook,* March, pp. 130–131.

Whole or ½ brain? (1986). (Advertisement). *New York Times,* July 3, p. 11.

Williamson, K. J., & Hudspeth, R. T. (1982). Teaching holistic thought through engineering design. *Engineering Education,* April, pp. 698–703.

Wonder, J., & Donovan, P. (1984). *Whole-Brain Thinking.* New York: Ballantine Books.

Young, A. W., & Ellis, A. W. (1981). Asymmetry of cerebral hemispheric function in normal and poor readers. *Psychological Bulletin, 89,* 183–190.

Young, G., Segalowitz, S. J., Corter, C. M., & Trehub, S. E. (Eds.). (1983). *Manual specialization and the developing brain.* New York: Academic Press.

Zaidel, E. (1985). Introduction. In D. F. Benson & E. Zaidel (Eds.), *The dual brain: Hemispheric specialization in humans* (pp. 307–318). New York: Guilford Press.

Zangwill, O. L. (1960). *Cerebral dominance and its relation to psychological function.* Edinburgh: Oliver & Boyd.

Zook, J. A., & Dwyer, J. H. (1976). Cultural differences in hemisphericity: A critique. *Bulletin of the Los Angeles Neurological Societies, 41,* 87–90.

9

The Effect of "Right Brain/Left Brain" Cognitive Profiles on School Achievement

HAROLD W. GORDON
University of Pittsburgh School of Medicine

DYSLEXIA

Clinical expediency has forced a formal definition of a learning-disabled child to be one who is otherwise neurologically sound and intellectually normal, but whose learning or achievement is 1 to 2 years below grade level. It is widely recognized that this designation is artificial, for reasons that include the controversial assessment of intelligence and an arbitrarily determined cutoff of 1 to 2 years for the intelligence–achievement discrepancy. Difficulties immediately arise. For one thing, the 2-year grade deficiency is necessarily different for a 2nd- or 3rd-grader than for a 5th- or 6th-grader, since the rate of learning and the nature of the deficit are not the same from year to year. Second, children whose achievement is at grade level, but whose intellect is considerably above, would not carry the label "dyslexic" even though the pattern of performance and the nature of the handicap would be the same as for the below-grade performers. The irony is that such students are smart enough to recognize their inadequacies relative to their peers, yet are passed over for special help because of their performance. It is almost as if such a subject is being punished for achieving grade-level success. Finally, children with normal or above-average intellect whose achievement is *less* than a year below grade level would just miss definitional boundaries. In other words, the difference between a learning-disabled student and a mainstream student may be more apparent than real. The problem is that although legal and some treatment purposes call for an arbitrary division into learning-disabled and "normal" groups, a truer distribution of the discrepancy between performance capability and academic achievement is continuous (Perfetti, 1985).

Research in clearly defined dyslexic populations suffers from efforts to characterize a disorder that is arbitrarily defined. The exclusion criteria may not be complete enough to limit cases to a "pure" diagnostic subgroup or subgroups. Subjects sharing etiological characteristics of the dyslexic group may be inappropriately excluded and may unwittingly become a part of the control group. For example, if one retained the requirement that there be a discrepancy of 2 years between intelligence and achievement, but dropped the requirement that individuals must achieve below grade level, then several more higher functioning "dyslexic" subjects would be added to the experimental pool and removed from the control group. On the other hand, if the 2-year discrepancy requirement were reduced to 1 year and the requirement for normal intelligence were relaxed, a lower functioning sample would result. There is no a priori reason to assume individuals with low IQs would be any less likely to have dyslexic etiology than those with superior intelligence. Results of investigations have already produced different conclusions about the nature of dyslexia depending on the definition of the population studied (Denckla, 1979; Myklebust, 1978; Pirozzolo, 1979).

The possibility that there are several dyslexic syndromes was recognized at least a decade ago and is still under study. An early method for recognizing these different groups was to set up arbitrary definitional criteria based on apparent patterns of performance on several neuropsychological tests (Mattis, French, & Rapin, 1975). In that study, three grouplings were defined according to previously observed deficit characteristics. Subjects referred for evaluation of learning and behavior disorders were then classified into them. Ninety percent of the subjects could be assigned to one of three groups; none fell into more than one group. It was therefore concluded that there were multiple forms of dyslexia, each of which was presumably related to its own cluster of specific deficits. Since the clusters were defined from a neuropsychological standpoint, the deficits were believed to be brain based. It was also shown, however, that these criteria did not distinguish between subjects with and without brain damage.

Another attempt to classify children on the basis of performance relied entirely on spelling errors (Boder, 1973). Although the specific criteria were not detailed, it appeared possible to separate the error types on a qualitative level. There were two types, defined as ''dyseidetic'' and ''dysphonetic,'' on the basis of primarily visual or primarily phonetic (auditory) misspellings. A third group committed errors of both types. Most subjects were classified into the dsyphonetic group, followed by the mixed and dyseidetic groups, respectively.

These are only examples of a number of studies that sought descriptive or subjective means by which to subtype children with learning disabilities. In recognition of the fact that objective subtyping would be more desirable, more recent studies have used sophisticated statistical methods to uncover objectively the nature of these subgroups (Doehring & Hoshko, 1977; Doehring, Trites, Patel, & Fiedorowicz, 1981). Starting from the assumption that subgroups of reading difficulties do exist, as is evident from different patterns of reading performance, a battery of reading tests was administered to a large sample of poor readers. Subgroups were determined statistically by a type of reverse factor analysis (*Q*-type) in which clusters of *subjects* are defined according to their pattern of performance on the reading tests. In one population of poor readers, three subgroups could be defined (Doehring & Hoshko, 1977), each with a characteristic pattern of performance on reading and other achievement tests. The result was replicated in another independent sample, thereby cross-validating the technique (Doehring *et al.*, 1981). Although the groups differed on their pattern of reading performance, however, they did not appear to differ on the basis of performance on specific language tests, nor were there unique neuropsychological profiles among the groups. Only a few of the comparisons among neuropsychological tests were significantly different between pairs of reading subgroups. The failure to find different cognitive profiles was confirmed by the *Q*-type factor analysis on the neuropsychological test variables themselves. Reliable subgroups could not be formed.

Despite the differences in achievement performance across three of the statistically defined reading groups, there were similarities in the cognitive profile. Visuospatial skills were performed a little better than average, and verbosequential skills a little worse. Although it is not specifically stated, these results suggest that the majority of reading-disabled children, regardless of their reading subtype, have similar cognitive profiles in which visuospatial tests, often associated with the right cerebral hemisphere, are performed better than average, whereas verbosequential tests, often associated with the left hemisphere, are performed below average. This dramatic similarity is depicted in Figure 9-1, where the difference between the Block Design and Digit Span subtests of the WISC is shown for each group. As far as these tests are concerned, the performance pattern of each subgroup is the same. In every subsample, the Block Design scaled score averaged above the norm;

A.

DIFFERENCE IN SCALED SCORES:

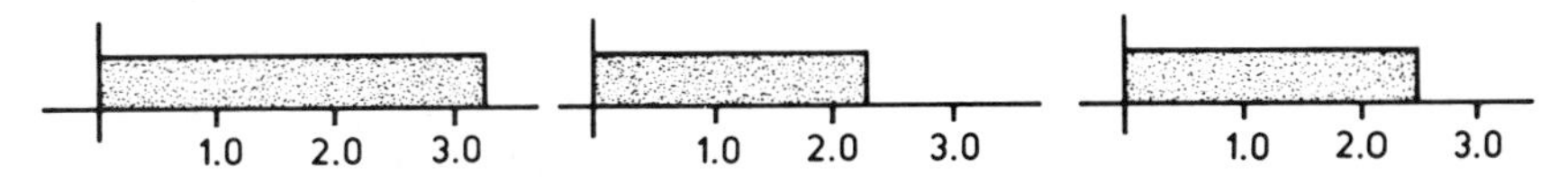

B.

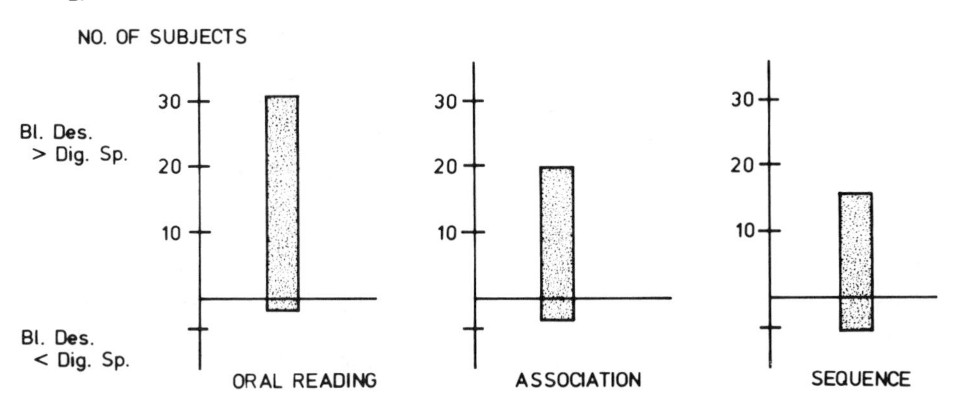

READING SUBTYPES

Figure 9-1. (A) Averaged difference in scaled score points (3 points = 1 standard deviation) between the Block Design and Digit Span subtests of the Wechsler Intelligence Scale for Children (WISC) in each of the groups of reading subtypes. (B) Number of subjects having higher Block Design scores than Digit Span scores or vice versa for the three reading subtypes. Data from Doehring, Trites, Patel, and Fiedorwicz (1981).

the Digit Span scaled score averaged below the norm. These are among the best examples of tests in the clinical repertory that have also been associated with assessment of right- and left-hemisphere function, respectively.

The association of clinical tests with brain function comes from repeated observations of selectively reduced scores on Performance IQ subtests, especially Block Design and Object Assembly, in patients with unilateral right-hemisphere damage, and reduced scores on Verbal IQ subtests, including Digit Span, in patients with unilateral left-hemisphere damage. In that regard, these subtests reflect a cognitive profile of performance superiorities as they relate to the right and left hemispheres. As can be seen, each subgroup, regardless of reading subtype, has the same profile favoring the associated right-hemisphere test. The differences would have been even more dramatic if Object Assembly and Arithmetic subtests, respectively, had been added to the Block Design and Digit Span comparisons.

Conclusions about hemispheric function drawn from performance on these IQ subtests have been confirmed in a study that tested the right–left-hemispheric dichotomy more directly (Harness, Epstein, & Gordon, 1984). A battery of tests designed to assess specialized functions associated with the left and right hemispheres (Bentin & Gordon, 1979; Gordon & Harness, 1977) was administered to over 100 children without neurological deficits referred during a one-year period to a clinic for reading disabilities. Nearly all (97%) of the referrals performed better on the visuospatial tests than on the verbosequential tests. On average, performance on the visuospatial tests was 0.5 standard deviation above average, whereas performance on the verbosequential tests was 0.5 standard deviation below. This 1 standard deviation difference between the visuospatial and verbosequential scores is the same as the three scaled score points that separated the subgroups depicted in Figure 9-1.

The implication from these studies is that the asymmetrical cognitive profile favoring visuospatial skills is a *necessary* condition for the majority of referred subjects with reading deficits. However, not everyone in the nonreferred population with a superiority for visuospatial skills has a reading problem, so the profile is not *sufficient* (Gordon, 1984). It can be hypothesized from these data that there is an underlying cognitive profile that is common to the majority of children with reading difficulties, but it has not been determined what compels some individuals with this profile to have learning difficulties and others not to report difficulties. We have proposed elsewhere that there is a cerebral "locking" mechanism that forces a visuospatial mode of thought in the dyslexics (Gordon, 1980). The biological nature of this mechanism, and whether it would be the factor more prevalent in males, remains to be determined.

The similarity of the cognitive profile among the majority of dyslexics does not ignore the presence of subtypes. Within the large population, there are undoubtedly additional factors that give rise to the observed differences in reading patterns. The argument put forth here is that these differences are secondary to the more salient feature of a predominant visuospatial profile in most dyslexics.

MAINSTREAM EDUCATION

It is an unresolved question whether the long history of the studies of learning-disabled children has implications for the educational mainstream population as well. Learning theories in general do not take cognitive profiles into consideration. Furthermore, dyslexia is considered to be a disorder at one end of a continuum of reading difficulties in the normal population. That is to say, the basics of learning and types of reading errors are presumed not to differ among dyslexic and normal groups (Perfetti, 1985).

The current theory derived from psycholinguistic research (Stanovich, 1980) is that individuals rely on a number of varied mechanisms while reading textual material. Phonetic encoding is one of the best known mechanisms that is sequential by nature. Other mechanisms, such as unitization—reading in units larger than letters—appear to rely more on "spatial" skills in which larger graphemic chunks are processed at one time (Healy, 1981). Although one school of thought divides reading into a dichotomy whereby the "sound it out" phonetic method is appropriate for some readers, and the "whole word" method is appropriate for others, a newer school of thought is that there is a single reading mechanism organized into different linguistic levels (Drewnowski & Healy, 1977).

In its most detailed description, the unitary reading strategy is an interactive process with a five-step hierarchical format, each level having its own set of mental representations of the text (Rumelhart, 1977). The most basic level is the feature level. "Features" are graphemes, segments of the printed letters, or the shapes of letters. The recognition of these features leads to the next higher level, the letter level. The letter level leads to the letter cluster (or letter pattern) level, which includes inflectional endings (e.g., *-ing*), short phrases, and small syntactic units. The final two levels are the lexical (or word) level and the semantic level, of which the latter is more abstract. The interaction among levels of the model suggest that simultaneously with the upward processing from features to words to meaning, there is a downward activation from words to features. For example, one would expect that words following each other will be appropriate according to the semantic content of the sentence. Also, well-known letter clusters will force predictions about letter and word shapes that should follow. Each of these interactions interplays from one level to another, the end result being reading.

How may the single unified mechanism of reading theory be related to the neuropsychological concept of cognitive profile? Theoretically, the relationship of reading to specialized cognitive performance should be synonymous with the relationship between mechanisms of reading and the cognitive profile. If individual differences in the pattern of cognitive ability affect different levels of the reading mechanism, then different reading patterns should be observed among subjects with different cognitive profiles. Since temporal or sequential ordering is one of the processes normally attributed to the left cerebral hemisphere, the fact that much of the reading mechanism is sequential in nature implies that individuals who excel on tests associated with the left hemisphere will also excel in reading. On the other hand, the right hemisphere has been shown to play a role in reading acquisition as well. All letters, words, and phrases are themselves patterns to the early reader. Accordingly, right-hemisphere dominance for word recognition has been demonstrated in children in the early grades by faster response times to words presented in the left visual field (Carmon, Nachshon, & Starinsky, 1976; Silverberg, Gordon, Pollack, & Bentin, 1980). In the later grades, faster response times shifted to the right field. Such results were not due to the age of the children, since a similar left-to-right visual field shift was observed during second language acquisition in a different (English) script by adolescents whose native tongue was Hebrew (Silverberg, Bentin, Gaziel, Obler, & Albert, 1979). It appears, then, that different levels within the reading hierarchy require different contributions of specialized functions from the right and left cerebral hemispheres. If so, the nature of the reading ability should differ according to differences in the cognitive profile.

The question of dyslexia can also be raised in the context of mechanistic levels of reading theory and cognitive profile. Is the failure of dyslexics to master the various levels within the theory of reading hierarchy an extreme disability along a continuum of reading failures, or are their patterns qualitatively different? Most dyslexics have a cognitive profile favoring visuospatial skills, so that their pattern of failure might resemble that of poor readers in the mainstream who also favor visuospatial skills. But poor readers with a verbosequential profile would not be expected to have the same qualitative difficulties. With respect to the reading hierarchical model, the theory has not been tested. With respect to reading achievement, however, we have collected some data.

Cognitive Profile and Achievement

Over the past several years we have undertaken to assess the consequences of a particular cognitive profile on performance of academic achievement tests (Gordon, 1983). In general, the methodology has been the same across several different studies. The cognitive profile is determined by a battery of tests (the Cognitive Laterality Battery, CLB), chosen to assess two main cognitive factors: visuospatial functions, associated with the right cerebral hemisphere, and verbosequential functions, associated with the left cerebral hemisphere. The cognitive profiles are defined according to better performance on either the visuospatial skills or the verbosequential skills. This performance bias can be considered a measure of hemisphericity (Bogen & Bogen, 1983). The definition is a functional one, however, and not necessarily related to hemispheric activation. The tests on the CLB were chosen from converging data in patients with unilateral cerebral lesions or complete forebrain commissurotomy, and in normal subjects. These data provided evidence that certain functions (assessed by particular tests) were attributable to the left or the right cerebral hemisphere. For the tests adapted for the CLB, factor analyses in several normal populations confirmed that the tests chosen for the left hemisphere loaded on one factor, whereas the right-hemisphere tests loaded on the second factor.

The CLB (described in detail in Gordon, 1986) is presented by audiotapes and 35mm slides on a sound/sync slide projector driven by a cue track on the audiotape. In a typical test session, students sit in their classrooms at desks arranged for best viewing of the projection screen. Testing lasts about 80 minutes, usually the equivalent of two regular class periods. Standard measures of achievement usually given as part of regularly scheduled assessments by the schools were used to compare among subjects with different cognitive profiles. A brief description of the subtests of the CLB follows:

VISUOSPATIAL TESTS:

1. *Localization:* An *x* appears within a rectangle on a screen and must be marked exactly in a blank rectangle. The score is the linear error.
2. *Orientation:* Two identical and one mirror image two-dimensional patterns ("flags") (Thurstone & Jeffrey, 1966) are presented in different orientations. The subject's task is to select the two identical patterns. There is a more complex version for adults using an L-shaped construction of about 10 cubes (Shepard & Metzler, 1971).
3. *Touching blocks* (MacQuarrie, 1953): In a construction made up of 7 to 10 rectangular blocks, the number of blocks touching a designated block must be reported.
4. *Form completion:* Incomplete silhouette drawings (Thurstone & Jeffrey, 1966; French, Ekstrom, & Price, 1962) must be identified.

SEQUENTIAL AND VERBAL TESTS:

1. *Serial sounds:* Familiar sounds (e.g., bugle, baby, bird) are presented in sequences of 2 to 7 in length, which are to be written in the same order. Scoring favors long sequences and allows partial credit.
2. *Serial numbers:* Number sequences 4 to 9 in length are presented for recall; scoring is like that for serial sounds.
3. *Word production, letters:* The maximum number of words that begin with a given letter must be listed in 1 minute. The score is the sum of three 1-minute trials with different letters.
4. *Word production, categories:* The same as letters, except that words in a category must be listed. The score is the sum of two 1-minute trials with different categories.

SCORING AND ANALYSIS

All the subtests have been previously administered to a randomly selected sample of over 750 elementary and secondary school children drawn from a metropolitan population, and 250 adults drawn mostly, but not entirely, from a college population. Factor analyses have confirmed the separate visuospatial and verbosequential groupings in both the child and adult populations. Using the scores of the random sample as norms, the scores of subjects in an experimental sample may be converted to standard scores. Since there are significant sex differences in performance on some tests, separate norms for all tests are used for males and females. An average visuospatial score is obtained by averaging the appropriate tests in this category; a verbosequential score is similarly obtained. Finally, a "cognitive profile" is defined as the difference between the visuospatial score and the verbosequential score, where a positive score for the cognitive profile reflects better performance on visuospatial tests and a negative score reflects better performance on verbosequential tests. Overall performance was assessed by the averaged performance on all tests.

The Cognitive Profile and School Achievement

The Cognitive Laterality Battery was administered to a number of different school populations in a continuing effort to see if cognitive profile measures are predictive of achievement scores beyond the prediction expected from general ability levels. Small studies on a rural and several international populations were undertaken to corroborate results in a small-scale metropolitan study (Gordon, 1983). Finally, a large-scale metropolitan study is described and related to the smaller studies.

NONMETROPOLITAN POPULATION

The study on nonmetropolitan children was performed on 111 4th, 5th, and 6th graders (51 males, 60 females), who constituted nearly all students in those grades at a rural district public school (McGranaghan, 1983). The children came from a fairly uniform background of miners' or steelworkers' families. In addition to the CLB, the Symbol–Digit Modalities Test (Smith, 1973) was given because it has been shown to load on both the verbosequential and visuospatial factors, making it a good measure of overall performance. Subjects were divided into two groups according to performance on the CLB. Those performing better on the visuospatial factor were compared with those performing better on the verbosequential factor on the Stanford Achievement Tests given each year at the school. The achievement tests include reading subtests; math subtests; and subtests of spelling, language, social studies, science, and listening comprehension.

The results demonstrated that subjects whose profile favored visuospatial skills performed significantly worse than those with the verbosequential profile on reading subtests (except vocabulary) and on the spelling and language subtests. But they did not differ on any of the math, science, or social studies tests. This was true only for the higher performing subjects, however; there was no difference between the lower performing profile groups for any of the tests. The fact that the cognitive profile specifically differentiated between groups for reading and language performance, and not for all achievement tests, suggests that the result is not trivial. That is, subjects with verbosequential profiles were not smarter, better test-takers, or better students than the visuospatial subjects. It also could not be said that preference for verbosequential skills significantly boosted scores for "traditionally verbal" material such as vocabulary or social studies. Finally, there was no difference between profile groups for performance on the Symbol–Digit Modalities Test, supporting the contention that the groups did not differ on overall ability. These results suggest that the cognitive profile was an important element for predicting achievement performance for this limited population. The next question was whether these findings can be extended to international populations.

INTERNATIONAL POPULATIONS

The first study was in a large Korean population (Koh, 1982; Koh & Gordon, 1983). The subjects were 729 students, aged 11 to 14, tested in classroom-size groups in four schools. The schools were one boys' and one girls' school in an urban and a rural district. The instructions for the Cognitive Laterality Battery were translated into Korean, and adjustments were made in the tests where necessary. Other than the language difference, administration and scoring were the same as for the English version of the test. Performance on the tests by the Korean students was, in general, better than that of U.S. students of comparable age. Two exceptions were verbal fluency (Word Production, Letters) and the closure test (Form Completion). The fluency tasks were performed at about the normative level; the closure test was performed significantly worse. However, the tests factored about the same as in the normative group, supporting their two-factor structure. The cognitive profiles were calculated according to the sample (Korean) norm. Achievement is traditionally assessed in these students by written examinations given at the end of the school year. These exams are given by the schools and are the only grades Korean students receive in their academic courses: language, math, English (foreign language), science, music, and art.

When the groups were split according to their cognitive profile—better performance on either the visuospatial or the verbosequential tests—those with the visuospatial profile performed significantly worse on all tests ($p < .05$). Actually, the difference between the groups for the (Korean) language test was the greatest ($t = 3.35$, $p < .001$). These results are supported by significant correlations between the cognitive *profile* (the difference score) and performance on each test (Table 9-1). The correlations were in the direction where a profile favoring visuospatial skills tended to predict worse achievement scores. It might seem counterintuitive for the scores on art and music to correlate in the same way as those on language and math, but these tests are knowledge-type, requiring a multiple choice response mode. It was true, however, that the correlations with these tests were the lowest. The correlations between the achievement test scores and the average visuospatial and verbosequential scores were also high (Table 9-1). As might be expected from the relationships with the cognitive profile, the achievement test scores were more highly correlated with scores on the verbosequential tests than with those on the visuospatial tests.

There was an indication that subjects who performed better overall on the CLB were more likely to have the verbosequential profile. Accordingly, the measure of overall performance, the Cognitive Performance Quotient (CPQ), was used as a covariate in comparing the two profile groups on the achievement tests. The results were the same for all the achievement tests except those on art and music, implying that the cognitive profile itself was an important dimension in addition to intellectual abilities alone. The Symbol–Digit Modalities Test was also given as an independent assessment of performance level. Using this score as a covariate, the differences between the profile groups were reduced; only the group difference for the language test remained significant. Finally, when the groups were divided according to above- or below-average performance on the CLB, significant group differences were most consistent for the above-average performers. This means that the cognitive profile was a less important variable for the lower performing subjects, a result found also in the rural U.S. group (McGranaghan, 1983).

A second group of international subjects was made up of 240 English-speaking high school students, ages 16 to 20, in Nigeria (Gwany, 1985). Since students must pass exams to matriculate in the Nigerian academic secondary schools, the subjects were among the better performers available in the population. Three government schools were chosen to participate in the study. Because assignment to these schools is somewhat arbitrary, they included students from all the major ethnic groups in Nigeria. Reflective of cultural factors, there were more males (137) in the sample than females (87). Achievement is traditionally measured by a nationwide standard examination, the results of which are used for college placement. The disciplines tested included languages (English plus others); general courses

Table 9-1. Correlations between School Achievement and Cognitive Profile for Korean Students

Subject area	Cognitive profile	Verbo-sequential	Visuo-spatial
Language	−0.31	0.49	0.25
Math	−0.21	0.38	0.25
English	−0.35	0.53	0.27
Science	−0.30	0.50	0.30
Music	−0.21	0.21	−0.04 (NS)
Art	−0.25	0.38	0.21

Pearson correlations; all significant at $p<.01$ except as indicated (from Koh, 1982).

(literature, religion, history, etc.); mathematics; science; arts and crafts; technical (e.g., applied electricity, auto mechanics); and commercial and secretarial courses. Tests are in the form of essay questions, multiple choice, and (for some subjects) laboratory skills. The CLB was given in the original (English) version, except that a sound/sync projector was not available. Therefore, instructions were presented on an audio cassette recorder while the slides were presented on a manual projector.

The cognitive profile was much less closely related to performance on the academic tests in this population than it had been in the Korean sample. There were the usual significant correlations with overall achievement and with English, mathematics, and language. But there were no relationships with the sciences (geography, physics, chemistry, biology), the arts, or social science and economics. As in the previous studies, the greater the visuospatial cognitive profile, the worse the academic test score. When the averaged visuospatial and verbosequential scores were compared separately, however, it was clear that the relationship was mostly driven in these subjects by strong correlations with the verbosequential score. The visuospatial score was also correlated with achievement in these subjects, but less so.

In general, visuospatial skills seemed to play minor roles in academic achievement in Nigerian secondary school students. For one thing, the students of this study did extremely poorly on the visuospatial tests (relative to the U.S. metropolitan, normative population). The reasons for this are not immediately obvious because there are no studies on this population. Performance on verbosequential tests was at the norm. It may be speculated that visuospatial skills are not favored for academic achievement in Nigerian society, as evidenced by the higher relationship with verbosequential skills.

METROPOLITAN POPULATION

The final study was a major effort in a large U.S. metropolitan public school district. The families of all children ($n>6{,}000$) in the 4th and 5th grades were contacted by mail requesting volunteers for a study entitled "Risk Factors in Learning Disabilities." Signed permission forms were received from 20% of those contacted, representing students from each of 57 elementary schools in the district. A testing schedule was arranged with each school during the winter months such that the subjects could be group-tested in classrooms in their own school. All subjects in attendance on the scheduled day of testing were given the CLB; there were no make-up days for absentees. A total of 1,042 children, 567 males and 475 females, completed the testing session.

All elementary and middle school students in the district are given the California

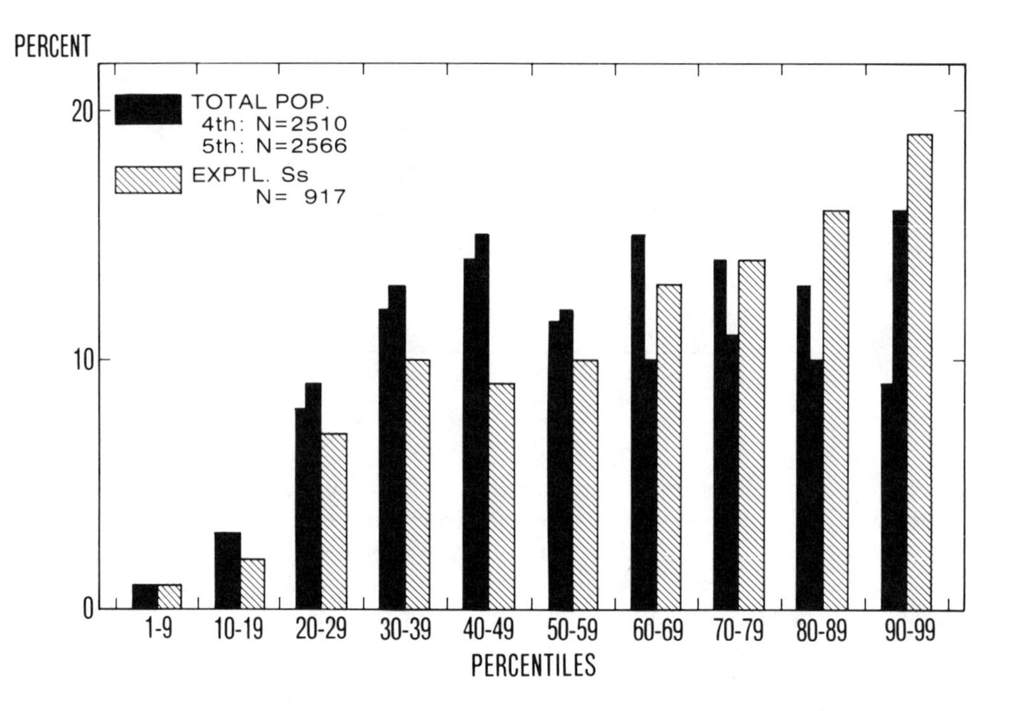

Figure 9-2. Distribution of California Achievement Scores for the total metropolitan population from which the sample was drawn (closed bars) and for the sample reported in the text (open bars).

Achievement Test (CAT) during April of the school year, 1 to 4 months after testing with the CLB. The CATs measure achievement in the academic areas of reading, language, and mathematics. Scores were collected for each of the subjects of the sample when they became available. Relative to national norms, the performance on the CAT by the entire school district was skewed to the higher percentiles. The distribution of scores by the subjects of this study was skewed even more (Figure 9-2). By contrast, the distribution of the overall performance (the Cognitive Performance Quotient or CPQ) as well as the cognitive profile (the difference between visuospatial and verbosequential scores, Cognitive Laterality Quotient, CLQ) was normal (Figures 9-3 and 9-4).

The relationship between the cognitive profile and achievement scores is, again, consistent with those of previous studies. There is a small but significantly negative correlation ($p<.001$; $df=929$) between the cognitive profile (visuospatial − verbosequential scores) and reading ($r=.19$; $t=5.89$) or language ($r=.13$; $t=3.99$) but not with math ($r=.07$; $t=2.14$) achievement. This suggests that a cognitive profile favoring visuospatial skills is associated with *lower* achievement in reading and language. The correlations in this sample were still significant when the Symbol–Digit Modalities Test was used as a covariate to control for overall performance level. Also, by accepting the alternative hypothesis that there is a correlation, the statistical power for the reading test is greater than 99% (for an α of .01) against making the Type II error.

The failure to find differences between the profile groups for arithmetic achievement in this group is consistent with the findings for the 111 rural children and for the Korean group. This finding, together with the saliency of the cognitive profile for its prediction of reading and language achievement in all the populations, cross-validates the initial report. Although skepticism, or at least wariness, would have been justified after the initial findings on the smaller group, replication of the general pattern of results in other diverse

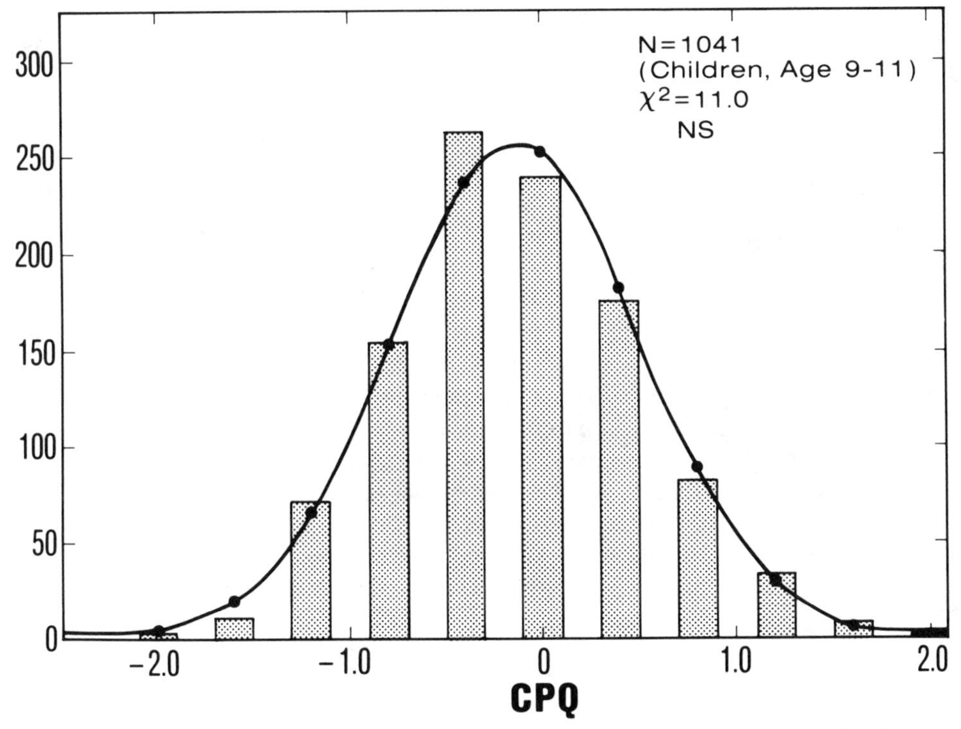

Figure 9-3. Distribution of overall performance on the Cognitive Laterality Battery for the experimental sample as calculated from a normative sample previously drawn from this same metropolitan population.

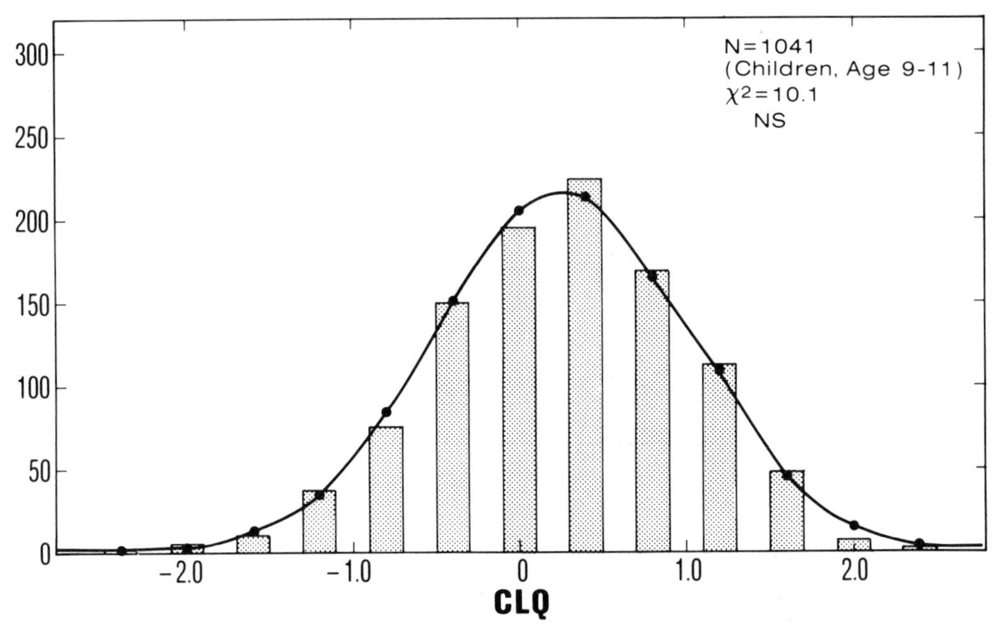

Figure 9-4. Distribution of the cognitive profile (the difference between the average visuospatial scores and the average verbosequential score) as calculated from a previously selected normative sample.

populations totaling nearly 2,000 subjects strengthens the conviction that the cognitive profile plays a role in academic achievement. Even with the variation in different types of achievement testing, the cognitive profile, as defined by the difference in performance on the visuospatial and verbosequential tests of the CLB, continues to be related to performance in reading and language. Simply stated, the effect size is small but robust.

Cognitive Profile and the Distribution of Achievement Scores

In addition to the overall difference in performance levels, the profile groups may differ in their distributions of achievement scores. In order to observe this, the number of subjects within each decile of the reading, language, and arithmetic achievement tests was plotted separately for the verbosequential and visuospatial profile groups (Figures 9-5, 9-6, and 9-7). For the reading and language achievement tests, the curves differed significantly, reflecting a greater number of subjects with the visuospatial profile in the lower decile categories and fewer of them in the higher categories (χ^2(Read) = 25.82, $p < .005$; χ^2(Lang) = 24.54, $p < .005$). These distributions reflect the same finding of inferior performance by the visuospatial group and negative correlation demonstrated between the reading and language achievement scores and the visuospatial cognitive profile. Also consistent with the previous result, the distribution of visuospatial and verbosequential profile groups

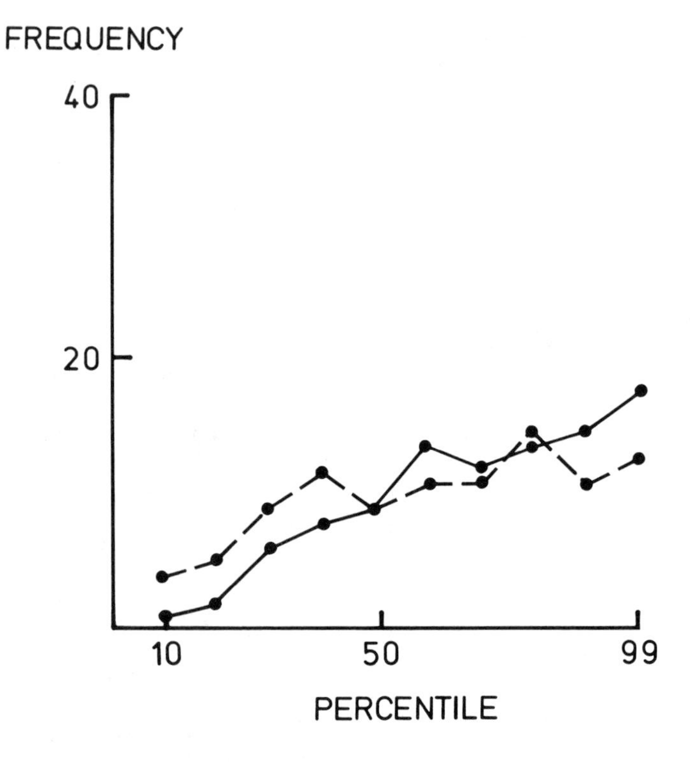

Figure 9-5. Distribution of Reading Achievement scores for subjects having a cognitive profile favoring visuospatial skills (dashed line) and subjects having a cognitive profile favoring verbosequential skills (solid line).

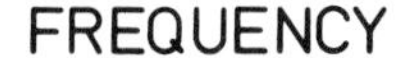

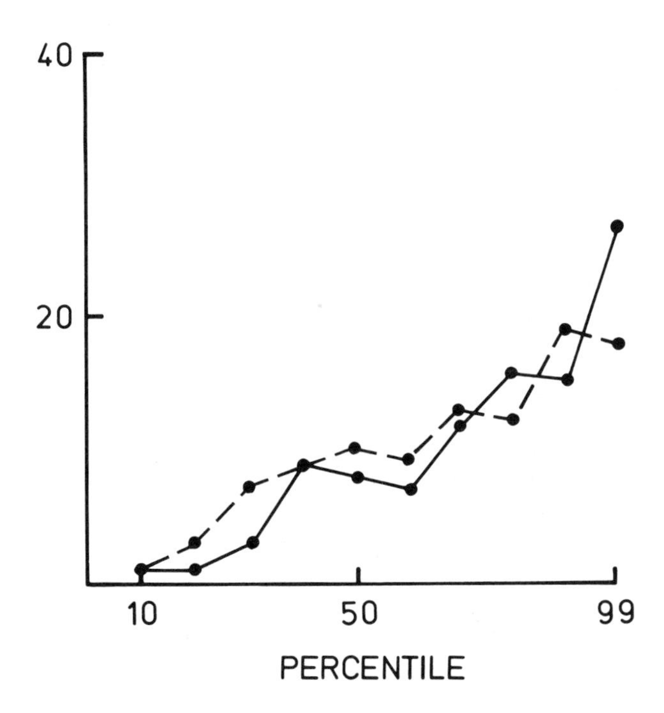

Figure 9-6. Distribution of Language Achievement scores for subjects having a cognitive profile favoring visuospatial skills (dashed line) and subjects having a cognitive profile favoring verbosequential skills (solid line).

did not differ for mathematics achievement (χ^2(Math) = 12.39, $p > .1$). This finding reinforces the notion that the cognitive profile affects specific skills, in this case reading and some language skills, but not mathematics.

Because of the skewed distributions toward the upper levels on the CAT, the two profile groups were again divided into two additional groups according to the average performances on the entire CLB. Since the cognitive tests had been standardized on a sample drawn from the same population as the present experimental group, the CLB distributions of total performance by experimental sample were centered around zero (Figure 9-3) and not much different from the normative group. Accordingly, the cutoff between the low- and high-performing groups was at the normative mean (CPQ = 0).

Only a few cognitively high-performing subjects had achievement percentile scores below the 50th percentile; most were above the 70th percentile. (Figures 9-8, 9-9, and 9-10) Continuing the previous trend, more subjects with the visuospatial profile performed at the lower percentiles, and more verbosequential subjects performed at the upper percentiles. The distributions for the language test differed significantly ($\chi^2 = 18.15$, $p < .05$).

In contrast to the higher performing subjects, the distributions were unusual for the achievement scores of the subjects who had performed below average on the CLB. For one thing, more than half of the subjects had percentile scores *above* the 50th percentile of achievement. Nevertheless, group differences were the same: Subjects with the visuospatial

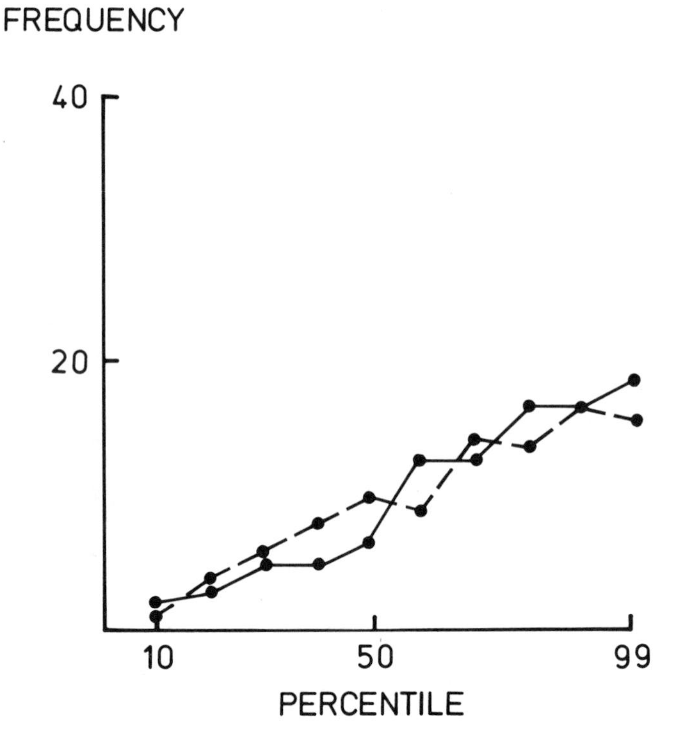

Figure 9-7. Distribution of Mathematics Achievement scores for subjects having a cognitive profile favoring visuospatial skills (dashed line) and subjects having a cognitive profile favoring verbosequential skills (solid line)

profile tended to have scores in the lower deciles. However, only the differences between the distributions for the Reading Achievement Test approached significance ($\chi^2 = 16.03$, $p < .07$) (Figure 9-8, bottom).

The second curious observation is the difference between the *shapes* of the curves for the two groups of lower performing children. For each of the achievement tests, the curves differed significantly (Kolmogorov-Smirnov two-sample, $p < .001$) although the differences were particularly striking for the reading achievement tests (Figure 9-8, bottom). The differences were not significant between the two high-performing profile groups for any achievement test. Also, within each profile group, the distributions did not differ between any pair of achievement tests. This seems to suggest that subjects falling in a particular percentile group for one achievement test will fall in the same percentile group for the other achievement tests. Nevertheless, there is some qualitative difference in the distributions for the reading test, compared to the other tests, that should be noted.

Bimodal Distribution

For the Reading Achievement Test, children with visuospatial profiles appeared to have scores distributed bimodally, with peaks at the 40th and 80th percentiles. By contrast, children with the verbosequential profile appeared to have a more unimodal curve, with

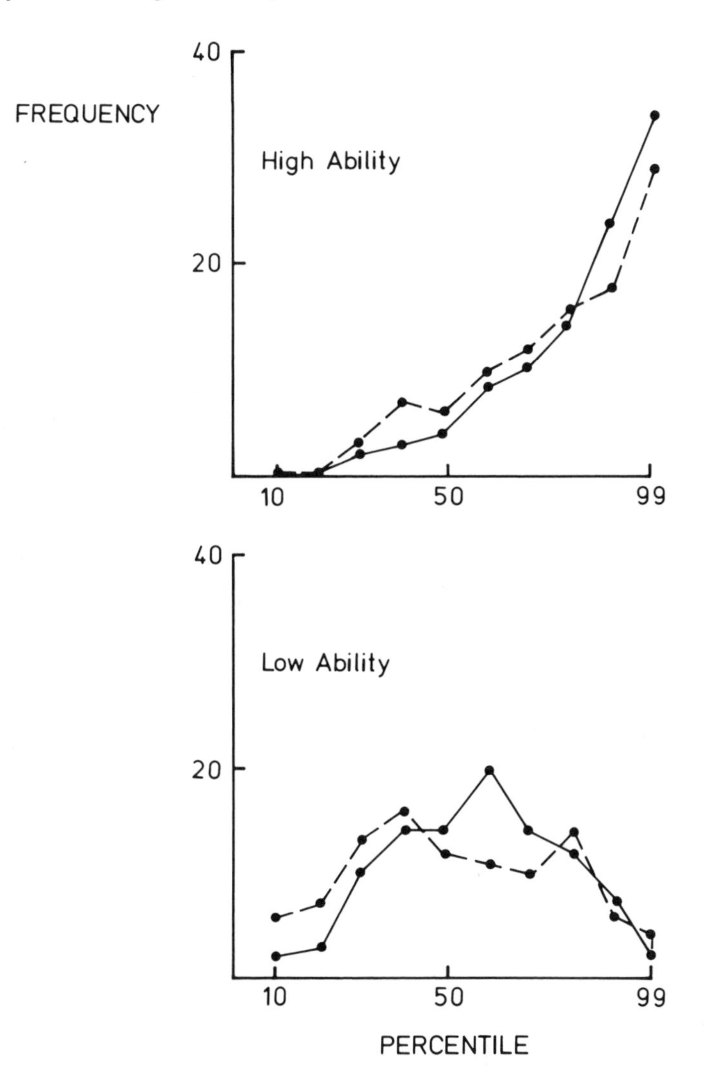

Figure 9-8. Distribution of Reading Achievement scores for subjects with above-average (high performers) and below-average (low performers) scores on the Cognitive Laterality Battery and with cognitive profiles favoring visuospatial (dashed line) or verbosequential (solid line) skills.

one peak at the 60th percentile, halfway between the two peaks in the visuospatial group. Consistent with the bimodal pattern for the lower performing visuospatial group, there was even a "blip" at the 40th percentile in the *high*-performing visuospatial subjects as well. On a qualitative level, the distributions of the other tests also appeared bimodal, but the curves were not as striking.

The language and mathematics distributions for the subjects with the visuospatial profile appear to be distorted versions of the bimodal curve observed for the reading test. The peak (i.e., the number of subjects) at the 40th percentile was reduced, and the upper percentile peak was increased. One interpretation is that fewer subjects are hurt by the visuospatial profile for language and mathematics achievement than for reading. For the verbosequential subjects, the change in the language and mathematics distributions is to broaden the peak at the 60th percentile. Qualitatively, this seems to result from a shift of

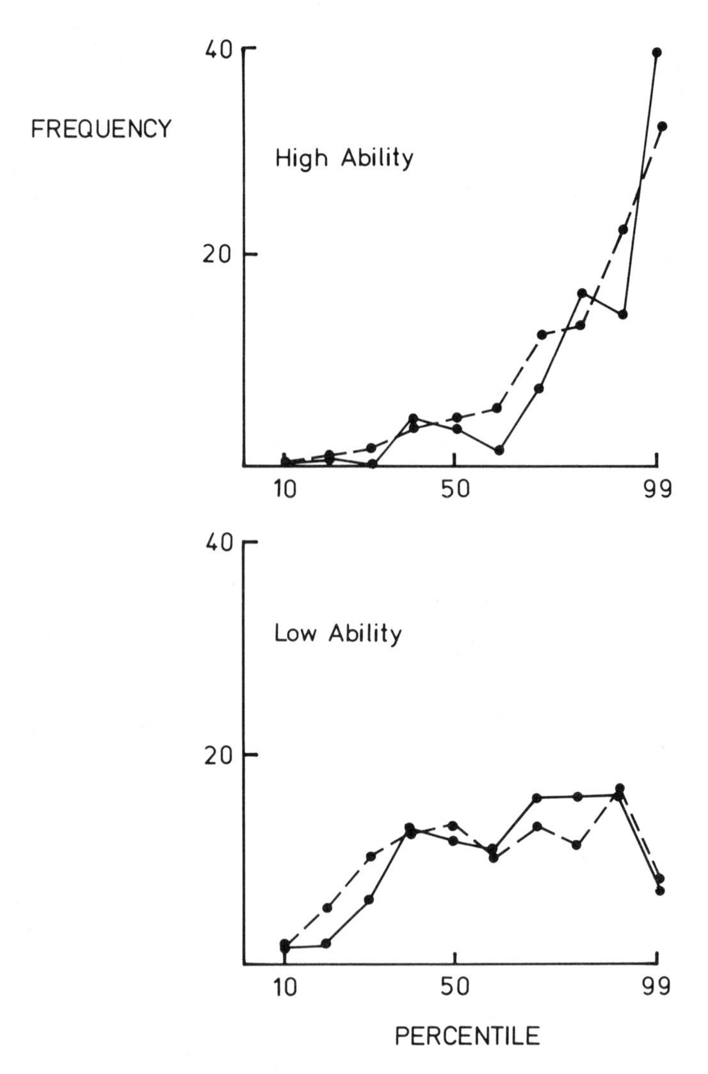

Figure 9-9. Distribution of Language Achievement scores for subjects with above-average (high performers) and below-average (low performers) scores on the Cognitive Laterality Battery and with cognitive profiles favoring visuospatial (dashed line) or verbosequential (solid line) skills.

some of the middle-percentile subjects to the upper percentiles. In addition, a group of lower percentile subjects appear to remain where they had been for the reading test, giving the appearance of a bimodal distribution for the verbosequential subjects in the language and mathematics tests.

CONCLUSION

The results on reading achievement for children in mainstream education, for diverse international populations as well as for a major metropolitan school district, reflect the conclusion often drawn for the reading disabled: Individuals having a visuospatial cognitive profile are at greater risk for lowered scores on reading and language achievement. The

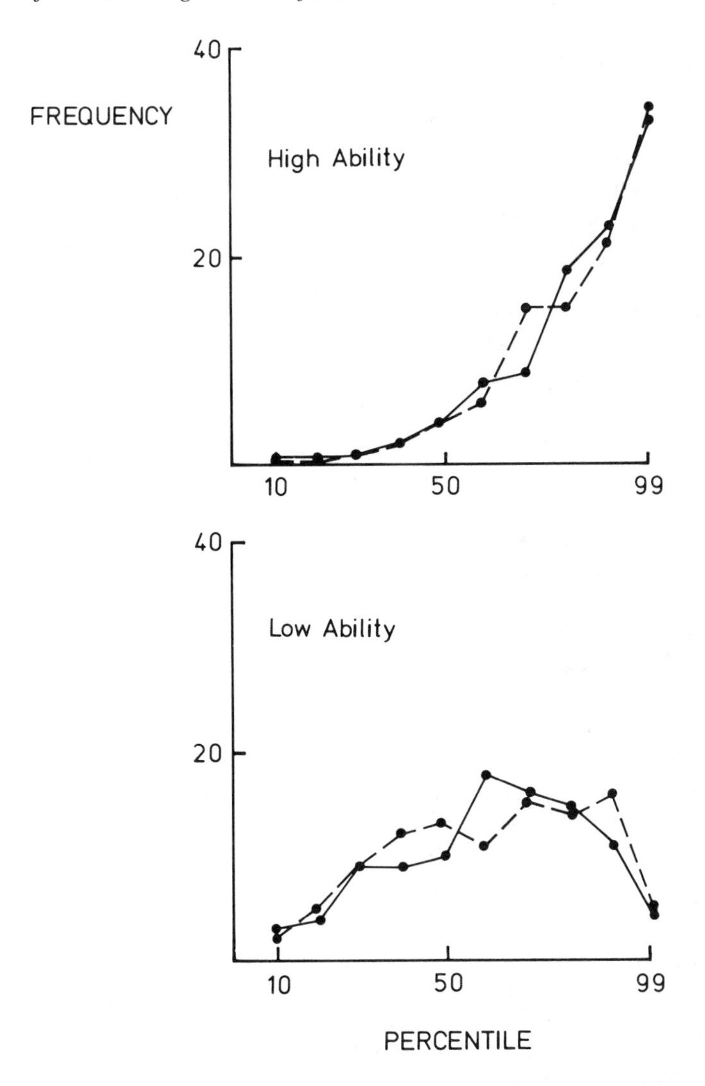

Figure 9-10. Distribution of Mathematics Achievement scores for subjects with above-average (high performers) and below-average (low performers) scores on the Cognitive Laterality Battery and with cognitive profiles favoring visuospatial (dashed line) or verbosequential (solid line) skills.

implication for performance in other disciplines, including mathematics, is more variable. When the differences in achievement performance between the cognitive groups are significant, however, the effect sizes (Cohen & Cohen, 1983) are small in terms of the amount of explained variance. The shapes of the curves for the better performing subjects were fairly uniform between the two cognitive profiles, but the subjects with the verbosequential scores dominated the highest percentile categories, whereas verbosequential subjects tended to be in the lower percentile categories. Group differences were found only for reading and language subjects, and not for mathematics. It was concluded, therefore, that the effect of the cognitive profile was specific to achievement requiring certain skills, but not to general overall ability. That is, one could not argue that children with a visuospatial profile were simply less capable.

Another reason for the small effect size is that the shapes of the curves for the lower performing subjects were not normally distributed. In fact, the differences between the two profile groups for any achievement was not significant in the lower performing group, as they had been for reading and language in the higher performing group. The odd, bimodal, or broadened shapes of the distributions both obscured performance differences and demonstrated that there are multiple factors contributing to achievement performance. If intellectual capacity alone accounted for the variance, the curves would have been Gaussian. Apparently, factors including the cognitive profile moderated performance, raising some scores and lowering others. These shape differences lend support to the idea that the cognitive profile is related to problem-solving schema that have differential effects on reading, language, mathematics, and other abilities.

Considerable research efforts have been devoted to subtyping learning-disabled children on the basis of performance on neuropsychological tests. Nevertheless, most of these children share a similar characteristic in that they perform well on visuospatial tests and poorly on verbosequential tests. Similarly, the evidence after testing children in the mainstream is that children with a cognitive profile favoring visuospatial skills are at greater risk for poor achievement performance in certain academic areas. The question is whether dyslexics may be "labeled" individuals who would have been in the lower peak in the reading distribution for the visuospatial subjects. Are the factors moderating intellectual ability similar in dyslexic and mainstream groups? Are factors that cause subtypes of performance among dyslexics similar to those that cause broadening of the distributions for mainstream students?

The data in this chapter are intended to focus on cognitive profiles in normal children, as defined by performance on specialized skills associated with the left or right cerebral hemisphere. Accordingly, a picture of individual differences of cognitive performance emerges that is based on brain function and may help explain performance patterns of more severely handicapped readers who are usually classified and studied separately from the mainstream.

ACKNOWLEDGMENTS

My gratitude to the Pittsburgh Public Schools for their cooperation in some of the studies reported here. Thanks also to Kathy McGranaghan, Young Hee Koh, and Danjuma Gwany for their hard work in data collection. Parts of this work were funded by a grant from the H. J. Heinz Foundation.

REFERENCES

Bentin, S., & Gordon, H. W. (1979). Assessment of cognitive asymmetries in brain damaged and normal subjects: validation of a test battery. *Journal of Neurology, Neurosurgery, and Psychiatry, 42*(8), 715–723.

Boder, E. (1973). Developmental dyslexias: A diagnostic approach based on three atypical reading–spelling patterns. *Developmental Medicine and Child Neurology, 15,* 663–687.

Bogen, J. E., & Bogen, G. M. (1983). Hemispheric specialization and cerebral quality. *Brain and Behavioral Sciences, 6,* 517–520.

Carmon, A., Nachshon, I., & Starinsky, R. (1976). Developmental aspects of visual hemifield differences in perception of verbal material. *Brain and Language, 3,* 463–469.

Cohen, J., & Cohen, P. (1983). *Applied multiple regression/correlation analysis for the behavioral sciences.* (2nd ed.). Hillsdale, NJ: Erlbaum.

Denckla, M. B. (1979). Childhood learning disabilities. In K. M. Heilman & E. Valenstein (Eds.), *Clinical neuropsychology* (pp. 535–573). New York: Oxford University Press.

Doehring, D. G., & Hoshko, I. M. (1977). Classification of reading problems by the *Q*-technique of factor analysis. *Cortex, 13,* 281–294.

Doehring, D. G., Trites, R. L., Patel, P. G., & Fiedorowicz, C. A. M. (1981). *Reading disabilities*. New York: Academic Press.

Drewnowski, A., & Healy, A. F. (1977). Detection errors on *the* and *and:* Evidence for reading units larger than the word. *Memory and Cognition, 5*(6), 636–647.

French, J. W., Ekstrom, R. B., & Price, L. A. (1962). *Kit of reference tests for cognitive factors*. Princeton, NJ: Educational Testing Service.

Gordon, H. W. (1980). Cognitive asymmetry in dyslexic families. *Neuropsychologia, 18,* 645–656.

Gordon, H. W. (1983). The assessment of cognitive functions for use in education. *Journal of Children in Contemporary Society, 16*(1–2), 207–218.

Gordon, H. W. (1984). Dyslexia. In Ralph E. Tarter (Ed.), *Advances in clinical neuropsychology* (Vol. 2, pp. 181–205). New York: Academic Press.

Gordon, H. W. (1986). The Cognitive Laterality Battery: Tests of specialized cognitive function. *International Journal of Neuroscience, 29*(3–4), 223–244.

Gordon, H. W., & Harness, B. Z. (1977). A test battery for diagnosis and treatment of developmental dyslexia. *DASH, Speech and Hearing Disabilities, 8,* 1–5.

Gwany, D. M. (1985). *Relationships between brain hemisphericity and academic achievement of Nigerian secondary school students*. Unpublished doctoral dissertation, School of Education, University of Pittsburgh.

Harness, B. Z., Epstein, R., & Gordon, H. W. (1984). Cognitive profile of children referred to a clinic for learning disabilities. *Journal of Learning Disabilities, 17*(6), 346–352.

Healy, A. F. (1981). The effects of visual similarity on proofreading for misspellings. *Memory and Cognition, 9*(5), 453–460.

Koh, Y. H. (1982). *An analysis of cognitive functioning of Korean middle school students*. Unpublished doctoral dissertation, School of Education, University of Pittsburgh.

Koh, Y. H., & Gordon, H. W. (1983). Hemispheric asymmetry in cognitive performance and school achievements. *The Journal of Korean Education, 10*(2), 97–107.

MacQuarrie, T. W. (1953). *Blocks*. MacQuarrie Test for Mechanical Ability. Monterey: California Test Bureau.

Mattis, S., French, J. H., & Rapin, I. (1975). Dyslexia in children and young adults: Three independent neuropsychological syndromes. *Developmental Medicine and Child Neurology, 17,* 150–163.

McGranaghan, K. M. (1983). *The relationship between cognitive profile and achievement test scores for elementary school students*. Unpublished master's thesis, School of Education, University of Pittsburgh.

Myklebust, H. R. (1978). Toward a science of dyslexiology. In H. R. Myklebust (Ed.), *Progress in learning disabilities* (pp. 1–39). New York: Grune and Stratton.

Perfetti, S. (1985). *Reading ability*. New York: Oxford University Press, Chapter 9.

Pirozzolo, F. J. (1979). *The neuropsychology of developmental reading disorders* (pp. 18–24). New York: Praeger.

Rumelhart, D. E. (1977). Toward an interactive model of reading. In S. Doronic (Ed.), *Attention and performance* (Vol. 6, pp. 119–126). Hillsdale, NJ: Erlbaum.

Shepard, R. M., & Metzler, J. (1971). Mental rotation of three-dimensional objects. *Science, 171,* 701–703.

Silverberg, R., Bentin, S., Gaziel, T., Obler, L. K., & Albert, M. L. (1979). Shift of visual field preference for English words in native Hebrew speakers. *Brain and Language, 8,* 184–190.

Silverberg, R., Gordon, H. W., Pollack, S., & Bentin, S. (1980). Shift of visual field preference for Hebrew words in native speakers learning to read. *Brain and Language, 11,* 99–105.

Smith, A. (1973). *Symbol–Digit Modalities Test*. Los Angeles: Western Psychological Services.

Stanovich, K. E. (1980). Toward an interactive–compensatory model of individual differences in the development of reading fluency. *Reading Research Quarterly, 16*(1), 32–71.

Thurstone, T. G., & Jeffrey, T. E. (1956). *Flags test*. Chicago: Industrial Relations Center.

Thurstone, L. L., & Jeffrey, T. E. (1966). *Closure speed*. Chicago: Industrial Relations Center.

PART THREE

Handedness and Intellectual Development

Left-handedness has enjoyed a special status in Western society for centuries, although "enjoyed" may be the wrong term to use. The history of discrimination against left-handers and negative attitudes toward left-handedness is well documented (Harris, 1983). Some of the ill will generated toward left-handers no doubt arose because of traditional distrust of nonconformity. Unfortunately, a commitment to educational pursuits certainly did not insulate scholars from taking up the prejudices of society at large, and even attempting to justify them.

But the presumption of recent decades that where there is so much smoke there must be no fire has been perhaps a hasty one. The historical relationship between handedness and developmental disability is certainly complex, as described in Chapter 12 by Harris and Carlson in this section. There has been a great deal of suggestion, interest, and theory, but we are still searching for the final resolution.

A prime issue is the definition of handedness. One view, offered by Satz, Soper, and Orsini in Chapter 10, suggests that three subtypes of non-right-handers should be distinguished. Each subtype, they argue, could well be associated with different cerebral mechanisms and organization. At some point, however, scientists need to go beyond the statistical level of association between handedness and the developmental symptoms. But what about the mechanisms that underlie hand preferences? Perhaps the right hemisphere is too dominant, causing left-hemispheric skills to be undeveloped; perhaps left-handedness correlates with atypical (and less efficient) brain organization; perhaps societal right-handedness confuses some left-handed children; and so on. One of the older treatises that earlier attempted an exhaustive review of the literature at that time (Wile, 1934, p. 76) sides with a social mechanism for the data, concluding that

> probably the groups arrested, convicted and in prisons comprise a large percentage of the poorly adjusted, and they certainly contain a larger percentage of the unadjusted, unstable, defectives and the like, by whom left-handedness is less readily rejected for social acceptance. The low positive correlation between left-handedness and social inadequacy only suggests concomitance. Concomitance is not causality; but for specific groups of people, their left-handedness becomes a dysgenic force that conduces to maladaptation in social living. The fact that the causal relationship does not exist is revealed by the large proportion of sinistrals who are highly intelligent, non-neurotic and wholly adapted to life in terms of a continued sinistrality or a socially acceptable ambidexterity.

Whatever one's view, it is clear that this issue of handedness and its relationship to cerebral organization is far from resolved.

REFERENCES

Harris, L. (1983). Laterality of function in the infant: Historical and contemporary trends in theory and research. In G. Young, S. J. Segalowitz, C. M. Corter, & S. E. Trehub (Eds.), Manual specialization and the developing brain (pp. 177–247). New York: Academic Press.

Wile, I. S. (1934). *Handedness, right and left.* Boston: Lothrop, Lee and Shepard.

10

Sinistrality, Brain Organization, and Cognitive Deficits

MARCEL KINSBOURNE
Eunice Kennedy Shriver Center, Waltham, Massachusetts, and Harvard Medical School, Boston, Massachusetts

NON-RIGHT-HANDEDNESS AS DEVIANCY

The mental skills of left-handers have been skeptically appraised for centuries, with an intensity of interest and persistence of effort that, on the face of it, seem surprising. The high level of interest in the issue is probably not completely explained by the factual evidence that certain disorders of mental development are more common in non-right-handers, as it is equally obvious that most non-right-handers develop mental skills in the normal manner. That it reflects the usual prejudice against an ever-present minority is also not a satisfying explanation, as there are many other physical variables that distinguish some people from most people (somatotype, skin and hair color, etc.) but have not attracted comparable interest. Rather, it would appear that when humans conceptualize the reasons that they outdo other animals in the subtlety and flexibility of behavioral control, they include right-handedness in that package.

The basic organization of the vertebrate, and certainly of the mammalian, central nervous system does not substantially depart from that of the human being. Certain animals outdo humans in sheer bulk of brain, and qualitatively there is no structure found in the human brain that is not to some extent represented in other animals. Recent concepts of what is presumably unique about the human brain have therefore invoked its organization. It has appeared plausible to suppose that what distinguishes humans' behavioral control from that of nonhumans is the functional asymmetry of brain organization: the lateralization of language and other sequential processes in one hemisphere, usually the left, and of certain spatial simultaneous skills in the other. This stereotype of what permits optimal mental functioning has often also been applied within the human species to distinguish between those who are thought of as fully human (adults) and those who are presumed not yet to be quite so (infants and young children). Even gender-related differences have been postulated, with the male allegedly more asymmetrically differentiated than the female (e.g., McGlone, 1980). In each of these contrasts it has been taken for granted that the more lateralized pattern of organization is functionally the more competent.

Non-right-handedness plays poorly in such a scenario. It is well known that non-right-handers are not simply mirror-image replicas of the dextral norm. To a varying extent they are less asymmetrical in bodily configuration and brain shape (Hicks & Kinsbourne, 1976a) and organization, as well as in how they distribute unimanual tasks between their hands. If peripheral and central asymmetry is a cardinal feature of the human condition, then non-right-handers should fall short in important ways. Investigators have searched for these important ways for many years.

Whereas stereotypes at best grossly exaggerate a factual situation and are often rationalized on the basis of preposterous theories, they customarily owe their existence to a kernel of truth. Non-right-handers are indeed overrepresented among the developmentally disabled: those with speech, language, and learning impairments as well as autism and frank mental retardation. Were left-handedness confined to such groups, it might be easy to explain that relationship. The puzzle, to which theorists are perpetually attracted, is that other non-right-handers, indeed most of them, appear to function as well as dextrals (Zangwill, 1969). An explanation is needed to clarify why left-handedness is associated with severe developmental deficits in so many cases and yet with no demonstrable deficit in still many more.

An obvious tactic in confronting these facts is to distinguish between two types of left-handedness: the biological, which is developmentally benign and fails to distinguish its owners from anyone else, and the pathological, which is a component of syndromes of developmental deficits. The former would reflect the "sinistral genotype," whereas the latter would be a phenocopy. From this vantage point theorists can then attempt to explain what mediates the relationship between being sinistral and being developmentally delayed.

An alternative proposition is that sinistrality in itself is not usually a component of a syndrome of neuropathology but, rather, is associated statistically with an otherwise unrelated pathogenic factor, by a relationship that could operate at a level of organization as remote from behavior as the chromosome.

It is the purpose of this discussion to organize findings with respect to mental skills of left-handers in order to evaluate the relative merits of these two radically different overarching approaches, and of suggested mediators between sinistrality and cognitive disability.

PATHOLOGICAL LEFT-HANDEDNESS

The concept of pathological left-handedness (Gordon, 1921; Satz, 1972) relies on the generally accepted view that right-handedness is a genetically determined trait. The pathological left-hander is assumed to be genotypically dextral but nevertheless to manifest a sinistral phenotype because of a hypothesized early lesion involving the left hemisphere. This lesion probably would have to implicate the left motor strip, as work with patients with early brain damage (Rasmussen & Milner, 1977) has shown that right-hand preference (and left language lateralization) is quite resistant to contralateral displacement unless significant early damage directly implicates the locus of manual control (or classical language areas). Olmstead and Villablanca (1979) have elicited analogous findings for peripheral laterality in an animal model.

Direct evidence of the hypothesized early left-sided brain damage is almost always lacking except in cases of explicit right-sided hemiplegic cerebral palsy, in which preference for the left hand is obviously dictated by overt impairment of right-sided motor control. Investigators have therefore searched for telltale associates of such damage. Bakan, Dibb, and Reid (1973) reported a higher incidence of signs of "birth stress" retrospectively attributed to themselves by those college students who were non-right-handed, and interpreted this finding to indicate that non-right-handedness in general is pathological. Attempts to confirm the relationship between sinistrality and birth stress have met with mixed results, but in any case such an association need neither be causal nor characterize all non-right-handers. It is compatible with the notion of pathological left-handedness as a sinistral subtype. It is also compatible with the view that familial sinistrality is a risk factor for a relatively high incidence of early brain damage in the family. The former and the latter account might even both be true. Perhaps sinistrals have a genetic vulnerability to factors causing birth trauma, and birth trauma might in turn set up more (pathological) sinistrality. Those sinistrals who are to be found in the general population evidently were not severely affected. Damaged populations would include those individuals in whom this risk factor had a more significant effect.

Bishop (1984) has focused attention on the relative agility of right and left index fingers, as reflected in their rate of speeded finger tapping. She postulated that pathological left-handers should have relatively depressed finger tapping rates in the nonpreferred hand (that is, in the hand from which they presumably switched on account of the alleged motor impairment). Based on data from a large-scale study, she estimated a prevalence of pathological left-handedness of about 1 percent in the general population. Gillberg, Waldenstrom, and Rasmussen (1984) have also identified clumsiness of the nonpreferred hand as particularly common in left-handers, and often associated with neurological dysfunction.

Silva and Satz (1979) have placed the pathological left-handedness syndrome on an objective basis in a special population. They studied patients with focal epilepsy, subgrouped in terms of side of dominant epileptic focus and early or late onset of the brain damage that caused the seizures. They found the subgroup with left-sided lesions of early onset to have by far the greatest incidence of non-right-handedness. Progressing from this demonstration, Satz and his colleagues have attempted to identify a syndrome of pathological left-handedness based on somatic asymmetry. In particular, they are looking for slightly smaller right than left palms of hands and soles of feet in these individuals (Satz, Orsini, Saslow, & Henry, 1985).

Pending validation of direct identifiers of pathologically left-handed individuals on lines such as these, studies must rely on inferences based on statistical analysis. For instance, if a particular neuropathological population incorporates a significantly higher proportion of non-right-handers than is found in their parents, the excess of non-right-handers in the sample under study could be made up by pathological non-right-handers. In such a case the correlation of hand preference between proband and parents, which is usually weakly significant (e.g., Hicks & Kinsbourne, 1976b), should be effectively zero.

Sinistrality has repeatedly been found to be disproportionately prevalent among the mentally retarded (e.g., Batheja & McManus, 1985); and Hicks and Barton (1975) and Bradshaw-McAnulty, Hicks, and Kinsbourne (1984) have shown that it is more prevalent among the severely than the more moderately affected. Does this reflect a cause of brain damage that disproportionately affects sinistrals, or is the sinistrality itself an effect of the insult that caused the mental retardation? If the personal sinistrality of the mentally retarded probands reflects familial sinistrality, then there should be a significant correlation between the hand preference of the proband and that of his or her parents. If familial sinistrality (as well as personal sinistrality) is a risk factor for brain damage, then parents of mentally retarded children should be more than usually sinistral. In addition, the more severe the proband's retardation, the greater should be the probability of non-right-handedness among the parents. This should apply to both dextral and sinistral mental retardates, if the brain damage causes pathological sinistrality some of the time. If the sinistrality is pathological, the sinistrality phenotype, not reflecting the familial genetic endowment, should not correlate significantly with mid-parent hand preference.

When they compared the hand preference of mentally retarded children to that of their parents, Bradshaw-McAnulty *et al.* (1984) found a negligible correlation. This is consistent with an interpretation in terms of pathological left-handedness. However, such an outcome can also be interpreted in another way. If personal and familial sinistrality additively indicate vulnerability to the effects of brain damage, then early adverse influences might take a greater toll on those who are personally sinistral than on those who are personally dextral, holding the degree of familial sinistrality constant. The more severely damaged subpopulation within a disease category would then be more likely to include a higher concentration of non-right-handers. Bradshaw-McAnulty *et al.* (1984) in fact found that the prevalence of non-right-handedness increased with increase in the severity of the mental deficiency.

In summary, several lines of circumstantial evidence suggest that pathological left-handedness contributes to the prevalence of left-handedness in the population. However, alternative explanations of each of these findings have not yet been ruled out.

EARLY LEFT-HEMISPHERE INSULT AND SINISTRALITY

As has been discussed, the explanatory value for developmental disabilities of the pathological left-handedness concept relies on the plausibility of the notion that the same antecedent cause could have determined both the sinistral phenotype and the developmental disability in question. Early brain damage of unspecified nature is usually incriminated, with the implicit assumption that the left hemisphere bears the brunt of such damage. A recent variant of this line of reasoning implicates not an externally imposed but an endogenous cause for this presumed left-hemisphere dysfunction.

Geschwind and Behan (1982) have suggested that testosterone generated by the fetus *in utero* depresses the rate of left-hemisphere maturation. A high level of testosterone gives the right hemisphere more opportunity to gain control of the preferred hand. Geschwind and Galaburda (1985) reiterate the suggestion that testosterone selectively inhibits prenatal development of the left hemisphere. They refer to autopsy data of Chi, Dooling, and Gilles (1977), indicating a slightly earlier forming of certain convolutions in the right than in the left hemisphere of the fetus. It follows that males, left-handers, and especially left-handed males, should exhibit a more pronounced lag of leftsided convolutional formation. Whether left-handedness has such an effect cannot be determined prenatally, as it is not possible to ascertain whether the fetus would have manifested sinistrality had it survived. But the prediction for gender finds a test in the data of Chi *et al.* and is disconfirmed. No sex difference was found in the right–left balance of emergence of convolutions.

Another prediction that follows from Geschwind's testosterone hypothesis is that the left-hander should be at risk for left-hemisphere syndromes only. This is perhaps more plausible with respect to allegedly left-hemisphere disorders such as developmental dysphasia, dyslexia, or stuttering than for mental retardation, in which dysfunction is bilateral, or autism, in which it can be variously distributed (Fein, Humes, Kaplan, Lucci, & Waterhouse, 1984). The left-hander should, if anything, exhibit enhanced right-hemisphere skills. Some studies have found dyslexics to be above the norm in visuospatial (right-hemisphere) skills (Gordon, 1980), but it is not clear whether this holds more for sinistral than for dextral dyslexics. Benbow (1985) has found an excess of sinistrality among children who are extremely gifted in either verbal or mathematical skills. The fact that verbal as well as mathematical precocity was associated with sinistrality makes overdevelopment of the right hemisphere an unattractive explanation for these outcomes. Of the large-scale psychometric studies of populations subdivided by hand preference, none has shown overall superiority in spatial skills in the sinistral subgroup.

The pathological left-handedness model does not make this strong prediction for selectivity of cognitive deficit. Even if a pathological left-hander's left hemisphere only is damaged, the right hemisphere might compensate for the language deficit. This might even "crowd out" spatial representation, as suggested by Levy (1969), resulting in an individual with adequate verbal but inferior spatial skills.

Geschwind and Behan's (1982) suggested testosterone antecedent links left-hand preference and language disorder not only in terms of their incidence but even in terms of their degree. It follows from this and any other pathological left-handedness theory (e.g., Bishop, 1983) that the more severe the left-hemisphere dysfunction, the greater should be the degree of left-hand preference. If the same agent that depresses left-hemisphere function impairs both its ability to control language and its ability to control the preferred hand, then it should be the extreme left-handers, rather than those who are more ambidextrous, whose language-related skills are most impaired. On the whole, studies do not support this prediction. For instance, among autists the ambidextrous subset is reported to show the more severe cognitive deficiency (Fein *et al.*, 1984). In dyslexia and learning disability it is more generally mixed-handers who are felt to be the more affected. In a general school-age population, Gutezeit (1982) found weakly and strongly left-handed children equally at a disadvantage in certain skills related to the acquisition of fluency in reading. In a recent study, Kinsbourne (1986) found the excess of non-right-handedness in a learning-disabled sample to be accounted for by mixed-handers rather than extreme sinistrals. This would be comprehensible if it took bilateral early brain damage to cause learning disability.

SINISTRALITY AND PSYCHOMETRIC FINDINGS IN THE GENERAL POPULATION

Unitary and subtype hypotheses of sinistrality differ in how they relate degree of personal sinistrality and amount of familial sinistrality to the emergence of intellectual functions. According to the unitary hypothesis of Bakan, sinistrality is one consequence of a factor inducing brain damage or maldevelopment. If this factor runs in families, one would expect to find more sinistrals (other individuals who are similarly brain damaged) in the families of sinistrals than in those of dextrals. Furthermore, the degree of familial sinistrality should index the severity of the adverse influence on left-brain development, and thus should correlate positively with the degree of cognitive impairment presumably caused by the same agent.

Thus, according to a unitary hypothesis, familial and sporadic left-handedness differ in degree only, whereas according to the subtype view, they differ in kind. According to the unitary view, the familial left-hander should exhibit the most explicit left-hand preference. According to subtypes, it will be the sporadic left-hander who is very left-handed (and exhibits decreased dexterity of the nonpreferred (right) hand, as claimed by Bishop (1984), or even exhibits measurable right-sided somatic underdeveloped quantifiable in terms of such dimensions as length of sole of foot or palm of hand—the pathological left-handedness syndrome of Satz *et al.* (1985). In the cognitive domain, the unitary hypothesis predicts that the familial left-hander will be at the greatest disadvantage, because his family has the maximum loading of the hypothesized adverse influence. According to pathological left-handedness, it is the sporadic left-hander who should be the most cognitively handicapped.

Whether the right-hander with familial sinistrality is more liable to have cognitive deficit than the dextral without familial sinistrality is differently predicted by the differing viewpoints: If the cognitive deficit is due to a familial factor that might find some, though less, expression in the dextral than in the sinistral family members, the familial right-hander will be more vulnerable. If the adverse factor is environmental and is limited in its impact to the proband, it will render him personally pathologically sinistral but leave those family members normal who are not thus affected. On such a view, the dextral relative of a cognitively deficient sinistral should have no more than the general population's probability of a developmental deficit.

In a psychometric study of undergraduates subgrouped by sex, hand preference, and presence or absence of familial sinistrality, Briggs, Nebes, and Kinsbourne (1976) found a minor diminution in Wechsler Adult Intelligence Scale (WAIS) IQ for the non-right-handed sample (less than 3 IQ points, distributed uniformly across the verbal and performance domains). Also, familial sinistral subjects were at a slight but significant disadvantage compared to subjects without sinistral family history, even when the subject himself was dextral. Not only were these differences minor, but on a variety of other mental tests no difference whatever was found, and none on Scholastic Aptitude Test (SAT) scores. Thus, if sinistrality incurs some cognitive penalty, this either is not enough to render the sinistral less competitive for higher education, or is amenable to compensation by additional studying. Otherwise one would also expect non-right-handers to be underrepresented in the college population, which appears not to be the case (Annett, 1970).

In the Briggs *et al.* study, the degree of non-right-handedness (whether ambidextrous or sinistral) did not significantly affect the degree of psychometric inferiority. This fits poorly with the Geschwind and Behan notion of an adverse influence with lateralized impact, which should render the person more left-handed in proportion to its intensity. On the basis of pathological left-handedness, one might also expect the most left-handed individuals to be the most cognitively affected; but, at least in this college sample, this was not so.

Sinistrality also seems to correlate with a greater vulnerability to certain diseases of the immune system, as Geschwind and Behan (1982) suggested and we (Kinsbourne, 1986) have confirmed. Again we find that this propensity is greatest in familial sinistrals, less so in sporadic ones, less again in familial dextrals, and least in dextrals without a family history of sinistrality (Kinsbourne, 1986).

The Time Frame of Cognitive Lag

The pathological mechanisms so far suggested would be expected to exert their influence early in cognitive development. The left-hemisphere underdevelopment hypothesized by Geschwind should show its effects as soon as left-hemisphere skills normally emerge. The heterogenous brain damage proposed by Bakan *et al.* (1973) would most probably show maximum effect early on and even manifest some catch-up or closing of the "cognitive gap" relative to the norm with increasing age, as this is the customary pattern in perinatal injury that is not particularly severe. The converse mechanism, by which cognitive development initially progresses relatively well, but later levels off at an unduly low plateau, has so far only been suggested for circumstances in which one hemisphere is compensating for major damage to the other (Kohn & Dennis, 1974). Yet, in the following study a hint of such a pattern was obtained for a small sample of non-right-handers who were generally cognitively intact and in the regular school system.

Swanson, Kinsbourne, and Horn (1980) presented mental test results on children who were tested longitudinally in fourth and seventh grade and subtyped by hand preference. The finding relevant to the present discussion was that whereas the dextrals maintained their IQ levels across successive testings, the non-right-handers (ambidextrous and sinistral) exhibited a drop in IQ. If this finding were validated with a much larger sample, it would suggest that sinistrality might be a marker for an earlier leveling off of mental growth.

Early Brain Damage and Compensation

The explanatory power of the notion of early left-hemisphere damage as a cause for developmental delay in the evolution of skills normally associated with that hemisphere may be less than would appear. The compensatory potential of the right hemisphere for early left-hemisphere cognitive deficit is known to be great. Even the total loss of a left hemisphere does not preclude the individual from developing language skills to within the normal range. That such a person is characterized by residual syntactic deficit is a real (Dennis, 1980), though not conclusively confirmed (Bishop, 1983), possibility. But it is questionable whether structural left-hemisphere damage so slight as to defy direct demonstration could profoundly impair the evolution of language and learning skills. For left-hemisphere impairment to have a major retarding effect on language development, it would have to be associated with a factor that precludes the right hemisphere (as well as intact areas of the left) from assuming their natural compensatory role. No such factor has been identified, or even suggested. This does not prove that it does not exist. It does, however, make it attractive to consider a different type of explanation. Such a one is afforded by the known departure from the dextral norm of cerebral organization in most left-handers.

Brain Organization in Sinistrals

In view of the evidence that sinistrals may have incurred some cognitive liability and the evidence for anomalous brain representation of cognitive functions in this group, it is now necessary to consider what is known about the localization of function in the brain of the non-right-hander. Sinistrals as a group have been known to differ from dextrals in brain organization almost since asymmetry of human cerebral function was first discovered. They have been thought either to have laterality relations the reverse of those of dextrals—that is, language right and spatial functions left lateralized (Broca, 1865)—or to have a more extensive cognitive cerebral territory, with substantial bilateralization of language and other functions that are lateralized in the dextral. The first of these ideas has been rarely supported (McManus, 1983). The second seems to be the rule for people who, before they acquired cerebral damage in adulthood, were apparently normal (Hecaen & Ajuriaguerra, 1964).

It has long been known that adult non-right-handers are apt to become aphasic after damage of either hemisphere, implying that they have deviant cerebral language representation (Goodglass & Quadfasel, 1954). The comprehensive data on the consequences of right- and left-brain injuries in right- and left-handers from Hecaen's case material in Paris (Bryden, Hecaen, & DeAgostini, 1983) makes it possible to derive reliable quantitative estimates of the prevalence of such deviant organization in non-right-handers. These authors, however, made an untenable assumption, which invalidates their data analysis and therefore their conclusions. They assumed that if a lesion of a hemisphere failed to cause a categorical cognitive deficit, that cognitive domain was not represented in the hemisphere in question. Such an assumption could be made only if the whole hemisphere were destroyed, a type of case not represented in the Hecaen patient material. My reanalysis of this data after discarding this assumption has indicated that some 70% of non-right-handers are bilateralized for language representation. Interestingly enough, most of the remaining 30% are left lateralized, just as are almost all right-handers. Very few appear to have the mirror image, right-lateralized type of organization. These conclusions are consonant with those of Gloning, Gloning, Haub, and Quatember (1969) and Carter, Hohenegger, and Satz

(1982). The finding conflicts only superficially with that of Rasmussen and Milner (1975), who find a substantial minority (15%) of right-language-lateralized left-handed patients as a result of their direct intracarotid amytal testing of hemispheric function.

The data of Rasmussen and Milner (1975) provide an interesting counterpoint to those derived from clinical samples of patients who acquired unilateral cortical disease during their adult years. Their population of left-handers who had suffered early brain damage exhibited left-hemisphere speech in 70% of cases (based on intracarotid amytal tests), right-hemisphere speech in 15%, and bilateral speech representation in only 15%. This suggests that only a relatively small minority of these individuals, those with bilateral speech representation, were genotypic sinistrals. The majority were presumably dextrals, all of whom had hand preference shifted to the left on account of left motor strip damage (i.e., they were pathological left-handers). A point of interest is that in most cases language dominance remained left-sided. Where it did shift, it shifted to the right; it did not become bilateral. This raises the possibility that bilateralized language representation differs qualitatively from unilateralized. In the unilateralized individual, damage of the language hemisphere either does or does not cause a shift in dominance, but does not result in a sharing of language control by two hemispheres. This inference is supported by the findings from hemispheric anesthesia by intracarotid amytal in right-handed adults who had become aphasic (Czopf, 1972; Kinsbourne, 1971). In most such cases, speech control remains unilateral, though more often shifted to the right hemisphere than remaining left-sided.

My interpretation of Hecaen's data suggests that double rightward shifting (of speech and hemisphere in control of the preferred hand) is very uncommon in the general population. Correspondingly, most laterality studies both of normally functioning left-handers and of individuals with developmental language and learning delays suggest that, if anomalous, their language representation is bilateralized rather than shifted to right-hemisphere control. This directs the focus of our interest to the question: Is there anything about bilateral language representation that either compromises the function of language areas or renders them more vulnerable to adverse influences of external origin?

Diffuse Brain Organization and Functional Insufficiency

An obvious way of relating anomalous language representation with the fact that left-handedness is a more than chance accompaniment of developmental deficits is through the more extensive language territory in the non-right-hander. My calculations based on Hecaen's data reveal that even within the left hemisphere, non-right-handers run a greater risk of sustaining aphasia, suggesting that within that hemisphere language representation involves a more extensive territory in the non-right-hander. Presumably a wider range of brain lesions would therefore encroach on language territory and impair its function, and this would be a simple explanation of the greater vulnerability of language.

As a corollary of this diffuse cerebral representation in non-right-handers, it appears that having sustained aphasia, they recover from it faster than right-handers do (Luria, 1966; Subirana, 1958). This consideration contradicts the explanation just given, as it would make for less rather than more language disorder in non-right-handers, at least in the long term. We therefore proceed to consider another way in which the sinistral pattern of cerebral representation of functions might be incriminated in developmental disabilities. This is based on the view that diffuse language representation inherently predisposes to relatively inefficient cerebral functioning.

Many take it for granted that lateralization is the optimal organization for language, and that "failure to lateralize" is pathological or at least indicates language immaturity. This viewpoint, inspired by the unsubstantiated assumption about central nervous system evolution mentioned in the introduction, was adopted by influential theorists such as Orton (1937) and Lenneberg (1967). Nevertheless, the evidence resoundingly rejects both contentions: that bilateral language representation can be considered immature and that it engenders inefficient language use. We have reviewed elsewhere (Kinsbourne & Hiscock, 1977, 1983) overwhelming evidence to the effect that bilateral representation does not represent the original state in the infant but, rather, that an individual's lateralization characteristics are early predetermined. Bilateral cerebral representation cannot be considered immature on ontogenetic grounds. As for it being inefficient, this lacks empirical support.

If overlapping specializations of cortex are detrimental, then left-handers should exhibit major psychometric deficits. In fact, such deficits as they have are either slight or nonexistent (Hardyck & Petrinovitch, 1977). This is evidence against the necessity of "hard-wiring" of cortex. It seems that wide cortical areas can be used for different purposes as long as this is done at different times. But the potential for cross-talk interference between simultaneously active cerebral loci might be amplified by overlapping cerebral representation. If so, the left-handers might do less well in certain dual-task situations (Kinsbourne, 1980). Dextral and sinistral groups that are matched in skill on a verbal and a spatial task when these are individually administered should yield dextral superiority when the tasks are done concurrently or when interference in the alternative mode is set up. These expectations have been confirmed by Berry, Hughes, and Jackson (1980) and partially by Nagae (1985). The mechanism of interference across cognitive domains could be neurological; incompatible concurrent patterns of activation causing interfering cross talk (Kinsbourne, 1980). Alternatively, interference could be due to inappropriate coding. Perhaps the diffuse representations foster dual coding by sinistral subjects, thereby rendering their processing subject to interference by a broad band of cognitive activity overlapping either mode (Nagae, 1985). The definitive study, which would determine whether when sinistrals do relatively poorly in a dual-task interfering situation they are indeed dual-coding, remains to be done.

Although the foregoing predictions are of theoretical interest, it is probable that very few situations in everyday life call for the kind of concurrent independent processing that in sinistrals is hypothesized to cause cross-talk interference. If this were the only situation in which sinistrals are at a disadvantage, one would conclude that even the dramatic difference in the representation of cerebral function between dextral and sinistral humans has little or no practical consequence for cognitive adaptive functioning. But there are suggestive indications of minor differences between hand preference groups in tests that do not call for dual-task performance. Studies by Briggs *et al.* (1976), Hicks and Beveridge (1978), and Bradshaw, Nettleton, and Taylor (1981) do show slightly inferior psychometric performance by a non-right-handed sample. These findings are perhaps consistent with Beaumont's (1974) suggestion that the more diffuse cerebral representation of many left-handers is less conducive to specificity and automatization in cognitive function. Presumably such differences could be overcome by more study and practice on the part of the weaker automatizers, so that the general finding that left-handers are as prevalent among college populations as in the general population is not necessarily contradictory. It might be instructive to compare right- and left-handers in how hard they find they have to study to achieve specific academic objectives. Left-handers might also diverge somewhat in their learning style, as implied by the suggestive findings of Cohen and Friedman crediting them with a more visual type of analysis in reading than is prevalent among right-handers. Beaumont's suggestion that the diffuse network is, in contrast, advantageous for integrative functions finds less support to date. Perhaps Benbow's (1985) finding of disproportionate numbers of left-handers among those with the very highest verbal and among those with the very highest mathematical SAT achievement is a case in point.

It still could be that whatever causes representation to be diffuse also at times imposes a penalty on efficient verbal thinking. There is much evidence that speech input occasions left-lateralized brain arousal even in preverbal infants (reviewed by Kinsbourne & Hiscock, 1983). This suggests that brain stem systems are specialized in advance (''prewired'') to activate the left hemisphere when language function is called for, and exhibit this tendency even before language competence has emerged. The non-right-hander may lack this brain stem asymmetry, and therefore be less able to maintain selective left-hemispheric orientation when this is called for by the demands of the task.

Ascending Activation and Handedness

The origin of hand preference has been traced back to the asymmetrical turning tendencies of the newborn (Gesell & Ames, 1947). Liederman and Kinsbourne (1980) observed spontaneous head turning of 1- and 2-day-old infants. They found the usual rightward turning bias (Gesell & Ames, 1950) in the offspring of dextral parents, but no such asymmetry in a group of 20 infants each of whom had one parent who was non-right-handed.

Turning tendencies of such early origin must be determined at brain stem level. As maturation proceeds, reaching, grasping (Goodwin & Michel, 1981), and perhaps pointing (Bates, O'Connell, Vaid, Sledge, & Oakes, 1986) are also each more frequently done with the right hand. The greater right-hand dexterity of most people must reflect an asymmetry at cerebral level. I have suggested (Kinsbourne, 1980) that hand preference (and cerebral asymmetry of function) are determined by asymmetrical ascending activation from brain stem to cortex. Absence of such asymmetry would lead to non-right-handedness, or at least a hand preference under the control of presumably environmental determinants (that would have been overridden by the biological ''right shift factor'' (Annett, 1970, 1973), had it been present). It might also lead to bilaterality in cerebral representation of function.

Perinatal asphyxia is known to abolish the newborn's rightward turning bias (Turkewitz, Moreau, & Birch, 1968). Whether this predicts absence of peripheral laterality throughout infancy has not been studied. If it does, we may conclude that the hypothesized asymmetry of ascending activation may be quite vulnerable to brain stem damage and that this is why peripheral asymmetry is lacking in many severely mentally retarded people.

An interesting case is that of the mentally retarded autist. Ambidextrous autists are generally lower functioning than are right- and left-handed ones (Fein *et al.*, 1984). There is also evidence that autistic symptomatology reflects overarousal (Hutt, Hutt, Lee, & Ounstead, 1964). Increased arousal has been shown in experimental animals to reduce asymmetries in behavior occasioned by lateral cerebral damage (Wolgin, 1984). Perhaps overarousal opposes the development of asymmetrical manual behavior (Kinsbourne, 1987). In the extreme case the overactivation might obstruct the emergence not only of a clear hand preference across tasks but also of one within tasks (a characteristic named ''ambiguous handedness'' by Soper and Satz (1984). Ambiguous handedness has recently been found also to be prevalent among the mentally retarded (Soper, Satz, Orsini, Van Dongen, & Green 1987). Whether overarousal, underarousal, or some other mechanism should be considered in this instance is unclear.

The diffuseness of cerebral representation in non-right-handers may be secondary to diffuseness of ascending activation. In some cases an intense ascending activation might therefore be insufficiently selective to enable the individual to adopt an effective selective verbal mental set when his language capabilities are challenged. Or the activation may even be misrouted to the right hemisphere, causing the individual to deploy inefficient right hemisphere strategies (Kinsbourne, 1980). This account of left-hemisphere inefficiency, though speculative, does find support in the work of Obrzut and colleagues (e.g., Obrzut, Hynd, Obrzut, & Pirozzolo, 1981). They have shown that reading-disabled children find it easier than normal readers to attend to the left ear in a verbal dichotic paradigm. Like normal adults (Treisman & Geffen, 1968), normal children cannot help but attend primarily to the right ear when exposed to competing left and right verbal input, a phenomenon I have attributed to the effect of left-hemisphere activation for purposes of instituting verbal mental set on the left frontal facility for shifting attention rightward (Kinsbourne, 1970, 1973). The absence of such a bias in non-right-handers would then imply that they were less selectively activating the left hemisphere, and this could also help explain why in some instances their verbal processing is less efficient.

An analogous rightward attentional bias appears to characterize dextrals but not sinistrals even in simple manual motor performance. In an imaginative experiment, Peters (1987) has demonstrated that right-handers exhibit an attentional bias toward their right hand in bimanual performance, whereas left-handers do not show an attentional bias toward either hand. Specifically, when tapping a bimanual two-to-one rhythm, right-handers did better when the attention-attracting faster rhythm was tapped by the right hand, whereas left-handers showed no asymmetry. The findings for the right-handers are enlightening with respect to two earlier results. In one, Kinsbourne and Hicks (1978) reported that pianists playing unrelated melodies simultaneously with the two hands made fewer errors when the performer hummed along with the right hand than when he hummed with the left. The humming would naturally guide attention to the hand it accompanied. Less obviously related but still possibly relevant is an unpublished finding by Kinsbourne and LaCasse. They examined the fingering for a set of well-known fugues. In a fugue, both hands play identical sequences of notes (though staggered in time). As specified on the score, the first finger to be used by the right hand was most commonly 1, 2, or 3. For the left hand it was equally distributed across all five fingers. I surmise that right-handers tend to acquire differential motor habits, using the right hand as the guiding instrument. Their left hands are less apt to acquire specific habits. Left-handers, being less differentiated, are presumably more flexible in how they do the same tasks.

SINISTRALITY AND READING DISABILITY: THE RELATIONSHIP

I now consider whether the concepts I have discussed might clarify the relationship between sinistrality and selective reading disability.

Different opinions have been voiced about the often asserted view that sinistrality is disproportionately prevalent among children with reading disability. Satz (1976) has noted that most claims for such a relationship are based on clinical samples (e.g., Denckla, 1978), whereas failures to verify it tend to characterize studies that sample good and poor readers in regular school systems. The diagnosis of dyslexia is usually based on a critical shortfall in reading and/or writing relative to chronological or mental age, but this is probably an insufficiently accurate approach. The true dyslexic (as opposed to the child whose reading backwardness is multiply determined) is one who not only is in retard but remains behind despite individualized remedial effort. Such individuals are to be found in clinical populations and in residential institutions for the learning disabled. Children retained in regular school systems may have milder and less specific reading problems.

We have recently confirmed a relationship between dyslexia and personal and familial sinistrality based on an institutional sample (Kinsbourne, 1986). In our questionnaire study we found that the incidence of dyslexia was greatest in familial sinistrals, less in sporadic sinistrals, less still in familial dextrals, and least in dextrals without a sinistral family history.

Geschwind and Behan (1982) have supposed that those fetuses in whom testosterone levels run relatively high are more prone to suffer from diseases of the immune system (as well as "left-hemispheric" cognitive deficits). We have confirmed the relationship between sinistrality and cognitive deficit including dyslexia, and immune disease. But there was no concordance between the cognitive and immune disorders in our data. They were distributed independently across the sample. This contradicts the possibility that a single agent (e.g., testosterone) causes both these manifestations. A recent analysis of our data revealed that cognitive deficit is predicted by immune disease in the mother, but not in the father. This suggests that the cognitive deficit was caused by maternal immune attack on the fetus.

SINISTRALITY AND READING DISABILITY: THE MECHANISM

Excess sinistrality in dyslexia (Orton, 1937) has been confirmed, but not Orton's suggested mechanism for the relationship. Bilateralization of language function is neither necessary nor sufficient to generate learning disability. When sinistrals exhibit cognitive deficit, it is a matter of undermaturation of specific cortical areas, or their underactivation, rather than of anomalous topography of cerebral representation of the behavior in question.

If a diffuse representation of function is less conducive to automatization, then this could well reflect on reading acquisition and cause the ranks of the dyslexics to be swelled by non-right-handers. A recent study by Gutezeit (1982) supports this point of view. Comparing 72 left-handed grade-school children with right-handed controls, he found signs of relative weakness on the part of the non-right-handers on a range of tasks calling for automatization. This finding alerts us to the fact that psychometric measures, not having been designed specifically to address the problem of differences in cognition between hand preference groups, may not adequately tap the automatization parameter and therefore not be sensitive to cognitive differences between right-handers and non-right-handers that in fact exist.

Although left-handedness is disproportionately prevalent among children with selective reading disability, the right-handers are still in the majority even in this group. But if left-handedness were to be a biological marker indicating probability of diffuse central nervous system organization, it would not follow that only left-handers tend to such brain organization. Dyslexic right-handers could be a dextral subgroup with more diffuse language representation than most dextrals have. As already mentioned, dextrals with familial sinistrality are more likely to suffer from dyslexia and related cognitive disorders than are dextrals without such family history (Kinsbourne, 1986). In view of the possibility that learning-disabled children represent a population in which brain organization to some extent lacks selectivity, it becomes interesting to determine whether dyslexics as a group will show a certain lack of specificity, or apparent immaturity, when performing tasks that have nothing whatever to do with reading, language processing in general, or functions possibly underlying language processing. In a recent study, Neff, Kinsbourne, and Languis (in preparation) used tasks of this type.

Each task subdivided into two conditions, one "within hemisphere" and one "between hemispheres." The "crossed" versus "uncrossed" design lends itself to interpretation in terms of hemispheric interrelations. As a preamble to discussing the results of this study, I now consider how the function of the corpus callosum might be measured by behavioral means in children, relative to tasks used by Neff and colleagues.

Test of Interhemispheric Transfer

The standard paradigm that purports to measure the function of the corpus callosum is conceptualized in terms of the efficiency or latency of interhemispheric information transfer. Subjects are presented with input to one hemisphere (the visual half-field, one ear with masking noise in the other, the skin surface of one hand), and a comparison is made of the latency or efficiency of some response to that input using an effector on the same or on the other side of the body. In children the following variant is more commonly used. Within a successive matching paradigm, input is presented to one side of the body for a match either on the same side or on the other. Any difference in efficiency to the detriment of the contralateral (crossed) comparison is attributed to information loss across the forebrain commissure. Guided by this logic, Galin and colleagues designed two procedures for the purpose of determining callosal function in young, normal children. In one they had children perform a successive texture match either within the same hand or across hands (Galin, Diamond, & Herron, 1974). In the other they had children localize a touched finger either on the touched hand or on the corresponding finger on the other hand (Galin, Johnson, Nakell, & Herron, 1979). There was the expected improvement of overall performance with increasing age. The youngest preschool children, however, also had greater difficulty across the midline than within the stimulated hand. This was interpreted as tapping the relative immaturity of the corpus callosum at that stage in the life span.

In the Neff *et al.* study, Galin's two procedures were modified to free them of confounding independent variables. In the original Galin texture-matching procedure (also used by Kletzkin, 1980), the same receptor surface was stimulated twice in the uncrossed condition, but in the crossed condition two different receptor surfaces were used. Therefore, in the former but not in the latter the child might have made use of lingering tactile memories of the first touch. These would tend to make the comparison to some extent "simultaneous" and correspondingly easier. We therefore confined the initial touch to one side of the hand surface and the subsequent match to the other side of that hand (or of the other hand). In the Galin finger localization paradigm, designating the finger on the other hand that corresponds to the one touched on the stimulated hand calls for a certain level of abstraction. This adds an uncontrolled element of increased difficulty to the crossed condition of the task. We therefore modified the task by having the child identify by touch the touched finger with either the ipsilateral or the contralateral thumb.

In a task of maze learning, children found their way through a finger maze twice in succession. The dependent variable was the amount of time saved in solving the maze a second time as compared to the first. Whereas in the uncrossed condition the child performed the maze successively with adjacent fingers, in the crossed condition the child used a finger from one hand, then a finger from the other.

Two associated movement tasks perhaps tap callosal function. When young children attempt discrete finger movements, they tend concurrently to make associated movements of adjacent fingers as well as movements of the mirror symmetrical finger on the other hand (Fog & Fog, 1963). Dennis (1977) observed that this propensity is particularly striking and enduring in individuals with agenesis of the corpus callosum (who, in contrast, do not show any striking information transmission deficit between the hemispheres). She made the reasonable suggestion that the corpus callosum might enhance the specificity of motor cortex action by helping suppress superfluous movement both ipsilaterally and contralaterally. This role of the corpus callosum would be inhibitory (Kinsbourne, 1974, 1982). The amplitude of associated movements diminishes with increasing age, both ipsilaterally and contralaterally (Lazarus & Todor, 1987).

Study of Dyslexics Using Nonlanguage Tests

The design of the study by Neff and colleagues focused on a cross-sectional comparison of groups of normal children of average age 3, 5, 7, 9, and 11, and two dyslexic groups aged 11 to 13, and 13 to 15, respectively. All children were right-handed. Five of the tasks used by Neff *et al.* had effectively no language component but were perceptual, motor, or visuospatial. For present purposes we confine the discussion to these tasks. They were a texture-matching task (modified from Galin *et al.*, 1979), two simple motor tasks involving differential finger movement (one according to Rey, 1941, the other according to Kinsbourne, 1973), a finger localization task (modified by Galin *et al.*, 1974), and a maze-learning task. In the first of these tasks, children were required to feel the texture of the surface of specially prepared "pillows" and perform successive same-or-different matches. In the Rey test children were asked to place their hands flat on the tabletop and lift only the indicated finger. The dependent variable was the number of other fingers inadvertently raised at the same time. In the other motor task, children held three sticks between the four fingers of each hand and were asked to drop only one at a time. The dependent variable was the number of any other sticks inadvertently dropped at the same time. In the maze task the subject is timed while negotiating a finger maze, and then while negotiating it a second time. The dependent variable is the time saved on repetition of the same maze.

Neff and colleagues found the expected performance increment with increasing age in the normal group for each of the three information transmission procedures, but also found that the ratio of error in the crossed versus uncrossed condition began in the youngest group at a value well above 1.0 and approximated to 1.0 with increasing age. The dyslexic children resembled younger normal children both in overall level of correct response and in the ratio of crossed to uncrossed errors. Typically, the reading-disabled children approximate normal children 4 to 6 years younger than themselves. The older reading-disabled children performed in a more "mature" manner than the younger ones. In the two associated movement tasks, uncrossed errors were always more frequent than crossed errors. But the age effect and ratio shift found for these two tasks across age and between normals and dyslexics was analogous to that in the other three.

Before venturing an interpretation of the results of Neff and colleagues, I will now summarize current understanding of the function of the corpus callosum.

The Forebrain Commissure and Cognition

The well-popularized literature on the effects of commissurotomy in humans (Gazzaniga, 1970) is presented mostly in terms of a disconnection model. The callosum is viewed as the structure that permits information presented to one hemisphere only to be made available to the other, in circumstances where the initially uninformed hemisphere is constrained by the nature of the task to participate in the expected response. Given the popularity of this concept, it is not surprising that a "functional disconnection" between the hemispheres, based on hypothesized callosal impairment or underdevelopment, has been proposed to explain a range of behavioral dysfunctions of controversial pathogenesis, ranging from schizophrenia (Dimond, 1979) to the focus of our present interest, dyslexia (Leslie, Davidson, & Batey, 1985). On the face of it, it is hard to see why disconnecting the two hemispheres would impair an individual's ability to learn to read, at any rate in the right half-field, and a selective reading difficulty confined to one (the left) half visual field has never been documented in children with selective reading disability. However, a somewhat more sophisticated version of this model would have it that in the early stages of reading acquisition, right-hemisphere participation is required for the purpose of decoding as yet unfamiliar letter and word shapes (Bakker, 1979), relying on the plausible notion that one of the specialized functions of the right hemisphere relates to the decoding of novel information (Goldberg & Costa, 1981). But dyslexia is notoriously persistent and by no means limited to the early stages of reading acquisition. Furthermore, there remains the obstacle that there is not direct evidence of callosal impairment in reading-disabled children, although some evidence, largely eletrophysiological, does suggest that interhemispheric relationships in reading-disabled children are not totally normal (Kletzkin, 1980; Leslie *et al.*, 1985). Direct anatomical evidence about the corpus callosum in the reading disabled is not available (except to the extent that anatomical examination of this structure in the few dyslexias recently autopsied appears not to have revealed any important abnormality—Galaburda, Sherman, Rosen, Aboitiz, & Geschwind, 1985). The corpus callosum has been reported to be thicker in left- than in right-handers (Witelson, 1985). If so, one could interpret this as being consonant with the generally more diffuse and extensive organization of the non-right-handed individuals that has already been commented on. However, the functional implication of differential thickens of this structure is simply unknown. It seems preferable for the time being to accept the fact that, like overall brain size itself, the size of components of the cerebrum, within the normal range, simply is not interpretable in terms of function (e.g., Passingham, 1979), and shift attention to studies of the interhemispheric commissure in action.

Although research on the function of the corpus callosum has overwhelmingly focused on its possible information-transmitting function, this attribution remains speculative, as most of the findings can be otherwise explained (Guiard, 1980; Guiard & Requin, 1978; Kinsbourne, 1974). But even if it were correct, the very split-brain subjects on whom it is based vividly illustrate the adaptively trivial nature of such a role for the callosum. In activities of daily living, these people are indistinguishable from normals as far as hemispheric coordination is concerned (Gazzaniga, 1970). It appears that alternative routes of hemispheric integration (whether within the brain, by bilateral projections, as in the auditory system, and communication through commissures at the brain stem level; or external, by looking from side to side and other forms of cross-cuing) amply compensate for any interruption in transcallosal information flow. Yet one cannot conceive that such a massive neural structure could have evolved in the absence of major adaptive pressures. A more significant role for the corpus callosum should be ascertainable.

Although they show behavioral evidence of hemisphere disconnection only in laboratory situations carefully contrived to confine input to one side, split-brain patients do appear intellectually handicapped in ways that have attracted comment (Sperry, 1968), but not systematic investigation. We can hypothesize the possible basis for such difficulties after considering callosal function in its biological context.

The corpus callosum is the most *cephalad* of an extensive system of transverse commissures that connects all segmental levels of the bisymmetric vertebrate nervous system. The basic function of these connections was definitively demonstrated by Sherrington (1906). They subserve the complementary aspect of bilateral activity. Laterally coordinated movement in nature is typically not symmetrical but reciprocal. A flexor response on one side is accompanied by inhibition of contralateral flexion and release of the opponent extensor synergy—the crossed extensor reflex. At the highest level of abstraction, this complementary function perhaps relates the feature-specifying activity of the left hemisphere to the constructing of a context by the right (Kinsbourne, 1982). Mirror image responses are primitive and potentially interfering, and their virtual elimination during development perhaps depends on callosal maturation (Dennis, 1977).

In the context of the present study, the ability to match successive inputs requires that two loci of patterned excitation be kept separate for comparison. Cortico-cortical connections, including the callosum, probably participate in this. At the cognitive level, inhibition is equally called for to enable component mental operations elaborated concurrently to be protected from interfering cross-talk until they are fully developed and ready to adopt specific relationships with one another within the total action program. On the basis of these considerations, one might look to the coordination (rather than intercommunication) of mental operations based on opposite hemispheres to explain cognitive weakness in split-brain patients.

In selective cognitive immaturities like dyslexia, there may be a general immaturity of cortico-cortical coordination, including but not limited to that implemented by the forebrain commissure.

Cerebral Differentiation Deficit in Dyslexics?

If, in the Neff *et al.* study, the dyslexics had performed normally in the uncrossed condition but exhibited disproportionate difficulty in the crossed, then it would have been natural to incriminate a callosal deficit in this condition (e.g., Klicpera, Wolff, & Drake, 1981; Leslie *et al.*, 1985). In fact, their deficit in the uncrossed condition was almost as great as in the crossed. To retain the callosal theory, one would need a second explanation for the uncrossed deficit. It is more parsimonious to see both as reflections of a single deficiency, perhaps an immaturity, on the part of the reading disabled. Behaviorally, this could be conceptualized as implicating the ability to manipulate generalization gradients. Neurologically, perhaps both within and between cerebral representations of the hands, dyslexics have more difficulty in maintaining comparable levels of activation for separate central loci for purposes of a successive match, and more difficulty selectively activating a single effector while leaving others within the same category in their activation base state. Rather than thinking in terms of a selective callosal deficit, we should bear in mind that the corpus callosum is simply the largest of an extensive set of cortico-cortical connections. Maybe these connections contribute to rendering cognition specific and differentiated, and perhaps it is in this rather general function that the reading-disabled children are in retard.

The findings presented here do not stand alone. Although she focused on the deficit in crossed performance and favored the construct of the selective callosal deficit, Kletzkin (1980) found a proportionately equally great deficit on uncrossed performance in the Galin tests by her dyslexic subjects. Badian and Wolff (1977) and Klicpera *et al.* (1981) found dyslexics to have difficulty in bimanual correlation (counterpoint to our associated movement results).

We are dealing here with performance deficits very remote from the problems in language and learning that brought the reading-disabled children to attention. Moving one's finger differentially is not obviously related to learning to read. But it is not necessary to assume that this or any other ability in which disabled readers prove inferior taps the source of the reading difficulty. As was postulated in the now unpopular concept of minimal cerebral dysfunction, multiple neurological immaturities with an impact on behavior could coexist. Nevertheless, a general function does conceivably link differential finger movement and differential word recognition: the ability to inhibit highly probable (compatible, familiar) responses in favor of less favorable but more specifically adaptive alternatives.

During reading acquisition, already acquired responses to letters and letter groupings are constantly being overridden as new words containing those letters are learned. The phonological referent of any letter grouping depends critically on other letters coexisting in the word. No sooner does the child learn how to pronounce a syllable than, in the context of a new word, he is told that it is pronounced differently. The impaired reader persists, for variable periods of time, with responses to letter groupings within a word that might be correct were these groupings present in isolation, but are incorrect or at least inadequate in the new context. The ability to override familiar in favor of more adaptive responses calls for neural inhibitory interactions generically related to those that enable one finger to be moved while the others are restrained from moving. The present results militate against the claim that developmental dyslexia (at least as currently diagnosed in rather large numbers of children) is a highly specific condition (Critchley, 1964) or even one limited to the language domain (Vellutino, 1978). The alleged selectivity of reading disability is still under experimental scrutiny. Matching disabled readers with controls on the WISC performance subscale does not suffice to demonstrate a pure "reading disability." Although occasional dyslexics might be fully capable on a wide range of measures, group comparisons reveal an inferiority of reading disabled, on a wide range of measures not readily encompassed by such global categorization as "linguistic" or even "left-hemispheric." Our data indicates a range of deficits overlapping not only the right-hemisphere domain (maze learning) but even sensorimotor functioning. That a quite general cognitive limitation underlies reading disability remains a serious possibility. The disorder may, at least in the majority of cases, reflect an immature state of cerebral neuronal circuitry, making for neuromotor immaturity and generating other signs of the type that used to be attributed to "minimal cerebral dysfunction," as well as the more specific and consequential cognitive deficits that preempt the educator's attention. The difficulty experienced by the older reading-disabled child is then comparable to that experienced by any younger normal child (although the assumption is not justified that therefore the dyslexic will ultimately mature sufficiently to "catch up"). In any case it would be easy to see why neuronal circuitry with a degree of underdifferentiation might lend itself only with difficulty to the higher levels of automatization (for left-handers, and presumably more particularly for left-handed dyslexics). The next reasonable step would seem to be to compare right- and non-right-handed normally reading children on procedures such as those used by Neff and colleagues to see whether even the normally reading non-right-hander can be distinguished from his age and reading-matched right-handed counterpart on parameters of this nature.

CONCLUSION

I have reviewed rival theoretical accounts of the relationship between sinistrality and cognitive immaturities or deficits. There is little empirical support for notions invoking the failure to lateralize or the anomalous brain organization. It is perhaps doubtful whether the pathological left-handedness concept, valid though it appears to be for certain children, fully accounts for the widespread phenomenon under scrutiny. Ingenious attempts have been made to rationalize the association between non-right-handedness and cerebral dysfunction in terms of a common antecedent cause. Hand preference and vulnerability to cognitive dysfunction of early origin might both derive from maternal immune disease. On such a view, non-right-handedness would be a biological marker indicating risk for immune dysfunction. Non-right-handers would then subdivide into those in whom that vulnerability translated into clinically significant cognitive deficit, and those in whom it remained latent. As for the mechanism of the cognitive dysfunction, support has been mustered for the notion of some genetic influence retarding or inhibiting the full differentiation of the cerebral neural network, perhaps secondary to incomplete specification by ascending activation from the brain stem. Such a deficit could generate a diverse array of cognitive and neurological immaturities or "soft signs," but only in a probabilistic fashion, apparently leaving many sinistrals unaffected.

REFERENCES

Annett, M. (1970). The growth of manual performance and speed. *British Journal of Psychology, 61,* 545–548.

Annett, M. (1973). Handedness in families. *Annals of Human Genetics, 37,* 93–105.

Badian, N. A., & Wolff, P. H. (1977). Manual asymmetries of motor sequencing in children with reading disability. *Cortex, 13,* 343–349.

Bakan, P., Dibb, G., & Reed, P. (1973). Handedness and birth stress. *Neuropsychologia, 11,* 363–366.

Bakker, D. J. (1979) Hemispheric differences and reading strategies: Two dyslexias? *Bulletin of the Orton Society, 29,* 84–100.

Bates, E., O'Connell, B., Vaid, J., Sledge, P., & Oakes, L. (1986). Language and hand preference in early development. *Developmental Neuropsychology, 2,* 1–15.

Batheja, J., & McManus, I. E. (1985). Handedness in the mentally handicapped. *Developmental Medicine and Child Neurology, 27,* 63–68.

Beaumont, J. G. (1974). Handedness and hemisphere function. In S. J. Dimond & J. G. Beaumont (Eds.), *Hemisphere function in the human brain* (pp. 89–120). New York: Wiley.

Benbow, C. P. (1985). The left hand of maths and verbal talent. *Science News, 127,* 263.

Berry, G. A., Hughes, R. V., & Jackson, L. D. (1980). Sex and handedness in simple and integrated task performance. *Perceptual and Motor Skills, 51,* 807–812.

Bishop, D. M. V. (1983). Linguistic impairment after left hemidecortication for infantile hemiplegia? A reappraisal. *Quarterly Journal of Experimental Psychology, 35A,* 199–208.

Bishop, D. M. V. (1984). Using non-preferred hand skill to investigate pathological left-handedness in an unselected population. *Developmental Medicine and Child Neurology, 26,* 214–226.

Bradshaw-McAnulty, G., Hicks, R. E., & Kinsbourne, M. (1984). Pathological left-handedness and familiial sinistrality in relation to degree of mental retardation. *Brain and Cognition, 3,* 349–356.

Bradshaw, J. L., Nettleton, N. C., & Taylor, M. J. (1981). Right hemisphere language and cognitive deficit in sinistrals? *Neuropsychologia, 19,* 113–131.

Briggs, G. G., Nebes, R. D., & Kinsbourne, M. (1976). Intellectual differences in relation to personal and family handedness. *Quarterly Journal of Experimental Psychology, 28,* 591–601.

Broca, P. (1865). Sur le siège de la faculté du language articulé. *Bulletin de Société Anthropol, 6,* 377–393.

Bryden, M. P., Hecaen, M., & DeAgostini, M. (1983). Patterns of cerebral organization. *Brain and Language, 20,* 249–262.

Carter, G. L., Hohenegger, M. K., & Satz, P. (1982). Aphasia and speech organization in children. *Science, 218,* 797–799.

Chi, J. G., Dooling, E. C., & Gilles, F. H. (1977). Gyral development of the human brain. *Annals of Neurology, 1,* 86–93.

Critchley, M. (1964). *Developmental dyslexia.* Springfield: IL: Thomas.

Czopf, J. (1972). Uber die Rolle der nicht dominanten Hemisphäre in der Restitution der Sprache der Aphasischen. *Archiv für Psychiatrie und Nervenkrankheiten, 216,* 162–171.

Denckla, M. (1978). Minimal brain dysfunction. In J. S. Chall & A. F. Mirsky (Eds.), *Education and the brain* (pp. 223–268). Seventy-seventh Yearbook of the National Society for the Study of Education, Part II. Chicago: University of Chicago Press.

Dennis, M. (1977). Impaired sensory and motor differentiation with corpus callosum agenesis: A lack of callosal inhibition during ontogeny? *Neuropsychologia, 14,* 455–459.

Dennis, M. (1980). Capacity and strategy for syntactic comprehension after left or right hemidecortification. *Brain and Language, 10,* 287–317.

Dimond, S. J. (1979). Disconnection and psychopathology. In J. Gruzelier & P. Flor-Henry (Eds.), *Hemispheric asymmetries of function in psychopathology* (pp. 35–46). Amsterdam: Elsevier.

Fein, D., Humes, M., Kappan, E., Lucci, D., & Waterhouse, L. (1984). The question of left hemisphere dysfunction in infantile autism. *Psychological Bulletin, 95,* 258–281.

Fog, E. & Fog, M. (1963). Cerebral inhibition examined by associated movements. In M. Bax & R. MacKeith (Eds.), *Minimal cerebral dysfunction.* Lavenham, Suffolk: Lavenham Press.

Galaburda, A. M., Sherman, G. F., Rosen, G. D., Aboitiz, F., & Geschwind, N. (1985). Developmental dyslexia: four consecutive patients with cortical anomalies. *Annals of Neurology, 18,* 222–233.

Galin, D., Diamond, R., & Herron, J. (1974). Development of crossed and uncrossed tactile localization on the fingers. *Brain and Language, 4,* 588–590.

Galin, D., Johnson, J., Nakell, L., & Herron, J. (1979). Development of the capacity for tactile information transfer between hemispheres in normal children. *Science, 204,* 1330–1332.

Gazzaniga, M. S. (1970). *The bisected brain.* New York: Appleton-Century-Crofts.

Geschwind, N., & Behan, P. (1982). Left-handedness: Association with immune disease, migraine, and developmental learning disorder. *Proceedings of the National Academy of Sciences, 79,* 5097–5100.

Geschwind, N., & Galaburda, A. M. (1985). Cerebral lateralization. Biological mechanisms, associations and pathology: II. A hypothesis and a program for research. *Archives of Neurology, 42,* 521–552.

Gesell, A., & Ames, L. B. (1947). The development of handedness. *Journal of General Psychology, 70,* 155–175.

Gesell, A., & Ames, L. B. (1950). Tonic-neck reflex and symmetro-tonic behavior. *Journal of Pediatrics, 36,* 165–178.

Gillberg, C., Waldenstrom, E., & Rasmussen, P. (1984). Handedness in Swedish 10-year-olds: Some background and associated factors. *Journal of Child Psychology and Psychiatry, 25,* 421–432.

Gloning, I., Gloning, K., Haub, G., & Quatember, R. (1969). Comparison of verbal behavior in right-handed and nonright-handed patients with anatomically verified lesions of one hemisphere. *Cortex 5,* 43–52.

Goodglass, H., & Quadfasel, F. A. (1954). Language laterality in left-handed aphasics. *Brain, 77,* 521–548.

Goodwin, R. S., & Michel, G. F. (1981). Head orientation position during birth and in infant neonatal period and hand preference at nineteen weeks. *Child Development, 52,* 819–826.

Goldberg, E., & Costa, L. (1981). Hemispheric differences in the acquisition and use of descriptive systems. *Brain and Language, 14,* 144–173.

Gordon, H. W. (1921). Left-handedness and mirror-writing, especially among defective children. *Brain, 43,* 313–368.

Gordon, H. W. (1980). Cognitive asymmetry in dyslexic families. *Neuropsychologia, 18,* 645–656.

Guiard, Y. (1980). Cerebral hemispheres and selective attention. *Acta Psychologica, 46,* 41–61.

Guiard, Y., & Requin, J. (1978). Between-hand versus within-hand choice–RT: A single channel of reduced capacity in the split-brain monkey. In J. Requin (Ed.), *Attention and performance* (Vol. 7, pp. 391–410). Hillsdale, NJ: Erlbaum.

Gutezeit, G. (1982). Linkshändigkeit und Lernstörungen? *Praxis der Kinderpsychologie und Kinderpsychiatrie, 31,* 277–283.

Hardyck, C., & Petrinovitch, L. F. (1977). Left handedness. *Psychological Bulletin, 84,* 405–411.

Hecaen, H., & Ajuriaguerra, J. de. (1964). *Left-handedness: Manual superiority and cerebral dominance.* New York: Grune and Stratton.

Hicks, R. E., & Barton, A. K. (1975). A note for left-handedness and severity of mental retardation. *Journal of Genetic Psychology, 127,* 323–324.

Hicks, R. A., & Beveridge, R. (1978). Handedness and intelligence. *Cortex, 14,* 304–307.

Hicks, R. E. & Kinsbourne, M. (1976a). On the genesis of human handedness: a review. *Journal of Motor Behavior, 8,* 257–266.

Hicks, R. E., & Kinsbourne, M. (1976b). Human handedness: a partial cross-fostering study. *Science, 192,* 908–910.

Hutt, C., Hutt, S. J., Lee, D., & Ounstead, C. (1964). Arousal and childhood autism. *Nature, 204,* 908–909.

Kinsbourne, M. (1970). The cerebral basis of lateral asymmetries in attention. *Acta Psychologica, 33,* 193–201. In A. F. Sanders (Ed.), *Attention and performance* (Vol. 3, pp. 193–204). Amsterdam: North Holland.

Kinsbourne, M. (1971). The minor cerebral hemisphere as a source of aphasic speech. *Archives of Neurology 25,* 302–306.

Kinsbourne, M. (1973). Minimal brain dysfunction as a neurodevelopmental lag. *Annals of the New York Academy of Sciences, 205,* 263–273.

Kinsbourne, M. (1974). Lateral interactions in the brain. In M. Kinsbourne & W. L. Smith (Eds.), *Hemispheric disconnection and cerebral function* (pp. 239–259). Springfield, IL: Thomas.

Kinsbourne, M. (1980). A model for the ontogeny of cerebral organization in nonright-handers. In J. Herron (Ed.), *Neuropsychology of left-handedness* (pp. 177–185). New York: Academic Press.

Kinsbourne, M. (1982). Hemispheric specialization and the growth of human understanding. *American Psychologist, 37,* 4111–4120.

Kinsbourne, M. (1986). Sinistrality and risk for immune diseases and learning disorders [poster]. Child Neurology Society meeting, Boston, MA.

Kinsbourne, M. (1987). Cerebral–brainstem interactions in infantile autism. In E. Schopler & G. Mesibov (Eds.), *Neurobiological theories of arousal and autism* (pp. 107–126). New York: Plenum.

Kinsbourne, M., & Hicks, R. E. (1978). Functional cerebral space: A model for overflow, transfer and interference effects in human performance: A tutorial review. In J. Requin (Ed.), *Attention and Performance* (Vol. 7, pp. 345–362). Hillsdale, NJ: Erlbaum.

Kinsbourne, M., & Hiscock, M. (1977). Does cerebral dominance develop? In S. Segalowitz & F. A. Gruber (Eds.), *Language development and neurological theory* (pp. 171–191). New York: Academic Press.

Kinsbourne, M., & Hiscock, M. (1983). The normal and deviant development of functional lateralization of the brain. In P. Mussen, M. Haith, & J. Campos (Eds.), *Handbook of child psychology* (pp. 157–280). New York: Wiley.

Kletzkin, D. (1980). *Electroencephalographic, neurologic and psychometric correlates of right and left cerebral hemisphere functions in on grade and below grade elementary school boys.* Unpublished doctoral dissertation, Rutgers University.

Klicpera, C., Wolff, P. H., & Drake, C. (1981). Bimanual co-ordination in adolescent boys with reading retardation. *Developmental Medicine and Neurology, 23,* 617–625.

Kohn, B., & Dennis, M. (1974). Selective impairments of visuo-spatial abilities in infantile hemiplegics after right cerebral hemidecortication. *Neuropsychologia, 12,* 505–512.

Lazarus, J. C., & Todor, J. I. (1987). Age differences in the magnitude of associated movements. *Developmental Medicine and Child Neurology, 29,* 726–733.

LeMay, M. (1984). Radiological developmental and fossil asymmetries. In N. Geschwind & A. M. Galaburda (Eds.), *Cerebral dominance: The biological foundations* (pp. 26–42). Cambridge, MA: Harvard University Press.

Lenneberg, E. H. (1967). *Biological foundations of language.* New York: Wiley.

Leslie, S. C., Davidson, R. J., & Batey, O. B. (1985). Purdue pegboard performance of disabled and normal readers: Unimanual versus bimanual differences. *Brain and language, 24,* 359–369.

Levy, J. (1969). Possible basis for the evolution of lateral specialization of the human brain. *Nature, 224,* 614–615.

Liederman, J., & Kinsbourne, M. (1980). Rightward motor bias in newborns depends upon paternal right-handedness. *Neuropsychologia, 18,* 579–584.

Luria, A. R. (1966). *Higher cortical functions in man.* New York: Basic Books.

McGlone, J. (1980). Sex differences in human brain asymmetry: A critical survey. *Behavioral and Brain Sciences, 3,* 215–264.

McManus, I. C. (1983). Pathological left-handedness: Does it exist? *Journal of Communication Disorders, 5,* 315–344.

Nagae, S. (1985). Handedness and sex differences in selective interference of verbal and spatial information. *Journal of Experimental Psychology: Human Perception and Performance, 11,* 346–354.

Neff, L. S., Kinsbourne, M., & Languis, M. (In preparation). Development of hemispheric interaction in normal and reading disabled children.

Obrzut, J. E., Hynd, G. W., Obrzut, A., & Pirozzolo, F. J. (1981). Effect of directed attention on cerebral asymmetries in normal and learning disabled children. *Developmental Psychology, 17,* 118–125.

Olmstead, C. E., & Villablanca, J. R. (1979). Effects on caudate nuclei of frontal cortical ablations in cats and kittens: Paw usage. *Experimental Neurology, 63,* 559–572.

Orton, S. T. (1937). *Reading, writing and speech problems in children.* New York: Norton.
Passingham, R. E., (1979). Brain size and intelligence in man. *Brain, Behavior and Evolution, 16,* 253–270.
Peters, M. (1987). A nontrivial motor performance difference between right handers and left handers: Attention as intervening variable in the expression of handedness. *Canadian Journal of Psychology, 41,* 91–99.
Rasmussen, T., & Milner, B. (1975). Clinical and surgical studies of the cerebral speech areas in man. In K. J. Zulch, O. Creutzfeld, & G. Galbraith (Eds.), *Cerebral localization* (pp. 238–257). Heidelberg: Springer.
Rasmussen, T., & Milner, B. (1977). The role of early left-brain injury in determining lateralization of cerebral speech functions. In S. Dimond & D. Blizard (Eds.), *Evolution and lateralization of the brain* (pp. 355–369). New York: New York Academy of Sciences.
Rey, A. (1941). L'examen psychologique dans les cas d'encephalopathie traumatique. *Archives de Psychologie, 28,* 286–340.
Satz, P. (1972). Pathological left-handedness: An explanatory model. *Cortex, 9,* 121–135.
Satz, P. (1976). Cerebral dominance and reading disability: An old problem revisited. In R. M. Knights & D. J. Bakker (Eds.), *The neuropsychology of learning disorders* (pp. 273–296). Baltimore: University Park Press.
Satz, P., Orsini, D., Saslow, E., & Henry, R. (1985). The pathological left-handedness syndrome. *Brain and Cognition, 4,* 27–46.
Sherrington, C. S. (1906). *The integrative action of the nervous system.* New Haven: Yale University Press.
Silva, D. A., & Satz, P. (1979). Pathological left-handedness: Evaluation of a model. *Brain and Language, 7,* 8–16.
Soper, H. V., and Satz, P. (1984). Pathological left-handedness and ambiguous handedness: A new explanatory model. *Neuropsychologia, 22,* 511–515.
Soper, H. V., Satz, P., Orsini, D., Van Dongen, W. G., & Green, W. (1987). Handedness distribution among the severely to profoundly mentally retarded. *American Journal of Mental Deficiency, 92,* 94–102.
Sperry, R. W. (1968). Hemispheric disconnection and unity in conscious awareness. *American Psychologist, 23,* 723–733.
Subirana, A. (1958). The prognosis of aphasia in relation to cerebral dominance and handedness. *Brain, 81,* 415–425.
Swanson, J. M., Kinsbourne, M., & Horn, J. M. (1980). Cognitive deficit and left-handedness: A cautionary note. In J. Herron (Ed.), *Neuropsychology of left-handedness* (pp. 281–292). New York: Academic Press.
Treisman, A., & Geffen, G. *(1968).* Selective attention and cerebral dominance in perceiving and responding to speech messages. *Quarterly Journal of Experimental Psychology, 20,* 139–150.
Turkewitz, G., Moreau, T., & Birch, H. G. (1968). Relation between birth condition and neuro-behavioral organization in the neonate. *Pediatric Research, 2,* 243–249.
Vellutino, F. R. (1978). Toward an understanding of dyslexia: Psychological factors in specific reading disorders. In A. Benton & D. Pearl (Eds.), *Dyslexia: An appraisal of current knowledge.* New York: Oxford University Press.
Witelson, S. F. (1985). The brain connection: The corpus callosum is larger in left handers. *Science, 229,* 665–667.
Wolgin, D. L. (1982). Motivation, activation and behavioral integration. In R. L. Isaacson & N. E. Spear (Eds.), *The expressions of knowledge* (pp. 243–290). New York: Plenum.
Zangwill, O. (1969). *Cerebral dominance and its relation to cerebral function.* London: Oliver and Boyd.

11

Human Hand Preference: Three Nondextral Subtypes

PAUL SATZ
HENRY V. SOPER
DONNA L. ORSINI
University of California, Los Angeles

Over the past century attempts have been made to link left-handedness with mental deficiency, dyslexia, speech disturbances, birth defects, epilepsy, emotional instability, motor awkwardness, and alcoholism (Hardyck & Petrinovich, 1977; Hardyck, Petrinovich, & Goldman, 1976). More recently, this list has grown to include disorders such as infantile autism (Fein, Humes, Kaplan, Lucci, & Waterhouse, 1984; Soper *et al.*, 1986; Aram, Eckelman, & Satz, 1986), schizophrenia (Dvirski, 1983; Gur, 1977; McCreadie, Crorie, Barron, & Winslow, 1982), early dementia of the Alzheimer type (Seltzer, Burres, & Sherwin, 1984), autoimmune disorder (Geschwind, 1983; Geschwind & Behan, 1982; Geschwind & Galaburda, 1985a, 1985b, 1985c), abnormal brain sensitivity to endocrines (Irwin, 1985), and tardive dyskinesia (McCreadie *et al.*, 1982).

The search for a putative link between sinistrality and various disorders if fostered by those who view dextrality as the dominant handedness trait in humans (approximately 90%) for at least the past five thousand years (Coren & Porac, 1977; Spennemann, 1984) and that any deviations from this "norm" must spring from nongenetic, neuropathological factors. Annett (1972) has proposed a single gene to account for left-hemisphere language dominance and dextrality. She contends that half of the proportion within the population in which this "right shift" bias gene is absent will develop, by chance, as left-handers.

Neuropathological explanations provide a more direct link between left-handedness and various disorders. Bakan (1977), for example, states that left-handedness represents a pathological phenotype that is caused by early injury to the left hemisphere, primarily during the perinatal period. More recently, Geschwind and his associates (Geschwind, 1983; Geschwind & Behan, 1982; Geschwind & Galaburda, 1985a, 1985b, 1985c) have proposed that sinistrality represents a form of anomalous dominance that springs from a combination of neuropathological, maturational, and hormonal alterations of the left hemisphere, occurring primarily during the prenatal period. Although this latter position represents a more heuristic and innovative attempt to account for the origins of left-handedness and its correlates (e.g., various disorders), it still basically postulates a neuropathological substrate in most, if not all, left-handers.

The purpose of this chapter is to argue that the search for a link between left-handedness and various disorders will continue to foster misleading statements about sinistrality as long as all nondextrals are subsumed under a unitary etiological category. We propose that at least three distinct nondextral subtypes exist in humans and that they should be identified in the search for putative links between handedness and brain disorders. In fact, much of the historical and contemporary controversy on this subject probably stems from this failure to identify different subtypes of nondextrals. The subtypes—(1) pathological left-handedness, (2) ambiguous handedness, and (3) natural left-handedness—which have not been reported together before, are described next.

PATHOLOGICAL LEFT-HANDEDNESS (PLH)

This subtype refers to a subset of natural right-handers who, because of early factors (injury or pathological growth) primarily affecting the left hemisphere, suffer a hypofunction of the contralateral hand, which in turn causes a shift in manual preference to the left (Hecaen & Ajuriaguerra, 1964; Satz, 1972). This subtype was first identified in epileptics, where a raised incidence of manifest left-handedness (MLH) (approximately 17%–20%) has long been reported. The model of PLH (Satz, 1972, 1973) also states that only a small proportion of natural right-handers (epileptic or otherwise) with early left-sided damage (before age 6) will shift handedness. This shift depends in part on whether the lesion encroaches on the critical zones and, possibly, on genotypic variables affecting the manual transfer threshold. The model also demonstrates that the occurrence of the converse trait—namely, pathological right-handedness (PRH)—is a rare event. The proportion of PRH to PLH would be approximately that of natural left- to right-handers in the normal population (1:10). The PLH subtype, which is caused by an early lesion primarily to the left hemisphere, has been reported in cases of stroke (Hardyck, Petrinovich, & Goldman, 1976), epilepsy (Hecaen & Ajuriaguerra, 1964; Orsini & Satz, 1986; Penfield & Robertson, 1959; Rasmussen & Milner, 1977; Satz, Orsini, Saslow, & Henry, 1985), hemiplegia (Tizard, Paine, & Crothers, 1954), and hemispherectomy (Dennis & Whitaker, 1977). Although the PLH subtype is more commonly observed in epileptics with early unilateral lesions, it has also been observed in subjects who are asymptomatic (Bishop, 1980; Orsini & Satz, 1986; Satz, Orsini, Saslow, & Henry, 1985). Note that this subtype refers to a subset of the natural *dextral* population who, because of early left-sided injury, masquerade as sinistrals. More recently, we have proposed that the lesion that produces this shift in manual preference may alter other levels of lateral organization that are beyond the scope of this chapter (Orsini & Satz, 1986; Satz, Orsini, Saslow, & Henry, 1985). The PLH subtype, though similar to that proposed by Geschwind (1983) and Bakan (1977) with respect to lesion substrate (i.e,, left-hemisphere), differs otherwise because it refers to only a subset of the left-handed population as pathological.

AMBIGUOUS HANDEDNESS (AH)

This subtype refers to a subset of the autistic population who have recently been found to have no established manual dominance (Satz, Soper, Orsini, Henry, & Zvi, 1985; Soper & Satz, 1984; Soper *et al.*, 1986). This phenomenon was observed by changing the assessment procedure typically used to measure hand preference or skill in humans. The subjects were asked to demonstrate their hand preference on items varying in level and type of skilled movement appropriate for a developmentally disabled sample [i.e., *eat* (spoon), *draw* (crayon), *pick up* (dime or candy), *drink* (half-filled cup), *brush teeth* (toothbrush, *throw* (ball), and *hammer* (hammer)]. The items were administered three times each in a quasi-random order within each of two sessions spaced a week apart in order to determine whether the response preference was stable or random and to minimize perseverative responding to an item. Using a 90% criterion for the classification of handedness, we found a subgroup (36%) in two samples unselected for handedness [University of California at Los Angeles (UCLA) and Camarillo State Hospital] who showed no consistency in hand preference within or between sessions or even within items. In contrast, subjects in the other handedness groups (left = 20%, right = 444%) showed consistent unilateral manual responses for the same items both within and between sessions. In fact, a one-year follow-up assessment of the Camarillo cohort revealed a dramatic stability for each of the handedness phenotypes, including the AH subtype. Although this type of assessment procedure (multiple presentation/retest) has seldom been used before (even with the developmentally disabled), other investigators have also reported a subgroup of autistics (approximately 35%) whose hand preference has been labeled incomplete, not established, or mixed (Barry & James, 1978; Colby & Parkison, 1977; Fein *et al.*, 1984; Tsai, 1982). Unfortunately, the use of a single presentation of each item (usually less than five) and the requirement of consistent directional preference for the classification of left- or right-handedness obscures whether such a "mixed" group is *ambidextrous* (inconsistent between items but consistent within items) or *ambiguous* (inconsistent within items). Despite this measurement concern, reports have continued to identify a subset of the autistic population (approximately 35%) whose hand preference is mixed or, more probably, ambiguous. We have hypothesized that this phenomenon of ambiguous handedness is due to severe early bilateral brain damage, primarily in natural right-handers (because of their predominance in the normal population), that prevents the establishment of manual dominance and cognitive development. Although the putative brain lesion remains to be confirmed by anatomic or metabolic imaging techniques, three recent studies have shown that this ambiguous or mixed dominant subtype represents a more cognitively impaired subgroup compared to autistic children with established dominance (left- or right-handed) (Fein *et al.*, 1984; Soper *et al.*, 1986; Tsai, 1982).

Is the AH subtype specific to autism, or is it a phenomenon observed in mental retardation in general? The fact that almost none of the mental retardation studies to date have reported this phenotype, despite consistent reports of a raised incidence of left-handedness (approximately twofold) (Bradshaw-McAnulty, Hicks, & Kinsbourne, 1984; Burt, 1937; Hicks & Barton, 1975; Silva & Satz, 1979; Wilson & Dolan, 1931), led us to hypothesize that ambiguous handedness may represent a subtype unique to infantile autism. [Curiously, one of the earliest such studies, conducted by Gordon (1920), reports a very few subjects who were inconsistent in handedness, but who were disregarded because they were very low functioning.] Unfortunately, this hypothesis was recently disconfirmed in a large-scale study (Soper, Satz, Orsini, Van Gorp, & Green, 1987) of nonautistic mentally retarded subjects at Camarillo State Hospital. Using the same test–retest assessment procedures as with the autistic subjects, we found that approximately 45% of the mentally retarded subjects fell in the AH group, 45% were right-handed, and 10% were left-handed. These handedness proportions approximate those of the autistic cohort at the same hospital. But if so, then why the discrepancy with earlier reports, which have uniformly noted an increased incidence of left-handedness among the mentally retarded? First, none of these earlier studies used a multiple presentation/retest procedure to determine item response consistency. Second, most of the mental retardation studies, including the excellent study by Bradshaw-McAnulty *et al.* (1984), have not defined the criteria for classifying handedness, which, if liberal (e.g., 60% consistent lateral preference), would spuriously elevate the incidence of left- or right-handedness and spuriously lower the incidence of AH. If the mentally retarded subjects from our study are reassigned using a very liberal and dichotomous criterion (50%), 23% fall into the left-handedness group. This proportion compares favorably with those found by others (Dennis & Whitaker, 1977).

We hypothesize that the AH subject represents a stable and reliable handedness phenotype that comprises a subset (approximately 40%) of the autistic and nonautistic mentally retarded population who, because of severe early bilateral brain injury, fail to establish manual dominance. This subtype is most compatible with Palmer's (1964) earlier concept of an undifferentiated handedness (ambilaterality), which he said should be distinguished from left-handedness. According to this theory, handedness develops from originally undifferentiated movement patterns of infancy to progressively more differentiated and asymmetrical skilled movement patterns of adulthood. In the present case, the AH subtype might possibly represent an arrest of this developmental/maturational process due to early brain injury. Interestingly, it was recently demonstrated in a follow-up assessment of normal infants between the ages of 18 and 42 months that in some cases hand preference can be inconsistent (Gottfried & Bathurst, 1983). Consistency of hand preference has virtually never been studied in normals before. Approximately half of the infant sample (47%) revealed inconsistent hand preference on the same item (i.e., draw) across five times probes, which approximates the percentage of AH reported for autistic and nonautistic mentally retarded samples. Also, this inconsistency in response preference is compatible with Palmer's (1964) developmental concept of an undifferentiated handedness. The comparability between the inconsistency observed in the young child and AH suggests the intriguing possibility that the AH, through whatever mechanisms, fail to develop normal manual dominance. Pilot data we have collected indicate a significantly lower rate of inconsistent handedness among normal 2-year-olds than among either our autistic or our nonautistic retarded samples. Hence, if AH does represent arrested development, it would be at a very early stage.

NATURAL LEFT-HANDEDNESS (NLH)

This subtype refers to a subset of the normal adult population whose hand preference is hypothesized to spring from genetic, accidental, and/or cultural factors that are not pathological (Annett, 1972; Bishop, 1980; Hardyck & Petrinovich, 1977; Hecaen & Ajuriaguerra, 1964; Kinsbourne, 1980; Satz, Orsini, Saslow, & Henry, 1985). The incidence of left-handedness, based on writing hand and/or self-report, appears to occur in approximately 8% to 12% of the population (Hardyck & Petrinovich, 1977; Hecaen & Ajuriaguerra, 1964). When assessed by questionnaire or demonstration method, the incidence of left-handedness will vary depending on the number of items and the method of classification used. If multiple items are employed, along with an extreme method of classification (100% of the items with the same hand), then three normal subtypes are typically observed, with a distribution of 5% left-handed, 30% mixed or ambidextrous, and 65% right-handed (Hardyck & Petrinovich, 1977). With fewer items and a less conservative method of classification (90% of items with the same hand), one observes an incidence of left-handedness that approximates that based on writing hand and/or self-report (8%–12%).

It should be noted that the term "mixed" or "ambidextrous" is largely an arbitrary designation based on the assessment and classification method employed. It refers to individuals within the handedness distribution who are less consistently left- or right-handed. Unlike individuals within the AH subtype, however, their hand preferences are consistent for the same task over time.

CONCLUSIONS

Because natural left-handedness (including both extreme and ambidextral left-handedness) is postulated to spring from genetic, accidental, and/or cultural factors, its origins are presumed to be nonpathological. Therefore, one would not predict an adverse outcome in terms of cognitive, achievement, and/or affective development. We propose that the putative link between left-handedness and brain dysfunction exists for only two of the three phenotypes discussed in this chapter, namely PLH and AH. According to this view, both represent neuropathological subtypes, one whose lesion is predominantly left-sided and mild to severe (PLH) and one whose lesion is predominantly bilateral and severe (AH). Note, however, that the PLH subtype represents, and the AH predominantly represents, genotypic dextrals who, because of early brain injury, masquerade as phenotypic nondextrals.

The advantage of this classification is that it partitions much of the variability associated with non-right-handedness into three distinct subtypes, each of which is hypothesized to spring from different etiological substrates. We hypothesize that the third handedness subtype, NLH, constitutes the largest and perhaps the most controversial subset of the nondextral population. Although its genotypic origins still remain unclear (Annett, 1972; Corballis, 1980), there is little evidence to support a neuropathological substrate (Hardyck & Petrinovich, 1977). Nor does the evidence lend much support for a link between left-handedness and cognitive or speech defects when results are based on more representative samples from the "normal" population (Hardyck & Petrinovich, 1977; Hardyck, Petrinovich, & Goldman, 1976). Similar null findings have been reported for reading and learning ability, especially when based on epidemiological surveys of total child populations (Belmont & Birch, 1965; Clark, 1970; Fennell, Satz, & Morris, 1983; Malmquist, 1958; Rutter, Tizard, & Whitmore, 1970; Satz & Fletcher, 1986).

Although these latter studies question a putative link between left-handedness and cognitive deficit for one subset of the nondextral population (NLH), is it possible that this subset represents a more heterogeneous phenotype than described in this chapter. If so, either the extreme left-hand tail of the handedness distribution or those sinistrals who exhibit a more variable hand preference (i.e., ambidexters) may make up an additional subgroup of individuals who, though free of brain damage, still may be at greater risk for autoimmune disorder (Geschwind & Behan, 1982), abnormal brain sensitivity to endocrines (Irwin, 1985), early dementia of the Alzheimer type (Seltzer *et al.*, 1984), and/or tardive dyskinesia (McCreadie *et al.*, 1982). Future studies should determine whether this link, if present, is associated with some of the preceding pathological subtypes and/or with a selected subset of the "normal" NLH subtype. It is unlikely that this search will advance significantly as long as one continues to view nondextrality as a unitary shift in the distribution of human hand preference.

ACKNOWLEDGMENTS

This research was supported, in part, by the following DSH funds: NIH (NS-18462) award to P.S., and NIMH Fellowship (1 F32 MH09082) to HVS. We gratefully acknowledge the help of Donna Gaier and James Stonich in the preparation of this chapter.

REFERENCES

Annett, M. (1972). The distribution of manual asymmetry. *British Journal of Psychology, 63,* 343–358.

Aram, D. M., Ekelman, B. L., & Satz, P. (1986). Tropic changes following early unilateral brain insult. *Developmental Medicine Child Neurology, 28,* 165–170.

Bakan, P. (1977). Left-handedness and birth order revisited. *Neuropsychologia, 15,* 837–839.

Barry, R. J., & James, A. L. (1978). Handedness in autistics, retardates, and normals of a wide age range. *Journal of Autism and Childhood Schizophrenia, 8,* 316–323.

Belmont, L., & Birch, H. G. (1965). Lateral dominance, lateral awareness, and reading disability. *Child Development, 36,* 57–71.
Bishop, D. V. M. (1980). Handedness, clumsiness and cognitive ability. *Developmental Medicine and Child Neurology, 22,* 569–579.
Bradshaw-McAnulty, G., Hicks, R. E., & Kinsbourne, M. (1984). Pathological left-handedness and familial sinistrality in relation to degree of mental retardation. *Brain and Cognition, 3,* 349–356.
Burt, C. (1937). *The backward child.* London: University of London Press.
Clark, M. M. (1970). *Reading difficulties in schools.* Harmondsworth: Penguin.
Colby, K. M., & Parkison, C. (1977). Handedness in autistic children. *Journal of Autism and Childhood Schizophrenia, 7,* 3–9.
Corballis, M. C. (1980). Is left-handedness genetically determined? In J. Herron (Ed.), *Neuropsychology of left-handedness* (pp. 159–176). New York: Academic Press.
Coren, S., & Porac, C. (1977). Fifty centuries of left-handedness: The historical record. *Science, 198,* 631–632.
Dennis, M., & Whitaker, H. A. (1977). Hemispheric equipotentiality and language acquisition. In S. J. Segalowitz & F. A. Gruber (Eds.), *Language development and neurologic theory* (pp. 95–157). New York: Academic Press.
Dvirski, A. E. (1983). Clinical manifestations of schizophrenia in right-handed and left-handed patients. *Zhurnal Neuropatologii i Psichiitri, 83,* 724–728.
Fein, D., Humes, M., Kaplan, E., Lucci, D., & Waterhouse, L. (1984). The question of left hemisphere dysfunction in infantile autism. *Psychological Bulletin, 95,* 258–281.
Fennell, E., Satz, P., & Morris, R. (1983). The development of handedness and dichotic ear listening asymmetries in relation to school achievement: A longitudinal study. *Journal of Experimental Child Psychology, 35,* 248–262.
Geschwind, N. (1983). Biological associations of left-handedness. *Annals of Dyslexia, 33,* 29–40.
Geschwind, N., & Behan, P. (1982). Left-handedness association with immune disease, migraine, and developmental disorder. *Proceedings of the National Academy of Sciences of the United States, 79,* 5097–5100.
Geschwind, N., & Galaburda, A. M. (1985a). Cerebral lateralization. Biological mechanisms, associations, and pathology: I. A hypothesis and a program of research. *Archives of Neurology, 42,* 428–459.
Geschwind, N., & Galaburda, A. M. (1985b). Cerebral lateralization. Biological mechanisms, associations, and pathology: II. A hypothesis and a program of research. *Archives of Neurology, 42,* 521–552.
Geschwind, N., & Galaburda, A. M. (1985c). Cerebral lateralization. Biological mechanisms, associations, and pathology: III. A hypothesis and a program of research. *Archives of Neurology, 42,* 634–654.
Gordon, H. (1920). Left-handedness and mirror writing, especially among defective children. *Brain, 43,* 313–368.
Gottfried, A. W., & Bathurst, K. (1983). Hand preference across time is related to intelligence in young girls, not boys. *Science, 221,* 1074–1076.
Gur, R. E. (1977). Motoric laterality imbalance in schizophrenics: A possible concomitant of left hemisphere dysfunction. *Archives of General Psychiatry, 34,* 33–37.
Hardyck, C., & Petrinovitch, L. F. (1977). Left-handedness. *Psychological Bulletin, 84,* 385–404.
Hardyck, C., Petrinovitch, L. F., & Goldman, R. D. (1976). Left-handedness and cognitive deficit. *Cortex, 12,* 266–279.
Hecaen, H., & Ajuriaguerra, J. D. (1964). *Left-handedness.* New York: Grune and Stratton.
Hicks, R., & Barton, A. (1975). A note on left-handedness and severity of mental retardation. *Journal of General Psychology, 127,* 323–324.
Irwin, P. (1985). Greater brain response of left-handers to drugs. *Neuropsychologia, 23,* 61–67.
Kinsbourne, M. (1980). A model for the ontogeny of cerebral organization in non-right-handers. In J. Herron (Ed.), *Neuropsychology of left-handedness.* New York: Academic Press.
Malmquist, E. (1958). *Factors related to reading disabilities in the first grade of elementary school.* Stockholm: Almqvist and Wiksell.
McCreadie, R. G., Crorie, J., Barron, E. T., & Winslow, G. S. (1982). The Nithsdale schizophrenia survey: III. Handedness and tardive dyskinesia. *British Journal of Psychiatry,* 591–594.
Orsini, D. L., & Satz, P. (1986). A syndrome of pathological left-handedness: Correlates of early left hemisphere injury. *Archives of Neurology, 43,* 333–337.
Palmer, D. (1964). Development of a differentiated handedness. *Psychological Bulletin, 62,* 257–273.
Penfield, W., & Roberts, H. L. (1959). *Speech and brain mechanisms.* Princeton, NJ: Princeton University Press.
Rasmussen, T., & Milner, B. (1977). The role of early brain injury in determining lateralization of cerebral speech functions. *Annals of the New York Academy of Sciences, 299,* 255–269.
Rutter, M., Tizard, J., & Whitmore, K. (1970). *Education, health, and behavior.* London: Longmans.
Satz, P. (1972). Pathological left-handedness: An explanatory model. *Cortex, 8,* 121–137.

Satz, P. (1973). Left-handedness and early brain insults: An explanation. *Neuropsychologia, 11,* 115–117.

Satz, P., & Fletcher, J. M. (1987). Left-handedness and dyslexia: An old myth revisited. *Pediatric Psychology, 12,* 291–298.

Satz, P., Orsini, D. L., Saslow, E., & Henry, R. R. (1985). Early brain injury and pathological left-handedness: Clues to a syndrome. In D. F. Benson & E. Zaidel (Eds.), *Dual brain: Hemispheric specialization in the human* (pp. 117–125). New York: Guilford Press.

Satz, P., Soper, H. V., Orsini, D. L., Henry, R. R., & Zvi, J. C. (1985). Handedness subtypes in autism. *Psychiatric Annals, 15,* 447–451.

Seltzer, B., Burres, M. S. K., & Sherwin, I. (1984). Left-handedness in early and late onset dementia. *Neurology, 34,* 367–369.

Silva, D., & Satz, P. (1979). Pathological left-handedness: Evaluation of a model. *Brain and Language, 7,* 8–16.

Soper, H. V., & Satz, P. (1984). Pathological left-handedness and ambiguous handedness: A new explanatory model. *Neuropsychologia, 22,* 511–515.

Soper, H. V., Satz, P., Orsini, D. L., Henry, R. R., Zvi, J. C., & Schulman, M. (1986). Handedness patterns in autism suggest subtypes. *Journal of Autism and Developmental Disorders, 16,* 155–167.

Soper, H. V., Satz, P., Orsini, D. L., Van Gorp, W. G., and Green, M. F. (1987). Handedness distribution in a residential population with severe or profound mental retardation. *American Journal of Mental Deficiency, 92,* 94–102.

Spennemann, D. R. (1984). Handedness data on the European Neolithic. *Neuropsychologia, 22,* 613–615.

Tizard, J. P. M., Paine, R. S., & Crothers, B. (1954). Disturbances of sensation in children with hemiplegia. *Journal of the American Medical Association. 155,* 628–632.

Tsai, L. Y. (1982). Handedness in autistic children and their families. *Journal of Autism and Developmental Disorders, 12,* 421–423.

Wilson, M. O., & Dolan, L. B. (1931). Handedness and ability. *American Journal of Psychology, 43,* 261–269.

12

Pathological Left-Handedness: An Analysis of Theories and Evidence

LAUREN JULIUS HARRIS
DOUGLAS F. CARLSON
Michigan State University

INTRODUCTION

Throughout history the evidence suggests that left-handers were always in the minority, ranging from only about 2% to 15%–20% of the population. Folk wisdom also linked left-handedness to a variety of undesirable personal characteristics. When left-handedness first came under scientific scrutiny, some of these notions appeared to find support (Harris, 1980a). For example, in 1903 Lombroso reported that left-handedness was three to five times more common in criminals than in law-abiding people. Over the years, the list grew to include degenerates and prostitutes (Audenino, 1907; Lattes, 1907); juvenile delinquents (Smith, 1917); people with "behavior disorders" (Wile, 1932) and "aggressive tendencies" (Burt, 1937, p. 317); and people, especially children, with speech and reading problems (e.g., Ballard, 1911–1912; Buchanan, 1908). Compared to the normal population, left-handedness also was reported to be roughly twice as common among mental retardates (Gordon, 1920; Hildreth, 1949) and epileptics (Mayet, 1902, cited in Gordon, 1920; Redlich, 1908; and Steiner, 1911, cited in Bingley, 1958).

New Studies of Characteristics Associated with Left-Handedness

Much of the old evidence consists of anecdotal reports, case histories, and surveys of perhaps questionable validity and reliability. Over the last two decades, however, a vast amount of new research has been completed. The result has been support for at least some of the old ideas. In at least two broad categories, epilepsy and mental retardation, the link to left-handedness appears reasonably well confirmed by a relatively large number of individual investigations (see Table 12-1).[1]

EPILEPSY

With respect to epilepsy (individuals with known CNS dysfunction), the newer evidence indicates that the percentage of left-handers is indeed roughly double that of control populations, as the early reports had said (e.g., Hecaen & Ajuriaguerra, 1964; Milner, Branch,

1. In making these assessments, we have *not* used the statistical technique that is the method of choice today for asking such questions, namely, meta-analysis. No one to date has carried out such analyses, although for several of the reported associations, the number of available studies is large enough for this statistical procedure. The data summary given in the text is for illustrative purposes only and does not constitute an exhaustive account of the literature. The references cited were chosen as representative of the research in that category.

Table 12-1. Characteristics Reported to Be Associated with Left-Handedness

Category and examples	Reviews or representative reports
Explicit neurological dysfunction:	
Epilepsy	Hecaen & Ajuriaguerra (1964); Penfield & Roberts (1959); Roberts (1958); Satz, Yanowitz, & Wilmore (1984)
Language/speech-related disorders:	
Reading disability (including dyslexia) and developmental language disorders)	Bishop (1983); Neils & Aram (1986)
Intellectual, academic achievement:	
Mental retardation	Bradshaw-McAnulty, Hicks, & Kinsbourne (1984); Ross, Lipper, & Auld (1987)
Grade repeaters	Hicks & Barton (1975)
Psychiatric disorders:	
Attempted suicide	Chayette & Smith (1981)
Psychosis	Lishman & McMeekan (1976)
Milder psychological problems:	
Anxiety	Hicks & Pelligrini (1978)
"Emotionality"	Orme (1970)
Neuroticism	Mascie-Taylor (1981)
Use of licit stimulant and depressive drugs:	
Alcohol	Harburg (1981); Lee-Feldstein & Harburg (1982)
Cigarettes	Harburg, Feldstein, & Papsdorf (1978)
Reactivity to drugs:	Irwin & Fink (1981); Irwin (1985)
Antisocial behavior:	
Aggression, delinquency	Gabrielli & Mednick (1980)
Physical ailments:	
Allergy	Geschwind & Behan (1982)
Autoimmune disorders	Kinsbourne & Bemporad (1984)
Migraine	

& Rasmussen, 1964; Penfield & Roberts, 1959; Roberts, 1958; Satz, Yanowitz, & Wilmore, 1984). The increase, however, is not invariable (e.g., see Bingley, 1958, p. 137; McManus, 1980).

MENTAL RETARDATION

Left-handedness also appears to be more frequent in mental retardates, many of whom presumably have CNS dysfunction (e.g., Bradshaw-McAnulty, Hicks, & Kinsbourne, 1984; Hicks & Barton, 1975; Batheja & McManus, 1985). As with the epilepsy data, the percentage is roughly double that found in the normal population (e.g., Batheja & McManus, 1985; Bradshaw-McAnulty *et al.*, 1984; Hicks & Barton, 1975). For example, in one study (Ross, Lipper, & Auld, 1987), 98 4-year-old children with IQs under 85 were compared with 54 children with normal IQs on a test of hand preference. In the under-85 IQ group, 19% were left-handed, compared to 11% of the normal controls. In these studies, however, the rise in the percentage of left-handers appears to be predominantly among the more severely retarded individuals (those more likely to have CNS dysfunction); among the mild or moderately retarded, the number of left-handers is scarcely different from that found in normal controls. In one study of 550 institutionalized mental retardates, most of whom were adolescents, only 13% of the mild to moderate retardates (36–67 IQ) were left-handed, compared to 28% among the severe and profoundly retarded (IQ below 20–35) (Hicks & Barton, 1975; see also Bradshaw-McAnulty *et al.*, 1984).

READING, SPEECH, AND LANGUAGE DISORDERS

For reading, speech, and language disorders, the data are inconsistent, both from direct comparisons of disabled and control subjects and from epidemiological surveys of total child populations, so that no strong conclusions seem possible at this time. In the case of reading disabilities, on the positive side, Bishop (1983) listed 17 separate studies in which retarded readers were compared to normal controls. By our count, in 12 studies, the percentage of left-handers was higher (average = 12.8%) among the retarded readers than among the normal controls (average = 6.8%)—thus a 90% surplus of left-handers among the retarded groups. On the negative side, in one of the remaining five studies in Bishop's review, the percentage of left-handers was equal (3%) in each group; and in the other four studies there were actually more left-handers in the control groups (11.25%) than in the retarded-reader groups (5.5%). Similar null findings have been reported by Belmont and Birch (1965); Fennell, Satz, and Morris (1983); Hardyck, Petrinovich, and Goldman (1976); Malmquist (1958); and Rutter, Tizard, and Whitmore (1970).

As for speech disorders, although some new studies have reported an association between left-handedness and speech and other articulatory problems, such as stuttering (e.g., Geschwind & Behan, 1982; see review in Bishop, 1983), the majority of new studies have not (e.g., Bishop, 1986; Calnan & Richardson, 1976; Douglas, Ross, & Cooper, 1967; Rosenfield, 1980; see review by Homzie & Lindsay, 1984). One potential confound in such comparisons is intelligence, since evidence suggests that where left-handedness is associated with speech problems, both are covariates of lower intelligence (Ross *et al.*, 1987). Another potential confound is the severity of the disorder. Neils and Aram (1986) found that non-right-handedness was more common only in children with severe language disorders (see Chapter 15 by Aram, this volume). Consistent with this possibility, an association between left-handedness and dyslexia seems to be clearest in dyslexics who also have a history of retardation in the development of speech, with difficulties in speech and sometimes also in comprehension as late as 4 or 5 years of age (Ingram, 1964).

AUTISM

It has been reported also that left-handedness is more common in young autistic children (e.g., Hauser, DeLong, & Rosman, 1975). More recent reports, however, have questioned these findings (see review in Fein, Humes, Kaplan, Lucci, & Waterhouse, 1984).

OTHER CATEGORIES

For still other categories, because of the small number of studies, no strong conclusions appear to be possible at this time, although the evidence is at least suggestive. These include reports of an association between left-handedness and certain psychiatric disorders (e.g., Chayette & Smith, 1981; Gur, 1977, Lishman & McMeekan, 1976; Shan-Ming *et al.*, 1985; but see McCreadie, Crorie, Barron, & Winslow, 1982, for a contrary view); the use of licit stimulant and depressive drugs such as cigarettes and alcohol (Harburg, 1981;

Harburg, Feldstein, & Papsdorf, 1978; Lee-Feldstein & Harburg, 1982); milder psychological disorders such as anxiety (Hicks & Pelligrini, 1978), "emotionality" (Orme, 1970), neuroticism (Mascie-Taylor, 1981), and difficulty in sleeping (Coren & Searleman, 1987); and antisocial behavior as indexed by juvenile delinquency (Gabrielli & Mednick, 1980). New reports also indicate that left-handers may be significantly more responsive than right-handers to neuroactive drugs (Irwin, 1985; Irwin & Fink, 1981).

PHYSICAL AILMENTS

Finally, Geschwind and Behan (1982) have proposed that the left-hander's problems might be physical and medical as well as psychological. They found that, in comparison to right-handers, left-handers suffer disproportionately more often from immune disorders, in particular disorders affecting the gastrointestinal tract such as regional ileitis (Crohn's disease), ulcerative colitis, and celiac disease. In strongly left-handed individuals those who gave only left-hand answers on the handedness questionnaire), such disorders were about three times more common than in strongly right-handed individuals. There also were about twice as many left-handers among individuals with well-diagnosed migraine headaches as in the general population. These original findings have been challenged on statistical grounds (Satz & Soper, 1986) and obviously need corroboration. To date, the evidence from new studies is inconclusive, with some reports positive (Bemporad & Kinsbourne, 1983; Searleman & Fugagli, 1987; also see Chapter 10 by Kinsbourne, this volume) and others negative (Bishop, 1986).

Left-Handedness and Psychological Performance in Nonclinical Populations

Lest we end this section on too bleak a note (at least so far as left-handers are concerned), we hasten to add that most of the positive evidence described thus far applies predominantly to clinical populations. Where left-handers and right-handers are compared in unselected samples of the general population, the evidence is far less clear that left-handers are psychologically impaired compared to right-handers. Reference already has been made to recent studies of reading and speech problems. Similar comparisons have failed to disclose any differences between right- and left-handers in intelligence, school performance, or other standard measures of intellectual achievement (Hardyck & Petrinovich, 1977). Indeed, some studies have suggested that left-handers actually excel in nonverbal or visual–spatial–constructional abilities (e.g., Annett & Kilshaw, 1982; Byrne & Sinclair, 1979; Deutsch, 1978; Mebert & Michel, 1980; Herrman & Van Dyke, 1978), although others have found just the reverse (Levy, 1969, 1974) (see review in Harshman, Hampson, & Berenbaum, 1983). Still other studies have suggested that left-handedness is over-represented among children with extremely high ability in mathematical reasoning (Benbow, 1986; Benbow & Benbow, 1984). The important point, then, is that there is no evidence that left-handers in the general population are intellectually *deficient* compared to right-handers.

THEORIES

At least a few of the old reports about left-handedness thus have been corroborated, and perhaps other old notions, as well as some new ones, are on the way to finding support as

Table 12-2. Explanations of Association between Left-Handedness (LH) and Psychological Problems and/or Neurological Dysfunction

Models	Explanation	Major advocate or representative analysis
Unilateral brain lesion	Rise in LH reflects contribution of PLH due to discrete lesion.	
Two-type model	Other LH is ''normal.''	Satz, Orsini, Saslow, & Henry (1985a, 1985b)
One-type model	All LH = PLH, whether or not it is associated with cognitive/behavioral disorders.	Bakan, Dibb, & Reed (1973)
Developmental neural dysfunction	LH is product of hormone-induced slowing of left-hemisphere maturation.	Geschwind & Behan (1982)
Neurobiological noise	Rise in LH reflects neurobiological insult at critical developmental period.	McManus (1984)
Left-handedness as a normal marker of higher risk	LH is not the result of pathological process but is biological marker of higher risk for psychological/physiological dysfunction.	Irwin & Fink (1981)
Social prejudice	Psychological problems arise from social prejudice against left-hand use.	Wile (1932); Young & Knapp (1966)

well. How, then, to account for these findings? Table 12-2 outlines five different explanations, or models.

Unilateral Brain Lesion Model of Pathological Left-Handedness (PLH)

One proposal is that left-handers are more common in certain *clinical* populations as a result of a discrete unilateral brain lesion. This possibility has been the major focus of attention among neuropsychologists today and will be the major focus of our analysis.

TWO-TYPE MODEL: SOME LEFT-HANDEDNESS IS PATHOLOGICAL

The unilateral brain lesion model has two variants. The first variant supposes that the surplus left-handers found in these clinical populations, in particular among epileptics and mental retardates, are actually genotypic right-handers whose left-handedness and associated symptoms both originate in injury to the left hemisphere of the cerebral cortex. These individuals thus are said to have pathological left-handedness (PLH), an *abnormal* condition initiated by injury or disease processes leading to certain structural and functional changes in the left hemisphere. In contrast, left-handers in the *general population* are presumed to be neurologically normal. We shall call this the *two-type* model.

The notion that there are two subtypes within the population of left-handers, one pathological (PLH), the other not, has precedents in 19th- and early-20th-century writings. For example, Lattes (1907) distinguished what he called ''constitutional'' left-handedness, which he assumed resulted from an inversion of normal cerebral asymmetry, from the pathological type, manifested after a left cerebral lesion. The latter, he believed, was the predominant type in epileptics and delinquents (cited in Jordan, 1911, p. 24). Gordon (1920) made a similar distinction to explain why, when twins were opposite in handedness and one twin was mentally retarded, the other normal, the retarded twin was far more often the left-hander. The left-handed twin, Gordon suggested, ''had been driven to the use of the left hand by some defect of the left hemisphere'' (Gordon, 1920, p. 362).

The same distinction has been made by more recent investigators, including Bingley

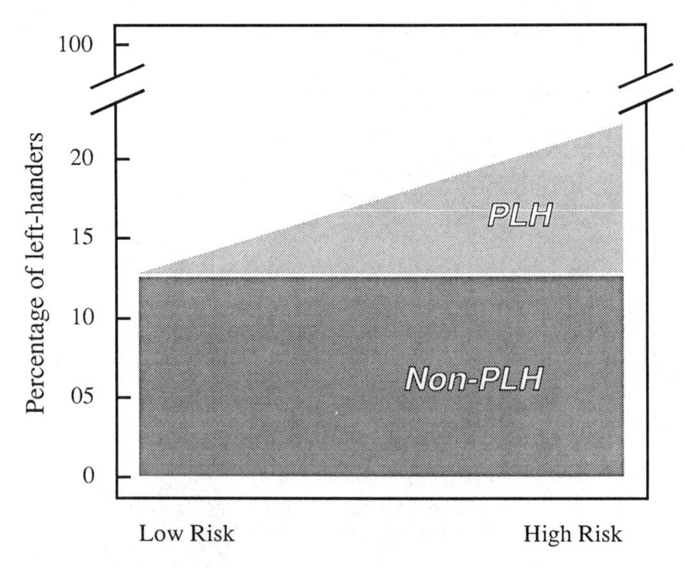

Figure 12-1. Hypothetical distribution of left-handers (PLH and non-PLH) along a continuum of risk for neurological insult: the two-type variant of the unilateral lesion model.

(1958); Schmidt and Wilder (1968); and, most prominently, Satz (e.g., 1972, 1973). Satz's version of the two-type model makes two basic assumptions: The first is that the location of brain lesions is a *random* process, just as likely to strike the left hemisphere as the right. Thus, in statistical terms, unilateral brain damage is a binomial function. Satz's second assumption is that *left*-hemisphere lesions lead to the greater incidence of *switched* handedness because there are far more right-handed people in the general population. Consequently, when early brain injury causes a change in hand dominance, the result more often will be pathological left-handedness (PLH) than pathological right-handedness (PRH).

We have illustrated this model in Figure 12-1, which shows a hypothetical distribution of the two kinds of left-handedness along a continuum of risk for neurological insult from low to high.[2] The bottom part of the figure represents the percentage of left-handers who would be expected to be non-PLH. We have set this figure arbitrarily at 12% (the approximate percentage of left-handers in the general normal population, to be discussed in the next section), and we have assumed that it does not change as a function of neurological risk. The top part of the figure represents the proportion of additional left-handers who would be expected to be PLH as a function of their position along the continuum of risk. Therefore, at the low-risk end, left-handedness should occur in about 12% of the population and should be of the nonpathological type. By contrast, at the high-risk end, where we would expect epilepsy and mental retardation, among other disorders, to be prevalent, the number of left-handers would be expected to rise, with the surplus being contributed by PLH and with the magnitude of the surplus depending on a variety of epidemiological factors.

2. As we shall see when we come to the second variant of the unilateral lesion model, the continuum of "risk for neurological insult" also can be cast in the form of a "continuum of reproductive casualty" to designate risk factors specifically associated with pregnancy and delivery (Pasamanick & Knobloch, 1961). We discuss this concept in greater detail in a later section.

We emphasize that this diagram is for illustrative purposes only. As we said, we have chosen a 12% base rate arbitrarily, and the slope shown in the top part of the figure implies a linear contribution of risk to PLH. The relationship might just as easily be curvilinear. Obviously, it depends on how risk is defined, where the threshold is set for its effect on hand use, and the possibility of a cumulative effect of multiple risk variables, among other factors (these questions will be addressed in a later section).

ONE-TYPE MODEL: ALL LEFT-HANDEDNESS IS PATHOLOGICAL

The second variant of the unilateral brain lesion model takes the notion of PLH to an extreme: It supposes that not just some, but *all,* left-handedness is pathological—that is, that all left-handers are actually genotypic right-handers. Therefore, in clinically asymptomatic left-handers (those who do *not* show any psychological dysfunction) the left-cerebral dysfunction was sufficiently mild so that left-handedness is the only symptom. We shall call this the *one-type* model.

In contrast to the two-type model, the one-type model seems to be without precedent in the early literature. Even those who regarded *all* left-handers as ''odd'' did not suggest that the left-handedness itself could result only from pathological process.

The originator of the one-type model is Bakan (e.g., Bakan, 1971; Bakan, Dibb, & Reed, 1973), according to whom left-handedness is probably the most prevalent and most benign of the conditions of neurological insult associated with birth stress. By this view, Bakan therefore adds left-handedness to the ''continuum of reproductive casuality'' (Pasamanick & Knobloch, 1961) as one of the ''minor effects of birth stress'' (Bakan, Dibb, & Reed, 1973, p. 365).

In Figure 12-2, we have illustrated the one-type model diagrammatically in terms of the same continuum of neurological risk as was shown in Figure 12-1 for the two-type model, except that now the risk factor is seen as associated with one's position along a ''continuum of reproductive casualty.'' Recall from the two-type model that at the low-

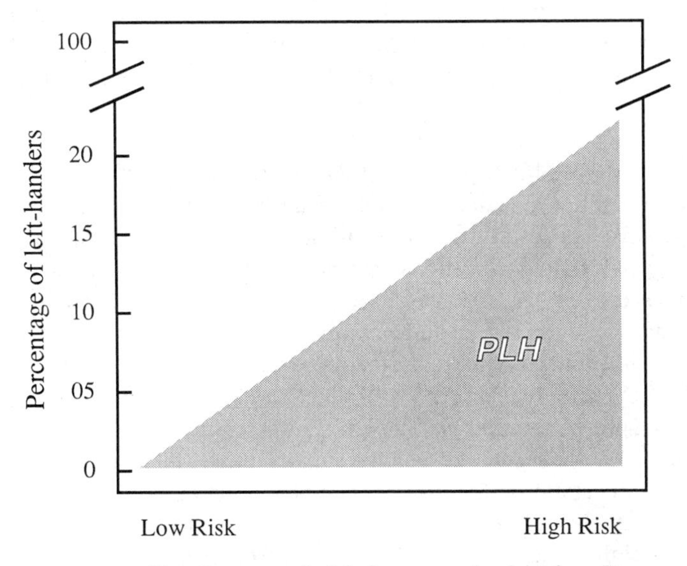

Figure 12-2. Hypothetical distribution of left-handers (all left-handedness = PLH) along a continuum of risk for neurologial insult: the one-type variant of the unilateral lesion model.

risk end of the continuum (which, in terms of the one-type model, encompasses the range from no birth stress to minor stress), we had expected left-handedness to appear in about 12% of the population, to be of the nonpathological type, and therefore to be psychologically unexceptional. By contrast, according to the one-type model, left-handedness should be absent altogether at the extreme low end of the continuum of risk (i.e., where birth stress itself is at the absolute minimum) and should appear with increasing frequency as birth stress increases. The models thus diverge at the low end of the continuum. They also diverge at the high end, where some evidence, as already noted, shows an approximate doubling of the percentage of left-handedness. Whereas the two-type model attributes the surplus to the cases of PLH, the one-type model implies that the left-handedness is PLH in *every* case, and thus the rise in the percentage of left-handedness is commensurate with the rise in the severity of birth stress. The one-type model thus must show that those left-handers who, by the two-type model, are neurologically normal, are in fact victims of left-hemisphere trauma sufficient to shift hand preference but without any associated neurological disorders. To do this, Bakan has argued that in left-handers who are asymptomatic and ostensibly neurologically normal (e.g., college students), the occurrence of minor neurological trauma, as indexed indirectly by birth stress, is significantly higher than among their right-handed counterparts.

The two models differ in still other ways. One implied difference is apparent in a comparison of the *slope* of the PLH distribution in Figures 12-1 and 12-2. To the extent that the models agree on the percentage of left-handers at the high end of the distribution, they must hold different assumptions about the cumulative effect of risk variables for PLH. Another difference is in the assumption about the probability of risk to each cerebral hemisphere. As already noted, Satz has assumed that the hemispheres are equally at risk for injury. Where hand preference is affected, however, the result more likely will be pathological left-handedness (PLH) than pathological right-handedness (PRH) because the base frequency of right-handers in the general population is greater than that of left-handers. Bakan, by contrast, assumes that the cerebral hemispheres are *not* equally at risk, and that the left hemisphere is the more susceptible. Because Bakan also denies that any left-handedness is "natural" and asserts instead that all individuals are genotypic *right*-handers, his model, in contrast to Satz's, seems to preclude the possibility of pathological *right*-handedness (PRH).

UNILATERAL LESION MODEL OF PLH AND LOCALIZATION OF LANGUAGE

A question relevant to both variants of the unilateral lesion model of PLH is the consequence of left-hemisphere injury on localization of language and the further implications for understanding psychological deficits associated with left-handedness. We can imagine several different scenarios. In each case, we use genotypic right-handers as our reference group because, as already noted, candidates for pathological handedness will come chiefly from their ranks. Only in this group, furthermore, can we be fairly sure of the pattern of speech lateralization, namely, that 95% to 99% of these individuals have speech lateralized to the left hemisphere (Lhermitte & Gautier, 1969; Rasmussen & Milner, 1977; Sperry, 1974). By contrast, the pattern of speech dominance in left-handers is less certain. If there is a consensus, it appears to be that the left hemisphere is predominant in speech functions in 60% to 70% of the cases (but see Satz, 1979, for a different estimate), with the rest either bilateral or right-lateralized, but with little agreement on the nature of or incidence of occurrence of the latter categories (Annett, 1975; Hecaen & Sauget, 1971; Kimura, 1983b; Milner, Branch, & Rasmussen, 1966; Rasmussen & Milner, 1977). The possibility also has been raised that certain verbal functions that are subserved by the same, that is, left, hemisphere in right-handers are laterally dissociated in left-handers, for example, visual and auditory verbal analysis (Herron, Galin, Johnstone, & Ornstein, 1979; McKeever & Hoff, 1979; Smith & Moscovitch, 1979; also see discussion in Levy, 1982).

If, for the sake of argument, we could assume that the known pattern of speech lateralization in genotypic *right-handers* conforms reasonably well to the pattern for language functions generally (a still open question, so far as we know), then injury to the left hemisphere could result hypothetically in any one of at least three outcomes with respect to PLH:

1. *Control for hand shifts from left to right hemisphere, while control for language remains on the left side, with no cognitive impairment.* The first possibility pertains to the PLH individual who is clinically asymptomatic. This implies that the lesion that forced a shift in hand control has not encroached on left-hemisphere language zones, so that language functions are not compromised. This, presumably, is the situation that Bakan would invoke to explain left-handedness among the general population.

2. *Control for hand shifts from left to right hemisphere, while control for language remains on the left side, with cognitive impairment.* We can imagine a variant on the first possibility according to which left-hemisphere injury causes a shift of hand control from left to right and encroaches on language zones sufficiently to cause language impairment, but without shifting language from left side to right. The result would be PLH associated with symptoms of left-hemisphere (language) dysfunction. This, presumably, is the condition that Bakan would invoke to explain any association found between, say, language disorders and left-handedness.

3. *Control for hand and language shifts from left to right hemisphere.* A third possibility is that the cerebral insult that causes hand control to change from the left hemisphere to the right will also tend to cause language control to shift to the extent that the lesion encroaches significantly on language zones of the left hemisphere. This is the situation that Satz (Satz, Orsini, Saslow, & Henry, 1985a, 1985b) appears to have called a prerequisite to any pathologically induced change in handedness. There is, in fact, some independent evidence for this joint outcome in cases of early left-hemisphere injury (Rasmussen & Milner, 1977), which we shall discuss later in the section evaluating the two-type unilateral lesion model. The question is: What would be the cognitive consequences? One possibility is that there would be language dysfunction in adulthood to the extent that the healthy right hemisphere is inherently a less adequate substrate for language than the left. Alternatively, the more prominent cognitive loss might be in spatial–perceptual functioning to the extent that the shifting of language to the right hemisphere compromises visual–spatial function through "cognitive crowding." Such a mechanism has already been invoked to account for this very pattern of deficits in clinical populations of genotypic right-handers with early left-hemisphere injury (Lansdell, 1969) but also to explain differences in the patterns of verbal and spatial skill between normal right-handers with unilateral speech representation and normal left-handers with presumptive bilateral speech representation (Levy, 1969, 1974). In this case, PLH would be associated with spatial dysfunction but not with language dysfunction, or at least the more prominent cognitive impairment would be nonlinguistic. Later, we shall discuss evidence pertaining to these two alternatives in cases of putative PLH.

In summary, there are at least three different scenarios in which left-hemisphere injury in genotypic right-handers might result in PLH with different, and even mutually exclusive, outcomes for cognitive performance.

PLH MODELS AND AFFECTIVE DYSFUNCTION

Can any of these three scenarios also account for the suggested link between left-handedness and affective dysfunctions? By now there is a growing consensus that the cortex plays an important role in the mediation of emotion (Heilman & Satz, 1983). Evidence suggests that the two hemispheres play somewhat different roles in this process, depending on whether the process is perceptual or expressive, and on whether the emotion is positive or negative. According to this new evidence, in perception the right hemisphere is more important, irrespective of emotional valence (e.g., Bryden & Ley, 1983; Carlson & Harris, 1985b). For expression, however, it has been suggested that the left hemisphere plays the leading role for positive emotions, or approach tendencies, and the right hemisphere for negative emotions, or avoidance tendencies (Kinsbourne & Bemporad, 1984; see also Chapter 7 by Davidson and Chapter 3 by Denenberg, this volume). The model supposes that the two hemispheres normally function in a state of mutual balance, with the negative expressive functions of the right hemisphere normally held in check through the inhibitory influences of the left hemisphere. According to the second scenario, we therefore could predict that left-hemisphere injury that causes dysfunction but without shifting language to the right side may reduce the capacity of the left hemisphere to inhibit the right hemisphere. If we can accept the still slim evidence, discussed earlier, associating left-handedness with emotional disorders, especially perhaps with disorders involving impulse control (e.g., delinquency), and if we assume further that at least some of these left-handers are PLH, might we be seeing the consequences of the release of the right hemisphere from inhibition by the left? Alternatively, following the third scenario, if a shift of language functions to the right hemisphere compromises spatial–perceptual skills, might right-hemisphere emotional functions be compromised as well, including those functions tied to language (e.g., prosody; see Ross & Mesulam, 1979)? If so, then the result in scenario 2 might be "acting-out" behavior; in scenario 3 it might be impaired emotional perception.

Developmental Neural Dysfunction Model

Model 2 is what we have chosen to call the "developmental neural dysfunction model." (It also could be called a "pathological" model, but with the understanding that, unlike the unilateral brain lesion models, the pathology is not assumed to stem from a brain lesion.) This model, proposed by Geschwind (Geschwind & Behan, 1982; Geschwind & Galaburda, 1985), was inspired by evidence that left-handedness as well as language disorders were more common in males than in females (see later sections on sex as a factor; pp. 311–312, 333). This led Geschwind to suggest that the mechanism for this sex difference is fetal testosterone, which is present in greater amounts in males than in females. According to the model, fetal testosterone slows *left*-hemispheric maturation, thereby giving the right hemisphere a lead in development and raising the likelihood of left-handedness, that is, of right-hemisphere dominance for movement of the limbs and for praxis. A further assumption is that in the extreme case, the slowing of left-hemisphere maturation may result in anomalous left-cerebral organization at a cellular level with associated cognitive dysfunction, including dyslexia. The model also has been invoked to explain the reported (but as we also said, disputed) link between left-handedness and autism on the assumption that the primary deficit in this disorder is linguistic-communicative, that is, in the left hemisphere (Geschwind & Galaburda, 1985; McCann, 1981). The model also attempts to account for the association of left-handedness with immune disorders of the sort listed earlier by postulating concomitant action of fetal testosterone on the developing thymus, a crucial organ in the immune system. The etiology of cognitive dysfunction in left-handers thus lies in neurodevelopmental processes that, during prenatal development, deviate sufficiently from the normal pattern to cause behavioral dysfunction.

There is one other important difference between the developmental neural dysfunction model and the two variants of the unilateral lesion model. Whereas both models seek to explain the behavioral and psychological deficits associated with left-handedness, the developmental neural dysfunction model also allows for the possibility that any deficits can be compensated by other, positive features. Specifically, Geschwind has predicted that left-handedness, if produced by a slowing of the growth of the left hemisphere, may be associated with superior right-hemisphere skills inasmuch as left-sided slowing allows compensatory cortical development on the right side. In support of this prediction, Geschwind cites reports of the kind described in the Introduction that normal left-handers excel over right-handers in visual–spatial skill. (The negative reports are ignored.) Geschwind also cites a report that dyslexic children have superior visual–spatial skills compared to non-dyslexic controls (Gordon, 1983). By contrast, neither variant of the unilateral lesion model, at least in their current forms, predicts any compensating feature in intellect. That is, neither variant predicts that individuals with PLH will be *superior* to right-handers (one-type model) or to either right-handers or nonpathological left-handers (two-type model).

"Neurobiological Noise" Model

Despite the differences between the two variants of the unilateral brain lesion model, and despite the further differences between this model and the developmental neural dysfunction model, both models see left-handedness arising from factors that act *directly* on the *left* hemisphere. In some cases, however, an increase in left-handedness has been found where unilateral brain injury seems unlikely. For example, in one of the studies of left-handedness and mental retardation cited earlier (Batheja & McManus, 1985), the incidence of left-handedness was 28.9% in a subgroup of retarded individuals with Down syndrome, 26.7% in a subgroup of non-Down retardates, and 10.6% in a group of normal children. As the authors pointed out, a unilateral injury is unlikely to have been the mechanism underlying the increased left-handedness in the Down syndrome group, since neuropathology in Down syndrome is usually diffuse and nonspecific (Crome, 1965, p. 225; see also Warkany, Lemire, & Cohen, 1981). Batheja and McManus (1985) therefore proposed an alternative explanation, not only for Down syndrome but for other clinical subgroups as well. According to this model, which we shall call a "neurobiological noise" model, a majority of the population early in development show directional asymmetry and hence become right-handed. Biological insults of any form at this critical early period can result in increased "biological noise" and hence a reversion to the more atavistic state of "fluctuating asymmetry," in the ultimate form of which 50% of the population is left-handed (p. 66). The difference from Satz's model "is that the individual has not acquired right-handedness and subsequently lost it as a result of an asymmetric lesion, but rather has never had it in the first place. It is not that there are more ex-right-handers; there are more left handers *de nova*" (Batheja & McManus, 1985, p. 66).[3]

3. Batheja & McManus seem to be implying that Satz has assumed that right-handedness is already established before the lesion occurs. We understand Satz to mean only that, were it not for the lesion, the child would become right-handed, that is, that the lesion has disrupted the phenotypic expression of a right-handed genotype. We therefore do not see Batheja and McManus's objection as referring to a critical part of Satz's (or Bakan's) model. For purposes of this review, we therefore have supposed that the *critical* difference between the "neurobiological noise" and the "unilateral lesion" model is the presumed necessity of a *unilateral* locus of pathology.

Left-Handedness as Normal Marker for Risk of Dysfunction

Some of the evidence that left-handers are "different" seems hard to reconcile with any of the aforementioned models. For example, if left-hemisphere dysfunction does underlie the association between left-handedness and certain language disorders, how could this also explain the left-hander's reportedly greater responsivity to neuroactive drugs or more frequent use of tobacco and alcohol, discussed earlier, unless we define "psychological disorder" so broadly as to rob the first three models of any usefulness whatsoever?

As an alternative, consider the possibility that left-handedness, even when associated with dysfunctional states, is itself *not* pathological, whether it is the result of a discrete unilateral lesion, a testosterone-initiated developmental neural dysfunction, or neurobiological noise at some critical developmental period. Perhaps left-handedness, like right-handedness, instead is an expression of a normal developmental process that, nevertheless, signifies one's membership in a subgroup of the population at higher risk, compared to right-handers, for psychological and physical dysfunction. By this same reasoning, we might suppose that at least some of the surplus left-handers in clinical populations (possibly more in some than in others) are "natural" rather than pathological left-handers but, as such, are more susceptible to whatever neural trauma has produced their dysfunction. Note that by this new model, the percentage of left-handers in the non-PLH population does not remain constant as a function of neurological risk as it does for the two-type unilateral lesion model (compare with Figure 12-1). Instead it *increases*.

The challenge for *this* model is to explain what there is about the normal developmental process whereby one becomes left-handed—whatever it may be—that puts the individual at higher risk for certain psychological, not to mention physical, disabilities. There may be several possibilities. For example, because left-handers as a group are far more heterogeneous in cerebral lateral organization than are right-handers (Milner, Branch, & Rasmussen, 1966), perhaps the cerebral organization of certain subgroups of left-handers puts them at greater risk for dysfunction for those cognitive and/or emotional functions best served by the modal form of laterality.

Social Prejudice Model

Finally, at least some of the psychological disorders associated with left-handedness, rather than signifying some abnormal condition of the nervous system, may instead be the result of social prejudice against left-handers (an issue to be discussed in the next section). To use the historically most familiar example, the left-handed child was said to be more at risk for stuttering because his parents and teachers were presumed to have interfered with his hand use at a critical period in his development of speech and manual skills. The assumption has been that similar prejudicial treatment can lead to emotional problems (see Young & Knapp, 1966). Eliminate this treatment and the left-handed child's "pathological" behavior disappears (see review in Harris, 1980a).

As we said, our analysis will be predominantly concerned with model 1, the unilateral brain lesion model in both of its variant forms, and less with the other models. Model 2 (developmental neurodysfunction) is discussed elsewhere (Chapter 10 by Kinsbourne, this volume), and the evidence pertaining to models 3, 4, and 5 is still sparse and would take us too far afield from our major topic. We also have not tried to review and analyze *all* of the empirical data bearing on either variant of model 1. Our emphasis instead will be on conceptual, methodological, and neuroanatomical issues that, to date, have received relatively little attention in connection with PLH theories. We believe, in any case, that until *these* issues are clarified, no definitive conclusions about *any* model are possible.

At the outset, we might note what should already be clear from the number and variety of dysfunctional, or at least unconventional, characteristics that have been linked to left-handedness: The answer is not likely to be found in any single explanatory model. We also note that, except for the difference between the two-type and one-type variants of the unilateral lesion model, none of the models should be regarded as mutually exclusive. As we proceed, some of the further similarities, and differences, will become apparent.

MEASUREMENT OF HANDEDNESS AND DISTRIBUTION IN THE GENERAL POPULATION

As we have seen, all the models assume that the percentage of left-handedness will vary according to certain conditions. Models 1 through 4 suppose that it will be higher in certain subgroups or clinical populations. Model 5 (social prejudice) supposes instead, as we shall see, that it might be lower, on the further assumption that certain social practices can *suppress* the manifestation of left-handedness. Before the unilateral lesion models, or for that matter any of the models, can be evaluated, several preliminary issues need to be addressed.

To begin with, we could not hope to undertake an analysis of PLH unless we understand and can measure handedness in its normative state. The first issue, then, is the definition and measurement of handedness, and the assessment of its distribution in the general population.

Definition of Handedness

By "handedness," we ordinarily mean that the arms and hands are asymmetrical in use and function so as to reliably favor one hand or the other across a range of skillful acts. Our reference point in this discussion will be the modal form, right-handedness.

"DOMINANT" RIGHT HAND

Manual asymmetry typically is manifested for acts that call for complex, coordinated sequences of movements involving the distal musculature—the hands and fingers. The dominant, or right, hand also is more skilled and more often used in acts calling for finely modulated application of force, such as hammering or drawing. Because of the structure of the hand–brain system (to be discussed later), this right-hand specialization is assumed to reflect the inherent specialization of the contralateral (left) cerebral hemisphere for analysis of sensory input as discrete, finely tuned stimuli within a temporal frame and for the programming of serially organized discrete movements (Bradshaw & Nettleton, 1981; Levy, 1974; Witelson, 1985).

"NONDOMINANT" LEFT HAND

The nondominant left hand, by contrast, is typically used for actions that support the role of the right hand, for example, holding while the right hand manipulates. Certain of these supportive roles, however, require specialized skills in which the *left* hand may truly excel—for example, in analyzing the spatial contours or configurational properties of objects prior to manipulation by the dominant hand (e.g., Harris, 1980b) and for controlling spatial positions of the effectors, as demonstrated by accuracy in open-loop ballistic aimed movements (Guiard, Diaz, & Beaubaton, 1983; but see Todor & Cisneros, 1985). These special functions may be seen as reflecting the inherent specialization of the contralateral (right) cerebral hemisphere for the synthesis of stimuli over the dimensions of time and space into holistic or gestaltlike configurations (Cohen, 1973; Levy, 1974).

We have begun with a characterization of hand skills in right-handers because it is the group from which any potential PLH individuals would come. With respect to the one-type variant of the unilateral lesion model, right-handers therefore would constitute the primary comparison group for the assessment of motor and cognitive function in PLH individuals. In the case of the two-type model, however, there must also be a way to distinguish the pathological from the nonpathological left-hander, meaning that we would have to rely on norms for hand skill in left-handers in the general population. Here, as already pointed out, the evidence is much less abundant, but what there is suggests that left-handers are not simply the mirror image of right-handers in hand skill. For example, in regularity and speed of finger tapping, left- and right-handers do not differ in skill with the preferred hand, but left-handers are superior to right-handers in performance with the nonpreferred hand, thus resulting in smaller between-hand differences (Peters & Durding, 1979).

Evaluation of Handedness in Adults

The preceding discussion implies that the complete characterization of handedness must consider both the distinct and the complementary specializations of both hands, and that the evaluation of handedness should include assessment of non-dominant-hand as well as dominant-hand skills. This has not been the practice. Instead, tests of handedness have compared the hands on only dominant-hand skills.

QUESTIONNAIRES AND PERFORMANCE TESTS

To assess handedness in normal adults, that is, in individuals whose handedness is presumed to be fully established, both questionnaires and tests of skill are commonly used.

In questionnaires (e.g., Crovitz & Zener, 1962; Healy, Liederman, & Geschwind, 1986; Oldfield, 1971; Provins, Milner, & Kerr, 1982), the respondent names the preferred hand for such familiar activities as eating, writing, drawing, hammering, throwing a ball, and the like, all of which are "primary-action" items according to factor analyses that show them loading on a single "handedness" factor (e.g., Bryden, 1977). Some inventories also include more idiosyncratic items. The respondent also may be asked to rate the consistency of hand use for each activity. There is still disagreement about scoring methods and about the optimal number and type of items (whether, for example, emphasis should be placed exclusively on primary-action items or whether other types should be considered).

Performance tests assess the actual skill of each hand. Like questionnaires, only presumptive dominant-hand skills are assessed. Because the tasks are chosen so as to diminish the influence of prior practice, the skills listed in questionnaires are not themselves assessed; instead, the tests are of such presumably less contaminated (because less specifically practiced) skills as peg moving (Annett, 1970), square drawing (Bishop, 1980), dot marking (Tapley & Bryden, 1985), and finger tapping (Peters & Durding, 1979).

DISTRIBUTION OF HANDEDNESS IN NORMAL ADULT POPULATION

Handedness questionnaires typically yield a J-shaped distribution, with the percentage of individuals showing a right-hand preference varying from one sample to another but with the bulk of the studies yielding estimates of 85% to 90% (e.g., Porac & Coren, 1981). On this basis, Annett (1972, 1976) has called questionnaires misleading because they fail to reflect what she believes is actually an underlying *continuous* distribution of handedness scores—the kind of distribution obtainable only, she believes, from performance tests.

Questionnaires and performance tests do, indeed, yield different distributions when compared within the same subjects, and there are further differences depending on the particular performance measure used (Borod, Caron, & Koff, 1984). For example, compare the speeded peg-moving task used by Annett with the dot-marking task (making pencil marks inside a sequence of small circles arranged in a sinusoidal pattern) used by Tapley and Bryden (1985). For both tasks, the distributions, on a scale from extreme right to extreme left, are bimodal, but in Annett's case the mean for the left-handers is zero, indicating no lateral bias, whereas for Tapley and Bryden the mean for the left-handers is negative, indicating a leftward bias. Thus, among those who agree that handedness is distributed continuously, and that a proficiency measure must be used, there is still uncertainty about the nature of the distribution, depending on which measure of hand skill is used. One could criticize Tapley and Bryden's measure on the grounds that dot marking shares many features with writing (e.g., making pencil marks), meaning that the skill being assessed is fundamentally similar to the well-practiced writing skill. On the other hand, it also resembles the finger-tapping test (which bears little or no resemblance to writing) in that it requires rapid rhythmic up and down movements. The point, in any case, is that, depending on the choice of decision rule and task, we could wind up with different handedness subgroups—in one case only "left-handers" and "right-handers," in the other case "left-handers," "right-handers," and various subgroups in between.

It is the subgroups in between who pose a particularly vexing problem for classification. In some studies they have been classified in a third group called "mixed handers," in others groups with left-handers and called "non-right-handers." In still other studies they have been called "weak left- (or weak right-) handers," with the strength of lateralization serving as the criterion. The problem of classification is compounded by the fact that any such classification may mean that the individual consistently uses the same hand on repeated trials of the same task, but not *across* tasks, or, instead, is inconsistent in hand use both within *and* across tasks. Soper and Satz (1984) suggest that the latter is more properly called "ambiguous handedness" rather than either mixed-handedness or weak handedness. To make the distinction would require a test–retest approach to the assessment of handedness, a method not yet in routine use.

DISTRIBUTION OF HANDEDNESS IN CLINICAL POPULATIONS: MIXED-HANDED VERSUS AMBIGUOUSLY HANDED

Questions about the definition and distribution of handedness are hard enough when our concern is only to characterize the nature and distribution of handedness types within the *general* population. They become crucial for deciding whether left-handedness is *more* common in certain subgroups of the population. In this light, at least some of the clinical literature cited earlier becomes problematical. For example, in Bishop's (1983) survey of left-handedness and reading retardation, we noted that only 12 of the 17 studies reported a higher percentage of left-handers among the retarded readers. Was this sampling error, or did different studies define left-handedness in different ways? We suspect the latter because 10 of the 17 studies also included the category of "mixed-handedness," which, in every case, included both retarded readers and normal controls. The percentages in retarded groups ranged from 2% to 49%, and in the controls from 2% to 56%. The average percentage of mixed-handers for the retarded groups was 28.75%, and for the control groups 26.75%, so there was no difference here. Given that only 10 studies included this category, whereas 7 did not, and given the extremely broad range of mixed-handers reported for these studies, it seems likely that the 17 studies used different measures of handedness and different decision rules for the classification of handedness. That is, children called left-handed in one study may have been called mixed-handed or weakly left-handed in another, and in some cases perhaps the most accurate classification would be ambiguously handed, in which case a diagnosis of PLH would be inappropriate, as would the inference of unilateral left cortical injury as the precipitating pathological condition. Soper and Satz (1984) have already applied the mixed-handed–ambiguous-handed distinction to the case of childhood autism and have found evidence that the reported higher percentage of left-handedness in this clinical population probably represents the contribution of ambiguous handedness, especially among the more retarded individuals. We note that a classification of autistic children as ambiguously handed is more consistent with the full clinical picture of autism, which includes both linguistic and social–affective disorders, as well as attentional and arousal disorders. It is also consistent with the view that the etiology is more likely to involve bilateral cortical (and subcortical) than unilateral cortical dysfunction (Fein *et al.*, 1984). In this light, the ambiguous handedness found in autistic individuals is more consistent with the neurobiological noise model (model 3) than with either variant of the unilateral lesion model.

Evaluation of Handedness in Infants and Children

As we shall see, a major method of testing PLH theories has been by determining whether presumptive evidence of early neurological insult, as indexed, say, by birth and neonatal status, predicts *adult* handedness. For this method, we must, of course, specify what we mean by handedness in adults and then determine the distribution of handedness types among adults. Researchers also have sought to establish whether such relationships exist in earlier periods, from immediately after birth through 3 to 5 years of age. To evaluate these empirical tests, two more things must be known. First, we must know whether, when, and how handedness is normally manifested during these early periods. That is, we need a handedness norm with which to compare the behavior of at-risk infants and children. Second, assuming that at-risk infants and children differ from normal individuals on these measures, we must know whether the differences foreshadow differences in adult handedness, or whether they are limited to the early period. In other words, if early risk factors are associated with deviations from modal laterality patterns in *early* development, we cannot assume that *adult* handedness will necessarily be affected. The point is that any test of a theory of pathological handedness that compares handedness of at-risk and not-at-risk infants and children can be valid only to the extent that we understand the development of handedness in the normal state. We hasten to add that a developmental analysis is prerequisite to any understanding of PLH even if tests were confined to adults, since the phenomenon itself is inherently developmental.

Like research on models of pathological handedness, research on the normal development of laterality and handedness has become a major focus of concern in the last 10 years (see Kinsbourne & Hiscock, 1983). In the discussion to follow, our aim was only to provide examples of major research trends (for more extensive reviews, see chapters in

Table 12-3. Examples of Tests of Motor Asymmetries, Birth through Early Childhood

Tests
Newborn to 2 months
Postural biases:
Head position
Grasp reflex
Stepping movements
Infancy: 2–3 months
Postural biases
Grasp duration
Infancy: 3–12 months
Reaching
Bimanual activities
Transition to early childhood: 1–2.5 years
Drawing
Hand used in free activity
Early childhood: 2–4 years
Unimanual tests:
Writing, drawing
Eating
Pointing
Use of tools
Throwing
Object manipulation
Finger tapping
Pegboard, formboard
Bimanual tests:
Threading beads
Winding thread
Nut and bolt
Removing container lid

Young, Segalowitz, Corter, & Trehub, 1983). We shall also comment on some of the empirical, methodological, and theoretical problems that arise when tests of models of pathological handedness use infant and childhood laterality scores as outcome measures.

Table 12-3 lists some of the motor behaviors and tasks for which lateral bias has been documented for different ages.

NEWBORN TO 2 MONTHS

From birth to about 2 months of age, normal infants show a variety of lateral motor and attentional biases. One of these is head position. More than a century ago, the physician and pioneer educator Edouard Séquin noted that infants "generally lie on their right sides" (1880, p. 32; see discussion in Harris, 1983, p. 186). Séquin's observation has been well supported. Numerous studies have shown that from 70% to 90% of newborns, while lying supine, keep their heads oriented to the right (e.g., Coryell & Michel, 1978; Harris & Fitzgerald, 1983; Liederman, 1977; Michel & Goodwin, 1979; Saling, 1979; Turkewitz, Gordon, & Birch, 1965; Turkewitz & Birch, 1971). Newborns also show a bias toward right turns after first having their heads held in either a midline or a left position (e.g., Cornwell, Barnes, Fitzgerald, & Harris, 1985; Goodwin & Michel, 1981; Michel & Goodwin, 1979; Saling, 1979).

INFANCY

The lateral biases in newborn infants most likely represent both motor and sensory biases mediated by subcortical rather than cortical mechanisms, since in the newborn infant myelination and PET-scan studies suggest that neocortical structures are functioning only at rudimentary levels (e.g., Chugani & Phelps, 1986). By 2 or 3 months of age, when the infant is cortically more mature and behavior starts to come under a greater measure of voluntary control, other kinds of lateral bias appear. For example, a rattle placed in the infant's hand is held longer with the right hand than with the left (Caplan & Kinsbourne, 1976; Hawn & Harris, 1983; Petrie & Peters, 1981). The 3-month-old also has begun to be capable of voluntary and skillful use of its arms and hands, thereby permitting direct assessment of hand preference for such behaviors as visually directed reaching. Initially, the infant's only response to the presentation of a target is to extend its arms. The earliest form of this behavior in neonates has been described as "prereaching" (see discussion in von Hofsten, 1986), and there have been reports of *left* bias at this early period (e.g., DiFranco, Muir, & Dodwell, 1978; McDonnell, 1979). With time, the response becomes more and more differentiated, and, by about the middle of the first year, most infants will begin to show a preference for the right hand for visually directed reaching (e.g., Baldwin, 1890 [see Harris, 1986]; Carlson & Harris, 1985a).

In the latter part of the first year, the infant also begins to use its hands discriminatively in bimanual manipulation using such objects as a plastic nut-and-bolt toy. Each hand assumes a qualitatively different function for the use or manipulation of the toy, with the left hand holding the nut while the right hand turns ("operates") the bolt (Ramsay, 1980; Ramsay, Campos, & Fenson, 1979).

Although group scores in studies of infant reaching lend an impression of increasing consolidation of hand-use preference in the first year, they also mask considerable individual variability both within and across age periods. For example, in our own longitudinal research (Carlson & Harris, 1985a), we tested 32 normal babies every 3 weeks from 18 to 52 weeks on a 27-trial visually directed reaching task. Although the infants as a group showed emerging right-hand preference, about 40% of these infants showed fluctuations from right-hand preference to left-hand preference and back again across testing periods. The performance of a typical infant is shown in Figure 12-3. This fluctuation was not likely to reflect unreliability of the measure because a majority of the babies showed high reliability on a repetition of the test sequence on the same testing day. We see, therefore, that before 18 months of age, at least certain lateralized behaviors show "fluctuating asymmetry," perhaps of the sort that Batheja and McManus (1985) had in mind when they characterized the "atavistic condition" in their model, as discussed earlier.

TRANSITION TO EARLY CHILDHOOD: 1 TO 4 YEARS

The period from 1 year on represents a developmental transition in motor skills related to hand use. Hand use increasingly can be indexed by fine motor manipulation in skilled tasks. Measurement of performance differences between the hands by tasks that place a demand on skill thus represents a more precise gauge of hand preference than the relatively crude approximations used for infants, such as visually directed reaching. Thus, handedness, in the sense that this term is applied to adults, might emerge only during the 1- to 4-year period, especially in the later part of this period. Although comparison across studies in this transitional period is complicated by terminological and methodological inconsistencies and by sampling problems, the data nonetheless again show a preponderant right-hand bias for such measures as writing and drawing (Annett, 1970; Brown, 1962; Flick, 1966; Gottfried & Bathurst, 1983), eating (Bruml, 1972; Gordon, 1931; Hildreth, 1949; Ingram, 1975), pointing (Annett, 1970; Bruml, 1972), throwing (Annett, 1970; Bruml, 1972; Hildreth, 1949), object manipulation (Annett, 1970; Bruml, 1972; Hildreth, 1949; Rice, Plomin, & De Fries, 1984; Updegraff, 1932), finger tapping (Bruml, 1972; Ingram, 1975; Tupper,

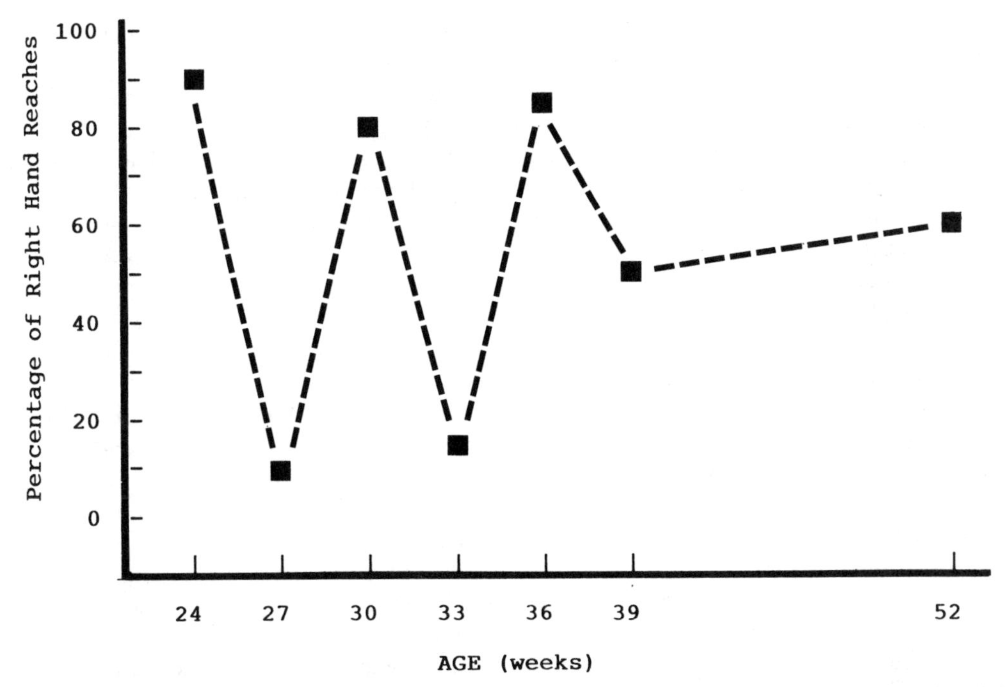

Figure 12-3. Variability in lateral preference across age in a voluntary reaching task by a familial right-handed boy.

1983), and pegboard or formboard performance (Annett, 1970; Flick, 1966; Heinlein, 1930; Tupper, 1983).

In summary, the evidence from normal infants and children shows that hand use takes some time to consolidate into a stable and consistent lateral preference, and that only later in the preschool period do we see evidence of hand preference in the adult sense. In this light, we might have reason to become suspicious when hand preference is highly consistent at a very early age, for example, under 9 to 12 months of age. Might it be a sign of neuropathology ipsilateral to the preferred hand? Clinical evidence supports this idea. A study of children with hemiparetic cerebral palsy revealed that one of the earliest signs in this group was their mother's report of "strong left- or right-handedness" by 4 to 6 months of age (Cohen & Duffner, 1981).[4] For this to be a good marker, however, we must know how "strong" is defined in such cases, and what are the associated signs. It seems clear enough that early strong handedness is pathognomonic in a child with obvious neurological signs, such as hemiplegia, but less clear where such signs are not apparent.

Continuity or Discontinuity from Infancy to Childhood?

In summary, we have reasonably consistent measures of laterality at different chronological ages from birth through early childhood. The next question is: On these measures, will at-risk individuals (whether infants or children) differ from normal individuals, and, if so,

4. Trehub, Corter, and Shosenburg (1983) make a similar point in distinguishing newborn reflex asymmetries that are overly strong and constant, and by implication, pathognomonic, from the kind of fluctuating asymmetries more typical of the normal infant.

will the differences foreshadow differences in adult handedness or will they be limited to the early period? We shall address the first part of this question later. As for the second part, there is not yet an answer because the necessary longitudinal studies have not yet been carried out even for *normal* infants. We still do not know whether, say, direction of head-turning bias in neonates predicts handedness in adulthood. Indeed, developmental psychologists have only just begun to try to answer the *more limited* question of whether the different measures of laterality are linked *within* the infancy and childhood period.

Because 2 months of age appears to mark a major transition from subcortical (reflexive) to cortical (voluntary) control, we might expect to find discontinuities in laterality across the 2-month transition age. In fact, the evidence is mixed.

On the continuity side, Goodwin and Michel (1980) found that neonates with a right head-position preference showed a right-hand reaching preference at 19 weeks, whereas neonates with a left-position preference showed a left-hand preference at 19 weeks. Michel (1981) went on to find, with a sample of 20 infants, that children with "consistent" lateral head-turning preferences at birth were significantly more likely to have same-side preference for *reaching* for a visual target at 19 weeks. Michel and Harkins (1986) found a similar continuity from birth to 74 weeks. To explain this continuity across age, the authors suggested that the early postural asymmetry had biased the infant's attention to that side, thereby affording the infant more opportunity to practice eye-hand coordination of the ipsilateral limb, eventuating in preference for that limb in a visually-directed reaching task.[5]

On the discontinuity side, we would note that, although the continuity between measures in these studies was impressive, it was not invariable. For example, 25 percent of the sample (5 of 20 infants) in Michel (1981) changed their laterality between the neonatal period, when orientation was assessed, and 19 weeks, when reaching was measured. Furthermore, as we have already mentioned, our own longitudinal study (Carlson & Harris, 1985a) showed discontinuities in the visually-directed reaching measure itself—the *outcome* measure in the aforementioned studies.

However these apparent discrepancies are resolved, we note that where the evidence brackets a still longer age period to include early childhood, the continuity is less clear. For example, J. Coryell (personal communication to Liederman, 1983, p. 75) compared the lateral bias of head position at 1, 2, 4, 6, 8, 10, and 12 weeks of age to hand preference of 8 children from 3 to 6 years of age. Only one correlation was significant (for the 6-week measure). Even assessments as late as the fifth month can label as a left-hander an infant who later will prefer the right hand (R. Goodwin, personal communication to Liederman, 1983, p. 75).

For studies that have assessed laterality from 3 years of age on, continuity across age appears to be much clearer, at least judging from cross-sectional studies. For example, Annett (1970) gave a series of hand preference tests (e.g., writing, drawing) and also a speeded peg-moving test to children ages 3½ to 15 years. On the preference tests, as well as the speed test, the majority of children (70% and 80%, respectively) showed a reliable right-hand bias, and on neither test did the direction of hand bias change with age. On the speed test, however, the margin of right-hand superiority increased with absolute differ-

5. This interpretation may put undue emphasis on visual attention alone, since it seems to imply different proportions of right- and left-handedness in the congenitally blind than in the sighted. The one study that we know of to compare these groups reported no differences (Ballard, 1911–1912). We could agree, however, that at least with respect to visually elicited reaching in infancy, *one* of the *proximate* conditions leading to hand preference might well be frequency of visual hand regard. For an analysis of the role of attentional mechanisms in the development of handedness, see Peters (1983).

ences favoring the right hand being larger in younger than older children, which Annett (1970) suggested was a result of the negative exponential shape of the curves. Annett, therefore, concluded that the distributions of hand preference and skill on a unimanual test are fairly constant across this age range and that the greater skill of the right hand is not the result of practice (Annett, 1985, pp. 338 ff.).

For her analysis of the preference data, Annett combined the 3½- to 8-year-olds into one group. Possible age changes within this period, therefore, could not be assessed. Tupper (1983) made a similar assessment across this same age period on a previously validated laterality preference inventory (Porac & Coren, 1981) and on three tests of unilateral motor skill. For the tests of lateral preference, approximately 80% of the sample at all ages from 3 to 8 years proved to be right-handed, with little age change in side, strength, or pattern of lateral preference. Motor skill on a peg-moving task, however, improved with age, but, as Annett (1970) found, the degree of dominant-hand advantage was constant across age, with the nondominant hand functioning at about 80% of dominant-hand performance at all ages.

The data from these two studies thus confirm our earlier impression that, depending on the measure used—writing, peg moving, drawing—only by about 3 to 4 years of age will children show differential hand use and hand skill of a kind comparable to adult measures. Although long-term reliability data are still either missing (as in the case of the peg-moving measure) or incomplete, our impression is that these hand differences are fairly reliable by about 3 to 4 years of age.

In summary, we have a better understanding today than only a decade ago of the development of handedness in the normal individual. This better picture, however, should make us cautious about how developmental data are used to test models of pathological handedness, since, at least for the neonatal period and infancy, the normative data show a system still in flux, with significant proportions of normal infants failing to show a rightward bias, and with lateral biases changing over time. In our estimation, any test of the pathogenic models that compares at-risk and not-at-risk individuals will have real significance only if the test embraces the age period through about 4 years. Comparisons of younger children may be useful, but we shall not know that until prospective, normative longitudinal data are available.

Other Factors Relevant to Evaluation of Hand Use and Handedness in Infants, Children, and Adults

Along with the points raised here, several other factors should be considered in the evaluation of laterality, whether we are using the still imperfectly validated measures used for infants and young children, or the more validated measures available for use in older children and adults. These factors also will be important in the evaluation of theories of pathological handedness.

FAMILIAL HANDEDNESS

One factor is familial handedness, that is, whether the individual is familial right-handed (FRH—all immediate biological relatives are right-handed) or familial left-handed (FLH—some are left-handed). Depending on the genetic model of handedness one follows, FLH may have different implications for the development of handedness and, thus, for theories of pathological handedness as well. A full explication of this question is beyond the scope of this chapter, but we shall provide some examples of issues that might be involved.

Among the genetic models that have been proposed, we shall consider only two. According to a two-gene, four-allele model (Levy & Nagylaki, 1972), both right- and left-handedness are genetically specified by two pairs of genes. The first pair determines which hemisphere will control speech. The second pair governs whether the preferred hand will be contralateral or ipsilateral to the speech hemisphere. By this model, FLH presumably signifies a higher probability that a "left-handed gene" is present in the individual.

So far, the two-gene model has not won broad support. The model that has achieved the broadest acceptance is Annett's (1978, 1981) single-gene model. According to this model, the vast majority of individuals inherit a gene that predisposes left-hemisphere control of speech, while incidentally increasing the chances of greater skill in the right hand as well as the right foot (a "right-shift" factor). All or nearly all of these individuals, therefore, become right-handed. A minority, however, lack this genotype, meaning that there is a lack of systematic bias to either side for speech or for hand use, so that any chance influences on the lateralization of speech and hand are independent. These individuals, therefore, become left- or right-handed with equal likelihood. In practice, however, there might be a slight preponderance of right-handers through environmental pressures, which, in principle, can include both social–cultural and biological influences.

Despite their differences, it is not clear that the two models make different predictions about the role of FLH in the development of handedness. It would seem that, whether FLH marks the presence of a left-handedness gene (by the two-gene model) or the absence of any directional gene (the right-shift, single-gene model), both models would predict a higher probability of left-handedness in an FLH infant than in an FRH infant. Adequate longitudinal data are still absent.

Both models, likewise, appear to make similar predictions about the ultimate strength of lateralization, namely that, on average, left-handers will be less clearly lateralized than right-handers. The evidence on this point is conflicting; some comparisons of FRH and FLH individuals, adults as well as infants, confirm the prediction (e.g., Hawn & Harris, 1983; McKeever & Van Deventer, 1977; Saling, 1983), whereas others do not (e.g., Orsini, Satz, Soper, & Light, 1984). In any case, to the extent that FLH raises a child's chance of being left-handed and to the extent that lateral preference in an infant test, such as visually directed reaching, foreshadows eventual handedness, we might expect to find more left-handed reaches in FLH than in FRH infants. In the case of the single-gene model, however, a second possible outcome might be predicted. In a prospective longitudinal study, we might expect that, in comparison to FRH infants, FLH infants, as a group, will show less clear development of hand preference, as indicated by, say, greater group scatter or variability. Finally, individual FLH infants might prove to be more variable in the hand used for reaching from one time to the next.

Let us consider, now, some possible implications of the FLH factor for the models of pathological handedness. The two-gene model obviously poses problems for Bakan's proposition that all left-handedness is pathological, since FLH presumably would reflect genotypic *left*-handedness. Later, when we consider the evidence for Bakan's hypothesis, we shall see that some studies, including one of Bakan's own (Bakan, Dibb, & Reed, 1973), found significant positive relationships between birth stress and FLH. Bakan deals with such findings by suggesting that the familial tendency to left-handedness is itself mediated by (or is a covariate of) a familial tendency to birth stress:

> A familial tendency to birth stress may be related to factors such as pelvic, uterine, or placental anatomy, hormonal factors, nutritional factors, vascular abnormalities, pain sensitivity influencing the need for anaesthesia, etc. These factors may have a genetic component or may be

> due to other biological or environmental factors. It has been pointed out that familial, but environmentally determined, deficits can be mistakenly interpreted as genetic in origin (Birch, Piñiero, Alcalde, Toca, & Cravioto, 1971). The notion of a gene for left-handedness may be too simple an explanation of the familial tendency for left-handedness. (Bakan *et al.*, 1973, p. 365)

This kind of reasoning sounds like special pleading; but, in the context of Annett's single-gene theory of handedness, there may be some bases for accommodation. That is, among the environmental factors contributing to handedness in cases where, by Annett's model, the right-shift factor is absent, we could reasonably include birth stress and other pathogenic factors of the sort proposed in Bakan's model.

Given all these considerations, it becomes clear that testing models of pathological handedness by comparing laterality scores of individuals with and without at-risk histories must take familial handedness into account. To find, for instance, that, among 6-month-old infants, those showing weaker lateralization on a test of visually directed reaching (or any other test) have a more positive history of birth stress than those who show stronger lateralization might not necessarily be evidence for nascant PLH if the infants showing weaker lateralization also were more likely to be FLH. That is, we could not determine whether the difference in lateralization pattern reflected the history of birth stress, whether it instead was a correlate of FLH, or whether it was a joint product of both variables. Obtaining full familial handedness data thus becomes crucial in any prospective longitudinal study and, for that matter, in any study with individuals of any age. Sample sizes also should be large enough to permit independent assessment of the influences of familial handedness and birth stress. We know of no such study to date.

SEX

Another possible contributor to the development of handedness is the sex of the individual. Girls show a faster rate of overall development than boys, as indexed by bone growth and other somatic measures (Tanner, 1978). In infancy, girls also reportedly show earlier development of left-hemisphere responsivity for language sounds (Shucard, Shucard, Cummins, & Campos, 1981), which may help to explain why girls lead boys in the rate of language acquisition (e.g., Harris, 1977; Wells, 1979). For these reasons, one might expect right-hand preference to emerge earlier in girls. This expectation was borne out in our longitudinal study (Carlson & Harris, 1985a) and was confirmed by Humphrey and Humphrey (1987).

In adults, evidence also suggests that the neural mechanisms underlying praxis and speech are more focally organized in the left hemisphere of women than is the case for men (Kimura & Harshman, 1984). According to Kimura (1983b), this may explain two other kinds of sex differences associated with handedness. First, the percentage of right-handers is slightly greater in women than in men, with the margin of difference in different surveys varying roughly from 1% to 3% or even 4%. Tapley and Bryden (1985) found that 91.4% of the women and 88.8% of the men in their college-age sample were right-handed. Other surveys have revealed similar differences, both in adults (e.g., Bryden, 1977; Oldfield, 1971; Porac & Coren, 1981) and in children (e.g., Calnan & Richardson, 1976; Peters, 1986; Peters & Pedersen, 1979; Porac & Coren, 1981). (Recall that this sex difference was predicted also from Geschwind's developmental neural dysfunction model.) Second, Kimura notes that the asymmetry in motor performance favoring the right hand is stronger in right-handed women than in right-handed men (e.g., Annett, 1970; Annett & Kilshaw, 1983, 1984), a difference that Annett interprets as indicating that the expression of the right-shift gene is greater in females than in males.

Finally, any or all of the sex effects might interact with familial handedness. This interaction appeared in our longitudinal study. In contrast to the FRH group, the male and female FLH infants did not show remarkably different patterns of hand use. Instead, for both sexes, the pattern over time was curvilinear, with a trend toward predominant left-hand use by 52 weeks (Carlson & Harris, 1985a).

In summary, the developmental pathway for handedness appears to be more "canalized" in females than in males in the sense of being a more clearly and directly specified outcome of developmental pressures. This calls to mind Tanner's (1978) remark about canalization—that "Regulation is better in females than in males" (p. 160). If so, girls also might be expected to show less variability in behavioral development than boys. This may be part of the complex of factors that place males at greater risk for suboptimal development, to be discussed later.

If sex and familial handedness contribute to the development of manual specialization in the ways suggested here, there may be implications for the understanding of pathological handedness. For example, if, following Annett's single-gene model, FLH decreases the likelihood that the infant has inherited the right-shift factor, and if the absence of this factor makes an infant's emerging hand preference more susceptible to environmental pressures, then this susceptibility should be maximized in the combination of maleness and FLH. Consequently, the determination that there is a "surplus" of left-handers in any particular clinical subgroup of the general population must be made in light of differences in frequency and strength of right- and left-handedness in the base populations of males and females. To date, we know of no study that has done this.

CULTURE

Assessment of handedness also must acknowledge cultural variations in the prevalence of left-handedness. Throughout the Muslim countries of the Middle East (Payne, 1987) as well as in China (Teng, Lee, Yang, & Chang, 1976), Japan (Hatta & Nakatsuka, 1976; Komai & Fukuoka, 1934), Italy (Salmaso & Longoni, 1983), Germany (Peters, 1986), the Soviet Union (Louis, 1983), and many nations of Africa (Brain, 1977; Dawson, 1972; Payne, 1981; Verhaegen & Ntumba, 1964), left-handers comprise a smaller percentage of the population—from approximately 1% to 8%—than the 10% to 15% figure reported for Western countries (e.g., Brackenridge, 1981; Spiegler & Yeni-Komshian, 1982). The evidence is that these variations reflect cultural differences in attitudes about use of the left hand, in particular for such public acts as eating and writing, since the cultural differences are weaker for other unimanual acts. Some of this same evidence also suggests that the effect of social training is stronger in girls than in boys (e.g., Brain, 1977; Komai & Fukuoka, 1934; Payne, 1981; Porac, Coren, & Searleman, 1986; Shimizu & Endo, 1983). It is not clear whether this is because of sex-related differences in training, in responsiveness to training, or in neurobiological organization.

How might the data on cultural variations bear on the testing of models of pathological handedness? One possibility is that an individual born with only mild hypofunction of the right hand would be *less* likely to develop *left*-hand preference if the environment discouraged left-hand use. Consequently, certain tests of handedness (e.g., eating and writing) that are valid in low-prejudice societies would be of doubtful validity in high-prejudice societies. One result might be an absence of the sort of PLH that figures in the "all left-handedness is pathological" variant of the unilateral lesion model, namely, PLH in the "normal" population. Perhaps even the surplus of left-handedness reportedly found in certain clinical populations (i.e., where presumed cortical injury was more severe) will be lowered. Alternatively, manifestation of PLH might be affected in both cases, for example, in "mild" cases the left hand might be used for actions other than those specifically proscribed for left-hand use. Finally, in each of these scenarios, the effects might differ for males and females because of possible sex differences in socialization for hand use.

SECULAR TRENDS

Finally, assessment of handedness must take into account secular trends in the prevalence of left-handedness. For example, with a British sample, Fleminger, Dalton, and Standage (1977) found that left-handedness for writing was inversely related to age, from 2.9% in 55- to 64-year-olds to 10.8% in 15- to 24-year-olds.

A similar relationship, also with a British sample, was reported by Smart, Jeffery, and Richards (1980), who examined handedness in three generations of biological relatives: grandparents, parents, and 6-year-old children. The percentage of left-handed writers was 6.2% among the grandparents, 10% among the parents, and 17.5% in the children. The authors suggest that the result "probably reflects the mellowing of school teachers' attitudes to sinistral writing from being punitive some 50 years ago to relatively liberal now" (p. 82). They also note that, therefore, there may be many "covert left-handers" among the parents and grandparents who are now right-handed writers but do not recollect their left-hand use being discouraged. If so, family history results would be of limited value for assessment of FLH and would suggest that measures other than handwriting should be used.

The existence of secular trends, by complicating the assessment of handedness, also complicates the evaluation of PLH models. That is, the statistical inference that there is a "surplus" of left-handers in any particular clinical subgroup of the general population must be made in light of these differences in the percentage of left- and right-handers in different age-cohort groups. If, indeed, these secular trends reflect the diminishing of culturally based biases against left-hand use, then we see here a point of contact between PLH theories and social-conditioning theories. Finally, the possibility of sex differences in socialization for hand use suggests that sex differences and secular trend effects must be considered together.

Does Obligatory Use of One Hand Count as Pathological Handedness?

There is one other question of definition to consider. If we can assume that a pathological condition can result in the predominant use of one hand that otherwise would not have been preferred, does this constitute "handedness" in the usual sense of the term? The problem can be made clearer with the following examples.

Imagine a 6-year-old child born with very modest hypofunction of the right upper limb, not enough to make the limb unusable but enough to give a slight advantage to the left hand as the child, over time, comes to develop hand motor skills. The child thus comes to use the left hand preferentially but does not show any obvious motor dysfunction of the right limb. Assume further that the child normally would have become right-handed. This is the sort of case that would seem to constitute a reasonably clear instance of PLH.

Imagine, now, a 6-year-old child born with hemiparetic cerebral palsy—the kind of child described by Cohen and Duffner (1981), mentioned earlier (see p. 307). If the hemiparesis involves the right side, this child also would come to use his left hand preferentially (and might even develop this preference abnormally early) but now clearly because the right hand was clinically impaired. For the same reasons, on a bimanual manipulation task, the child would not be likely to use his right hand with the same skill shown by the first child. Or consider another 6-year-old with established *right*-handedness who, at 4 years of age, suffers a left-hemisphere injury that results in severe right hemiplegia, in consequence of which the child is forced to shift from his right hand to his left. These last two cases are examples of what Gordon (1920, p. 339) called "left-handers of necessity." Do they also constitute legitimate instances of PLH, or does the clearly more obligatory nature of the outcome make such cases trivial with respect to PLH theory? McManus (1983), who has raised this issue, regards such instances as indeed trivial, even meaningless, and would exclude them from the data base. For McManus, PLH (or PRH) could be inferred only if it could be shown to "occur in the absence of signs of a hemiplegia, hemiparesis, lower-motor neuron weakness or other defect of the limb, or lack of control due to tremor, athetosis, ataxia, etc." (McManus, 1983, p. 316), and where the individual, presumably, is not obligated or constrained to use one hand rather than the other. For the same reason, McManus presumably would exclude from consideration the child in our first example inasmuch as that child also was constrained, although more subtly. (McManus also regards as "trivial" those cases in which hand-use preference is the result of damage to *peripheral* structures, that is, to the hand directly.)

On the basis of such arguments, McManus has concluded that the evidence for PLH (e.g., in epilepsy) rests on just such "obligatory" cases. Indeed, he contends that "there is not a single case in the literature that can be regarded as acceptable proof of the existence of the phenomenon" (p. 316). He also has added the stipulation that handedness *alone* must be altered by a lesion (p. 339)—a requirement, therefore, that would preclude any case where a change of handedness accompanied a change in localization for speech, irrespective (presumably) of whether there is associated hemiparesis or not.

With respect to McManus's second point regarding a change in localization for speech, we confess that we do not understand why the definition of PLH should be restricted in this way. We are more in sympathy with his first point. As we understand McManus's argument, someone who has lost his right hand not only cannot be regarded as pathologically *left*-handed, but, indeed, cannot even be regarded as *handed.* The concept of handedness implies that there are two hands, either of which, in principle, is capable of being used, but that one hand comes to assume priority for certain acts or skills. So we agree that it is meaningless to speak of pathological handedness in cases where the individual is functionally (or physically) one-handed. We are less in sympathy with McManus's apparent intention to preclude any instance of hand preference that would be mediated by contralateral peripheral factors, however mild, even when they originate in CNS damage. We find this precondition unduly restrictive. Although McManus appears open to the possibility of PLH, provided his criteria could be met, he believes that no such demonstration has been made. But with such criteria, could it ever be made? In the absence of peripheral symptoms, is it likely that the individual will voluntarily use the other hand in a fashion that approximates what is usually meant by handedness?

Still, McManus raises a very useful question: What are the proximate factors underlying the development of hand use after cerebral injury? To what extent are sensory or motor impairments required for phenotypic hand preference to deviate from the genotype? Here, we are obviously on a slippery slope. Where, on the continuum from mild to severe, should the line be drawn? At present, we have no answer. When we consider the empirical evidence, however, we shall be concerned to identify the nature and extent of the functional deficit of the nonpreferred hand. We then shall be in a better position to decide whether PLH can develop in individuals who are *not* suffering from overt motor (or sensory) disorders, and we shall be better able to understand the proximate factors underlying the development of PLH, for example, whether or not sensory or motor impairment in any degree is required.

ANATOMICAL AND PHYSIOLOGICAL FOUNDATIONS OF HAND CONTROL AND HANDEDNESS

Definition and measurement of handedness is one prerequisite to the evaluation of pathogenic models of left-handedness. Another is to take account of the anatomical and physiological foundations of hand control and handedness. After all, it is pointless to speculate about the effects of injury on handedness unless the injured area is involved in upper-limb and hand control or in attentional mechanisms. In this section, we focus our review on the anatomy and physiology of this control system and then on the factors in this system that may underlie handedness.

In broad overview, voluntary control of the upper limbs and hands represents the operation of cortical and subcortical mechanisms effected through monosynaptic and multisynaptic tracts that originate in cortical gray matter and descend to synapse on spinal neurons. The hand–brain system, furthermore, is predominantly crossed, with nerve fibers making connections between the spinal cord and the contralateral hemisphere. This is why we conventionally say that each half of the brain controls the opposite side of the body.

Motor Systems

A variety of neural systems are involved in the control of voluntary movement of the upper limbs. One major category, the motor system, consists of three descending systems that originate in cerebral cortex.

DIRECT CORTICOSPINAL SYSTEM

One descending system is the corticospinal or pyramidal tract. Approximately two-thirds of the fibers making up the pyramidal tract arise from "motor" areas in precentral cortex, predominantly in the motor strip (Brodmann's area 4) and in premotor area 6; the remaining third originate in portions of the postcentral cortex (areas 3, 1, and 2, and possibly area 5) (Kuypers, 1985).

It is frequently assumed that the giant cells of Betz in this system are of special importance for hand control, but this is a mistaken view, evidently based on an outmoded notion that Betz cells are the predominant source of the fibers in the corticospinal tract (see discussion by Brodal, 1981, pp. 184–185). In fact, Betz cells make up only 3% to 5% of cells in the motor strip, with most fibers from the motor strip originating in cells other than Betz cells (Brodal, 1981, p. 185).[6]

From their origins in cortex, corticospinal fibers descend to the medullary pyramid, where they decussate, or cross to the opposite side, and continue to terminations in the spinal cord. The system, however, is not completely crossed; a significant minority of fibers terminate *ipsilateral* to their side of origin (see Witelson, 1980, for discussion).

6. Differential cell counts (Lassek, 1954) also show that 75% of human Betz cells are located in motor areas supplying the *leg* or foot, compared to 17.9% in the arm region and 6.6% in the "head" area, despite the dedication of far more extensive cortical areas to head and arm than to leg, as shown in the motor homunculus. As in laboratory animals, the massive dendritic arborization characteristic of these Betz cell systems is not present in the newborn infant but begins to develop rapidly as the organism attempts to bear weight on its extremities and to initiate standing–walking–playing activities. As Scheibel (1979, p. 392) has noted in a discussion of this point, a positive correlation thereby is suggested between Betz elements and muscle mass or antigravity status, or both: "The major responsibility for maintenance of antigravity tonus in bipeds is, of course, localized to the lower extremities and back" (p. 392).

Kuypers (1984) has shown that significant control of the limbs is retained in the absence of crossed cortico-spinal pathways.

Lesion studies with monkeys have shown that sectioning the direct corticospinal tract with bilateral pyramidotomy abolishes the capacity to execute relatively independent hand and finger movements (Lawrence & Hopkins, 1972; Lawrence & Kuypers, 1968). Most of the fibers in this tract terminate on spinal interneurons that innervate many motor neurons. A restricted number, however, appear to make connections with motoneurons that innervate a single or small number of distal muscles, making possible the independent control of fractionated finger movements.

The result of this design is that the individual movement of the digits depends almost entirely for control on the fiber systems from the contralateral cerebral hemisphere. If, by handedness, we mean hand differences in the proficiency for fine manipulation with the fingers, then the motor control afforded by the direct cortico-spinal fibers would seem crucial. As we have already seen, those measures of handedness in adults that make up the primary factors in handedness tests make precisely these demands (Bryden, 1977; Healy, Liederman, & Geschwind, 1986).

The direct corticospinal pyramidal tracts develop only gradually early in postnatal life (Kuypers, 1962; Lawrence & Hopkins, 1976). In humans, the pyramidal fibers that are present in the perinatal period are not myelinated (Yakovlev & Rakic, 1966). Postnatally, corticospinal synaptogenesis and the extended process of myelination parallel the emergence of hand use in the human infant. Given this correspondence, Kuypers (1985) argues that a strong link exists between developing anatomy and developing behavior.

VENTROMEDIAL BRAIN STEM SYSTEM

The second descending system, the ventromedial system, is a phylogenetically older and more basic motor system by which the brain controls motility and posture. This system is crucial for control of proximal and axial muscles, especially for maintenance of erect posture, orientation, movement integration, and synergy of limbs. The reticulo-spinal and vestibulospinal tracts are two of the most prominent descending pathways in this system (Kuypers, 1985). In contrast to the largely contralateral corticospinal pathways, the ventromedial system projects bilaterally (Brinkman & Kuypers, 1973). With respect to the question of handedness, the ventromedial system controls the movements of the arm, especially the upper, or proximal, muscles, and thus is important for positioning of the hand and fingers for manipulation. To the extent that a test of handedness involves use of the whole arm rather than only the hands and fingers, then this bilateral system will be involved. This in turn raises questions about the proper interpretation of handedness when it is indexed by tests involving a high degree of arm movement, for example, use of visually directed reaching in tests with infants and perhaps even the use of a pegboard test with children and adults to the extent that the arm, and not just the hand and fingers, is important for execution.

LATERAL BRAIN STEM SYSTEM

The third descending system, the lateral brain stem system, appears to increase the resolution of the ventromedial system and to add a capacity for independent use of the extremities. The major component of this system is the rubrospinal tract, which is almost entirely crossed (Brodal, 1981, p. 195). The rubrospinal tract decussates in the mesencephalon and establishes connections with motor neurons that innervate muscles of each distal extremity. Following sectioning of the direct corticospinal fibers, the capacity for fractionated finger movements is lost, but the use of the hand is maintained, and the hand can still be used for grasping (Lawrence & Kuypers, 1968). The fact that grasping is spared after lesions to the direct corticospinal tract is attributable to the role of the rubrospinal pathway in the lateral brain stem system. With respect to the question of handedness, this third descending system may play an important role in any test involving simple reaching or grasping, for example, a reaching test used for young infants.

Sensory Systems

For both functional and anatomical reasons, a motor system should not be considered in the absence of a sensory system. Even though many gross movements are possible in the absence of sensory information, the successful completion of the kinds of skilled discrete motor acts assessed in handedness tests must be guided by sensory feedback. As Jung and Hassler (1960) have said, "a motor system without sensory control is a fiction, not even a useful fiction" (p. 864).

The primary somatosensory cortex, Brodmann's areas 3, 1, and 2, occupies the postcentral gyrus. Its somatotopic organization, the sensory homunculus, parallels the proportionate representation of the body surface in the motor homunculus. As already noted, postcentral areas (Brodmann's area 6) also contribute some fibers to the corticospinal system, but their primary terminations in the spinal dorsal horn (Coulter & Janes, 1977; Kuypers, 1960) suggest a direct sensorimotor feedback loop rather than a motor role.

The analysis of motor control thus must involve systems wherein sensory information regarding movement is conveyed to cortex. This sensory information arises from specialized receptor cells in the periphery and ascends via the spinothalamic tracts to the medulla, where the tracts are known collectively as the medial lemniscus. At this level the tracts decussate, mirroring the predominantly crossed structure of the descending motor tracts, and ascend to terminate in modality-specific relay nuclei of the thalamus. Direct projections from the thalamus convey sensory information to the primary sensory areas of the cortex in the last leg of the spinothalamocortical system. The system is less restricted than this description implies, since many reciprocal connections are made with the brain stem reticular formation and various subcortical structures. Extensive reciprocal connections also exist between thalamic nuclei and the cerebral cortex.

Sensorimotor Integration

The anatomical evidence thus implies a high degree of integration of motor and sensory systems in hand control, and functional analyses support this conclusion. For example, many studies, including regional cerebral blood flow studies, indicate a major role for nonprimary motor cortex in the guidance of and, particularly, in the preparation for movement (Wise, 1984). Even the "simple" act of reaching for an object is controlled by an intricate interaction of precentral, postcentral, and subcortical structures. For the control of visually directed reaching, Humphrey (1979, 1983) emphasizes the importance of connections among postcentral areas 5 and 7 in the parietal lobe, the frontal eye field, and portions of "premotor" and supplementary motor areas, all acting in concert with primary motor cortex and subcortical structures. Other evidence from the animal literature supports the idea that *both* sensory and motor processes are crucial for the fine control of limb movement. Experimental lesions of forelimb sensory fibers (deafferentation) in monkeys cause an apparent *paralysis* of that limb and dysfunction as serious as that ensuing from damage to descending motor systems (Taub & Berman, 1968). As a result, the animal makes do with the other limb, much as individuals with hemiparesis do.

Commissural Systems

We also should consider the contributions of the extensive systems of reciprocal connections between the cerebral hemispheres—the corpus callosum. The important role of the corpus callosum in the integration of bihemispheric processing in the normal brain is well known (see discussion by Levy, 1985, and Selnes, 1974). One way to achieve this integration and unity may be through reciprocal inhibitory function to the contralateral hemisphere. Reciprocal inhibition, by preventing the two hemispheres from working at cross purposes, can sharpen processing in each, analogous to the way lateral inhibition in the retina sharpens the perception of edges (Denenberg, 1980).

Electrophysiological evidence suggests that the corpus callosum also plays a role in the control of movement. Kornhuber (1974, 1984) describes three cerebral potentials that precede and accompany unilateral finger movement. The first potential, called *Bereitschaftpotential,* or readiness potential, is a widespread *bilateral* brain wave pattern, predominantly in parietal and precentral regions, that precedes movement. The second potential, the pre-motion positivity, is also bilateral and widespread. The third potential appears just before actual movement of a finger or hand. This is a unilateral motor potential and can be detected over the hand area of the contralateral precentral motor cortex. Thus, in contrast to the conventional anatomical view that hand control is predominantly contralateral, the electrophysiological evidence indicates that the contralateral initiation and control of movement come in only after an earlier period of bilateral activation. These patterns therefore suggest an important rule for the corpus callosum in early stages of preparation for movement. Early bilateral activation of both hemispheres seems to ready the brain for movement, even movement of a single digit.

Subcortical Sensory and Motor Systems

Elsewhere, we have alluded to the role of subcortical structures in the coordination of voluntary movement. Prominently involved are the basal ganglia (BG), a bilateral collection of interconnected structures. Although there has long been disagreement about the totality of structures making up the BG, most recent accounts (Anderson, 1981) include the putamen, globus pallidus, and caudate nucleus, and also, according to some authorities, the subthalamic nucleus and substantia nigra. In the classical view, movement was controlled by two supraspinal motor systems, pyramidal and extrapyramidal (Nieuwenhuys, 1977), with the BG regarded as part of the extrapyramidal system. In contrast to the direct, monosynaptic spinal connections of the pyramidal system, the extrapyramidal system was regarded as a multisynaptic, indirect descending route for motor impulses that included relays through subcortical and brain stem structures. This view is now seen as too simple and as incorrect on several points.

The anatomical connections of the BG suggest that the BG nuclei are more than components of the motor system. The BG contribute few fibers to descending motor systems and do not connect in a chain-like fashion to the other parts of the so-called extrapyramidal system. Although the putamen and caudate receive unilateral projections from all cortical regions (Divac, 1972), including motor cortex, the somatosensory regions contribute more fibers than do other sensory areas (Nieuwenhuys, 1977). These BG structures also receive innervation via the corpus callosum from *contralateral* sensorimotor and supplementary motor areas (Kunzle, 1975). The primary efferent targets of the BG structures are thalamic nuclei that, in turn, project not to primary motor cortex (area 4) but to premotor, supplementary motor, and prefrontal association areas (DeLong & Georgopoulos, 1981). The BG, interposed between sensory and integrative cortical areas and the primary motor system, constitute a number of interrelated circuits that converge very indirectly on motor cortex.[7]

In summary, the anatomical bases of control of the upper limbs cannot be relegated to any single neural system. Humphrey (1979) expressed it best when he said, describing the simple act of visually directed reaching, ". . . what may appear to the observer of a coordinated movement of body and hand to be the output of a single, movement-generating system, may in fact be a *multi-channel* output from a much more complex central processor" (p. 103). Much work remains to identify the "channels," or components, that contribute to hand control.

Physiological Processes

Discussion of the development of possible cortical mechanisms underlying hand control customarily begins with the brain of the newborn, consistent with the general emphasis in neurobiology on postnatal processes. Of course, the importance of prenatal processes for postnatal behavior has always been appreciated, but much more strongly in recent times than in the past (see Chapter 1 by Best, this volume; see also Lund, 1978; Parmelee & Sigman, 1983; Rakic, 1984). The earliest influences on the mechanisms of hand control therefore might be sought in any of a variety of embryonic processes. These include neurogenesis, which is thought to be completed during prenatal and possibly very early postnatal life (Clarke, 1985; Cowan, 1978; Purves & Lichtman, 1985); cell migration (Sigman & Rakic, 1973); dendritic maturation, the outgrowth of dendritic surfaces that become the primary sites for synaptic connections from other axons; and synapse formation, which Goldman-Rakic (1986, p. 244) calls "the *sine qua non* of functional maturity." Synapse formation begins prenatally, with synaptic density increasing well into childhood. An early overproduction of synapses appears to be followed by a period of consolidation, possibly influenced by experiential factors, in which synapses are "pruned" to adult levels. Rakic, Bourgeois, Eckenhoff, Zecevic, and Goldman-Rakic (1986) regard synaptic density as a strong correlate of functional capacity. This normal process of selective pruning of surplus synapses, as well as axons and neurons, which appears to play an important role in the formation and regulation of the precision of cortical connections (Clarke, 1985; Oppenheim, 1984; Rakic, 1986).

7. Lidsky, Manetto, and Schneider (1985) have challenged the conventional view of the BG as primarily a motor system. They point out that a large body of evidence shows BG involvement in behavior that is not congruent with a motor system or that plays only an indirect role in movement. Like the transcortical connections discussed in the section on sensorimotor integration (see p. 317), BG may function as a sensory modulator for motor systems. Afferent, receptor-oriented information is translated by the BG into a form that is directly relevant for motor control, that is, attentional orientation. The BG influence movement by regulating the ease with which sensory afference gains access to motoneurons, that is, by gating sensory inputs into other motor areas rather than by directly affecting these areas. Kornhuber (1984) sees the BG as the locus for the generation of programs of voluntary movement. Both Divac (1977) and Lidsky *et al.* (1985) argue that the BG are implicated in a system that translates cognition into action.

The postnatal organization of the brain builds on all of the aforementioned prenatal physiological processes, some of which extend well into postnatal life. For example, myelination proceeds at different rates in different regions of the prenatal and postnatal brain (Yakovlev & Lecours, 1967). Developmental changes in regional metabolism, another index of functional maturity, also show a cortical progression that is strongly correlated with the postnatal pattern of myelinogenesis (Chugani & Phelps, 1986) and probably with synaptic density as well.

Finally, cytoarchitectonic parcellation and fissuration of the cerebral surface occur in the last third of gestation and seem to coincide with the cortical invasion of thalamocortical fibers. As these processes proceed, the mature sulcal pattern appears with the growth of intracortical connections.

Foundations of Functional Asymmetry (Handedness)

If analysis of the anatomical and physiological factors underlying hand control is well advanced (although our review hardly plumbs all of the complexities in this system), much less is known of the underlying influence of these factors for handedness. Our guiding presumption is that there is some asymmetry in one or more of the systems already mentioned. We shall identify only a few possibilities.

CORTEX

At the level of the cortex, many structural asymmetries have been reported in gross anatomy (Geschwind & Levitsky, 1968; LeMay, 1977) and, more recently, in fine anatomy (e.g., Scheibel *et al.*, 1985). The inference that these asymmetries somehow underlie lateral specialization and handedness is based largely on further evidence that they are less clear in left-handers than in right-handers (e.g., Witelson, 1980; see also Witelson, Chapter 2, this volume).

SUBCORTICAL STRUCTURES

Because cortical and subcortical processes are not independent in the intact brain, functional asymmetries in cortical structures will be accompanied by, and perhaps even driven by, asymmetries in subcortical structures. The subcortical structure receiving the most attention is the thalamus, which also has been shown to be functionally asymmetrical and to contribute to lateral specialization for speech (Ojemann, 1983). It is also possible that the thalamic relay nuclei for lemniscal and cranial nerve sensory systems mediate sensory feedback differently on the right than on the left. If so, thalamic asymmetries may be important for asymmetries in motor control by modulating sensory feedback for motor functions.

The role of the thalamus goes far beyond service as a relay of sensory signals from peripheral receptors to cerebral cortex. As discussed earlier, certain thalamic nuclei also are anatomically interposed between the basal ganglia and motor areas of the cortex. One source of functional asymmetries, in turn, may be asymmetrical concentrations of neurotransmitters in thalamus or basal ganglia (e.g., Glick, Ross, & Hough, 1982; Oke, Keller, Mefford, & Adams, 1978). Whether asymmetries in neurotransmitters are related to lateral specialization of higher functions or to handedness remains to be seen.

CORTICOSPINAL TRACTS

As a last example, since hand control depends ultimately on the innervation of peripheral muscles by descending fibers, it also might be reasonable to search for the structural underpinnings of handedness in the corticofugal systems, most notably the pyramidal tract. As discussed earlier in this section, the pyramidal tract is a predominantly but not totally crossed system. Yakovlev and Rakic (1966) examined 130 fetal and neonatal brains for patterns of pyramidal tract decussation and their termination in the spinal cord. In 87% of the cases the left pyramidal tract was larger and decussated at a higher level than fibers from the right. The spinal moto-neuronal pool on the right side also was found to receive more fibers from both the left and the right hemisphere than was the case for the neuronal pool on the left side.

In this study, the handedness of the subjects was not known (a moot point in fetuses and neonates, anyhow). Assuming, however, that the sample was representative, then 85% to 90% of these individuals would have become right-handed, meaning that the percentage of cases in which the right hand receives more fibers than the left approximates the percentage of right-handers in the population.

Nyberg-Hansen and Rinvik (1963) reviewed the literature documenting individual variations in patterns of the pyramidal system. Variation was maximal at the decussation of the tract in the medullary pyramids, where all conditions intermediate between complete crossing and noncrossing of pyramidal fibers were found. The functional significance of these variations is not clear.

What is needed, of course, is to correlate asymmetries in patterns of pyramidal decussation to known handedness. We know of one such study. Kertesz and Geschwind (1971) conducted a postmortem examination of the medullae of 125 individuals, all of whom were right-handed according to survivors' accounts. Instead of counting the number of fibers, however, the authors examined the level of the neuroaxis at which left and right pyramidal tracts cross the mid-saggital plane. Of the 125 medullae, 73% showed a higher left-to-right than right-to-left crossing, 17% showed a higher right-to-left, and for the remaining 10% there was no clear difference. Because the fibers were not counted (as had been done in the studies reviewed by Nyberg-Hansen and Rinvik, 1963, keeping in mind that these studies did not assess handedness), we do not know whether these percentages agree with those from the fiber count studies. If they did, this would provide strong converging evidence that central motor tracts play a major role in handedness. What is needed are similar comparisons with an adequate sample of left-handers. Kertesz and Geschwind (1971) found only seven, far too few for any firm conclusions, especially given the greater heterogeneity of lateral functional specialization in left-handers.[8]

All things considered, the evidence of asymmetries in motor innervation is impressive, but such asymmetries, with certain qualifications (see footnote 8), would explain only the "dominant-hand" specialization for motor control, not the superiority of the nondominant hand for configurational–spatial functions. Since we cannot see how *less* motor innervation could confer an *advantage* on the nondominant hand for these sensory functions, we are forced to consider that the structural underpinnings of handedness also must be sought in higher structures, such as the basal ganglia, thalamus, and cortex, as mentioned earlier.

8. From the perspective of functional analysis, it is also unclear what parameter(s) of the pyramidal system should be considered in relation to manual dexterity—for example, tract size, number of fibers in the tract, diameter of larger fibers, average fiber size, depth of termination in the spinal cord, or deepest termination within the spinal gray. For example, morphometric analyses of the pyramidal tract's relation to digital dexterity in different mammals show that variations in dexterity correspond most closely to the place of termination of pyramidal tract fibers within the spinal cord and correspond less closely to variations in the size of the tract itself (Heffner & Masterton, 1975, 1983). If these comparative analyses are correct and if they also have any implications for understanding lateral differences in dexterity within a species, it suggests that it may have been more revealing if Kertesz and Geschwind (1971) had examined the inferior rather than the superior end of the pyramidal tract.

NATURE, SITE, AND TIMING OF PATHOLOGY

With this background in the anatomy and physiology of hand control and handedness, we turn to a third prerequisite for the evaluation of a theory of pathological handedness—consideration of the *nature, site,* and *timing* of the presumptive pathological agents for affecting limb preference. In the by now voluminous literature on PLH, the common practice (in the case of the unilateral lesion model) is to suppose that the neural insult occurs between the perinatal period and sometime in early childhood and that it affects areas in the (left) cerebral cortex presumptively critical for hand control. (The neurobiological noise model, as already noted, merely supposes that there is some neurological insult, not necessarily unilateral in locus or in effect.) Given what we know about the neuroanatomy of hand control and handedness as outlined in the preceding section, it seems to us that the actual story could be far more complicated—and far more interesting. Injury could be of different types, act at different loci, and occur at different developmental periods from embryogenesis at least through the early childhood period; finally, depending on the type, locus, and timing of injury, it could have very different functional consequences for hand preference. The functional consequences could appear in different ways and at different postnatal periods depending, again, on the type, locus, and timing of neural insult. Because the range of possible neurological sites or functional consequences is so broad, we shall mention just a few of the more obvious possibilities. These are listed in Table 12-4.

We note at the outset that some of these possibilities fall more within the scope of the unilateral lesion model because they pertain to unilateral damage. Others fall more within the scope of the developmental dysfunction model because they pertain to anomalies, also lateralized, of prenatal developmental processes. And still others fall more within the scope of the neurobiological noise model because they pertain to injuries or developmental anomalies of either diffuse or uncertain lateral locus or to injuries or anomalies in the midline.

Maturational Processes

As already mentioned, the cerebral cortex is nearly always named as the site of pathology in the unilateral brain lesion and developmental neurodysfunction models. Cortical pathol-

Table 12-4. Developmental Processes and Structural Sites Potentially Vulnerable to Pathology That Could Affect Limb Preference

Maturational processes:
Neurogenesis and cell migration
Dendritic maturation
Synapse formation
Development and organization of connections
Myelination
Cytoarchitectonic parcellation and fissuration of the cerebral surface
Structures and sites of injuries that could affect limb preference:
Intracortical
Intercortical (commissures)
Corticofugal pathways
Subcortical sites:
Thalamic
Midbrain
Basal ganglia

ogy, however, could take different forms depending on its developmental timing. In several cases (see Table 12-4), the effect could be on sensitive periods of normal brain maturation, notably embryonic and fetal processes. Although some of these processes extend into postnatal life (see the preceding section), neuroembryological evidence suggests that the prenatal period should not be neglected in theorizing about the origin of PLH. For instance, Lemire, Loeser, Leech, and Alvord (1975) provide many examples of anomalies of the postnatal nervous system that can be traced to interference with specific stages of embryonic or fetal development. Most examples are of severe and even life-threatening malformations (e.g., anencephaly); but, in principle, similar but far milder pathologies also might lead to the development of anomalous hand control. Thus PLH might result from alterations of normal embryonic or fetal maturation. Although the connection between prenatal maturational processes and anatomical substrates for handedness is conjectural, any of the processes named earlier could be subjected to pathology. To name but one possibility, distortions in some of these processes may eliminate neurons that have survived the normal pruning process.

Sites of Injuries That Could Affect Limb Preference

INTRACORTICAL SITES

Where injury is to cortex, some writers, following Bakan (1978a), have assumed that the primary site for affecting handedness will be the motor strip, given its presumptively crucial role for *motor* control of the hand. A corollary assumption, as Bakan himself (1977, p. 838) has assumed, is that Betz cells in the left motor cortex are more important to this development than are other classes of cells. Bakan calls these the ''cells controlling fine motor coordination'' of the hands (Bakan, 1978b, p. 3).

It should be clear from the section on anatomy that it is questionable to focus only on the Betz cells and the motor strip. As already noted, Betz cells constitute only a small percentage of the cells in the motor strip and appear to be concentrated in areas controlling the lower limbs. Focusing exclusively on the motor strip, in any case, assumes that preference for what otherwise would be the nonpreferred hand would be induced only by hypofunction in *motor* control of the other hand. A *sensory* deficit, however, might be just as important in inducing hand preference, as demonstrations with experimentally deafferented monkeys have made dramatically clear (Taub & Berman, 1968). We therefore should be alert to the importance of lesions to sensory as well as to motor systems. Indeed, if our focus is on the pyramidal system, we must consider both motor and sensory functions, since, as already noted, the pyramidal system is composed of fibers originating in *both* pre- and postcentral areas. Here, again, recall Jung and Hassler's (1960) remark that ''a motor system without sensory control is a fiction'' (p. 864).

INTERCORTICAL SITES

The corpus callosum and other interhemispheric commissures are other potential sites of pathology with possible consequences for development of pathological handedness. One kind of clinical evidence for this possibility would be an increased percentage of left-handedness in patients with congenital absence (agenesis) of the corpus callosum. The evidence at first seems quite impressive. For example, in a summary of 24 cases of agenesis in the clinical literature, Levy (1985) found 12 instances (50%) of left-handedness or ambilaterality. Chiarello (1980) reported a lower but still elevated percentage in a review of 29 cases, which included most of the same cases summarized by Levy (1985). There were only 9 non-right-handers (32%), of whom 4 (14%) were left-handed and 5 (18%) were mixed-handed or ambilateral. The difference between the two estimates appears to be related to the use of different sampling criteria. Levy included only cases of total agenesis, whereas Chiarello added cases of partial agenesis, and Chiarello notes that individuals with total agenesis (two-thirds of her sample) were more likely to be non-right-handed than were patients with partial agenesis. Chiarello also excluded all individuals with IQs below 70. At least 2 of these cases were non-right-handed, and both of these were included in Levy's analysis. The evidence thus suggests that both the degree of agenesis and the presence of mental retardation may contribute to the effect. Chiarello, however, also notes another factor that makes any definite conclusions suspect: Individuals with total agenesis were not only more likely to be non-right-handed, but also more likely to have signs of *left-hemisphere* damage. Our reading of the literature confirms this pattern. For example, in one study (Ettlinger, Blakemore, Milner, & Wilson, 1972), of 4 patients with total agenesis, hand preference was reported for 2 patients, both of whom were left-handed. In one, the right arm was slightly smaller and clumsier than the left, and hypotonia was more marked on the right side. The other patient showed a mild right hemiparesis and marked synkinetic movements on the right side. If, therefore, left-handedness is more prevalent in individuals with callosal agenesis, it is unclear whether the primary cause is the agenesis or the cortical dysfunction.[9]

In this connection, a speculation by Levy (1974, Levy & Reid, 1978) is worth noting, namely, that where anomalies of inter-cortical or other midline structures (culminating possibly in partial agenesis of the corpus callosum) are associated with left-handedness, a potential behavioral sign might be hand posture for writing. The left-hander in question uses an inverted hand posture (left inverters: LI) in contrast to those left-handers who write in the normal noninverted position (LN). Levy (1982) also has speculated that, as a possible consequence of a midline anomaly, the central linguistic motor programs in the LI individual might be ipsilateral to the writing hand, meaning that hand control would be mediated either by trans-commissural pathways or via the uncrossed motor tracts. In other words, LI may mark one's membership in that subgroup of left-handers with ipsilateral (left hemisphere) control for language functions, in particular, those functions that are visually rather than auditorily mediated (Herron *et al.*, 1979; McKeever & Hoff, 1979).

Finally, on the basis of reports that LI individuals scored lower than either LN or right-handers on reading tests (Allen & Wellman, 1980) and (for nonfamilial left-handers) on neuropsychological tests known to be sensitive to left-hemisphere lesions (Gregory & Paul, 1980), Levy has made the tentative proposal that there may be two groups of LI individuals, one being a normal variant indicated by familial sinistrality, the other representing "pathological sinistrality arising from early damage to the hand-control regions of the left hemisphere" (Levy, 1982, p. 604). We recognize that the question of the neurological significance of handwriting posture is controversial (see exchange between Weber & Bradshaw, 1981, and Levy, 1982). However, assuming that the findings of an association between handwriting posture and psychological variation can be confirmed, Levy's

9. Assuming that the handedness effect is reliable and is due to callosal agenesis and not to lateralized pathology, then what is the underlying mechanism? Among the possibilities mentioned by Levy (1985), one is that normal lateralization depends on normal interhemispheric communication, which in turn depends on callosal integration. Another is that callosal agenesis is a reflection rather than a cause of disordered lateral development, which entails "a diminished specification of bodily coordinates during embryogenesis. The result is poor expression of normal mechanisms controlling lateral differentiation, with the consequence that handedness and other lateralized traits would be randomly determined (Levy, 1985, p. 17).

suggestion of variant forms poses an interesting possibility. The reason is that, if we assume that the pathological variant is the one derived from the midline anomaly, then the proposal is consistent with Chiarello's conclusion (1980) that midline dysfunction alone is rare in the absence of associated cortical damage, and that the cortical dysfunction is more likely to be on the left side than on the right.

Gross callosal agenesis is an infrequent congenital abnormality in clinical populations (Jeret, Serur, Wisniewski, & Fisch, 1985–1986) and, on its own, could hardly constitute a major basis for PLH, even if the evidence linking agenesis with left-handedness (e.g., Chiarello, 1980) were adequate. Most of that evidence, however, comes from clinical populations, which raises the possibility that subtle or mild forms of agenesis may go undetected in nonclinical or asymptomatic individuals. In any case, the evidence, such as it is, at least alerts us to the possibility that the pathology in PLH need not be exclusively in cortex proper, and that where cortical pathology is associated with commissural abnormalities of a sort that can disrupt interhemispheric communication (for example, commissural lesions), both may contribute to PLH. Note, too, that pathological abnormalities involving the corpus callosum are, by definition, abnormalities of a midline structure, not of a lateral structure (as in the case of unilateral cortical lesions). Consequently, if left-handedness proves to be associated with such midline developmental anomalies, such an outcome would seem to be more consistent with the neurobiological noise model (see p. 299), as were the data on left-handedness and Down syndrome (Batheja & McManus, 1985), than with either variant of the unilateral lesion model.

CORTICOFUGAL PATHWAYS

As just noted, one way that commissural lesions could promote left-handedness is by promoting anomalous development in the motor pathways (corticofugal system), in particular by promoting growth of the usually smaller ipsilateral pathways. Alternatively, anomalous development might occur as a direct result of a lesion in the motor system or motor pathways, although we know of no evidence. The most likely sites of such injuries would be associated with nuclei lying in the path of indirect descending systems.

SUBCORTICAL SITES

Finally, motor and/or sensory effects on developing limb preference might result from lesions at various subcortical levels—including thalamus, midbrain, and basal ganglia.

Like cortical injuries, subcortical injuries could have consequences for the assessment of laterality at *different chronological* periods. For example, as mentioned earlier, the kinds of asymmetries found in neonates, such as postural asymmetries and stepping movements, are, in all likelihood, subcortically rather than cortically controlled, whereas the asymmetries found in older infants, such as visually directed reaching movements, are under more voluntary (cortical) control. Therefore, injuries to subcortical regions might be expected to have more effects on the more primitive reflexive behaviors characteristic of the neonatal and early infancy period (recall the discussion of the role of the ventromedial descending pathways for limb positioning; p. 316), but less effect on the more voluntary and skilled behaviors that enter the child's repertoire later in development. Lesions in certain *cortical* regions, on the other hand, might be expected to be functionally "silent" early in development and to become manifest only later. Such a developmental change is well documented for the effects of early versus late prefrontal lesions in discrimination learning in monkeys (Goldman, 1974; Goldman-Rakic, Isseroff, Schwartz, & Bugbee, 1983).

Where hand preference is concerned, this scenario itself might be too simple. For example, if the predominant right postural bias in early infancy affords the infant more opportunities for practicing eye–hand coordination with the right hand than with the left, and if this experience is functionally linked to the infant's later preferential use of its right hand for visually directed reaching (Michel, 1981; Michel & Harkins, 1986), then subcortical lesions that disrupt the reflexive postural bias could indirectly disrupt the later, more voluntary behavior as well.

Pathology That Could Lead to Associated Behavioral Dysfunction

So far, we have identified only the disease conditions that could promote PLH. Since the theory also must account for the behavioral (cognitive and affective–emotional) dysfunctions (or characteristics) associated with PLH, then either the pathological condition that affects hand preference is also the necessary and sufficient cause of the behavioral characteristics, or there would have to be additional neurological damage beyond that affecting hand preference. We have already discussed this question in considering the possible cognitive and affective consequences of damage to left-hemisphere language zones. Here, too, the pathological processes could be of different types, act at different loci within both cortical and subcortical structures, and occur at different developmental periods. As in the case of those pathological processes that merely affect hand preference, changes in cognitive and affective functions could take different forms and could appear at different postnatal developmental periods depending, again, on the type, locus, and timing of neural insult.

Can Pathological Handedness Be Caused by Other than Neural Insult?

All the examples offered so far pertain to pathological conditions affecting the central nervous system (brain and spinal cord). What about peripheral sites? For example, certain *in utero* positions can cause congenital dislocation of the hip (Dunn, 1976). Similarly, certain *in utero* positions could injure one limb and thus influence hand preference directly rather than through the indirect neurological route involving pressure on the head (see Harris, 1980a, pp. 32–34).

Upper-limb preference also could be affected *postnatally* through trauma to one upper limb (arm, hand, or fingers) that restricts the use of that limb. A dramatic demonstration of the power of even a mild, nontraumatic peripheral interference on hand use is shown in a study by Umansky (1973). Simply placing a sock on one forearm of 4- to 12-month-old infants led to rapid disuse, not only for prehension, which would be understandable, but also for reaching, which was not mechanically hindered by the sock. We agree with Umansky that this relatively minor peripheral handicap provides a potential behavioral parallel of neurologic dysfunction in infancy.

Time of Injury

Finally, whether or not injury at any particular anatomical site affects handedness should depend on the time of the injury. The question of the exact effect of timing is hard to answer. Presumably we could invoke the general proposition in developmental neurobiology that recovery of function is usually better after early lesions than after later lesions

(Finger & Stein, 1982). With respect to PLH, this could mean that the earlier the left-hemisphere lesion, the greater the capacity of the left hemisphere to reorganize and to assume its normal function for control of the dominant hand. Early injury, therefore, might not generally be expected to lead to PLH. On the other hand, it could mean that the earlier the left-hemisphere lesion, the greater the capacity of the right hemisphere to assume functions normally controlled by the left hemisphere. With respect to hand control, this may mean only that the right hemisphere has assumed the role of dominant hand control strictly by default, in which case early injury would lead to PLH. In both cases, however, the eventual handedness would be less likely to look obligatory because of any associated hemiparesis (see pp. 313–314) than would the outcome following a later injury. It seems clear that the choice between these two alternatives can be made only on the basis of further empirical work. Whether or not there is a shift of control from left to right hemisphere or simply a reorganization of left-hemisphere function thus may depend on the timing as well as the anatomical site of the injury.

However these questions are answered, the issue of timing raises the further question of whether certain points in development could be used to demarcate major transitions in effects of lesions. As we shall see, some researchers have divided their clinical samples into prenatal (congenital) and postnatal (acquired) injury groups (Varga-Khadem, O'Gorman, & Watters, 1985) on the grounds that birth, though not marking a clear discontinuity in development between prenatal and early postnatal brains, is coincident with the completion of a variety of intrauterine stages (Humphrey, 1964, 1969).

We think there are other good reasons to distinguish postnatal lesions from neuropathology that may be traced to prenatal processes. Because the fetus is relatively well buffered from insults to which the infant and young child are exposed, prenatal pathology may represent a qualitatively different type of injury. In particular, the effects of prenatal developmental anomalies may be more likely to represent systemic CNS dysfunction than would postnatal unilateral lesions. One reason may be the very speed of development of cellular mechanisms, especially during early stages (Schneider, 1979). Cerebral palsy and some forms of mental retardation (without unilateral lesions) may be examples of this kind. To this extent, prenatal injuries would fall more within the purview of a developmental dysfunction model.

Despite the potential usefulness of the distinction between prenatal and postnatal sources of pathology, identification of prenatal injury is complicated by the fact that pathological processes often escape detection until after birth. This may be why many CNS injuries attributed to parturition are misclassified. Towbin (1970) even contends that the concept of "birth injury" is misguided and that such terms as "cerebral trauma," "hemorrhage," and "anoxia" are used ambiguously to suggest that brain damage in the newborn is generally the result of labor and delivery. Such descriptions of CNS injury are "pathologically inconclusive and plainly circumvent the problem of etiology" (p. 529). In Towbin's view, the pathological evidence instead indicates that a major portion of CNS lesions present at birth "are due to latent processes having origin prenatally and may be well advanced prior to labor" (p. 541). In a study of children with hemiparetic cerebral palsy, Cohen and Duffner (1981) reported that substantial prenatal pathology often did not result in noticeable distress at birth. Most of these children showed no perinatal problems and were discharged as normal infants. It was not until 4 to 6 months of age that any abnormalities were detected. Recall that the earliest sign of problems in this group was their mother's report of unusually strong left- or right-handedness. Towbin's analysis therefore implies that birth injury may not be among the primary etiological factors in PLH, as the one-type unilateral lesion model assumes. Instead, the sources of CNS injury generally seen for the first time at birth also should be sought in physiological and anatomical factors during embryonic and fetal development.

In the case where lesions are clearly acquired postnatally, it also has been common practice to suppose that the neural events leading to PLH occur sometime between the perinatal period and some period following the end of infancy, in some cases the second year, in other cases as late as the sixth year. For this reason, clinical populations with postnatal injuries often have been divided into subgroups—those with injuries before 2 to 6 years and those with later injuries.

Assuming that the timing of the lesion is known, apart from questions about age-related changes in neural plasticity, any consequences for hand preference must take into account the child's hand preference at the time of injury. In other words, a unilateral lesion that occurs before a consolidation of manual preference might have quite different consequences than afterwards because the system is less well established. Again, Umansky's study (1973) provides an illustration of this point because the character of hand disuse after covering with a sock changed with the age of the infant. Although infants at all ages showed the disuse effect, older infants appeared capable of eventually discovering that prehension with the sock-covered hand was still possible, whereas younger infants did not.

Still another complication in the determination of the time of injury is that prenatal and early postnatal cortical injuries do not always have immediate behavioral consequences. Indeed, as Lenneberg (1968) has argued, that is more the rule than the exception. He notes, for example, that in studies of hemiplegia, all four extremities move well and symmetrically at first, and growth is as yet entirely unaffected. When higher centers, probably the cortex, begin to exert an influence on the behavior of the normal infant (at about 3 months of age), the first signs of abnormality make their appearance in the hemiplegic child, but, as Lenneberg goes on to say, they often are so inconspicuous as to escape parents' attention. In summary, "the child with a perinatal cerebral injury only gradually 'grows into his symptoms' and . . . both lesions and symptoms have their own ramified consequences, often affecting distant structures years after the primary injury" (Lenneberg, 1968, p. 165).

IS THE LEFT HEMISPHERE MORE AT RISK THAN THE RIGHT?

In the preceding section we discussed the nature, site, and timing of the pathology that may influence hand preference. The next question is whether, as Bakan has supposed, the left cerebral hemisphere is at greater risk of injury than the right hemisphere, or whether both hemispheres are at equal risk, as Satz has presumed. As far as we can see, the resolution of this question will not help us choose between the two variants of the unilateral lesion model. That is, if the left hemisphere proves to be more at risk, it would not logically follow that all left-handedness must be PLH. Likewise, if the hemispheres are at equal risk it would not follow that there must be two kinds of left-handedness, one PLH and one non-PLH. The existence of risk differences, however, is crucial to the *statistical* assumptions underlying the two-type model, since any prediction about the relative proportions of PLH versus PRH in a population of individuals with unilateral injury must take into account the ratio of left-to-right lesions; on the other hand, it would appear to be irrelevant to statistical assumptions underlying the 1-type model, since that model does not recognize the possibility of PRH in the first place.

Evidence

There are several ways to determine whether the cerebral hemispheres are at different risk for dysfunction.

RATIO OF RIGHT-TO-LEFT VERSUS LEFT-TO-RIGHT HEMIPLEGIA

One way is to compare the ratios of left-to-right hemiplegias in the clinical literature. If the left hemisphere is more at risk—in this case for the kinds of injury that result in contralateral paralysis—then right hemiplegia should be more prevalent than left hemiplegia. We know of six studies that provide evidence on this question: Five support the prediction, with the ratio of right–left hemiplegia ranging from 1.5:1 to a high of 4:1 (Annett, 1973; Eastman, Kohl, Maisel, & Kavaler, 1962; Hood & Perlstein, 1955; Levine, Huttenlocher, Banich, & Duda, 1987; Mitchell, 1961). In the one negative case (Woods, 1957), no differences were found. The difference seems to be clearest in the case of congenital lesions. Levine *et al.* (1987) found that the ratio of left–right injury was 3:1 for congenital lesions but 1:1 for acquired lesions, even with a control for lesion size.

EFFECTS OF EXPERIMENTALLY INDUCED HYPOXIA

Evidence of greater left-hemisphere vulnerability *in utero* also is suggested in an experiment by Brann and Myers (1975). Hypoxia was induced by brief anesthetization in 8 rhesus monkeys pregnant with fetuses within days before birth. At the end of the period of asphyxia, each fetus was surgically delivered. At least 10 minutes of mechanical ventilation were required before any of the fetuses began to breathe.

All of the 8 asphyxiated fetuses showed brain edema, in 6 instances the swelling being accompanied by zones of hemorrhagic or nonhemorrhagic cortical softening (3 animals each). The zones affected in each case were the middle third of the paracentral region. Of these 6 animals, in 3 cases the softening effect was asymmetrical, and it was the left hemisphere that was the more affected in every instance.

Brann and Myers note the similarity of the clinical findings to those observed in human newborns who have suffered severe intrapartum asphyxia and who die within the first days of life (see Desmond, Rudolph, & Phitaksphraiwan, 1966).

LATERAL DIFFERENCES IN EEG ABNORMALITIES

If greater left-hemisphere risk in early development proves to be more closely connected to congenital than to acquired lesions (Levine *et al.*, 1987), the left hemisphere also appears at greater risk for the kind of neurological injuries to which adults are largely susceptible. For example, Paoluzzi and Bravaccio (1967, cited in Subirana, 1969) examined over 4,000 EEG records of adult patients with diagnosed exclusive or prevalent localized pathology in a single hemisphere and found evidence of more frequent pathology in the left than in the right hemisphere by a ratio of 7:3. Similar differences have been reported in certain abnormalities in EEG records in persons not having explicit cerebral pathology and whose EEGs otherwise tend not to be seriously disturbed. The abnormalities are paroxysms of more or less regular slow waves, predominantly in the derivations of the temporal lobe. These waves have been called an "electroclinical pseudo-tumoral syndrome of vascular origin" (Paillas, Bonnal, & Gastaut, 1953; cited in Bruens, Gastaut, & Giove, 1960, p. 283) and, according to Bruens *et al.* (1960, p. 291), are likely to represent the effects of an arteriosclerotic narrowing of the cerebral vessels, with its resultant reduction of cerebral circulation. When the slow waves appear unilaterally, it is more frequently on the left side than the right. In a large group of elderly people having no medical complaint, the slow-wave activity was found in nearly half the cases, with a left-temporal locus in 75% of the cases. Similar differences have been reported with other patient groups (see Meyer, Liederman, & Denny-Brown, 1956; Tucker, 1958).

Why Is the Left Hemisphere More Vulnerable? Some Possibilities

If the left hemisphere is more vulnerable throughout the life span, it may be for several different reasons.

BLOOD SUPPLY

One possibility has to do with the design of the cerebral arteries. The right cerebral hemisphere is supplied from the brachiocephalic artery that it shares with the right upper extremity, whereas the left hemisphere is supplied directly from the aortic arch. Brann and Myers (1975) suggest that, under asphyxial conditions, the blood shunted to the left carotid artery therefore will be less well oxygenated than the blood to the right carotid artery (p. 338). Brann and Myers presumably mean that because less blood is supplied along this artery, the tissues served will be less oxygenated.

ARTERIOSCLEROTIC NARROWING

The left cerebral arteries, perhaps because of their asymmetrical design, also may be more likely to show arteriosclerotic narrowing, thereby diminishing blood supply to the left side directly. Bruens *et al.* (1960) raise and then dismiss this possibility. We know of no direct evidence either way.

METABOLIC REQUIREMENTS

Bakan *et al.* (1973) have suggested that the left hemisphere may be at greater risk because it has greater metabolic requirements. This was how Bruens *et al.* (1960) explained the preponderance of slow waves in the left hemisphere in their EEG records. The asymmetry, rather than necessarily being related to a preponderance of arteriosclerotic narrowing on the left side, instead is attributed "to a greater sensibility of the dominant hemisphere which has the greatest need of oxygen. Therefore, a generalized cerebral ischemia will manifest itself first in dysfunction of the left Sylvian area" (p. 292).

MECHANICAL FACTORS

Simple mechanical factors also may be at work. Hood and Perlstein (1955) suggested that the higher percentage of left-sided injury (right hemiplegia) found in their survey was the result of the more common birth presentation of the left occipital anterior (LOA) head position. In this position, the left side of the head (and left cerebral hemisphere) during passage through the birth canal could be compressed by the left sacral promontory. Consistent with this proposal, Hood and Perlstein (1955) found that the higher ratio of right-to-left hemiplegia occurred only in full-term, not preterm, infants. Preterm infants, presumably because of their smaller heads, would be at less risk for cranial compression during delivery (although other interpretations may be possible, as will be discussed in the next section). Consequently, if preterm infants (and perhaps all constitutionally small full-term infants) were to show differences in the incidence of left and right cerebral injury, it may be for other reasons.

As Liederman (1983, p. 86) has pointed out in a discussion of Hood and Perlstein's data, the predominance of left-hemisphere lesions cannot be solely a consequence of the large number of births delivered from an LOA position because evidence shows that the left hemisphere is more vulnerable when the occiput is right rather than left (Churchill, 1966). These cases consisted primarily of patients with unilateral focal epilepsy or hemiplegic hemiepilepsy. A left-hemisphere focus was associated with a right occiput anterior (ROA) position in 67% of the cases; a right-hemisphere focus was associated with an LOA position in 85% of the cases. Even though proportionately fewer children were born from an ROA than from an LOA position, the majority of the lesions were left-sided. We agree with Liederman that this suggests that the left hemisphere is inherently more vulnerable to damage than the right hemisphere.

MATURATIONAL FACTORS

Finally, it has been suggested that the left hemisphere is more at risk because it matures earlier than the right hemispehre (Geschwind & Galaburda, 1985). This hypothesis is hard to evaluate. First, the question of the relationship between risk and rate of maturation is itself vexed. The evidence is unclear whether greater risk or vulnerability attends to slower or to more rapid maturation. Second, rate of maturation and length of maturational period are rarely distinguished, partly because of the difficulty in identifying markers of maturation. Third, the premise that one hemisphere matures before the other itself has been questioned, with some arguing that any such differences in growth would be cyclic, favoring first one side and then the other (e.g., Mittwoch, 1978), and with others arguing that no single growth or maturation gradient can reasonably account for the known complexities of development (e.g., Kraft, 1980). For further discussion, see Corballis and Morgan, target article and commentaries (1978); also see Best, Chapter 1, this volume.

POTENTIAL RISK VARIABLES FOR PLH

This overview of anatomical and functional details bearing on the question of handedness gives some idea of the range of issues that any theory of pathological handedness must try to embrace. The only issue remaining before we are ready to evaluate the two variants of the unilateral lesion model is that of the potential risk variables for PLH.

Prenatal, Intrapartum, and Postnatal Variables

Table 12-5 lists variables that, according to standard epidemiological science, constitute risk variables for the developing fetus and newborn infant. This list is not definitive. We chose it for illustrative purposes and because it was used in one test of the PLH model to be discussed later (Speigler & Yeni-Komshian, 1982). Some of these variables apply to the prenatal period, others to the intrapartum period, and still others to the postnatal period. Each variable is weighted on the basis of its estimated individual contribution to overall risk. Some variables also are likely to be more influential than others, depending on when they occur and on the individual's age at the time laterality measures are made.

Continuum of Reproductive Casualty

Following Pasamanick and Knobloch's (1961, 1966) concept of a continuum of reproductive casualty, we can suppose that, depending on the number and severity of reproductive

Table 12-5. Examples of Variables Indicative of Varying Degrees of Risk

Risk age periods	Risk weight points
Prenatal variables:	
1. Diabetes	10
2. Multiple pregnancy (twins)	10
3. Minor heart disease	5
4. Mild toxemia	5
5. Vaginal spotting	5
6. Viral infection	5
7. Anemia	5
8. Maternal age: <16 or >34	5
9. Smoking, >20 cigarettes per day	1
Intrapartum variables:	
1. Placenta previa	10
2. Abruptio placentae	10
3. Prolapsed cord	10
4. Gestation over 42 weeks	10
5. Meconium staining	7
6. Labor: <4 hr, >20 hr	5
7. Medical induction of labor	5
8. Forceps (mid)	5
9. Forceps (outlet)	1
Neonatal variables:	
1. Weight at birth: <2,000 g	10
2. Multiple apneic episodes	10
3. Respiratory distress syndrome (definite)	10
4. Five-minute Apgar: <5	5
5. One-minute Apgar: <5	5
6. Respiratory distress syndrome (suspected)	5
7. Presumed anoxia	5
8. Cyanosis	5
9. Resuscitation at birth	5

Source: Spiegler and Yeni-Komshian (1982).

complications in any given child, there will be a range in the likelihood and severity of abnormality in development. Relatively minor perceptual, attentional, motor, and behavioral disabilities will occur toward the lower and middle parts of the continuum; gross anomalies, such as cerebral palsy, will occur at the high end (see Figure 12-2, p. 295). As mentioned earlier in the section on theories, we can consider the models of PLH in terms of this continuum.

Proximate Causes of Neural Insult

The variables listed in Table 12-5 are only clues to, or indirect measures of, the *proximate* causes of neural insult or injury. At least two major categories of proximate causes can be contemplated:

DIRECT MECHANICAL MEANS

Injury may come through direct mechanical means, such as deformation of the skull and brain. The injury could occur at different developmental periods and hence by different means. *In utero* injuries could arise from anomalous *in utero* positions, birth injuries from difficult passage through the birth canal, and postnatal injuries from either exogenous or endogenous sources. As already noted, the left hemisphere appears to be at greater risk, but not in every circumstance. For example, we would not necessarily expect any lateral difference in risk for postnatal exogenous head injury.

HYPOXIA

There also may be injury through hypoxia, either through direct mechanical means of the sort just listed or by other means.

Other Risk Variables

PARITY

Another variable that has figured importantly in tests of PLH is parity, where primiparity—first live pregnancy—is ordinarily regarded as a higher risk condition than later pregnancies. Risk differences presumably arise in a variety of ways, for example, through mechanical trauma at delivery and/or through fetal hypoxia consequent upon longer first labors, which, in turn, are commoner among first-born infants. The relationship is not necessarily straightforward. For example, Eastman *et al.* (1962, p. 466) found that the percentage of primiparas in normal children was significantly higher than in children with cerebral palsy (43% versus 37.4%, $p < .04$) but only after certain cases of "hemolytic disease" had been deleted from the sample.

Fourth and later births also are associated with raised risks, although for different reasons, including the greater age of the mother. The reported result has been a U-shaped relationship between parity and perinatal mortality (e.g., Bakketeig & Hoffman, 1979).

SEX

Many or all of the risk factors named above also could have statistically different consequences for males and females. Males generally are regarded as being at greater biological risk than females. For example, proportionately more males than females are lost through miscarriage, stillbirth, or death in the perinatal period. More males also are conceived—a reproductive "strategy" that presumably compensates for the lesser male viability (McMillen, 1979). To the extent, then, that nonlethal pathological factors can affect hand preference, males should be at greater risk than females. If so, greater male vulnerability might partly underlie the higher percentage of left-handers among males as well, perhaps, as the greater number of language-related behavioral and cognitive disorders in males. By the one-type "all left-handedness is pathological" model, the male "surplus," therefore, would suggest that the factors causing PLH are more effective for males than for females. By the two-type "some left-handedness is pathological" model, the sex difference, instead, might represent only or predominantly those males with PLH.

SEASON OF BIRTH

Another potential risk variable for PLH may be season of birth. For reasons still unclear, there are well-established seasonal variations in congenital malformations in the United States by climatic regions. This suggests that teratogenic factors may be more potent in certain climatic regions (Torrey, Torrey, & Peterson, 1977; Wehrung & Hay, 1970).

Cultural and Temporal Variations in Reproductive Casualty

The existence of PLH, in principle, may be able to explain more than the higher percentage of left-handers among males. It also might account, at least in part, for variations in the numbers of left-handers in different cultures and generations. For example, the rise in left-handedness over the last several decades in the United States (Fleminger *et al.*, 1977) and Great Britain (Smart *et al.*, 1980), which we suggested earlier reflects the diminution of cultural pressures against use of the left hand, also might be viewed against secular trends in neonatal mortality. Since proportionately more infants are surviving today than in the past because of better nutrition, medical care, and the like (at least among those social–ethnic groups having access to these advances), the number of individuals with PLH might be expected to change as well.

What is harder to predict is the direction of the change. On the one hand, a decline in mortality may bring a decline in the absolute number of individuals with PLH paralleling the overall decline in the number of infants with birth injuries generally. Alternatively, a decline in mortality could bring an *increase* in the absolute number of individuals with PLH if PLH is actually a symptom of an impairment that, previously, would *not* have been expressed because the children destined to show PLH did not survive.

The analysis of the role of cultural and temporal variations for pathological handedness has implications for the analysis of sex difference, too, in that sex differences in left-handedness might be related to changes in the number and severity of risk factors. Again, the direction of the effect may not be straightforward. Because males are more at risk, then as overall mortality declines (i.e., viability improves), we might expect the sex difference to decline as well. Epidemiological data, however, suggest that precisely the reverse will occur, with mortality growing proportionately larger for males as overall mortality declines (Abramowicz & Barnett, 1970). That is, in the last century, the decline in overall mortality has resulted in an increase in the male:female ratio. This finding is consistent with the principle that "sexual dimorphism in diseases is revealed only when the nosogenic agent is not overwhelming" (Glücksmann, 1981, p. 135). In other words, sex differences would not be expected in, say, virulent epidemics except if the chance of contact with the infecting agent is greater for one sex than for the other. The same applies to near-instantaneous death following accidents and major mechanical, physical, or chemical trauma. "Sex differences are to be expected in less severe diseases due to endogenous abnormalities, exogenous causations or the combination of the two: the reaction of males and females to environmental agents" (Glücksmann, 1981, p. 135). The implication would seem to be that, if the risk factors decline (because of improved obstetrical, gynecological, and pediatric care) so that environmental stresses are substantially reduced, and if that leads to a decline in the absolute number of pathological cases of left-handedness, that should only *increase* the male: female ratio of left-handers.

This already complex scenario may be still more complex because epidemiological evidence indicates that female infants are more likely to survive *serious* developmental problems than male infants. One piece of evidence is Leck's (1974) finding that although the sex ratio of affected births (for neural tube defects) is always very low, even in "epidemics," the increase is largely due to *girls*. Therefore, at the upper end of the birth risk continuum, where we are looking at children who have survived very serious problems, we might expect to find proportionately *more* girls than boys and therefore proportionately more *PLH* girls than *PLH* boys. Where PLH predominates in males, therefore, may be instead at the low-risk end of the continuum (including the low end of the high-risk area).

Thus, with improved viability, meaning that the more devastating (killer) diseases have declined, the male:female ratio would *increase*. In other words, only with improved viability, when a sufficiently large number of infants survive, is the inherently greater male weakness permitted full expression. But as applied to the continuum of reproductive casualty, it means that at the lower end (greater viability), there will be a larger male:female ratio, whereas at the higher end (poorer viability), among the survivors, the sex ratio will be smaller, perhaps even reversing in direction.

Social–Cultural Variables: The Continuum of Caretaker Casualty

The foregoing points about the potential modifying influences of medical and socioeconomic factors on the likelihood of poor development illustrate what Sameroff and Chandler (1975) have called a fundamental weakness of the concept of a continuum of reproductive casualty. They suggest that, in order to predict the actual developmental course of such disorders—*one* of which, according to pathogenic models, will be left-handedness—we must consider the *transactions* between the continuum of reproductive casualty and what they call the "continuum of caretaker casualty."

The continuum of caretaker casualty ranges from an environmental and family situation having few adverse factors to one having multiple, deleterious factors. As an example of the interaction of the continua of reproductive casualty and caretaker casualty, consider that, although nearly 10% of all children are born with some kind of handicap or anomaly (see reports in Niswander & Gordon, 1982), many of these defects decrease or disappear with age. Why do many children overcome their deficits whereas others do not? As Sameroff and Chandler (1975) point out,

> Self-righting influences are powerful forces toward normal human development, so that protracted developmental disorders are typically found only in the presence of equally protracted, distorting influences. . . . Even if one continues to believe that a continuum of reproductive casualty exists, its importance pales in comparison to the massive influences of socio-economic factors in both prenatal and postnatal development. (p. 189)

For another example, consider the variable of parity, which, as we said earlier, has figured importantly in tests of the PLH model. Eastman *et al.* (1962), in their study of the relationship between parity and cerebral palsy, noted that, for the percentage of first births among cerebral palsy to be meaningful, the figure must be carefully controlled by a series of patients in the same social, economic, and intelligence strata distributed equally among the same hospitals in the same period of time. Similarly, the reported U-shaped relationship between parity and perinatal mortality has been the subject of controversy, since parity in most studies has been confounded with birth interval and with socioeconomic variables (Bakketeig & Hoffman, 1979).

As a last example, consider the risk variables of birth order and maternal age. Ordinarily, first-born infants (primiparas) are at greater risk than later-born infants, but the difference probably will be greater if the mother is 14 years old than if she is 24 years old because of the younger mother's physiological and psychological immaturity and because of associated differences in prenatal, perinatal, and postnatal care. All these differences, in turn, may be associated with socioeconomic and educational status. Consequently, any surplus of PLH among first-borns may prove to be due disproportionately to very young mothers (or to very old mothers—but here for different reasons).

One general point to note is that any prediction of later development from neonatal condition must take into account the transactions between multiple measures of infant state and the environmental conditions in which the child will develop, and as this applies to motor development generally (as it does to cognitive development), we might reasonably expect it to apply to the development of limb preference and manual specialization as well. Consequently, as the concept of a continuum of caretaker casualty implies, certain demographic variables are often used as indirect—and imperfect—indices of risk. These include such variables as parental education, income, and other variables associated with socioeconomic status and, by implication, pre-, peri-, and postnatal care. The relationship among variables might be very complex. For instance, whereas low socioeconomic status may be associated with factors that put the infant at higher risk, both on the continuum of reproductive casualty and on that of caretaker casualty, and in this respect could raise the likelihood of PLH, low socioeconomic status also could be associated (especially in certain cultural–ethnic groups) with lower social tolerance for left-handedness. Thus, left-handedness might be less prevalent in these groups. Depending, then, on how we construe the role of socioeconomic variables, we could predict either *more* or *less* left-handedness.

Risk Variables and Causal Mechanisms for PLH

Finally, to the extent that we can identify the particular risk variables involved in any particular instance of supposed PLH, we may be able to improve our understanding of the actual contributing conditions, that is, the proximate variables, or disease conditions, that led to this pathological condition. The epidemiological considerations, however, are complex. For example, consider the risk factor of low birth weight (the small-for-term infant). (In Table 12-5, a birth weight under 2,000 grams is regarded as constituting a birth risk with a weighting equal to 10). From one perspective, the small infant might be expected to be at lower risk for cerebral injury due to deformation of the skull during passage through the birth canal because the infant's small size protects it against this kind of injury. By this view, whatever risk low birth weight might pose in connection with PLH (or any change in lateral preference) is *not* likely to come in the form of mechanical injuries during vaginal passage. Rather, those at risk would be very large infants, especially when the mother has a small birth canal. From a different perspective, however, if the low birth weight is associated with prematurity, then any advantage of small size may be offset by the lesser readiness, meaning lesser elasticity, of the birth canal for parturition. In evaluating an infant for birth stress, we therefore should not assume that all the individual risk factors are simply additive. If, for example, low birth weight is a risk factor, the likelihood of mechanical deformation during delivery will depend, at least in part, on whether the low birth weight is due to prematurity or to some other factor.

Birth position presents another example of the problem of identification of risk variables. Breech-delivered infants should be more at risk for head pressure and deformation than vertex infants; at least, forces on the head would be different from those associated with vertex presentation.

As a last example, consider the use of a caesarian (C-section) delivery. C-section delivery ordinarily signals the presence of risk variables. Given the nature of the procedure, however, it should preclude that category of risk associated with head pressure during delivery.

CAN LEFT-HEMISPHERE INJURY CAUSE PLH? EVALUATION OF THE TWO-TYPE UNILATERAL LESION MODEL

The clinical and experimental evidence both suggest that the left hemisphere is at greater risk than the right hemisphere for injury or dysfunction, although the circumstances and reasons are still unclear. The next question is, whatever else may prove to be the behavioral sequence of such injuries, do they include PLH?

We begin with the two-type model because, if PLH cannot be demonstrated where associated neurological signs are clear, then no further consideration need be paid to the more extreme view that all left-handedness is PLH, including left-handedness in the clinically *asymptomatic* population.

Prevalence of Left-Handedness in Clinical Groups with Unilateral Brain Injuries

Earlier, we cited empirical studies that document the raised frequency of left-handedness in populations with brain dysfunction compared with that found in nonclinical populations. Recall that these were studies of epileptic and mentally retarded groups. Similar findings have been reported in patients with unilateral brain injuries but without seizure disorders. For example, in a study of 17 children with left lesions, 12 were left-handed, whereas of 12 children with right lesions, all were right-handed (Aram, Ekelman, & Satz, 1986).

Once the fact of this increase in left-handedness is established, several questions occur, some of which were raised earlier.

Locus of Neural Abnormality

UNILATERAL VERSUS BILATERAL

One question is whether the increase in left-handedness predicted by the two-type model for cases of unilateral left-side abnormality also would be found under conditions of bilateral abnormality. The evidence is that it would not. In one study, Silva and Satz (1979) examined EEGs in 572 mentally retarded patients and classified the EEGs as normal (n = 96) or abnormal (n = 476). Of those with abnormal EEGs, 17% (82/476) were left-handed. In contrast, only 9% (9/96) of those with normal EEGs were left-handed.[10] Of the patients with abnormal EEGs, in 136 patients the abnormality was either unilateral or bilateral asymmetric. Among these patients, left-handedness was primarily associated with unilateral (left-sided) abnormalities.

CORTICAL LOCI

In the section on anatomy, we outlined the cortical systems contributing to motor control of the hands. Does the clinical evidence show that some of these areas are more critical than others in cases of PLH? We shall consider three studies. In the Rasmussen and Milner study (1977) cited earlier, the cortical injuries associated with a rise in left-handedness were located in inferior frontal and temporoparietal regions on the left side. As the authors noted, these also were primary language zones, so that in this patient group there also was an associated shift in language lateralization from left hemisphere to right. By contrast,

10. As Silva and Satz (1979) note, 9% is very close to the percentage of left-handers found in normal samples. Unless there is some associated measurement error in this study, this result would seem to mean that in MR populations, any increase in left-handedness will occur only in the presence of unilateral injury. If so, then the results suggest that the mechanism driving the positive relationship between left-handedness and degree of mental retardation reported in earlier studies (Bradshaw-McAnulty, Hicks, & Kinsbourne, 1984; Hicks & Barton, 1975; see Introduction), may be unilateral left-hemisphere abnormality. The earlier studies, in turn, imply that the subset of mentally retarded individuals with normal EEGs in Silva and Satz's (1979) study were *less severely* retarded than those with abnormal EEGs.

even major lesions to areas outside the language zones "rarely seem to affect the subsequent lateralization of speech" (p. 363), the implication presumably being that such lesions also failed to effect a change in handedness. Rasmussen and Milner therefore concluded that "an early lesion that does not modify hand preference is on the whole unlikely to change the side of speech representation" (p. 359).

Satz and his collaborators make little mention of the precise location of lesions, even when CT data are available (as in Satz *et al.*, 1985b). Instead, most of the descriptions are qualitative (e.g., "cortical atrophy"). However, inasmuch as Satz sees his data as consistent with those of Rasmussen and Milner (1977) in associating PLH with a shift in language lateralization, we presumably can infer that most of his PLH patients likewise had injuries that encroached on frontotemporoparietal language zones.

Somewhat better information, at least with respect to location along the anterior–posterior axis, is provided in the study by Aram *et al.* (1986), mentioned earlier. Of the 12 children with left-hemisphere lesions who were left-handed, 11 had "postcentral" damage, and 7 of those also had "precentral" damage. The 12th child had precentral damage only, but with associated basal ganglia damage. By contrast, of the remaining 5 children in the left-lesion group who were not left-handed, in only 2 cases did injury extend to postcentral areas.

In summary, the evidence suggests that when language zones were involved, handedness is more likely to be affected, with damage to postcentral areas possibly being more important than damage to precentral areas.

CORTICAL VERSUS SUBCORTICAL

In the section on anatomy, we also noted the important role of subcortical systems, in particular the basal ganglia, in motor control. We therefore were interested to see to what extent PLH would be associated with injuries to these areas in addition to cerebral cortex. This information is hard to glean from the clinical literature on PLH because data on subcortical injury either are not reported (e.g., Satz *et al.*, 1985b) or, if reported, are not discussed (Aram *et al.*, 1986). One reason may be the presupposition that it is cortical sites that are paramount. Another reason (in the case of the older literature) is that most investigators lacked the sophisticated imaging techniques, such as CT scan, that would help localize the injury. Finally, because these have been clinical rather than postmortem investigations, researchers have not been able to precisely relate behavioral and anatomical data in the same individuals.

Whatever the reason, our suspicion that these structures may play a role in PLH is supported by the CT scan data provided in the report by Aram *et al.* (1986). Of the 17 individuals with left-side lesions (12 left-handers, 5 right-handers), 6 of the 12 left-handers (by our count) had injuries confined to cortex, 5 had cortical injuries with basal ganglia involvement, and 1 had subcortical injuries only. In contrast, of the 5 right-handers (those presumably who did not shift handedness), 4 had cortical injuries alone, and only 1 had cortical injuries with basal ganglia involvement (Aram *et al.*, 1986, Table 1, pp. 166–167). The numbers are too small to be statistically significant, but, if we put together the findings on the cortical area involved along with basal ganglia, the numbers at least suggest that hand preference is more likely to be affected after left-hemisphere injury when a postcentral lesion includes the basal ganglia.

The anatomical data also fail to support the notion (in the one-type model) that injury to motor strip alone is the predominant cause of PLH. This is not to say that motor strip injuries could *not* affect hand preference, but only that where there *is* presumptive evidence of PLH, the injury almost invariably is to larger regions, most frequently postcentral. This supports our view that sensory areas are crucial in the development of hand control and therefore would also figure in PLH.

Associated Clinical Signs of Brain Pathology in PLH

In the Introduction, we identified several of the psychological characteristics associated with left-handedness of possible pathological origin. Satz and his colleagues have addressed this question in their own clinical groups and have proposed that the lesion that produces PLH also may produce associated cognitive, as well as somatic, changes with sufficient consistency to constitute a true clinical syndrome. They suggest that previous efforts to identify cases of PLH were limited by a failure to recognize these correlative signs.

The first sign, to which we have already made reference, (see p. 297) is altered hemispheric specialization for language, specifically a change from left-hemisphere specialization to right- or bilateral specialization. Prior to their own new clinical reports, the strongest evidence to date, as Satz *et al.* (1985b) note, came from Rasmussen and Milner's (1977) study of epileptic patients, mentioned earlier. Before surgery for temporal lobe resection, all of these patients were assessed for side of speech dominance with the sodium amytal procedure. Of the patients *without* clinical evidence of early left-sided injury, 53% were right-handed and 47% were left- or mixed-handed. Of the right-handed patients, 96% showed unilateral left-sided representation of speech, compared with a more variable representation among the left-handers or mixed-handers (left-sided in 70%, right-sided in 15%, and bilateral in 15%). By contrast, the results in patients *with* evidence of early left-sided injury indicated an increase in the percentage of left- or mixed-handers (from 47% to 69%), together with more than a tripling of the incidence of right-hemispheric speech dominance (53%) in this group.

As Satz *et al.* (1985b, p. 29) point out, no reference was made to PLH in Rasmussen and Milner's study, but they suggest that the rise in the percentage of left-handers in combination with right-sided speech strongly implicates this phenomenon. To test this idea, Orsini and Satz (1986) looked for evidence of right-sided language dominance (as indexed by a left-ear advantage for speech sounds on a dichotic listening test) in four groups: a group with suspected PLH, these being left-handers with early (under age 6) unilateral left or predominantly left lesions, and three control groups: (1) left-handers with late left-or right-sided lesions; (2) normal left-handers with no history of brain injury; and (3) right-handers with early left-sided lesions. Of the patients with suspected PLH, 10 were examined for language dominance, of whom 90% (9 subjects) showed right-hemisphere dominance, compared to 29% in control group 1, 13% in control group 2, and 13% in control group 3. We have strong misgivings, in the absence of any converging evidence, about interpreting a left-ear advantage on a dichotic listening test to indicate anomalous right-hemisphere dominance for language, but the results nonetheless are consistent with the sodium amytal data (Rasmussen & Milner, 1977).

The second correlative sign of PLH is a cognitive change directly related to the change in language lateralization. Recall that we earlier (p. 297) identified two possible alternative consequences to this change—impaired language skill or impaired visuospatial/constructional ability. Satz *et al.* (1985b, p. 29 ff.) have suggested that the latter alternative is the more likely, and they cite several earlier studies in support, the first being the study by Lansdell (1969), mentioned earlier. Lansdell tested 15 left-brain-injured epileptics, 12 of whom sustained their lesions before age 5. Twelve of these patients were left-handed, which Satz *et al.* suggest was most probably PLH, and 3 were right-handed. All 15 patients had right-hemisphere speech as indexed by the sodium amytal test. Lansdell then studied the association between age when the first neurological symptoms appeared and the difference between verbal and nonverbal scores on the Weschler Bellevue Scale, and found that verbal performance suffered less with earlier lesions, nonverbal factors less with later lesions (i.e., after 5 years). Lansdell, therefore, suggested that the relative sparing of verbal cognitive functions in the early left-injured group was the result of commitment of right-hemisphere tissue to displaced language functions, which then interfered with the development of nonverbal abilities normally served by the right hemisphere. Satz *et al.* (1985b, p. 30) also cite, in indirect support, an early study by Tizard, Paine, and Crothers (1954). Satz *et al.* (1985b) provided further corroboration in their own clinical sample of 12 patients, all of whom showed impaired performance on clinical tests of spatial constructional ability together with a pattern of poorer Wechsler Performance Intelligence Quotient (PIQ) relative to normal Verbal Intelligence Quotient (VIQ).

To this point, the evidence for impaired spatial performance looks convincing. However, in the more recent study by Orsini and Satz (1986), which reported only Wechsler Scale scores, the association is less clear. Of the patients with suspected PLH, 12 of whom were given Wechsler IQ tests, only 6 (50%) showed a lower PIQ than VIQ, which was a higher percentage of patients than control group 1 (left-handers with late left or right lesions), but lower than control group 3 (right-handers with early left lesions). No data were available from control group 2, normal left-handers.

The status of the "cognitive crowding" hypothesis thus is uncertain. What is needed now are more refined tests. For one thing, the Performance and Verbal scales of the Wechsler tests are composed of subtests with very different processing demands (e.g., see Kimura, 1987; Linn & Petersen, 1985), not all of which fall neatly into right versus left hemisphere categories. Future tests of the model should use spatial tests with better validation as measures of right-hemisphere spatial functions (e.g., see Lewis & Kamptner, 1987). Similarly, more refined assessments of linguistic ability need to be carried out along the lines used by Dennis in her detailed psycholinguistic analyses of language function in brain-damaged children (e.g., Dennis, 1987; Dennis & Kohn, 1985).

Future tests also should make careful use of normal left-handers as a control group, since only by this means could we determine whether a particular pattern of cognitive deficit (lower spatial than verbal) is peculiar to PLH, as Satz *et al.* (1985a, p. 123) have contended, or whether it also appears in some normal left-handers, as Levy (1969, 1975) has proposed.

Finally, we recommend that studies expand the number of psychological tests to include tests of affect and emotion, since, as we suggested in the section on theories, "cognitive crowding" in the right hemisphere might be expected to have consequences for affect or emotion as well as for spatial ability. We note, however, that if left-handedness proves to be associated with affective problems, including problems in emotion and interpersonal relationships, a very different explanation is possible. We may instead be seeing non-PLH left-handers with *right*-hemisphere dysfunction. Weintraub and Mesulam (1983) described 14 patients who showed a consistent pattern of emotional, interpersonal, and cognitive dysfunction as well as left-sided signs (e.g., asymmetrical left-arm posturing during complex gait) indicative of right-hemisphere injury. In fact, only two of these patients were left-handed (those presumably lacking the left-sided *motor* signs), whereas the rest were right-handed. In terms of the two-type model, the possibility arises that some of the right-handers, especially those with left-sided motor signs, originally were left-handed, meaning that now they are pathological *right*-handers (PRH).

The third proposed correlative sign of PLH is right hemihypoplasia. The assumption is that early injury to the left hemisphere can affect not only hand preference but also (depending on the location and nature of injury) physical growth of the contralateral limb. If the surplus left-handers among individuals with known neurological injury are indeed PLH, then we might expect associated trophic characteristics either for the now nondominant hand or for the foot on the nondominant side.[11]

Early evidence on this point was reported by Landauer (1939), who reviewed 22 cases of congenital hemiatrophy (i.e., hemihypoplasia) involving the arm and/or the leg but without hemiplegia. Of the 22 cases, 16 involved the left side of the body, 6 the right side. Of the 6 cases of right hemiatrophy, 5 were left-handed, whereas only 2 of the 16 cases of left hemiatrophy were left-handed. Landauer was puzzled by this relationship, but Satz *et al.* (1985b) see it as consistent with their proposal that right-sided skeletal undergrowth represents a somatic marker of PLH. A similar suggestion was made by Schmidt and Wilder (1968) in their discussion of soft signs in the neurological examination of epileptics. Recall that these authors, along with Satz, also posited a two-type PLH model. They also suggested that early acquired defects of one cerebral hemisphere may lead to "a reduction in somatic growth on the opposite side of the body, resulting in shorter and smaller limbs" (Schmidt & Wilder, 1968, p. 126; see also Penfield & Robertson, 1943).

To put the trophic change hypothesis to a thorough test, Satz, Yanowitz, and Willmore (1984) studied groups of epileptics and a group of mental retardates. The results were positive, indicating that left-hemisphere injury sustained before 2 years of age retards skeletal growth in the right foot, producing a pedal asymmetry, and that, under certain circumstances, significant underdevelopment of the right foot and PLH may be causally related: "Presumably, injury before two years of age to the left hemisphere, which includes the anterior parietal region, produces a partial failure of unilateral somatic development along with a change in hand preference" (Henry, Satz, & Saslow, 1984, p. 268).

Similar effects for feet were reported by Orsini and Satz (1986) and for both hands and feet by Aram *et al.* (1986). Furthermore, although the results agree with the data from epileptic groups that lesions incurred before age 2 were most reliably associated with trophic shortfall, 2 years did not prove to be an absolute demarcation. Instead, changes were evident even in a child whose lesion was acquired as late as 6 years of age.

Severity of Lesion and Age of Injury

The adult clinical data presented by Satz and his co-workers show that left-handedness is more prevalent in individuals who have sustained early unilateral left-brain damage. What

11. Certain cerebral injuries are known to cause underdevelopment, or "trophic shortfall," of the contralateral limb, either the upper or the lower limb depending on the precise area of cerebral injury (see Lenneberg, 1968). Injury to postcentral gyrus, for instance, is associated with underdevelopment of the bones of the foot. The reasons are still unclear. Satz *et al.* (1984, pp. 103–104) mention several possibilities. Among them are bone changes resulting from motor weakness (Dreifuss, 1956) and changes in blood supply to the limbs (Grinker, Bucy, & Sahs, 1959). Given our own comments on the role of sensory systems in motor control (pp. 317–318), we would add that even a deficit confined to sensory systems may have similar effects on limb growth. As noted earlier, experimental evidence with monkeys has shown that sensory denervation alone of the forelimb produces disuse of the limb (Taub & Berman, 1968). The result, therefore, could be physical atrophy in an adult animal or undergrowth in a still developing animal.

the data do not yet reveal is whether an effect on handedness is related to the severity, or size, of the lesion—or, to put it another way, whether there is a minimum level of severity for handedness to be affected.

Earlier (pp. 326-328), we raised the related question of whether a lesion has different consequences for the development of PLH according to the time of injury. As we have just pointed out, Satz sees his data as consistent with Rasmussen and Milner (1977) in associating PLH with a shift in language lateralization. Since the evidence on language lateralization suggests that such shifts are much less likely with later lesions (after 6 years of age), we can expect changes in handedness to follow a similar time course. Satz's data, however, do not address the question of whether birth is another important demarcation, that is, whether prenatal (congenital) and postnatal (acquired) injuries have different consequences even when the postnatal injuries are very early.

Both variables—severity and timing over the prenatal to postnatal periods—recently have been tested by Vargha-Khadem *et al.* (1985). They studied 28 patients with left-hemisphere lesions, 25 with right hemisphere lesions, and 15 normal control subjects. All of the patients were children ranging in age from 66 to 17 years at the time of testing. The two clinical groups were divided into three groups on the basis of age at injury: prenatal, early postnatal (2 months to 5 years), and late postnatal (5 to 14 years). Lesions ranged from mild to severe, as indicated on CT scan by the size of ventricular dilation and extent of tissue damage. Hand preference was evaluated by questionnaire, an adaptation of Crovitz and Zener (1962). Preference was assessed for 18 common unimanual and bimanual actions, permitting a range of scores from "strong right-handed" to "strong left-handed" (following Milner, 1975). The younger children could not reliably indicate their hand preference and were asked to make the appropriate gestures.

To determine the relationship between handedness and the variables of side of cerebral injury, age at injury, and severity of lesion (as indicated by CT scan indices together with results on somatosensory and motor tests), tests of correlation were carried out for the left- and right-hemisphere-injury groups separately. For the left-hemisphere-injury group, *all* of the patients with prenatal and early postnatal left-hemisphere lesions proved to be strongly left-handed, but more so in the prenatal lesion group than in the early postnatal lesion group. By contrast, all four children in the late postnatal left-hemisphere lesion group were right-handed. Of these four, three were right-handed prior to the lesion and remained so afterward. The fourth child was right-handed before injury and, following brain injury (at 5.2 years), became left-handed. For the *right*-hemisphere lesion group, all were right-handed, and there was no significant relationship between age of injury and hand dominance.

In the left-hemisphere injury group, there was no relationship between severity of cerebral lesion and left-hand preference, at least within the range of severity encompassed by these clinical cases. The data, that is, do not define a lower limit of severity. The authors concluded that, in light of the nature of their cerebral lesions, patients in these groups could be considered to be PLH, and their left-handedness may be indicative of bilateral or right-hemisphere representation of language consistent with Rasmussen & Milner (1977). Perhaps it is not surprising that lesion size was not more predictive of hand preference, since, as we already mentioned, smaller lesions may sometimes produce greater functional deficits than larger lesions (see Irle, 1987). The clinical and animal literature suggests that the effects of lesion size may be difficult to predict without considering many other variables, including those discussed in this section.

More evidence on the importance of timing is provided by Woods and Carey (1979), who compared 11 individuals who had suffered from *perinatal* left-hemisphere lesions with

16 individuals with left-hemisphere lesions incurred from 1 year to 15 years of age. At the time of the observations, the subjects ranged in age from 8 through the mid-20s. In the perinatal group, 10 of the 11 individuals were left-handed (91%), whereas in the later-lesion group, 12 of the 16 (75%) were left-handed. Within the later lesion group, 6 individuals had lesions before age 3, and all were left-handed, including 3 known to have been right-handed prior to injury. Of the 4 subjects with lesions acquired between 3 and 6 years of age, 3 were left-handed. Finally, of the remaining 6 subjects with lesions after age 7, all of whom were known to have been right-handed prior to injury, 3 switched following injury.

Further evidence on the prenatal–postnatal difference also comes from the study by Aram *et al.* (1986). Of 5 children who had suffered prenatal left-hemisphere lesions, all were left-handed when assessed at 4 and 11 years of age. Of 8 other children (3 to 7 years of age) who acquired their lesions postnatally but before age 2, 6 were left-handed. Finally, of 4 children (4 to 11 years of age) who acquired their lesions after age 2, only one was left-handed (a boy whose lesion was at 6.2 years and who was assessed at age 10).

Sex and Familial Handedness Effects

Earlier we discussed the possibility that males may be at greater risk for PLH than females, and we mentioned the implication that the known sex differences in left-handedness might represent only or predominantly those males with PLH. Ther is some "soft" evidence for this proposition in a report that the rise in the number of left-handers among psychiatric patients was virtually confined to males (Lishman & McMeekan, 1976). Without direct evidence of lesions, however, such an association could just as well mean that left-handedness is a normal marker for risk of psychiatric dysfunction, especially for males.

The sex difference hypothesis is more appropriately tested with clinical data of the sort reported in the current section because we now have actual lesion data. In practice, however, the test is hard to make because sex differences are rarely reported in these studies.

The omission of data on sex differences is unfortunate for still another reason. In light of evidence of possible sex-related differences in cerebral organization for certain language and spatial functions in both clinical and in normal non-clinical populations (Harris, 1978; Kimura, 1983a, 1987; Kimura & Harshman, 1984), consideration of the sex of the patient in putative PLH populations may help clarify the data on cognitive functions associated with PLH. The interactions may well be very complex given still other evidence that patterns of performance on verbal and spatial–constructional tests interact with sex and handedness as well as with reasoning ability (Harshman, Hampson, & Berenbaum, 1983; Lewis & Harris, 1985; Lewis & Kamptner, 1987). Some evidence consistent with this possibility has been reported by Novelly and Naugle (1986). In 22- to 29-year-old epileptic patients with early-onset seizures (before age 6) and with *right*-hemisphere dominance for speech (as indexed by a sodium amytal test), only the males showed significantly reduced scores on the Performance Scale of the WAIS relative to Verbal Scale scores. The results also support our suggestion that certain subtests of the WAIS would be more suitable than others for testing the crowding hypothesis. Novelly and Naugle (1986) found that only the Picture Completion and Object Assembly subtests figured in the effect.

Orsini and Satz's (1986) study also was one of the few clinical studies to have examined the potential role of familial handedness for PLH. The results failed to indicate that FLH had played a significant role in changing the likelihood of PLH.

Was Left-Hand Use Obligatory Because of Right-Hand Sensory or Motor Impairment?

Finally, was the PLH observed in early-lesion groups necessitated by paresis of the right upper limb? Were the patients "left-handers of necessity"? McManus's (1983) own evaluation of the clinical evidence has convinced him that hemiparesis is indeed invariably present in cases of putative PLH and that where motor impairments are likely to be absent (e.g., in less severe childhood epilepsy), the frequency of left-handedness is not significantly raised. On these grounds, McManus not only appears to have rejected all the empirical evidence put forth in support of the PLH model but also has rejected PLH itself as a nosological entity. We have not examined case histories in all of the studies reported to date, but judging from those we have seen, the evidence looks reasonably clear that hemiparesis is frequently associated with PLH. For example, Rutter, Graham, and Yule (1970) found a high percentage (23%–25%) of left-handedness among two groups of 5- to 15-year-old children with neurological impairments (Table 12, p. 66), but 35% of the children in one group and 55% in the other also had limb "dyspraxia" and other signs of motor impairment (Table 12, pp. 67–68). Martin, Friedrich, Mottier, and Guignard (1968, cited by Bishop, 1983, p. 170) found an association between left-sided abnormality on neuroradiography and left-handedness, but, as Bishop (1983, p. 170) pointed out, the association looked "much less impressive" once the hemiplegic cases were excluded. Penfield and Roberts (1959) did not say how many of their epileptic subjects had motor handicaps, but they noted that *many* of those with early injuries were hemiparetic, and it is precisely in *this* group that left-handedness was more prevalent.

The picture appears to be largely the same in the more recent studies described earlier in this section. In the Satz *et al.* (1985b) report, of 12 case histories of PLH, right hemiplegia was reported to be present in 5 cases at the time of observation and to be absent in 6 others. No mention was made in the remaining case. In the Orsini and Satz (1986) report, hemiplegia also figured in the clinical picture, although we should point out that this was inevitable inasmuch as hemiplegia was one of the clinical signs on the basis of which patients were selected for the sample. The results, in any case, revealed that among the patients with suspected PLH (left-handers with early left-hemisphere injury), there was motor impairment as indexed by a tapping text with the nondominant (right) hand in 7 of 12 patients given this test, a higher proportion than in either control group 1 or control group 2.

Similarly, hemiparesis (as indicated by a variety of somatosensory tests) was one of the signs of neuropathology used by Vargha-Khadem *et al.* (1985) to classify their individual patients as brain-injured. From our reading, hemiparesis was involved in every instance. For the prenatal group, the determination that the injury was, in fact, prenatal was made partly on the evidence, during an examination before 6 months of age, of unilateral deficits in motor coordination or of asymmetry in limb size, together with an early reliance on one hand for most actions (which, as we already have noted, is atypical for this age). (see p. 307). In addition, there was no evidence of perinatal or postnatal episodes that may have been responsible for the hemiparesis (Cohen & Duffner, 1981; Michaelis, Rooschuz, & Dopper, 1980). The unilateral motor weakness in these patients was usually noted by parents and/or pediatricians during routine activities and was documented during the first 6 to 9 months of life. The patients in the postnatal group, by contrast, all showed hemiparesis only after a single well-documented, distinct, and nonprogressive episode, usually involving admission to the hospital. The episode in some cases occurred before

5 years (early postnatal group), in other cases between 5 and 14 years (late postnatal group). Before the episode, all the patients had been neurologically normal infants and children. The hemiparesis apparently was still evident in the left-handed (left-hemisphere lesion) group at the time of testing, even though some patients exhibited only "minimal hemiparesis affecting only the lower limb and not motor or sensory impairment in the right hand" (Vargha-Khadem *et al.*, 1985, p. 693).

In the Woods and Carey (1979) study, among the 22 left-handers from the total sample of 27 in both the perinatal and postnatal groups, all were characterized as hemiparetic at time of observation, with injuries ranging from mild to severe. Subjects with no hemiparesis were right-handed.

In the Aram *et al.* (1986) study, hemiparesis was assessed for both upper and lower extremities in only 8 of the 17 cases of left-brain lesion. Of the 8 cases, 7 were left-handed, and hemiparesis was rated as moderate to severe in all cases but 1, this latter showing no sign of hemiparesis. Furthermore, wherever hemiparesis was apparent, it was stronger for the arm than for the leg.[12]

In summary, compared to control groups, left-handedness clearly is more frequent in individuals with explicit left-hemisphere injury, injury that is identifiable either directly from brain scan or other monitoring measures or indirectly through associated neurological signs. The timing is important, the upper age limit being approximately 6 years. The presence of pedal asymmetries, in combination with cognitive measures, provides converging evidence of PLH in these individuals. Finally, the left-handedness in these cases is associated more often than not with right hemiparesis, albeit sometimes in only a mild form. To this extent, we would agree with McManus that the left-handedness often was obligatory. Depending on the degree of hemiparesis (not always reported), the question may be raised whether such individuals are properly called "handed" in the first place. The fact that hemiparesis was not detected in *every* case, however, suggests that it is not a *necessary* condition for PLH.

IS ALL LEFT-HANDEDNESS PLH? EVALUATION OF THE ONE-TYPE MODEL

The clinical evidence thus indicates that the surplus of left-handers in certain clinical populations may indeed represent the contribution of PLH, keeping in mind the qualifications pertaining to hemiparesis. Now, what of the proposal that all left-handedness is PLH, even in clinically asymptomatic individuals?

12. In the case of the study by Vargha-Khadem *et al.* (1985), let us assume, for the sake of argument, that, even though by later childhood no motor or sensory impairment of the right hand was discernible, there nevertheless *had* been sensory–motor impairment (brought on by explicit unilateral cortical injury) at some initial period, and that it was this early impairment that had initiated preferential use of the contralateral (left) hand. If so, it would suggest the not unreasonable possibility that an early *obligatory* preference for the left hand persists and becomes consolidated into left-handedness in later life even though the initial reasons for left-hand preference are no longer operative. Under these circumstances, the *initial* use of the left hand, having been obligatory, means that the demonstration presumably would still fail to meet McManus's requirement for PLH. What would still be needed, then, would be a demonstration of PLH where no such obligatory use of the left hand can be reasonably assumed (at any developmental period) but where some sign of neuropathological origin can be reasonably inferred nonetheless.

As already noted in the section on theories, the one-type hypothesis assumes that the primary source of pathology that underlies PLH (in the nonclinical population) comes from birth stress, so that the major test of this model has been to assess the relationship between birth risk factors and subsequent limb preference. Before proceeding, we would only repeat our earlier caution that diagnoses such as "birth injury" and "cerebral trauma" not only are used ambiguously with regard to specific pathology but also may be misleading as to etiology, since a major proportion of CNS injuries are due to processes that occur prenatally. Therefore, to the extent that "birth stress" is used as a presumptive indication of cerebral injury, any relationship found between "birth stress" and handedness may represent the contributions of prenatal events and not simply of labor and parturition. We also would repeat our earlier caution that the effects of prenatal and perinatal cortical lesions are often delayed until after 3 months, thus *after* the very developmental period assessed by many of the "birth stress" studies. This means that the kind of screening methods used in the first category of studies to be reviewed (for example, Apgar scores) are not likely to pick up all positive cases.

The hypothesis has been tested in two ways. In one, the relationship is assessed during infancy itself. All such studies have been prospective, and all have drawn on medical records directly and consequently are more trustworthy in that respect, but they are valid tests of the PLH model only with the qualifications just raised and to the extent that the infant measures foreshadow later handedness. As noted in the section on measurement, this latter question is still open.

In the other kind of test, the relationship is assessed when the subjects are either adults or school-age children, meaning that handedness is reliably established and can be measured by conventional means. In most of these studies, information about pregnancy and birth status has been drawn from interviews with the mothers or, in some cases, with the individuals themselves rather than from medical records directly. In all such instances, particularly the latter, the validity of data can be questioned.

Relationship between Birth Status and Laterality within Neonatal and Infancy Periods

We begin with studies of the relation between birth status and laterality within the neonatal and infancy periods. Perhaps the first to address this question were Turkewitz, Moreau, and Birch (1968). Using Apgar scores as an index of neonatal status (Apgar, 1953; Apgar & James, 1962), Turkewitz *et al.* compared neonates with high scores (9 or 10, where 10 is maximum) with neonates with medium (7–8) and low (under 6) scores on a test of head turning in response to somesthetic stimulation of the perioral region on each side of the face. In this test, the infants lay supine. Infants with intermediate to high scores showed a rightward bias (i.e., turned to the right in response to right-side stimulation significantly more often than they turned to the left in response to left-side stimulation), whereas infants with low scores either showed no bias in either direction or were slightly more responsive to left-side stimulation. Not all infants with low Apgar scores showed atypical lateral differentiation, but even those with typical overall patterns showed weaker lateral differentiation than did infants with normal Apgar scores.

More recent studies have been generally consistent with these early results. For example, where the measure of laterality is spontaneous supine head position, prematurity is associated with a decrease in right bias (Gardner, Lewkowicz, & Turkewitz, 1977; Kurtzberg *et al.*, 1979).[13] The picture, however, may be more complex than this account implies. Fox and Lewis (1982) compared normal-term infants with preterm infants (gestational age ≤ 33 weeks) who had suffered from respiratory distress syndrome. This comparison, made when the preterm infants were 38 conceptional weeks of age, showed differences *not* in the tendency to spontaneously assume the head-right posture but only in the speed with which the affected infants resumed the head-right posture after their heads had been held in midline. Initially, only 20% of the affected infants turned to the right, compared with 70% of the term infants. However, after 15 minutes, 80% of the affected infants and 90% of the normal-term infants had assumed the right position. Evidently, postnatal illness in premature infants can slow the lateral head-turn response after midline placement but without disrupting the maintenance of the right postural asymmetry itself.

The evidence thus indicates that perinatal and postnatal status does have certain consequences for neonatal laterality. What about the other factors of potential relevance to the evaluation of handedness in infants (see pp. 309–313)? To date, there has not been much systematic study of these variables, but what there is suggests that they do play a role. For example, a study by Saling (1983) has implicated familial handedness as well as a new variable—parental sex—as contributing factors. The subjects were 210 full-term infants. All were observed on day 3. Instead of examining their responsiveness to lateral somesthetic stimulation of the mouth area, Saling assessed the infants' spontaneous head position while the infants lay supine. The results showed that birth risk (on a scale derived in part from Littman and Parmelee, 1974a, 1974b) contributed to lateral differentiation, but the relationship was complex. The only significant contributor to lateral differentiation (LD) was the interaction of familial handedness (parents' handedness) and birth risk. For offspring of two right-handed parents, birth risk was unrelated to LD; for offspring with one or both parents left-handed, the relationship was positive, implying that increments in birth stress are linearly and continuously associated with increasing leftward bias in neonatal position. Separate analyses disclosed that this interaction was primarily attributable to an interaction of *paternal* handedness and birth risk. The interaction of *maternal* handedness and birth risk did not account for additional variance.

Some or even all of the effects in neonatal studies may, of course, reflect only the interference effects of transient state variables at the time of delivery rather than a persistent change in neural organization. To clarify the picture, we must know whether differences like those shown in newborns and neonates also appear in older infants, when transient state variables are less likely to be operating. Evidence on this point has been reported by Liederman and Coryell (1982). They compared 16 infants between 4 and 10 weeks of age, all with a history of perinatal complications (PC), with an equal number of infants having no such history, matched carefully for sex, age, and parental handedness. To be assigned to the PC group, an infant had to have one or more of the following perinatal complications: C-section, nonvertex delivery, nuchal cords, toxemia, fetal distress, prematurity (37 weeks gestation), or postmaturity (43 weeks gestation). The behavior examined was spontaneous turning preference while the infants were lying supine, and the in-

13. Saling (1983, p. 277) sees the effect as the result of "neurological nonoptimalities, rather than immaturity itself" and supports this conclusion by pointing to the findings of Prechtl, Fargel, Weinmann, and Bakker (1979): Preterm infants, selected on the basis of an undamaged nervous system, showed the rightward bias in spontaneous head position; preterm infants with nervous system dysfunctions did not. Similarly, an absence of rightward bias in spontaneous head position was found in full-term neonates with three or more nonoptimal neurological signs during the first few days of postnatal life (Saling & Abkeiwicz, no date; cited in Saling, 1983, pp. 277–278).

cidence, strength, and tonicity of the asymmetric tonic neck reflex (ATNR) as affected by head position.

The result was that PC infants demonstrated a different lateral organization from the no perinatal complications (NPC) group. As a group, the PC infants lacked the usual right-turning bias showed by the NPC infants as well as the lateralization of the ATNR. The question of sex differences was not raised, so we do not know whether, in either the PC or the NPC group, the absence of the right-turning bias was commoner in boys than in girls.

The fact that these differences occurred 4 to 10 weeks after delivery suggests a relatively stable change in neural organization and not merely the interference of transient state variables at the time of delivery.

Liederman and Coryell also assessed parental handedness, but the results were the reverse of Saling's (1983). Where Saling found that birth stress was associated with lateral differences only in FLH infants (with the father's contribution playing the main role), Liederman and Coryell (1982) found a relationship between perinatal insult and leftward head position preference only in their FRH subjects (both parents right-handed), but *not* in FLH infants (with at least one parent left-handed).[14]

In summary, the neonatal and early-infancy studies reveal that unusual patterns of lateral asymmetry *are* associated with a history of birth complications. However, Liederman and Coryell (1982) also found several instances of non-right preference in children whose births had been free of complications. This means that not all deviations from right preference can be laid to damage as a result of birth complications. Liederman and Coryell, therefore, see their results as supporting the two-type, but not the one-type, model.

The still scanty evidence thus suggests that birth status *does* have certain consequences for laterality within the neonatal and early infancy period for certain infants, but not for others. It also suggests that whether or not a particular infant shows an effect may depend on parental handedness, although the direction of the contribution is less certain. Saling's data suggest that the effect is more likely in individuals with FLH, whereas Liederman and Coryell's data suggest the reverse.

The next question is, will these effects (e.g., weaker or absent postural right bias) have any consequences for lateral preference over the longer term whether or not the absence of lateral bias can be said to have stemmed from perinatal stress? Liederman (1983, pp. 84–85), in a discussion of the Liederman and Coryell (1982) study, takes a cautious view. She regards the kind of perinatal injury likely to have occurred in the PC group as being very mild, for example, brief episodes of oxygen deprivation during labor and delivery. The effect would be temporary disruption of function within the left hemisphere (which Liederman assumes is more vulnerable than the right) and therefore possibly a temporary shift of control to the intact right hemisphere. The result then would be only transient leftward behavioral bias (or no bias at all). The answer to this question lies in prospective longitudinal studies, that is, where the same individuals who show disturbances in laterality in infancy are examined repeatedly until about 4 to 5 years of age, when their true handedness can be compared with that of children who did not show disturbances in laterality in infancy. So far we know of no such investigation. All we have, instead, are studies that

14. Saling (1983) sees his own findings as having greater reliability, noting Liederman and Coryell's small sample size (only 9 of the 32 infants were FLH) as well as their (in Saling's view) questionable criterion for normal birth weight. Liederman and Coryell used 4,500 grams to indicate normality, a value that actually extends into the high-risk range (Lubchenko, 1976; cited in Saling, 1983, p. 282), leading, possibly, to errors in classification (Saling, 1983, p. 282).

simply extend the time span of the relationship between birth status and handedness in childhood and adulthood, but where no actual assessment of laterality in infancy is made. These studies nevertheless are useful in determining whether any such relationship exists, even if they do not permit us to chart the course of development of any individual child.

Relationship between Birth Status and Laterality in Childhood (4 Years and Older) and Adulthood

BIRTH STRESS AS INDEXED BY PARITY

Studies of the relationship between infant risk and adult (or child) handedness have used several different measures of birth stress. Following Bakan, one of the measures assessed has been birth order on the assumption that primiparity (and also fourth or later births) poses the greatest risk for perinatal stress (see p. 333).

It seems fair to say that, except for Bakan's own studies of college students, along with one or two others (e.g., Bakan, 1971, 1977; Bakan *et al.*, 1973; Leviton & Kilty, 1976), the results are negative, or at best inconclusive. Left-handers do not appear to be significantly overrepresented among either first- or fourth- or later-born individuals (e.g., Annett & Ockwell, 1980; Ehrlichman, Zoccolotti, & Owen, 1982; Hicks, Elliot, Garbesi, & Martin, 1979; Hicks, Evans, & Pellegrini, 1978; Hubbard, 1971; Leiber & Axelrod, 1981; Nachson & Denno, 1986; Schwartz, 1977; Tan & Nettleton, 1980; Teng *et al.*, 1976). Indeed, in at least one instance, the reverse relationship was found (Hubbard, 1971).

Several of the early studies failed to consider the possibility that the birth order–handedness relationship is moderated by other risk variables. One of these would be maleness, on the view that males are more likely than females to be affected by untoward environmental events. The evidence is inconclusive. Bakan himself (1971) found the birth order effect only for males, as did Leviton and Kilty (1976). In the negative reports cited earlier, the effects of sex generally were not reported. Hicks, Pellegrini, and Evans (1978) made such an examination but found no evidence, contra Bakan, that sex, in and of itself, was a moderator variable.

Bakan (1977, 1978a) himself has responded to the negative reports by noting that birth order by itself would not be a valid index of pregnancy and birth complications until variables such as socioeconomic status, infant morality, nutritional factors, and medical care are taken into account. We agree, and we recall that Eastman *et al.* (1962) made a similar point in discussing the relationship between parity and cerebral palsy (see p. 333). Nevertheless, Bakan's attempts to save the parity explanation by appeal to such correlated variables seems forced and unpersuasive. The consensus in the neuropsychological literature appears to be that parity has little, if any, relationship to adult handedness, at least in college populations where, presumably, intelligence is normal or above, and where other sequelae of presumed PLH most likely are absent. Still, in light of two other studies, perhaps we should not give up on the parity variable just yet.

Unlike the aforementioned studies of adults, mostly college students, both of these investigations examined the relationship between parity and handedness in children—6-year-olds in a study by Smart *et al.* (1980), 4-year-olds in a study by Badian (1983).

Smart *et al.*'s (1980) sample consisted of 1,094 children, for all of whom birth medical records were available. Each family answered a mail questionnaire about the child's and family's handedness for writing or drawing (we earlier reported on the secular trends found; p. 313). A relationship between parity and non-right-handedness was found, but it was neither simple nor direct. The group with the highest percentage of non-right-handedness was fourth- and later-born boys (23.7%), but non-right-handedness also was higher in boys overall (19.9% versus 13.6% in girls), and this percentage for fourth- and later-born boys was not significantly different from those in other male birth order groups. Where a sex effect was evident was in mode of delivery. Forty percent of boys born by breech delivery were non-right-handed, compared with only 13% of boys delivered by C-section. No such effect was seen for girls.

Straightforward parity effects, then, were absent. Earlier, however, we pointed out that parity effects might well be moderated by maternal age, (see p. 335), so that primiparity would have very different significance for a young teenage mother than for a woman in her mid-20s. This possibility is borne out in Smart *et al.*'s data. Considering all mothers, those aged 39 years or older produced more non-right-handed children than did younger mothers, but this relationship was significant only for primiparae and not for multiparae. Of 21 children of "elderly" primiparae, 9 were non-right-handed (43%). If, then, the parity variable has any influence, it would be only in combination with maternal age, although the mechanism moderating such a relationship is not revealed.

Badian's (1983) study also implicates the parity variable, but more directly. Her subjects (592 boys, 594 girls) represented approximately 90% of the children about to enter kindergarten in a small school system over an 8-year period. The median age was 4 years, 9 months, with almost all children between 4 years, 3 months and 5 years, 3 months. Handedness in this study was defined as right or left if only one hand was used on these tasks, or as mixed if the child switched hands between tasks or in the middle of a task. Birth order information was obtained for 1,097 children (92.5%) of the sample.

To assess the relationship between birth order and handedness, Badian divided her sample into right-handers and non-right-handers, with the latter group consisting of the left- and mixed-handed children. For boys, the result was significantly more non-right-handers for birth positions 1 and 4 or later than for 2 or 3. In contrast to Smart *et al.*'s (1980) results, this difference also was apparent for each maternal age as well as for the total group of boys. Non-right-handedness occurred in 19.9% of the 282 boys in birth orders 1 and 4 or later, compared with 11.3% of the 266 second- or third-born boys. For girls, the two groups were not significantly different. In fact, the percentage of non-right-handed girls for birth positions 2 and 3 was slightly higher (15.98%) than for positions 1 or 4 or later (13.2%).

Like Smart *et al.*, Badian also assessed the role of maternal age. First- and later-born (4+) children of mothers <20 years or >30 years (group A) were compared with the second- and third-born children of mothers aged 20 to 29 years (group B). For boys, the groups differed significantly, with 20.7% of group A being non-right-handed, compared with 9.9% of group B. For girls, the two groups were not significantly different in the percentage of non-right-handers (group A = 13.9%; group B = 14.6%).

If it is the so-called mixed-handers who are mainly contributing to Badian's effect, this is certainly interesting, but it may not have any bearing on the PLH hypothesis because we do not yet have any data on the developmental outcome of the mixed-handers. What we are seeing may actually be a *delay* in the establishment of handedness in the first- and later-born boys, rather than true non-right-handedness. If, say, 2 years later, the "mixed-handed" boys showed a ratio of right- to left-handedness about the same as in the second and third birth order groups, then all we could say is that parity was related to circumstances or conditions that slowed the establishment of handedness. The sex effect, then, would be reinterpreted to mean not that boys were more at risk for PLH but that they were more at risk for a developmental delay.

Until these questions about Smart *et al.*'s (1980) and Badian's (1983) studies are resolved, we think the wiser conclusion is the more conservative: The proposed relationship between parity and left-handedness, even as moderated by maternal age and sex, remains unproved.

BIRTH STRESS AS INDEXED BY CONDITIONS OF PREGNANCY AND DELIVERY

Recognizing that parity provides, at best, a most imperfect index of birth stress, many researchers have sought to measure birth stress more directly by the use of such criteria as were listed earlier (pp. 331–336). This information has been obtained in different ways.

Retrospective Accounts of Birth Stress by Subjects. One way has been to ask the subjects themselves. In the first such study, by Bakan *et al.* (1973), 510 university students were divided, by means of a 12-item handedness questionnaire, into three handedness groups (58 left-handers, 58 "ambilaterals," and 282 right-handers). Each subject also answered a birth stress questionnaire, which included the conditions "multiple birth, prolonged labor, caesarian birth, breech birth, blue baby, breathing difficulty at birth, other." Subjects reporting one or more stress conditions constituted the stress group; subjects reporting no birth stress or "don't know" constituted the "normal" group. The result was that birth stress was reported by 40% of the left-handers, 41% of the ambilaterals, and only 22% of the right-handers. Bakan *et al.* (1973) concluded that their results supported the PLH model.[15]

In a study of similar design, Schwartz (1977) gave 600 university undergraduates a 14-item handedness questionnaire and a questionnaire about the nature of their mother's pregnancy. (The only example provided in Schwartz's report was, "Was your birth normal in terms of labor, and no complications during pregnancy or delivery?") Schwartz divided the subjects into four handedness groups—strong and weak left- and right-handers—a more rigorous procedure for classification than Bakan *et al.* (1973) had used. The results failed to show any increase in left-handedness in students as a result of any complication in their mother's pregnancy or delivery, and this was so for all four handedness classifications. The results of subsequent investigations also have been negative (e.g., Searleman, Tsao, & Balzer, 1980).[16]

15. An immediate problem for the model, as Bakan himself understood (Bakan *et al.*, 1973), was the additional finding of a familial factor associated with left-handedness, and the relationship between FLH and birth stress. Regardless of the handedness of the subject, subjects who reported left-handedness or ambilaterality in the family also reported more birth stress in their own births. The relationship was statistically significant for both the left-handers and the right-handers but failed to reach significance for the ambilaterals. Insofar as this finding is consistent with a genetic model of left-handedness, it would challenge the PLH model. Recall, however, that Bakan *et al.* (1973) suggested that the familial tendency to left-handedness is itself mediated by a familial tendency to birth stress. (pp. 310–311). Annett and Ockwell (1980) tested this possibility by personally interviewing the mothers themselves. If left-handers are more likely than right-handers to experience stress in giving birth, then left-handed mothers should report more stressful births for their children than right-handed mothers. The results were to the contrary: Left-handed mothers reported stressful births in 23% of their children, right-handed mothers in 30%.

16. In one sense, even if further investigations agreed with Bakan *et al.* (1973), we would question the findings simply because the data base is suspect. Why would one trust college students, or anyone else for that matter, to have accurate knowledge of such medical details? Even supposing that the recollections of the left-handers and ambilaterals in Bakan *et al.*'s (1973) report were accurate, perhaps when medical histories are positive for stress, this information (for whatever reason) is more likely to be communicated to left-handers and ambilaterals than to right-handers. This would artificially lower the percentage of non-right-handers reporting difficult pregnancies and births. Alternatively, perhaps the tendency of non-right-handers to report problems in birth history simply represents a generalized negative response bias on their part.

Measures of Birth Stress as Provided by the Mother or by the Medical Record Directly. A better approach has been to use information either provided by the mother herself or, preferably, from the medical records directly. For example, for a sample of 245 children, Schwartz (1986) derived seven different measures of high-risk pregnancy and birth from medical records directly and from the mother herself. None of the measures was associated with an increase in left-handedness (assessed by a variety of preference and performance measures) when the children were 2 years old.

Because we had recommended 4 years as the minimum age for evaluation of the birth stress hypothesis), it is possible that handedness differences might appear at later ages, at least in some children. The evidence, however, is to the contrary. At least five such studies based on national survey data have been reported, two in Great Britain (Bishop, 1984; McManus, 1981), three in the United States (Ehrlichman *et al.*, 1982; Nachson & Denno, 1987; Spiegler & Yeni-Komshian, 1982). We shall mention just two of the studies.[17]

The subjects in the American national survey were children who had been participants in the National Collaborative Perinatal Project (NCPP) conducted by the (United States) National Institute of Neurological and Childhood Diseases in the 1950s and 1960s (for a description of the sample and research design, see Broman, Nichols, & Kennedy, 1975; Niswander & Gordon, 1972). Along with many other measures, the children's handedness was assessed at 7 years of age. In using the NCPP data to test the PLH model, Spiegler and Yeni-Komshian (1982) deliberately limited their analysis in three ways. First, to test the applicability of the PLH model to a population of ostensibly normal children, they included only those children whose 7-year-old IQ scores were equal to or greater than 80. There were 17,733 cases that met this criterion.

Second, although three different measures of hand preference were available in the data pool, only one measure was used—a test in which the child was required to mark an X on paper on three successive trials. (The other measures were observed writing hand and self-report of hand preference for three different unimanual tasks—throwing a ball, using a spoon, and writing.)

Third, the analysis included only those children who used the same hand across the three trials of the X-making test, or, failing this criterion, were consistent on two additional trials for a total of four out of five. Thus, children with what we would call ambiguous handedness (at least on this one measure) were excluded. By this criterion, approximately 2% of the 17,333 cases were excluded, leaving a total sample of 17,220 children, with 12.5% of the boys and 10.3% of the girls left-handed, a statistically significant difference consistent with other reports.

Birth risk was derived from a classification system (Hobel, Hyvarinen, Okada, & Oh, 1973) designed to predict neonatal morbidity and mortality. The system permitted division of the perinatal period into three phases: prenatal (beginning of pregnancy to onset of labor), intrapartum (labor and delivery), and neonatal (birth to discharge from hospital). Risk was assessed by simple summing of scores on each variable (see Table 12-4, p. 322).

The results failed to support Bakan's hypothesis. There were not proportionately more left-handed children, either boys or girls, among the high-risk cases, and this was so for each of the three perinatal phases.

17. The reports for each country actually have drawn on the same national survey data, one British, one American, but because they have asked somewhat different questions, they have defined the dependent variables in somewhat different ways and have used somewhat different selection criteria. In the case of the American studies, the one by Spiegler and Yeni-Komshian (1982) drew on the entire national data base pool, whereas the others drew on sub-groups of this pool. Nevertheless, all of the studies come to essentially the same conclusions. We therefore have focused on only one report from each national survey.

Because the children represented a broad range of socioeconomic groups, perhaps the variables associated with high socioeconomic status had mitigated any long-term effects of early trauma. In other words, risk status on the continuum of reproductive casualty may have been influenced by risk status on the continuum of caretaker casualty (see pp. 335). If so, "surplus" left-handedness (presumed PLH) might be expected only among those high-risk infants who came from poorer families. To find out, Spiegler and Yeni-Komshian defined a subgroup consisting of children whose families were among the lowest 20% of the socioeconomic distribution. Socioeconomic class was determined by combining scores of education, family income, and occupation into a single score. Within this subgroup, the subjects then were separated into low- and high-risk groups according to the same criteria as previously described. Again, the results were negative: Birth complications were not related to left-handedness.

The British study was a longitudinal survey of medical, education, and social aspects of development from a 1958 cohort. McManus (1981) concentrated on a subgroup of 11,029 children for whom there were adequate hand preference data at ages 7 and 11 years. Data were collected on 19 variables, including factors related to mother's medical history, apart from her pregnancy, and to prenatal, perinatal, and postnatal variables similar to those used in the U.S. survey. Like the American survey, the evidence, considered individually and collectively, failed to show any relationship between left-handedness and birth stress at any of the stages related to parturition.

Given the known heterogeneity for cerebral organization in ostensibly normal left-handers, none of these studies seem to have considered the possibility that the birth stress-handedness association might be more likely in some subgroups of left-handers than others. At least one attempt has been made to take this possibility into consideration. Searleman, Porac, and Coren (1982) found a positive association between maternal report of birth complications and left-handedness in college-age subjects, but only in males and predominantly in those with inverted handwriting posture. We recall Levy's (1974; Levy & Reid, 1978) hypothesis that the inverted posture may be a possible marker for that subcategory of left-handers with left hemisphere control for visually-mediated language functions. Given Levy's speculation that this condition originates in embryonic or fetal disturbances in the development of midline structures (see p. 324), we would not be inclined to accept Searleman *et al.*'s supposition that birth stress (that is, *perinatal* factors) are the primary cause. Here, instead, would be a possible example of misclassification of prenatal CNS injuries attributed to parturition (Towbin, 1970; see earlier discussion, pp. 327–328). Nonetheless, the possibility that inverted writing posture may be a marker for pathology is worth pursuing, especially because Searleman *et al.*'s findings are consistent with the evidence that males are at greater risk for pathology than females; because, in the studies reviewed in the current section, the scant evidence linking birth stress with handedness nonetheless implicates mostly males; because the inverted posture is far more common in males than females (McKeever, 1979; Peters & Pedersen, 1978); and, finally, in light of reports mentioned earlier in this chapter that the inverted writing posture was associated with lowered scores on reading and neuropsychological tests.

Birth Stress and Handedness in Intellectually Subnormal Individuals

In all the studies reviewed in this section, the subjects were at least of normal intelligence. As we have noted, this was necessary for testing the hypothesis that left-handedness is actually PLH even in the absence of any other clinical signs. As we have seen, with a few provocative exceptions where males are concerned, the evidence did not support the hypothesis: "Normal" left-handers and right-handers were *not* positioned differently on the continuum of risk. As we also have seen, left-handedness *is* overrepresented among individuals with mental retardation. This suggests that, if we were to sample from those populations, we might begin to find the relationship between birth conditions and handedness that was so clearly lacking among the normal populations. This was the case in the study by Ross *et al.* (1987), discussed in the Introduction, which found a doubling of the percentage of left-handers in 4-year-old children with IQs below 85 compared with children with IQs above 85. In that study, *all* of the below-85 IQ children had been premature infants with low birth weight. What is especially revealing about this study in the current context is that a certain proportion of the premature children had *normal* intelligence. Among those children, there was no significant difference from the controls (all full-term births) either in the percentage of left-handers or in performance on language and speech measures. In other words, where prematurity, as a risk factor, is actually associated with a rise in left-handedness, there also must be associated neurological signs (namely, mental retardation and other cognitive deficits). Thus, where left-handedness *is* a sign of PLH, it is highly improbable that it is the only sign.

Independent Markers of PLH in Ostensibly Normal Individuals

The statistical evidence thus fails to support the one-type PLH model. Whereas the surplus of left-handers in certain clinical populations can be attributed to PLH, there is no convincing evidence that all ostensibly normal left-handers are actually PLH. The evidence, however, *is* consistent with the possibility that the PLH phenotype exists in some small proportion of the population of clinically asymptomatic left-handers, and that there are proportionally more males than females among them. But if this subgroup exists, then, as Henry *et al.* (1984) have pointed out, we need a reliable way to identify it—some independent marker. In addition to the still largely untested speculation regarding inverted writing posture, two possibilities have been suggested.

HIGHLY DISCREPANT SKILL FAVORING THE DOMINANT HAND: BISHOP'S EXTENDED PLH MODEL

One possible marker has been suggested by Bishop (1980, 1984). As noted earlier, the dominant hand is normally more skillful than the non-dominant hand. The extent of this difference, however, varies across individuals such that in some persons the dominant hand is only slightly better than the nondominant hand, whereas in other persons the advantage is considerably greater, although not to such an extent that the nondominant hand is considered pathologically clumsy. In other words, nothing in the overt behavior of these individuals suggests a history of brain injury. Nonetheless, the question is whether very marked inferiority of the nonpreferred hand may constitute a unilateral "soft" neurological sign.

Bishop's proposal is that it can, and that the left-hander who is actually PLH ought to be less skillful with his *right* hand than his left hand to a markedly greater degree than a left-hander whose handedness is not pathological. Her reasoning is that PLH could be the result of a brain abnormality too mild to produce epilepsy, mental retardation, or gross neurological signs but sufficient to make the genotypically preferred hand clumsy, thus forcing a preference for the other hand in most cases. Such individuals therefore could be identified not by the performance of their preferred hand but by the poor performance, relative to unaffected individuals, of their *nonpreferred hand.* This idea has now been tested in three separate studies of nonclinical populations of schoolchildren (Bishop, 1980, 1984; Gillberg, Waldenstrom, & Rasmussen, 1983). In each study, left-handedness was significantly more common among those children with poorest nonpreferred hand performance (the high-risk or target group). Target group children, however, performed just as well as non–target group children with their *preferred* hand. The higher number of left-handers in the target group thus does not mean that left-handers generally are simply clumsier than right-handers. In light of some of the new data reported on hand skills in left-handers in the general population, (see p. 302), Bishop's results may even underestimate the extent to which the pathological left-hander may differ from the nonpathological left-hander. Recall that in normal left-handers, left-hand scores are equal to right-handers' right-hand scores, whereas left-handers' right-hand scores are superior to the right-handers' left-hand scores. The implication would seem to be that the difference is skill between the hands in PLH individuals is even more different from that found in their non-PLH counterparts than it is from that of normal right-handers. These hypothesized differences are shown in Figure 12-4.

Bishop also reasoned that if poor performance by the nonpreferred hand is a marker of unilateral dysfunction that leads to PLH in the case of the genotypic right-hander, then poor nonpreferred hand performance also would be associated with inferior cognitive performance, even in subclinical children. The evidence confirmed this prediction: among left-handers in the target group there were more speech problems than there were among non–target group children (both right- and left-handers).

In summary, Bishop's data suggest that PLH, though not at all a common condition, can arise in children who do *not* have gross motor impairment, much less hemiplegia. Therefore, to the extent that left-hand preference is obligatory because of right-sided peripheral dysfunction (even if associated with brain injury), the threshold need not be so high as McManus (1983) has suggested (see pp. 299). Instead, even so mild a dysfunction

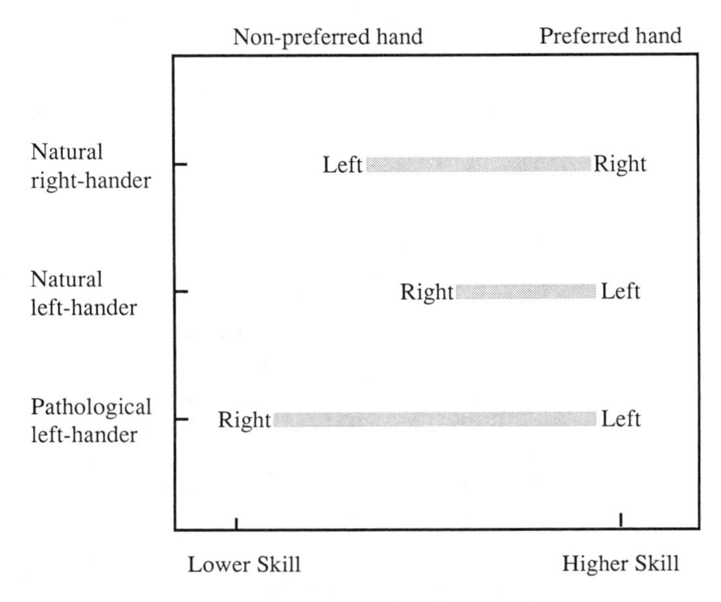

Figure 12-4. Hypothetical differences in skilled performance between the hands in normal right-handers, normal left-handers, and pathological left-handers.

as clinically asymptomatic clumsiness of the right hand may be sufficient to induce preference for the left hand.

Although Bishop's work supports and extends Satz's model, there is an interesting discrepancy between the bodies of data. Satz, we recall, suggests that PLH in individuals with explicit unilateral neurological injury will be associated with impaired visual–spatial but normal language ability. The reason is the shift of language to the right hemisphere, which comes at the expense of spatial skills (with the caution, as noted earlier, that the evidence for this last outcome is still uncertain). Recall that the supposition behind this model is that hand preference is most likely to shift when neurological injury occurs early, encroaches on the language zones of the left hemisphere, and shifts language to the right hemisphere. Bishop (1984, p. 224) sees her data as consistent with this interpretation. We would like to suggest a further possibility. As we have just seen, Bishop's data indicate PLH in clinically asymptomatic children who proved to have associated language problems, whereas one of the associated signs of PLH in at least some of Satz's patients was *normal* language with associated visual–spatial problems. This suggests to us that the neurological injury causing PLH in Bishop's target children encroached on left-hemisphere language zones with sufficient severity to cause right-hand clumsiness and a shift of *hand* control to the right hemisphere, but *not* with sufficient severity to force a shift of *language* function. Therefore, in these children, the implication would seem to be that the left hemisphere is still mediating language functions, although at a mildly impaired subclinical level. This is precisely what one could expect on the assumption that the threshold for shifting hand preference is lower than the threshold for shifting language. Bishop's data therefore fit the second of the three scenarios outlined earlier (p. 297), whereas Satz's, as already noted, provide a better fit with the third scenario.

PEDAL ASYMMETRY

Another possible marker of PLH in subclinical populations is pedal asymmetry. Earlier, we reviewed evidence that suggested that pedal asymmetry can be a biological marker for PLH in individuals of known early neural injury, namely, in epileptic and mentally retarded individuals. A study by Yanowitz, Satz, and Heilman (1981) of pedal asymmetries in normal persons raises the possibility that such a physical asymmetry also might serve as a marker of PLH in clinically asymptomatic individuals. Although they did not find any significant differences in foot length in their subjects, there was an incidental finding that bears on the question of PLH. Left-handed males showed a larger variability in foot length asymmetry than did any of the other subgroups (left- or right-handed females or right-handed males). This variability was due largely to four left-handed men whose foot length differences exceeded two standard deviations compared to the study sample as a whole, suggesting something more than normal variance. For three of these four men, the difference significantly favored the left foot (>1.3 cm). Yanowitz *et al.* (1981) suggested that the result was consistent with trophic changes in the extremities that have been reported in clinical cases with known early birth trauma. They also concluded that the presence of a markedly shorter right foot in left-handers indirectly suggests the presence of PLH and noted that the appearance of the effect only in males is consistent with known sex differences in risk for birth injury and disease. Henry *et al.* (1984, p. 266) urge a cautious view of this finding, since the subjects in Yanowitz *et al.*'s study were neurologically intact. Nevertheless, they thought it "tempting and reasonable" to speculate that these subjects were asymptomatic individuals who had experienced early left-hemisphere trauma that had two effects: manual transfer, resulting in PLH, and underdevelopment of the bones of the right foot due to involvement of the left postcentral gyrus. They went on to warn that the relationship between handedness and trophic changes in subjects with known brain injury must first be examined before this interpretation can be accepted. Assuming that this prior question is satisfactorily answered and that trophic shortfall can be used as a marker variable in clinical populations (as the data cited in the previous section already suggest), then limb size may prove to be a useful marker of PLH in clinically asymptomatic (''normal'') individuals as well, especially if combined with Bishop's (1980) measure of highly discrepant hand skill. That is, the group of ''asymptomatic'' left-handed individuals most likely to show trophic shortfall of the nondominant lower limb should be those individuals whose performance on tests of hand skill shows the largest discrepancy favoring the dominant hand. If, then, pedal asymmetry is an anatomical marker of PLH, here may be a basis for distinguishing subgroups of left-handers within the ''normal'' population for comparison on, say, Bishop's (1980, 1984) tests of skill of the nondominant hand. We also might suggest additional tests of foot performance, since many of the performance asymmetries found in the hands are also found in the feet (see Peters, 1988). Might there be a pathological left-footedness that is associated with pathological left-handedness?

CONCLUSIONS AND SUGGESTIONS FOR FURTHER RESEARCH

We hope that we have succeeded in laying out some of the questions and issues that arise in connection with theories of pathological handedness. What general conclusions can be drawn from our review and analysis? Throughout the text we have already made many observations and suggestions pertaining to both conceptual and empirical questions, so we shall not repeat them here. Instead, we shall conclude by emphasizing some of the more important points, particularly those relevant for further research.

Throughout this analysis we have focused on the unilateral lesion model and each of its variants. We feel confident that we can dismiss the one-type variant. The notion that *all* left-handedness arises from lateralized injury to the left cerebral hemisphere finds no support from a large number of studies that have put the hypothesis to a fair and rigorous test. The evidence, however, does support the two-type model, with such qualifications as we have already mentioned. The question is: Where do we go from here?

There continues to be a need for better and more comprehensive empirical studies of the relationship between handedness and psychological characteristics in both normal and clinical populations. As we have noted, the picture looks clearer for some characteristics than for others. In some cases, the data base is simply insufficient to tell, either because of an inadequate number of empirical investigations or because the populations studied are not specified carefully enough. There are recent signs of progress—for example, in distinguishing populations of mental retardates by degree and kind of retardation—but much more could be done. An answer to these questions will help us to assess the explanatory power of current models and to generate better ones.

At the heart of gaining a clearer picture of the psychological correlates of left- and right-handedness, we also must resolve questions about the definition and measurement of handedness. In particular, the distinction between ambiguous handedness and mixed-handedness needs to be further addressed both in populations with severe disorders and in populations with less severe disorders, for example, across the spectrum of mental retardation. This can be done only by assessing the reliability of hand use with repeated measures, a procedure that, as we have noted, is not routine. The kind of assessment used (performance or questionnaire), particularly in clinical populations, also may be crucial. More attention also should be paid to the evaluation of nondominant hand skills as part of the measurement and definition of handedness. This could have important implications for the evaluation of PLH. For example, if compromised visuospatial ability proves to be associated with PLH, then what would be predicted about left-hand performance by PLH individuals on spatial tasks using such methods as dichhaptic discrimination?

Much work remains in charting the natural history of handedness, since handedness, pathological or not, is fundamentally a developmental phenomenon and can be fully understood only within a developmental perspective. Only in this way, too, shall we have norms with which to test pathological handedness models through comparisons of normal with at-risk infants and children. As we noted, some clinical evidence suggests that a strong hand preference before about 6 months of age may be pathognomonic, but any such diagnosis depends on good developmental norms, especially where associated neurological signs are not evident. We also still have only a fragmentary understanding of the role of familial handedness, sex, and cultural context in the development of normal handedness, much less in the development of pathological handedness. The variable of sex, in particular, shows some promise as a moderating factor in the analysis of pathological handedness.

In individuals with brain injury (those at risk for pathological handedness), the clinical literature provides us with little or no information about the actual processes in the development of hand preference. How soon after injury is one hand favored? How quickly and how effectively do different levels of sensory or motor impairment begin to affect preference? What role is played by parents, teachers, or rehabilitation specialists in the remediation of deficits and restoration of function? We also would like to see more experimental modeling of these pathological processes in normal individuals. A variety of methods might be used. One example is Umansky's (1973) demonstration of the effects of peripheral interference (placing a sock over the infant's forearm) on hand preference. Furthermore, if, as has been argued recently (MacNeilage, Studdert-Kennedy, & Lindblom, 1987), handedness is not a uniquely human phenomenon, then the use of animal models also can contribute importantly to our understanding of central as well as peripheral mechanisms in the development of pathological handedness.

We took some pains to discuss the anatomy and developmental physiology of motor control because we saw them as crucial to any speculation about the effects of injury to any particular anatomical site. Unfortunately, we are still in the dark with respect to the neurological loci that might set a bias toward left- or right-handedness in the normal individual. In other words, we still are far from understanding the neuroanatomical means by which, in the case of the genotypic right-hander, the normal right-shift factor is expressed. Until we do, we shall not understand anomalous handedness either. In the clinical literature, we also would hope to see much more attention given to precise localization of lesions, both cortical and subcortical, in cases of suspected PLH. Along with a more refined evaluation of hand skill, this also would help to test the strength of the association between the pathological induction of hand preference and changes in language lateralization. In this same connection, we also need more accurate estimates of the relative frequencies of left- and right-hemisphere injuries in the population. The evidence strongly suggests that the left hemisphere is more at risk than the right, but how much more, and does the risk difference occur at developmental periods and anatomical sites that are more or less likely to affect hand preference? Such information is necessary for estimation of the population of brain-injured persons who will constitute the pool of candidates for pathological handedness.

One of the most promising of recent developments in the analysis of pathological handedness has been the identification of associated clinical signs. As already noted, what is needed now is to assess these signs with cognitive tests that have been validated as measures of left- and right-hemispheric functions. Only in this way could we hope to resolve the inconsistent findings pertaining to the pattern of cognitive impairment in individuals suspected of PLH. This also would help to distinguish PLH from non-PLH. We also would like to see attention paid to the question of associated clinical signs in pathological right-handedness (PRH). As noted, such signs might be quite different in the two groups.

In light of the scope of the further research needs, as we see them, there clearly is a need for cooperation among laboratories for both normal developmental and clinical studies. Only by such means could we assemble a clinical data base adequate to assess the mutual contributions to pathological handedness of such variables as timing of injury, site of injury, and degree of motor or sensory impairment, and of subject variables such as sex and familial handedness. Furthermore, because so many factors must enter into the equation and because we cannot assume that they are related to each other in a linear fashion, we no longer should rely on univariate methods of data analysis—the method used in many previous studies. A multivariate problem needs multivariate procedures.

Although we have focused on the unilateral lesion model, we want to re-emphasize our conviction that a full understanding of the psychological profile of left-handedness must look beyond a single model. The other models outlined earlier also deserve continued study, and no doubt even they do not exhaust the possibilities.

Finally, we wish to emphasize that we see the resolution of these questions as having implications that go far beyond clinical issues. Both from a neurophysiological perspective and from a psychobiological perspective, the explication of the phenomenon of pathological handedness can teach us a great deal about the normal development of the nervous system.

ACKNOWLEDGMENTS

Some of the empirical research reported herein was supported by a grant to L. J. H. from the Michigan State University Foundation and the Spencer Foundation. We are grateful to Michael Peters, Richard S. Lewis, and Juliet Vogel for their helpful comments on an earlier version of this chapter.

REFERENCES

Abramowicz, M., & Barnett, H. L. (1970). Sex ratio of infant mortality: Trends of change. *American Journal of Diseases of Children, 119,* 314–325.

Allen, M., & Wellman, M. M. (1980). Hand position during writing, cerebral laterality and reading: Age and sex differences. *Neuropsychologia, 18,* 33–40.

Anderson, M. E. (1981). The basal ganglia and movement. In A. L. Towe & E. S. Luschei (Eds.), *Handbook of behavioral neurobiology: Vol. 5. Motor coordination* (pp. 367–399). New York: Plenum.

Annett, M. (1970). The growth of manual preference and speed. *British Journal of Psychology, 61,* 545–558.

Annett, M. (1972). The distribution of manual asymmetry. *British Journal of Psychology, 63,* 343–358.

Annett, M. (1973). Laterally of childhood hemiphegia and the growth of speech and intelligence. *Cortex, 9,* 4–33.

Annett, M. (1975). Hand preference and the laterality of cerebral speech. *Cortex, 11,* 305–328.

Annett, M. (1976). A coordination of hand preference and skill replicated. *British Journal of Psychology, 67,* 587–592.

Annett, M. (1978). Genetic and nongenetic influences on handedness. *Behavior Genetics, 8,* 227–249.

Annett, M. (1981). The genetics of handedness. *Trends in Neurosciences, 2,* 256–258.

Annett, M. (1985). *Left, right, hand and brain: The right shift theory.* London: Lawrence Erlbaum Associates.

Annett, M., & Kilshaw, D. (1982). Mathematical ability and lateral asymmetries. *Cortex, 18,* 547–568.
Annett, M., & Kilshaw, D. (1983). Right- and left-hand skill II: Estimating the parameters of the distribution of left-right differences in males and females. *British Journal of Psychology, 24,* 269–283.
Annett, M., & Kilshaw, D. (1984). Lateral preference and skill in dyslexics: Implications of the right-shift theory. *British Journal of Psychology, 25,* 357–377.
Annett, M., & Ockwell, A. (1980). Birth order, birth stress, and handedness. *Cortex, 16,* 181–187.
Apgar, V. (1953). Proposal for a new method of evaluation of newborn infants. *Current Researches in Anesthesia and Analgesia, 32,* 260–267.
Apgar, V., & James, L. S. (1962). Further observations on the newborn scoring system. *American Journal of Diseases of Children, 104,* 419.
Aram, D. M., Ekelman, B. L., & Satz, P. (1986). Trophic changes following early unilateral injury to the brain. *Developmental Medicine and Child Neurology, 28,* 165–170.
Audenino, E. (1907). L'homme droit, l'homme gauche et l'homme ambidextre. *Archivio di Psichiatria, Neuropatologia, Antropologia, Antropologia Criminale e Medicina Legale* (Torino), *28,* 23–31.
Badian, N. A. (1983). Birth order, maternal age, season of birth, and handedness. *Cortex, 19,* 451–463.
Bakan, P. (1971). Handedness and birth order. *Nature* (London), *229,* 195.
Bakan, P. (1977). Left handedness and birth order revisited. *Neuropsychologia, 15,* 837–839.
Bakan, P. (1978a). Handedness and birth order: A critical note on a critical note. *Perceptual and Motor Skills, 46,* 556.
Bakan, P. (1978b). Handedness of offspring and maternal cigarette smoking during pregnancy. Paper presented at the 86th annual meeting of the American Psychological Association, August, Toronto, Canada.
Bakan, P., Dibb, G., & Reed, P. (1973). Handedness and birth stress. *Neuropsychologia, 11,* 363–366.
Bakketeig, L. S., & Hoffman, H. J. (1979). Perinatal morality by birth order within cohorts based on sibship size. *British Medical Journal, ii,* 693–696.
Baldwin, J. M. (1890). Origin of right or lefthandedness. *Science, 16,* 247–248.
Ballard, P. B. (1911–1912). Sinistrality and speech. *Journal of Experimental Pedagogy and Training College Record* (London), *1,* 298–310.
Basso, A., & Della Sala, S. (1986). Ideomotor apraxia arising from a purely deep lesion. *Journal of Neurology, Neurosurgery, and Psychiatry, 49,* 458.
Batheja, M., & McManus, I. C. (1985). Handedness in the mentally handicapped. *Developmental Medicine and Child Neurology, 27,* 63–68.
Belmont, L., & Birch, H. G. (1965). Lateral dominance, lateral awareness, and reading disability. *Child Development, 36,* 57–71.
Bemporad, B., & Kinsbourne, M. (1983). Sinistrality and dyslexia: A possible relationship between subtypes. In M. Kinsbourne (Ed.), Brain basis of learning disabilities, *Topics in Learning and Learning Disabilities, 3,* 48–65.
Benbow, C. P. (1986). Psychological correlates of extreme intellectual precocity. *Neuropsychologia, 24,* 719–725.
Benbow, C. P., & Benbow, R. M. (1984). Biological correlates of high mathematical reasoning ability. In G. J. De Vries, J. P. C. De Bruin, H. B. M. Uylings, & M. A. Corner (Eds.), *Sex differences in the brain: The relation between structure and function: Vol. 61. Progress in brain research* (pp. 469–490). Amsterdam: Elsevier Science.
Bingley, T. (1958). Mental symptoms in temporal lobe epilepsy and temporal lobe glioma. *Acta Psychologica Neurologica Scandinavia, 33,* Suppl. 120.
Birch, H. G., Piñiero, C., Alcalde, T., Toca, T., & Cravioto, J. (1971). Relation of kwashiorkor in early childhood and intelligence at school age. *Pediatric Research, 5,* 579–585.
Bishop, D. V. M. (1980). Handedness, clumsiness and cognitive ability. *Developmental Medicine and Child Neurology, 22,* 569–579.
Bishop, D. V. M. (1983). How sinister is sinistrality? *Journal of the Royal College of Physicians of London, 17,* 161–172.
Bishop, D. V. M. (1984). Using non-preferred hand skill to investigate pathological left-handedness in an unselected population. *Development Medicine and Child Neurology, 26,* 214–226.
Bishop, D. V. M. (1986). Note: Is there a link between handedness and hypersensitivity? *Cortex, 22,* 289–296.
Borod, J. C., Caron, H. S., & Koff, E. (1984). Left-handers and right-handers compared on performance and preference measures of lateral dominance. *British Journal of Psychology, 75,* 177–186.
Brackenridge, C. J. (1981). Secular variation in handedness over ninety years. *Neuropsychologia, 19,* 459–462.
Bradshaw, J. L., & Nettleton, N. C. (1981). The nature of hemispheric specialization in man (target article with commentaries). *The Behavioral and Brain Sciences, 4,* 51–91.

Bradshaw-McAnulty, G., Hicks, R. E., & Kinsbourne, M. (1984). Pathological left-handedness and familial sinistrality in relation to degree of mental retardation. *Brain and Cognition, 3,* 349–356.

Brain, J. L. (1977). Handedness in Tanzania: The physiological aspect. *Anthropos, 72,* 180–192.

Brann, A. W., Jr., & Myers, R. E. (1975). Central nervous system findings in the newborn monkey following severe in utero partial asphyxia. *Neurology, 25,* 327–338.

Brinkman, J., & Kuypers, H. (1973). Cerebral control of contralateral and ipsilateral arm, hand, and finger movements in the split-brain rhesus monkey. *Brain, 96,* 653–674.

Brodal, A. (1981). *Neurological anatomy in relation to clinical medicine* (3rd ed.). New York: Oxford University Press.

Broman, S. H., Nichols, P. L., & Kennedy, W. A. (1975). *Preschool IQ: Prenatal and early developmental correlates.* Hillsdale. NJ: Erlbaum.

Brown, J. L. (1962). Differential hand usage in three-year-old children. *Journal of Genetic Psychology, 100,* 167–175.

Bruens, J. H., Gastaut, H., & Giove, G. (1960). Electroencephalographic study of the signs of chronic vascular insufficiency of the sylvian region in aged people. *Electroencephalography and Clinical Neurophysiology, 12,* 283–295.

Bruml, H. (1972). Age changes in preference and still measures of handedness. *Perceptual and Motor Skills, 34,* 3–14.

Bryden, M. P. (1977). Measuring handedness with questionnaires. *Neuropsychologia, 15,* 617–624.

Bryden, M. P., & Ley, R. G. (1983). Right-hemisphere involvement in the perception and expression of emotion in normal humans. In K. M. Heilman & P. Satz (Eds.), *Neuropsychology of human emotion* (pp. 6–44). New York: Guilford Press.

Buchanan, L. (1908). Mirror-writing with notes on a case. *Opthalamoscope, 6,* 156–159.

Byrne, B., & Sinclair, J. (1979). Memory for tonal sequence and timbre: A correlation with familial handedness. *Neuropsychologia, 17,* 539–542.

Calnan, M., & Richardson, K. (1976). Developmental correlates of handedness in a national sample of 11-year-olds. *Annals of Human Biology, 3,* 329–342.

Caplan, P. J., & Kinsbourne, M. (1976). Baby drops the rattle: Asymmetry of duration of grasp by infants. *Child Development, 47,* 532–534.

Carlson, D. F., & Harris, L. J. (1985a). Development of the infant's hand preference for visually directed reaching: Preliminary report of a longitudinal study. *Infant Mental Health Journal, 6,* 158–172.

Carlson, D. F., & Harris, L. J. (1985b). Perception of happiness and sadness in free-viewing of chimeric faces (abstract). *Journal of Clinical and Experimental Neuropsychology, 7,* 636.

Chayette, C., & Smith, V. (1981). Brain asymmetry predicts suicide among navy alcohol abusers. *Military Medicine, 146,* 277–278.

Chiarello, C. (1980). A house divided? Cognitive functioning with callosal agenesis. *Brain and Language, 11,* 128–158.

Chugani, H. T., & Phelps, M. E. (1986). Maturational changes in cerebral function in infants determined by ^{18}FDG positron emission tomography. *Science, 231,* 840–843.

Churchill, J. (1966). On the origin of focal motor epilepsy. *Neurology, 16,* 49–58.

Clarke, P. G. H. (1985). Neuronal death in the development of the vertebrate nervous system. *Trends in Neuroscience, 8,* 345–349.

Cohen, G. (1973). Hemispheric differences in serial versus parallel processing. *Journal of Experimental Psychology, 97,* 349–356.

Cohen, M. E., & Duffner, P. K. (1981). Prognostic indicators of hemiparetic cerebral palsy. *Annals of Neurology, 9,* 353–357.

Colby, K. M., & Parkison, C. (1977). Handedness in autistic children. *Journal of Autism and Childhood Schizophrenia, 7,* 3–9.

Corballis, M. C., & Morgan, M. J. (1978). On the biological basis of human laterality: I. Evidence for a maturational left–right gradient (target article with commentaries). *The Behavioral and Brain Sciences, 2,* 261–336.

Coren, S., & Searleman, A. (1987). Left sidedness and sleep difficulty: The alinormal syndrome. *Brain and Cognition, 6,* 184–192.

Cornwell, K., Barnes, C., Fitzgerald, H. E., & Harris, L. J. (1985). Neurobehavioral reorganization in early infancy: Patterns of head orientation following lateral and midline holds. *Infant Mental Health Journal, 6,* 126–136.

Coryell, J. F., & Michel, G. F. (1978). How supine postural preferences can contribute toward the development of handedness. *Infant Behavior and Development, 1,* 245–257.

Coulter, J. D., & Janes, E. G. (1977). Differential distribution of corticospinal projections from individual cytoarchitectonic fields in the monkey. *Brain Research, 129,* 235–240.

Cowan, M. W. (1978). Aspects of neural development. In R. Porter (Ed.), *International review of physiology: Neurophysiology III* (Vol. 17, pp. 149–191). Baltimore: University Park Press.

Crome, L. (1965). Pathology of certain syndromes. In L. T. Hilliard & B. H. Kirman (Eds.), *Mental deficiency,* (2nd ed.) (pp. 225–273). London: Churchill.

Crovitz, H. F., & Zener, K. (1962). A group test for assessing hand and eye dominance. *American Journal of Psychology, 75,* 271–276.

Dawson, J. L. M. (1972). Temne-Arunta hand–eye dominance and cognitive style. *International Journal of Psychology, 7,* 219–233.

DeLong, M. R., & Georgopoulos, A. P. (1981). Motor functions of the basal ganglia. In J. M. Brookhart & V. B. Mountcastle (Eds.), *Handbook of physiology: Sec. 1. Motor Control: Vol. 2, Part 2.* Bethesda, MD: American Physiological Society.

Denenberg, V. H. (1980). General systems theory, brain organization, and early experiences. *American Journal of Physiology: Regulatory, Integrative and Comparative Physiology, 7,* R3–R13.

Dennis, M. (1987). Using language to parse the young damaged brain. *Journal of Clinical and Experimental Neuropsychology, 9,* 723–753.

Dennis, M., & Kohn, B. (1985). The active–passive test: An age-referenced clinical test of syntactic discrimination. *Developmental Neuropsychology, 1,* 113–137.

Desmond, M. M., Rudolph, A. J., & Phitaksphraiwan, P. (1966). The transitional care nursery: A mechanism for preventive medicine in the newborn. *Pediatric Clinics of North America, 13,* 651–668.

Deutsch, D. (1978). Pitch memory: An advantage for the left-handed. *Science, 199,* 559–560.

DiFranco, D., Muir, D., & Dodwell, P. (1978). Reaching in very young infants. *Perception, 7,* 385–392.

Divac, I. (1972). Neostriatum and functions of prefrontal cortex. *Acta Neurobiologica Experimentalis, 32,* 461–477.

Divac, I. (1977). Does the neostriatum operate as a functional entity? In A. R. Cools, A. H. M. Lohman, & J. H. L. Van den Berkcken (Eds.), *Psychobiology of the striatum* (pp. 21–30). Amsterdam: North-Holland.

Douglas, J. W. B., Ross, J. M., & Cooper, J. E. (1967). The relationship between handedness, attainment, and adjustment in a national sample of school children. *Educational Research, 9,* 223–232.

Dreifuss, F. E. (1956). Bone changes in hemiplegia of early onset. *British Journal of Radiology, 29,* 601–604.

Dunn, P. M. (1976). Congenital postural deformities. *British Medical Bulletin, 32,* 71–76.

Eastman, N. J., Kohl, S. G., Maisel, J. E., & Kavaler, F. (1962). The obstetrical background of 753 cases of cerebral palsy. *Obstetrical and Gynecological Survey, 17,* 459–500.

Ehrlichman, H., Zoccolotti, P., & Owen, D. (1982). Perinatal factors in hand and eye preference: Data from the Collaborative Perinatal Project. *International Journal of Neuroscience, 17,* 17–22.

Ettlinger, G., Blakemore, C. B., Milner, A. D., & Wilson, J. (1972). Agenesis of the corpus callosum: A behavioural investigation. *Brain, 95,* 327–346.

Fein, G., Humes, M., Kaplan, E., Lucci, D., & Waterhouse, L. (1984). The question of left hemisphere function in infantile autism. *Psychological Bulletin, 95,* 258–281.

Fennell, E., Satz, P., & Morris, P. (1983). The development of handedness and dichotic ear listening asymmetries in relation to school achievement: A longitudinal study. *Journal of Experimental Child Psychology, 35,* 248–262.

Finger, S., & Stein, D. G. (1982). *Brain damage and recovery: Research and clinical perspectives.* New York: Academic Press.

Fleminger, J. J., Dalton, R., & Standage, K. F. (1977). Age as a factor in the handedness of adults. *Neuropsychologia, 15,* 471–473.

Flick, G. L. (1966). Sinistrality revisited: A perceptual–motor approach. *Child Development, 37,* 613–622.

Fox, N., & Lewis, M. (1982). Motor asymmetries in preterm infants: Effects of prematurity and illness. *Developmental Psychobiology, 15,* 19–23.

Gabrielli, W. F., Jr., & Mednick, S. A. (1980). Sinistrality and delinquency. *Journal of Abnormal Psychology, 89,* 654–661.

Gardner, J., Lewkowicz, D., & Turkewitz, G. (1977). Development of postural asymmetry in premature infants. *Developmental Psychobiology, 10,* 471–480.

Geschwind, N., & Behan, P. (1982). Left-handedness: Association with immune disease, migraine, and developmental learning disorder. *Proceedings of the National Academy of Science, 79,* 5097–5100.

Geschwind, N., & Galaburda, A. M. (1985). Cerebral lateralization: Biological mechanisms, associations and pathology: A hypothesis and a program for research, I, II, III. *Archives of Neurology, 42,* 426–457, 521–552, 634–654.

Geschwind, N., & Levitsky, W. (1968). Left/right asymmetries in temporal speech region. *Science, 161,* 186–187.

Gillberg, C., Waldenstrom, E., & Rasmussen, P. (1983). Handedness in Swedish 10-year-olds: Some background and associated factors. *Journal of Child Psychology and Psychiatry, 25,* 421–432.

Glick, S. D., Ross, D. A., & Hough, L. B. (1982). Lateral asymmetry of neurotransmitters in human brain. *Brain Research, 234,* 53–63.

Glücksmann, A. (1981). *Sexual dimorphism in human and mammalian biology and pathology.* London: Academic Press.

Goldman, P. S. (1974). An alternative to developmental plasticity: Heterology of CNS structures in infants and children. In D. G. Stein, J. J. Rosen, & N. Butters (Eds.), *Plasticity and recovery of function in the central nervous system* (pp. 149–174). New York: Academic Press.

Goldman-Rakic, P. S. (1986). Setting the stage: Neural development before birth. In S. L. Friedman, K. A. Klivington, & R. W. Peterson (Eds.), *The brain, cognition, and education* (pp. 233–258). Orlando, FL: Academic Press.

Goldman-Rakic, P. S., Isseroff, A., Schwartz, M. L., & Bugbee, N. M. (1983). The neurobiology of cognitive development. In M. M. Haith & J. J. Campos (Eds.), *Infancy and developmental psychology* (pp. 281–344). Vol. II of P. H. Mussen (Ed.), *Handbook of child psychology.* New York: Wiley.

Goodwin, R., & Michel, G. F. (1981). Head orientation position during birth, in neonatal period, and hand preference at 19 weeks. *Child Development, 52,* 819–826.

Gordon, H. (1920). Left-handedness and mirror writing, especially among defective children. *Brain, 43,* 313–368.

Gordon, H. W. (1983). The learning disabled are cognitively right. In M. Kinsbourne (Ed.), Brain basis of learning disabilities. *Topics in Learning and Learning Disabilities, 3,* 29–39.

Gordon, K. (1931). Brief reports: A study of hand and eye preference. *Child Development, 2,* 321–324.

Gottfried, A. W., & Bathurst, K. (1983). Hand preference across time is related to intelligence in young girls, not boys. *Science, 221,* 1074–1076.

Gregory, R., & Paul, J. (1980). The effects of handedness and writing posture on neuropsychological test results. *Neuropsychologia, 18,* 231–235.

Grinker, R. R., Bucy, P. C., & Sahs, A. L. (1959). *Neurology.* Springfield, IL: Thomas.

Guiard, Y., Diaz, G., & Beaubaton, D. (1983). Left-hand advantage in right-handers for spatial constant error: Preliminary evidence in a unimanual ballistic aimed movement. *Neuropsychologia, 21,* 111–115.

Gur, R. E. (1977). Motor laterality imbalance in schizophrenia: A possible concomitant of left hemisphere dysfunction. *Archives of Psychiatry, 34,* 33–37.

Harburg, E. (1981). Handedness and drinking–smoking types. *Perceptual and Motor Skills, 52,* 279–282.

Harburg, E., Feldstein, A., & Papsdorf, J. (1978). Handedness and smoking. *Perceptual Motor Skills, 47,* 1171–1174.

Hardyck, C., & Petrinovich, L. F. (1977). Left-handedness. *Psychological Bulletin, 84,* 385–404.

Hardyck, C., Petrinovich, L. F., & Goldman, R. D. (1976). Left-handedness and cognitive deficit. *Cortex, 12,* 266–279.

Harris, L. J. (1977). Sex differences in the growth and use of language. In E. Donelson & J. Gullahorn (Eds.), *Women: A psychological perspective* (pp. 79–94). New York: Wiley.

Harris, L. J. (1978). Sex differences in spatial ability: Possible environmental, genetic, and neurological factors. In M. Kinsbourne (Ed.), *Asymmetrical function of the brain* (pp. 405–522). Cambridge: Cambridge University Press.

Harris, L. J. (1980a). Left-handedness: Early theories, facts, and fancies. In J. Herron (Ed.), *Neuropsychology of left-handedness* (pp. 3–78). New York: Academic Press.

Harris, L. J. (1980b). Which hand is the "eye" of the blind? A new look at an old question. In J. Herron (Ed.), *Neuropsychology of left-handedness* (pp. 303–329). New York: Academic Press.

Harris, L. J. (1983). Laterality of function in the infant: Historical and contemporary trends in theory and research. In G. Young, S. J. Segalowitz, C. M. Corter, & S. E. Trehub, (Eds.), *Manual specialization and the developing brain* (pp. 177–247). New York: Academic Press.

Harris, L. J. (1986). James Mark Baldwin on the origins of right- and left-handedness: The story of an experiment that mattered. In A. B. Smuts & J. W. Hagen (Eds.), *History of research in child development.* Monographs of the Society for Research in Child Development (pp. 44–64). Special Issue in Celebration of the Fiftieth Anniversary of the Society, Serial No. 211, *50,* Nos. 4–5.

Harris, L. J., & Fitzgerald, H. E. (1983). Postural orientation in human infants: Changes from birth to three months. In G. Young, S. J. Segalowitz, C. M. Corter, S. E. Trehub (Eds.), *Manual specialization and the developing brain* (pp. 285–305). New York: Academic Press.

Harshman, R. A., Hampson, R., & Berenbaum, S. A. (1983). Individual differences in cognitive abilities and brain organization: Part I. Sex and handedness differences in ability. *Canadian Journal of Psychology, 37,* 144–192.

Hatta, T., & Nakatsuka, Z. (1976). Note on hand preference of the Japanese people. *Perceptual and Motor Skills, 42,* 530.

Hauser, S. L., DeLong, G. R., & Rosman, N. P. (1975), Pneumographic studies in the infantile autism syndrome. *Brain, 98,* 667–688.

Hawn, P. R. & Harris, L. J. (1983). Hand differences in grasp duration and reaching in two- and five-month-old infants. In G. Young, S. J. Segalowitz, C. M. Corter, & S. E. Trehub (Eds.), *Manual specialization and the developing brain* (pp. 331–348). New York: Academic Press.

Healy, J. M., Liederman, J., & Geschwind, N. (1986). Handedness is not a unidimensional trait. *Cortex, 22,* 33–53.

Hécaen, H., & Ajuriaguerra, J. de. (1964). *Left-handedness,* New York: Grune and Stratton.

Hécaen, H., & Sauget, J. (1971). Cerebral dominance in left-handed subjects. *Cortex, 7,* 19–48.

Heffner, R. S., & Masterton, R. B. (1975). Variation in form of the pyramidal tract and its relationship to digital dexterity. *Brain, Behavior, and Evolution, 12,* 161–200.

Heffner, R. S., & Masterton, R. B. (1983). The role of the corticospinal tract in the evolution of human digital dexterity. *Brain, Behavior, and Evolution, 23,* 165–183.

Heilman, K. M., & Satz, P. (Eds.). (1983). *Neuropsychology of human emotion.* New York: Guilford Press.

Heinlein, J. H. (1930). Preferential manipulation in children. *Comparative Psychology Monographs, 7,* 1–121.

Henry, R., Satz, P., & Saslow, E. (1984). Early brain damage and the ontogenesis of functional asymmetry. In C. R. Almi & S. Finger (Eds.), *Early brain damage: Vol. 1. Research orientations and clinical observations,* (pp. 253–276). Orlando, FL: Academic Press.

Herrman, D. J., & Van Dyke, K. (1978). Handedness and the mental rotation of perceived patterns. *Cortex, 14,* 521–529.

Herron, J., Galin, D., Johnstone, J., & Ornstein, R. E. (1979). Cerebral specialization, writing posture, and motor control of writing in left-handers. *Science, 205,* 1285–1289.

Hicks, R. E., & Barton, A. K. (1975). A note on left-handedness and severity of mental retardation. *Journal of Genetic Psychology, 127,* 323–324.

Hicks, R. E., Elliott, D., Garbesi, L., & Martin, S. (1979). Note: Multiple birth factors and the distribution of handedness. *Cortex, 15,* 135–137.

Hicks, R. E., Evans, E. A., & Pelligrini, R. J. (1978). Correlation between handedness and birth order: Compilation of five studies. *Perceptual and Motor Skills, 46,* 53–54.

Hicks, R. E., & Pelligrini, R. J. (1978). Handedness and anxiety, *Cortex, 14,* 119–121.

Hicks, R. E., Pelligrini, R. J., & Evans, E. A. (1978). Note: Handedness and birth risk. *Neuropsychologia, 16,* 243–245.

Hildreth, G. (1949). The development and training of hand dominance: II. Developmental tendencies in handedness. *Journal of Genetic Psychology, 75,* 221–275.

Hobel, C. J., Hyvarinen, M. A., Okada, D. M., & Oh, W. (1973). Prenatal and intrapartum high risk screening: I. Prediction of the high risk neonate. *American Journal of Obstetrics and Gynecology, 117,* 1–9.

Hofsten, C. von. (1986). The emergence of manual skills. In M. G. Wade & H. T. A. Whiting (Eds.), *Motor development in children: Aspects of coordination and control* (pp. 167–185). Dordrecht: Martinus Nijhoff.

Homzie, M. J., & Lindsay, J. E. (1984). Language and the young stutterer: A new look at old theories and findings. *Brain and Language, 22,* 232–252.

Hood, P. N., & Perlstein, M. A. (1955). Infantile spastic hemiplegia: II. Laterality of involvement. *Journal of Physiological Medicine, 34,* 457–466.

Hubbard, J. I. (1971). Handedness is not a function of birth order. *Nature, 232,* 276–277.

Humphrey, D. E., & Humphrey, G. K. (1987). Sex differences in infant reaching. *Neuropsychologia, 25,* 971–975.

Humphrey, D. R. (1979). On the cortical control of visually directed reaching: Contributions by nonprecentral motor areas. In R. E. Talbott & D. R. Humphrey (Eds.), *Posture and movement* (pp. 51–112). New York: Raven Press.

Humphrey, D. R. (1983). Corticospinal systems and their control by premotor cortex, basal ganglia, and cerebellum. In W. D. Willis (Ed.), *The clinical neurosciences: Vol. 5. Neurobiology* (pp. V:547–V:587). New York: Churchill Livingstone.

Humphrey, T. (1964). Some correlations between the appearance of human fetal reflexes and the development of the nervous system. In D. P. Purpura (Ed.), *Growth and maturation of the brain: Progress in Brain Research* (Vol. 4, pp. 93–135). Amsterdam: Elsevier Science.

Humphrey, T. (1969). Postnatal repetition of human prenatal activity sequences with some suggestions of their neuroanatomical basis. In R. J. Robinson (Ed.), *Brain and early behavior: Development in the fetus and infant* (pp. 43–71). London: Academic Press.

Ingram, D. (1975). Motor asymmetries in young children. *Neuropsychologia, 13,* 95–102.

Ingram, T. T. S. (1964). The dyslexic child. *The Practitioner, 192,* 503–516.

Irle, E. (1987). Lesion size and recovery of function: Some new perspectives. *Brain Research Reviews, 12,* 307–320.

Irwin, P. (1985). Greater brain response of left-handers to drugs. *Neuropsychologia, 23,* 61–67.

Irwin, P., & Fink, M. (1981). Do psychoactive drugs affect the EEG from the cerebral hemispheres differently? *Advances in Biological Psychiatry, 6,* 121–125.

Jeret, J. S., Serur, D., Wisniewski, K., & Fisch, C. (1985–1986). Frequency of agenesis of the corpus callosum in the developmentally disabled as determined by computerized tomography. *Pediatric Neuroscience, 12,* 101–103.

Jordan, H. E. (1911). The inheritance of left-handedness. *American Breeder's Magazine, 2,* 19–28, 113–124.

Jung, R., & Hassler, R. (1960). The extrapyramidal motor systems. In J. Field, H. W. Magoun, & V. E. Hall. (Eds.), *Handbook of physiology* (Sec. 1, Vol. II, pp. 863–927). Washington, DC: American Physiological Society.

Kertesz, A., & Geschwind, N. (1971). Patterns of pyramidal decussation and their relationship to handedness. *Archives of Neurology, 24,* 326–332.

Kimura, D. (1983a). Sex differences in cerebral organization for speech and praxic function. *Canadian Journal of Psychology, 37,* 19–35.

Kimura, D. (1983b). Speech representation in an unbiased sample of left-handers. *Human Neurobiology, 2,* 147–154.

Kimura, D. (1987). Are men's and women's brains really different? *Canadian Psychology, 28,* 133–147.

Kimura, D., & Harshman, R. A. (1984). Sex differences in brain organization for verbal and non-verbal functions. In G. J. De Vries, J. P. C. De Bruin, H. B. M. Uylings, & M. A. Corner (Eds.), *Sex differences in the brain: The relation between structure and function: Vol. 61. Progress in brain research* (pp. 423–441). Amsterdam: Elsevier Science.

Kinsbourne, M., & Bemporad, B. (1984). Lateralization of emotion: A model and the evidence. In N. A. Fox & R. J. Davidson (Eds.), *The psychobiology of affective development* (pp. 259–291). Hillsdale, NJ: Erlbaum.

Kinsbourne, M., & Hiscock, M. (1983). The normal and deviant development of functional lateralization of the brain. In M. M. Haith & J. J. Campos (Eds.), *Infancy and developmental psychology* (pp. 157–280). Vol. II of P. H. Mussen (Ed.), *Handbook of child psychology.* New York: Wiley.

Komai, T., & Fukuoka, G. (1934). A study of the frequency of left-handedness and left-footedness among Japanese school children. *Human Biology, 6,* 33–42.

Kornhuber, H. H. (1974). Cerebral cortex, cerebellum, and basal ganglia: An introduction to their motor functions. In F. O. Schmitt & F. G. Worden (Eds.), *The neurosciences: Third study program* (pp. 267–280). Cambridge, MA: MIT Press.

Kornhuber, H. H. (1984). Mechanisms of voluntary movement. In W. Prinz & A. F. Sanders (Eds.), *Cognition and motor processes* (pp. 163–173). Berlin: Springer-Verlag.

Kraft, A. von. (1980). On the problem on the origin of asymmetric organs and human laterality. *The Behavioral and Brain Sciences, 3,* 478–479.

Kunzle, H. (1975). Bilateral projections from precentral motor cortex to the putamen and other parts of the basal ganglia: An autoradiographic study in *Macacca fasicularis. Brain Research, 88,* 195–209.

Kurtzberg, D., Vaughan, H. G., Daum, C., Grellong, B. A., Albin, S., & Rotkin, L. (1979). Neurobehavioral performance of low-birthweight infants at 40 weeks conceptional age: Comparison with normal fullterm infants. *Developmental Medicine and Child Neurology, 21,* 590–607.

Kuypers, H. G. J. M. (1960). Central cortical projections to motor and somatosensory cell groups: An experimental study in the rhesus monkey. *Brain, 83,* 161–184.

Kuypers, H. G. J. M. (1962). Corticospinal connections: Postnatal development in the rhesus monkey. *Science, 138,* 678–680.

Kuypers, H. G. J. M. (1984). *Brain systems providing motor control.* Paper presented at the 12th annual meeting of the International Neuropsychological Society, Houston, February.

Kuypers, H. G. J. M. (1985). The anatomical and functional organization of the motor system. In M. Swash & C. Kennard (Eds.), *Scientific basis of clinical neurology* (pp. 3–18), Edinburgh: Churchill Livingstone.

Landauer, W. (1939). Supermammary nipples, congenital hemihypertrophy, and congenital hematrophy. *Human Biology, 11,* 447–472.

Lansdell, H. (1969). Verbal and nonverbal factors in right hemisphere speech: Relation to early neurological history. *Journal of Comparative and Physiological Psychology, 69,* 734–738.

Lassek, A. M. (1954). *The pyramidal tract: Its status in medecine*. Springfield, IL: Thomas.
Lattes, L. (1907). Destrismo e mancinismo in relazione colle asimmetrie funzionali del cervello. *Archivio di Psichiatria, Neuropatologia, Antropologia criminale e medicina legale,* Torino, *28,* 281–303. (Currently *Minerva Medicolegale.*)
Lawrence, D. G., & Hopkins, D. A. (1972). Developmental aspects of pyramidal motor control in the rhesus monkey. *Brain Research, 40,* 117–118.
Lawrence, D. G., & D. A. Hopkins, (1976). The development of motor control in the rhesus monkey: Evidence concerning the role of corticomotoneuronal connections. *Brain, 99,* 235–254.
Lawrence, D. G., & Kuypers, H. G. J. M. (1968). The functional organization of the motor system in monkey: I. The effects of bilateral pyramidal lesions. *Brain, 91,* 1–14.
Leck, I. (1974). Causation of neural tube defects: Clues from epidemiology. *British Medical Bulletin, 30,* 158–163.
Lee-Feldstein, A., & Harburg, E. (1982). Alcohol use among right- and left-handed persons in a small community. *Journal of Studies on Alcohol, 43,* 824–829.
Leiber, L., & Axelrod, S. (1981). Not all sinistrality is pathological. *Cortex, 17,* 259–272.
LeMay, M. (1977). Asymmetries of the skull and handedness. *Journal of the Neurological Sciences, 32,* 243–253.
Lemire, R. J., Loeser, J. D., Leech, R. W., & Alvord, E. C. (1975). *Normal and abnormal development of the human nervous system.* Hagerstown, MD: Harper and Row.
Lenneberg, E. H. (1968). The effect of age on the outcome of central nervous system disease in children. In R. L. Isaacson (Ed.), *The neuropsychology of development.* New York: Wiley.
Levine, S. C., Huttenlocher, P., Banich, M. T., & Duda, E. (1987). Factors affecting cognitive functioning of hemiplegic children. *Developmental Medicine and Child Neurology, 29,* 27–35.
Leviton, A., & Kilty, T. (1976). Birth order and left-handedness. *Archives of Neurology, 33,* 664.
Levy, J. (1969). Possible basis for the evolution of lateral specialization of the human brain. *Nature, 224,* 614–615.
Levy, J. (1974). Psychobiological implications of bilateral asymmetry. In S. J. Dimond & J. G. Beaumont (Eds.), *Hemisphere function in the human brain* (pp. 121–183). New York: Wiley.
Levy J. (1982). Handwriting posture and cerebral organization: How are they related? *Psychological Bulletin, 91,* 589–608.
Levy, J. (1985). Interhemispheric collaboration: Single-mindedness in the asymmetrical brain. In C. T. Best (Ed.), *Hemispheric function and collaboration in the child* (pp. 11–31). Orlando, FL: Academic Press.
Levy, J., & Nagylaki, T. (1972), A model for the genetics of handedness. *Genetics, 72,* 117–128.
Levy, J., & Reid, M. (1978). Variations in cerebral organization as a function of handedness, hand posture in writing, and sex. *Journal of Experimental Psychology: General, 107,* 109–144.
Lewis, R. S., & Harris, L. J. (1985). *Relationship between cerebral hemisphere specialization and visual–spatial and verbal ability in young adults of superior reasoning ability.* Paper presented at the 13th annual meeting of the International Neuropsychological Society, San Diego, California.
Lewis, R. S., & Kamptner, N. L. (1987). Sex differences in spatial task performance of patients with and without unilateral lesions. *Brain and Cognition, 6,* 142–152.
Lhermitte, F., & Gautier, J-C. (1969). Aphasia. In P. J. Vinken & G. W. Bruyn (Eds.), *Handbook of clinical neurology: Vol. 4. Disorders of speech, perception, and symbolic behavior* (pp. 84–104). Amsterdam: North-Holland.
Lidsky, T. I., Manetto, C., & Schneider, J. S. (1985). A consideration of sensory factors involved in motor functions of the basal ganglia. *Brain Research Reviews, 9,* 133–146.
Lieber, L., & Axelrod, S. (1981). Not all sinistrality is pathological. *Cortex, 17,* 259–272.
Liederman, J. (1977). *Lateral head-turning asymmetries in human infants: Hereditary, organismic, and environmental influences.* Unpublished doctoral dissertation, University of Rochester.
Liederman, J. (1983). Mechanisms underlying instability in the development of hand preference. In G. Young, S. J. Segalowitz, C. M. Corter, & S. E. Trehub (Eds.), *Manual specialization and the developing brain* (pp. 71–92). New York: Academic Press.
Liederman, J., & Coryell, J. (1982). The origin of left hand preference: Pathological and non-pathological influences. *Neuropsychologia, 20,* 721–725.
Linn, M. C., & Petersen, A. C. (1985). Emergence and characterization of sex differences in spatial ability: A meta-analysis. *Child Development, 56,* 1479–1498.
Lishman, W. A., & McMeekan, E. R. L. (1976). Hand preference patterns in psychiatric patients. *British Journal of Psychiatry, 129,* 158–166.
Littman, B., & Parmelee, A. H. (1974a). *Manual for obstetrical complications scale.* Mental Retardation Center, Neuropsychiatric Institute, University of California at Los Angeles.

Littman, B., & Parmelee, A. H. (1974b). *Manual for postnatal complications scale.* Mental Retardation Center, Neuropsychiatric Institute, University of California at Los Angeles.

Lombroso, C. (1903). Left-handedness and left-sidedness. *North American Review, 177,* 440–444.

Louis, J. (1983). The trouble with being a lefty in Russia. *The Times* (London), Educational Supplement, February 11, No. 3476, p. 16.

Lubchenko, L. O. (1976). *The high risk infant.* Philadelphia: Saunders.

Lund, R. D. (1978). *Development and plasticity of the brain: An introduction.* New York: Oxford University Press.

Malmquist, E. (1958). *Factors relating to reading disabilities in the first grade of elementary school.* Stockholm: Almqvist and Wiksell.

Martin, F., Friedrich, G., Mottier, C. H., & Guignard, F. (1968). La lateralité chez l'epileptique. *Annals Medico-Psycholoqiques, 2,* 665–692.

Mascie-Taylor, C. G. N. (1981). Hand preference and personality traits. *Cortex, 17,* 319–332.

Mayet, L. (1902). Les stigmates anatomiques et physiologiques de la dégénérescence et les pseudo-stigmates anatomiques et physiologiques de la criminalité. Lyon, France. Cited in Gordon (1920).

MacNeilage, P. F., Studdert-Kennedy, M. G., & Lindblom, B. (1987). Primate handedness reconsidered (target article with commentaries). *The Behavioral and Brain Sciences, 10,* 247–303.

McCann, B. S. (1981). Hemispheric asymmetries and early infantile autism. *Journal of Autism and Developmental Disorders, 11,* 401–411.

McCreadie, J., Crorie, J., Barron, E. T., & Winslow, G. S. (1982). The Nithsdale schizophrenia study: III. Handedness and tardive dyskinesia. *British Journal of Psychiatry, 140,* 591–594.

McDonnell, P. M. (1979). Patterns of eye–hand coordination in the first year of life. *Canadian Journal of Psychology, 33,* 253–267.

McKeever, W. F. (1979). Handwriting posture in left-handers: Sex, familial sinistrality, and language laterality correlates. *Neuropsychologia, 17,* 429–444.

McKeever, W. F., & Hoff, L. A. (1979). Evidence of a possible isolation of left hemisphere visual and motor areas in sinistrals employing an inverted handwriting posture. *Neuropsychologia, 17,* 445–454.

McKeever, W. F., & Van Deventer, A. D. (1977). Familial sinistrality and degree of left handedness. *British Journal of Psychology, 68,* 469–471.

McManus, I. C. (1980). Left-handedness and epilepsy. *Cortex, 16,* 487–492.

McManus, I. C. (1981). Handedness and birth stress. *Psychological Medicine, 11,* 485–496.

McManus, I. C. (1983). Pathological left-handedness: Does it exist? *Journal of Communication Disorders, 16,* 315–344.

McMillen, M. M. (1979). Differential mortality by sex in fetal and neonatal deaths. *Science, 204,* 89–91.

Mebert, C. J., & Michel, G. F. (1980). Handedness in artists. In J. Herron (Ed.), *Neuropsychology of left-handedness* (pp. 273–279). New York: Academic Press.

Meyer, J. S., Leidermann, H., & Denny-Brown, D. (1956). Electroencephalographic study of insufficiency of the basilar and carotid arteries in man. *Neurology, 6,* 455–477.

Michaelis, R., Rooschuz, B., & Dopper, R. (1980). Prenatal origin of congenital spastic hemiparesis. *Early Human Development, 4,* 243–255.

Michel, G. F. (1981). Right handedness: A consequence of infant supine head-orientation preference. *Science, 212,* 685–687.

Michel, G. F., & Goodwin, R. (1979). Intrauterine birth position predicts newborn supine head position preferences. *Infant Behavior and Development, 2,* 29–38.

Michel, G. F. & Harkins, D. A. (1986). Postural and lateral asymmetries in the ontogeny of handedness during infancy. *Developmental Psychobiology, 19,* 247–258.

Milner, B. (1975). Psychological aspects of focal epilepsy and its neurosurgical management. *Advances in Neurology, 8,* 299–321.

Milner, B., Branch, C., & Rasmussen, T. (1964). Observations on cerebral dominance. In A. V. S. de Rueck & M. O'Connor (Eds.), Ciba Foundation Symposium, *Disorders of language,* 200–214. London: Churchill.

Milner, B., Branch, C., & Rasmussen, T. (1966). Evidence for bilateral speech representation in some non-right handers. *Transactions of the American Neurological Association, 91,* 306–308.

Mitchell, R. B. (1961). Analysis of each type of cerebral palsy. In J. I. Henderson (Ed.), *Cerebral palsy in childhood and adolescence: A medical, psychological, and social study* (pp. 73–121). Edinburgh: E & S Livingston.

Mittwoch, U. (1978). Changes in the direction of the lateral growth gradient in human development—left to right and right to left. *The Behavioral and Brain Sciences, 2,* 306–307.

Nachson, I., & Denno, D. (1986). Birth order and lateral preferences. *Cortex, 22,* 567–578.

Nachson, I., & Denno, C. (1987). Birth stress and lateral preferences. *Cortex, 23,* 45–58.

Neils, J. R., & Aram, D. M. (1986). Handedness and sex of children with developmental language disorders. *Brain and Language, 28,* 53–65.

Nieuwenhuys, R. (1977). Aspects of the morphology of the striatum. In A. R. Cools, A. H. M. Lohman, & J. H. L. Van den Berkcken (Eds.), *Psychology of the striatum* (pp. 1–19). Amsterdam: North-Holland.

Niswander, K. R., & Gordon, M. (1972). *The women and their pregnancies.* Washington, D.C.: U.S. Department of Health, Education and Welfare.

Niswander, K. R., & Gordon, M. (Eds.), (1982). *The collaborative perinatal study of the National Institute of Neurological Diseases and Stroke: The women and their pregnancies.* Philadelphia: Saunders.

Novelly, R. A., & Naugle, R. (1986). *Acquired right hemisphere speech: Gender specific effects on VIQ vs. PIQ.* Paper presented at the 14th annual meeting of the International Neuropsychological Society, Denver, Colorado, February.

Nyberg-Hansen, R., & Rinvik, E. (1963). Some comments on the pyramidal tract, with special reference to its individual variations in man. *Acta Neurologica Scandinavica, 39,* 1–30.

Ojemann, G. (1983). Brain organization for language from the perspective of electrical stimulation mapping (target article with commentaries). *The Behavioral and Brain Sciences, 2,* 189–230.

Oke, A., Keller, R., Mefford, I., & Adams, R. N. (1978). Lateralization of norepinephrine in human thalamus. *Science, 200,* 1411–1413.

Oldfield, R. C. (1971). The assessment and analysis of handedness: The Edinburgh Inventory. *Neuropsychologia, 9,* 97–111.

Oppenheim, R. W. (1984). Cellular interactions and the survival and maintenance of neurons during development. In S. C. Sharma (Ed.), *Organizing principles of of neural development* (pp. 49–80). New York: Plenum.

Orme, J. E. (1970). Left-handedness, ability, and emotional instability. *British Journal of Social and Clinical Psychology, 9,* 87–88.

Orsini, D. L., & Satz, P. (1986). A syndrome of pathological left-handedness: Correlates of early left hemisphere injury. *Archives of Neurology, 43,* 333–337.

Orsini, D. L., Satz, P., Soper, H. V., & Light, R. K. (1984). The role of familial sinistrality in cerebral organization. *Neuropsychologia, 23,* 223–232.

Paillas, J. E., Bonnal, J., & Gastaut, Y. (1953). L'epreuve de la compression de la carotide saine au cours de la thrombose de la carotide interne opposée. *Seminaire de Hôpital, 29,* 889–893.

Paoluzzi, C., & Bravaccio, F. (1967). Ripartizione tra i due emisferi delle anomalita EEG focalizzate. *Atti XVI Congress Nazionale Neurologia* (Vol. 3, pp. 367–372). Rome: Il Pensiero Scientifico.

Parmelee, A. H., & Sigman, M. (1983). Perinatal brain development and behavior. In M. M. Haith & J. J. Campos (Eds.), *Infancy and developmental psychology* (pp. 95–155), Vol. II of P. H. Mussen (Ed.), *Handbook of child psychology.* New York: Wiley.

Pasamanick, B., & Knobloch, H. (1961). Epidemiologic studies on the complications of pregnancy and the birth process. In G. Caplan (Ed.), *Prevention of mental disorders in children* (pp. 74–94). New York: Basic Books.

Pasamanick, B., & Knobloch, H. (1966). Retrospective studies on the epidemiology of reproductive casualty: Old and new. *Merrill-Palmer Quarterly, 12,* 7–26.

Payne, M. A. (1981). Incidence of left-handedness for writing: A study of Nigerian primary schoolchildren. *Journal of Cross Cultural Psychology, 12,* 233–239.

Payne, M. A. (1987). Impact of cultural pressures on self-reports of actual and approved hand use. *Neuropsychologia, 25,* 247–258.

Penfield, W., & Roberts, L. (1959). *Speech and brain mechanisms.* Princeton, NJ: Princeton University Press.

Penfield, W., & Robertson, J. S. M. (1943). Growth asymmetries due to lesions of the postcentral cortex. *Archives of Neurology, 50,* 405–430.

Peters, M. (1983). Differentiation and lateral specialization in motor development. In G. Young, S. J. Segalowitz, C. M. Corter, & S. E. Trehub (Eds.), *Manual specialization and the developing brain* (pp. 141–159). New York: Academic Press.

Peters, M. (1986). Incidence of left-handed writers and the inverted writing position in a sample of 2,194 German elementary school children. *Neuropsychologia, 24,* 429–443.

Peters, M. (1988). Footedness: Asymmetries in foot preference and skill and neuropsychological measurement of foot movement. *Psychological Bulletin, 103,* 179–192.

Peters, M., & Durding, B. (1979). Left-handers and right-handers compared on a motor task. *Journal of Motor Behavior, 11,* 103–111.

Peters, M., & Pedersen, K. (1978). Incidence of left-handers and noninverted writing position in a population of 5910 elementary school children. *Neuropsychologia, 16,* 743–746.

Petrie, B. F., & Peters, M. (1981). Handedness: Left/right differences in intensity of response and duration of rattle holding in infants. *Infant Behavior and Development, 3,* 215–221.

Porac, C., & Coren, S. (1981). *Lateral preferences and human behavior.* New York: Springer-Verlag.

Porac, C., Coren, S., & Searleman, A. (1986). Environmental factors in hand preference formation: Evidence from attempts to switch the preferred hand. *Behavior Genetics, 16,* 251–261.

Prechtl, H. R. R., Fargel, J. W., Weinmann, H. M., & Bakker, H. H. (1979). Postures, motility, and respiration of low-risk pre-term infants. *Developmental Medicine and Child Neurology, 21,* 3–27.

Provins, K. A., Milner, A., & Kerr, P. (1982). Asymmetry of manual preference and performance. *Perceptual and Motor Skills, 54,* 179–194.

Purves, D., & Lichtman, J. W. (1985). *Principles of neural development.* Sunderland, MA: Sinauer Associates.

Rakic, P. (1984). Organizing principles for development of primate cerebral cortex. In S. C. Sharma (Ed.), *Organizing principles of neural development* (pp. 21–48). New York: Plenum.

Rakic, P. (1986). *The role of competition in the formation of synapses.* Paper presented at the First Biennial Developmental Biology Symposium, University of Michigan, Ann Arbor, June 11–14.

Rakic, P., Bourgeois, J-P., Eckenhoff, M. F., Zecevic, N. & Goldman-Rakic, P. S. (1986). Concurrent over-production of synapses in diverse regions of the primate cerebral cortex. *Science, 232,* 232–235.

Ramsay, D. S. (1980). Beginnings of bimanual handedness and speech in infants. *Infant Behavior and Development, 3,* 67–77.

Ramsay, D. S., Campos, J. J., & Fenson, L. (1979). Onset of bimanual handedness in infants. *Infant Behavior and Development, 2,* 71–76.

Rasmussen, T., & Milner, B. (1977). The role of early left-brain injury in determining lateralization of cerebral speech functions. *Annals of the New York Academy of Sciences, 299,* 355–369.

Redlich, (1908). Cited without reference in T. Bingley (1958). Mental symptoms in temporal lobe epilepsy and temporal lobe glioma. *Acta Psychologica Neurologica Scandinavia, 33,* Supplement 120.

Rice, T., Plomin, R., & De Fries, J. C. (1984). Development of hand preference in the Colorado Adoption Project. *Perceptual and Motor Skills, 58,* 683–689.

Roberts, L. H. (1958). Functional plasticity in cortical speech areas and integration of speech. *Archives of Neurology and Psychiatry, 79,* 275–283.

Rosenfield, D. R. (1980). Cerebral dominance and stuttering. *Journal of Fluency Disorders, 5,* 171–185.

Ross, E. D., & Mesulam, M.-M. (1979). Dominant language functions of the right hemisphere? Prosody and emotional gesturing. *Archives of Neurology, 36,* 144–148.

Ross, G., Lipper, E. G., & Auld, P. A. M. (1987). Hand preference in four-year-old children: Its relationship in premature birth and neurodevelopmental outcome. *Developmental Medicine and Child Neurology, 29,* 615–622.

Rutter, M., Graham, P., & Yule, W. (1970). A neuro-psychiatric study in childhood. *Clinics in Developmental Medicine, 35–36.* Philadelphia: Lippincott.

Rutter, M., Tizard, J., & Whitmore, K. (Eds.). (1970). *Education, health, and behavior.* London: Longmans.

Saling, M. (1979). Lateral differentiation of the neonatal head turning response: A replication. *Journal of Genetic Psychology, 135,* 307–308.

Saling, M. (1983). Familial handedness, prenatal environmental adversity, and neonatal lateral organization. In G. Young, S. J. Segalowitz, C. M. Corter, & S. E. Trehub (Eds.), *Manual specialization and the developing brain* (pp. 275–284). New York: Academic Press.

Saling, M., & Abkiewicz, C. (no date). Neurological risk and head position preferences in newborns. Unpublished data. (Cited in Saling, 1983, pp. 277–278.)

Salmaso, D., & Longoni, A. M. (1983). Hand preference in an Italian sample. *Perceptual and Motor Skills, 57,* 1039–1042.

Sameroff, A. J., & Chandler, M. J. (1975). Reproductive risk and the continuum of caretaking casualty. In F. D. Horowitz, E. M. Hetherington, S. Scarr-Salapatek, & G. M. Siegel, (Eds.), *Review of child development research* (Vol. 4, pp. 187–244). Chicago: University of Chicago Press.

Satz, P. (1972). Pathological left-handedness: An explanatory model. *Cortex, 8,* 121–135.

Satz, P. (1973). Left-handedness and early brain insult: An explanation. *Neuropsychologia, 11,* 115–117.

Satz, P. (1979). A test of some models of hemispheric speech organization in the left- and right-handed. *Science, 203,* 1131–1133.

Satz, P., Orsini, D. L., Saslow, E., & Henry, R. (1985a). Early brain injury and pathological left-handedness: Clues to a syndrome. In D. F. Benson & E. Zaidel (Eds.), *The dual brain: Hemispheric specialization in humans* (pp. 117–125). New York: Guilford Press.

Satz, P., Orsini, D. L., Saslow, E., & Henry, R. (1985b). The pathological left-handedness syndrome. *Brain and Cognition, 4,* 27–46.

Satz, P., & Soper, H. V. (1986). Left-handedness, dyslexia, and autoimmune disorder: A critique. *Journal of Clinical and Experimental Neuropsychology, 8,* 453–458.

Satz, P., Yanowitz, J., & Wilmore, J. (1984). Early brain damage and lateral development. In R. Bell, J. Elias, R. Green, & J. Harvey (Eds.), *Interfaces in psychology* (pp. 87–107). Lubbock: Texas Tech Press.

Scheibel, A. B. (1979). Development of axonal and dendritic neuropil as a function of evolving behavior. In F. O. Schmitt & F. G. Worden (Eds.), *The neurosciences: Third study program* (pp. 381–398). Cambridge, MA: MIT Press.

Scheibel, A. B., Fried, I., Paul, L., Forsythe, A., Tomiyasu, U., Wechsler, A., Kao, A., & Slotnick, J. (1985). Differentiating characteristics of the human speech cortex: A quantitative golgi study. In D. F. Benson & E. Zaidel (Eds.), *The dual brain: Hemispheric specialization in humans* (pp. 65–74). New York: Guilford Press.

Schmidt, R., & Wilder, B. J. (1968). *Epilepsy.* Philadelphia: Davis.

Schneider, G. E. (1979). Is it really better to have your brain lesion early? A revision of the "Kennard Principle." *Neuropsychologia, 17,* 557–584.

Schwartz, M. (1977). Left-handedness and high-risk pregnancy. *Neuropsychologia, 15,* 341–344.

Schwartz, M. (1986). *Handedness, prenatal stress, and pregnancy complications.* Paper presented at the 14th meeting of the International Neuropsychological Society, Denver, Colorado, February.

Searleman, A., Porac, C., & Coren, S. (1982). The relationship between birth stress and writing hand posture. *Brain and Cognition, 1,* 158–164.

Searleman, A., & Fugagli, A. K. (1987). Suspected autoimmune disorders and left-handedness: Evidence from individuals with diabetes, Crohn's disease, and ulcerative colitis. *Neuropsychologia, 25,* 367–374.

Searleman, A., Tsao, Y.-C., & Balzer, W. (1980). A re-examination of the relationship between birth stress and handedness. *Clinical Neuropsychology, 2,* 124–128.

Selnes, O. A. (1974). The corpus callosum: Some anatomical and functional considerations with special reference to language. *Brain and Language, 1,* 111–139.

Séquin, E. (1880). *Report on education* (2nd ed.). Milwaukee, WI: Doerflinger Book & Publishing Company (photo reproduction: Delmar, NY: Scholars' Facsimiles & Reprints, 1976.) (First published 1875.)

Shan-Ming, Y., Flor-Henry, P., Dayi, C., Tiangi, L., Shuguang, Q., & Zenxiang, M. (1985). Imbalance of hemispheric functions in the major psychoses: A study of handedness in the People's Republic of China. *Biological Psychiatry, 20,* 906–917.

Shimizu, A., & Endo, M. (1983). Handedness and familial sinistrality in a Japanese student population. *Cortex, 19,* 265–272.

Shucard, J. L., Shucard, D. W., Cummins, K. R., & Campos, J. J. (1981). Auditory evoked potentials and sex related differences in brain development. *Brain and Language, 13,* 91–102.

Sidman, R. L., & Rakic, P. (1973). Neuronal migration, with special reference to developing human brain: A review. *Brain Research, 62,* 1–35.

Silva, D. A., & Satz, P. (1979). Pathological left-handedness: Evaluation of a model. *Brain and Language, 7,* 8–16.

Smart, J. L., Jeffrey, C., & Richards, B. (1980). A retrospective study of the relationship between birth history and handedness at six years. *Early Human Development, 4,* 79–88.

Smith, L. C., & Moscovitch, M. (1979). Writing posture, hemispheric control of movement, and cerebral dominance in individuals with inverted and noninverted hand postures during writing. *Neuropsychologia, 17,* 637–644.

Smith, L. G. (1917). A brief survey of right- and left-handedness. *Pedagogical Seminary, 24,* 19–35.

Soper, H. V., & Satz, P. (1984). Pathological left-handedness and ambiguous handedness: A new explanatory model. *Neuropsychologia, 22,* 511–515.

Spiegler, B., & Yeni-Komshian, G. H. (1982). *Birth trauma and left-handedness: Test of a theory.* Paper presented at the 10th annual meeting of the International Neuropsychological Society, Pittsburgh, February.

Sperry, R. W. (1974). Lateral specialization in the surgically separated hemispheres. In F. O. Schmitt & F. G. Worden (Eds.), *The neurosciences: Third study program* (pp. 5–19). Cambridge, MA: MIT Press.

Subirana, A. (1969). Handedness and cerebral dominance. In P. J. Vinken & G. W. Bruyn (Eds.), *Handbook of clinical neurology: Vol. 4. Disorders of speech, perception, and symbolic behavior* (pp. 248–272). Amsterdam: North-Holland.

Tan, L. E., & Nettleton, N. C. (1980). Left handedness, birth order and birth stress. *Cortex, 16,* 363–374.

Tanner, J. M. (1978). *Fetus into man: Physical growth from conception to maturity.* Cambridge, MA: Harvard University Press.

Tapley, S. M., & Bryden, M. P. (1985). A group test for the assessment of performance between the hands. *Neuropsychologia, 23,* 215–221.

Taub, E., & Berman, A. J. (1968). Movement and learning in the absence of sensory feedback. In S. J. Freeman (Ed.), *The neuropsychology of spatially oriented behavior* (pp. 173–192). Homewood, IL: Dorsey Press.

Teng, E. L., Lee, P. H., Yang, K., & Chang, P. C. (1976). Handedness in a Chinese population: Biological, social, and pathological factors. *Science, 193,* 1148–1150.

Tizard, J. P. M., Paine, R. S., & Crothers, B. (1954). Disturbances of sensation in children with hemiplegia. *Journal of the American Medical Association, 155,* 628–632.

Todor, J. I., & Cisneros, J. (1985). Accommodation to increased accuracy demands by the right and left hands. *Journal of Motor Behavior, 17,* 355–372.

Torrey, E. F., Torrey, B. B., & Peterson, M. R. (1977). Seasonality of schizophrenic births in the United States. *Archives of General Psychiatry, 34,* 1065–1070.

Towbin, A. (1970), Central nervous system damage in the human fetus and newborn infant: Mechanical and hypoxic injury incurred in the fetal–neonatal period. *American Journal of Diseases of Children, 119,* 529–542.

Trehub, S. E., Corter, C. M., & Shosenberg, N. (1983). Neonatal reflexes: A search for lateral asymmetries. In G. Young, S. J. Segalowitz, C. M. Corter, & S. E. Trehub (Eds.), *Manual specialization and the developing brain* (pp. 257–272). New York: Academic Press.

Tucker, J. S. (1958). The electroencephalogram in brain stem vascular diseases. *EEG and Clinical Neurophysiology, 10,* 405–416.

Tupper, D. E. (1983). *The pattern of lateral preference and motor dominance in children ages 3 to 8.* Paper presented at the 11th annual meeting of the International Neuropsychological Society, Mexico City, February.

Turkewitz, G., & Birch, H. G. (1971). Neurobehavioral organization of the human newborn. In J. Hellmuth (Ed.), *Exceptional infant* (Vol. 2, pp. 24–40). New York: Brunner/Mazel.

Turkewitz, G., Gordon, E. W., & Birch, H. G. (1965). Head turning in the human neonatae: Spontaneous patterns. *Journal of Genetic Psychology, 107,* 143–148.

Turkewitz, G., Moreau, T., & Birch, H. G. (1968). Relationship between birth condition and neuro-behavioral organization in the neonate. *Pediatric Research, 2,* 243–249.

Umansky, R. (1973). Effect of a hand sock on prehension in infancy. *Developmental Psychobiology, 7,* 407–419.

Updegraff, R. (1932). Preferential handedness in young children. *Journal of Experimental Education, 1,* 134–139.

Vargha-Khadem, F., O'Gorman, A. M., & Watters, G. V. (1985). Aphasia and handedness in relation to hemispheric side, age at injury, and severity of cerebral lesion during childhood. *Brain, 108,* 677–696.

Verhagen, P., & Ntumba, A. (1964). Note on the frequency of left-handedness in African children. *Journal of Educational Psychology, 55,* 89–90.

Warkany, J., Lemire, R. J., & Cohen, M. M., Jr. (1981). *Mental retardation and congenital malformations of the central nervous system.* Chicago and London: Year Book Medical Publishers.

Weber, A. M., & Bradshaw, J. (1981). Levy and Reid's neurological model in relation to writing hand/posture: An evaluation. *Psychological Bulletin, 90,* 74–88.

Weintraub, S., & Mesulam, M.-M. (1983). Developmental learning disabilities of the right hemisphere. *Archives of Neurology, 40,* 463–468.

Wells, G. (1979). Variation in child language. In P. Fletcher & M. Garman (Eds.), *Language acquisition: Studies in first language development* (pp. 377–395). Cambridge: Cambridge University Press.

Wehrung, D. A., & Hay, S. (1970), A study of seasonal incidence of genital malformations in the United States. *British Journal of Preventive Social Medicine, 24,* 24–32.

Wile, I. S. (1932). Relation of left-handedness to behavior disorders. *American Journal of Orthopsychiatry, 2,* 44–57.

Wise, S. P. (1984). The nonprimary motor cortex and its role in the cerebral control of movement. In G. E. Edelman, W. E. Gall, & W. M. Cowan (Eds.), *Dynamic aspects of neocortical function* (pp. 525–555). New York: Wiley.

Witelson, S. F. (1980). Neuroanatomical asymmetry in left-handers: A review and implications for functional asymmetry. In J. Herron (Ed.), *Neuropsychology of left-handedness* (pp. 79–113). New York: Academic Press.

Witelson, S. (1985). On hemispheric specialization and cerebral plasticity: Mark II. In C. T. Best (Ed.), *Hemispheric function and collaboration in the child* (pp. 33–85). Orlando, FL: Academic Press.

Woods, B. T., & Carey, S. (1979). Language deficits after apparent clinical recovery from childhood aphasia. *Annals of Neurology, 6,* 405–409.

Woods, G. E. (1957). *Cerebral palsy in childhood.* Bristol, England: John Wright & Sons.

Yakovlev, P. I., Lecours, A.-R. (1967). The myelogenetic cycles of regional maturation in the brain. In A. Minkowski (Ed.), *Regional development of the brain in early life* (pp. 3–70). Oxford: Blackwell.

Yakovlev, P. I., & Rakic, P. (1966). Patterns of decussation of bulbar pyramids and distribution of pyramidal tracts on two sides of the spinal cord. *Transactions of the American Neurological Association, 91,* 366–367.

Yanowitz, J., Satz, P., & Heilman, K. (1981). Hemispheric laterality and body asymmetries. *Science, 212,* 1418.

Young, G., Segalowitz, S. J., Corter, C. M., & Trehub, S. E. (1983). *Manual specialization and the developing brain.* New York: Academic Press.

Young, H. B., & Knapp, R. (1966). Personality characteristics of converted left handers. *Perceptual and Motor Skills, 23,* 35–40.

PART FOUR

Lateralization and Atypical Development

Whereas the initial three sections of this book focused on the development of lateralization in ''normal'' populations of infants and young children, this section and the one that follows address the relationship between what are viewed as abnormal patterns of functional lateralization and a variety of abnormal developmental patterns. In this section the abnormal forms of lateralization are associated with X-chromosome abnormalities, unilateral childhood lesions, autism, and childhood depression. In general, as the reader is well aware, the relationship between abnormal forms of behavior and aberrant forms of lateralization is not an easy one to make and, as Liederman notes in Chapter 13, is further obscured by preconceived and untested hypotheses that have little foundation from the existing scientific literature. As a way of addressing this problem, Liederman identifies and attempts to correct what she views as widespread misconceptions concerning early brain damage, hemispheric asymmetries, and the child's behavior. Several chapters, such as Chapter 15 by Aram and Whitaker on unilateral lesions and Chapter 16 by Dawson concerning autism, point out that research in these areas, while providing a basis for our current thinking, is fraught with methodological and conceptual problems. In Chapter 15, Aram and Whitaker provide a review of case and group studies investigating the effects of unilateral lesions during childhood on cognitive abilities such as central auditory processing, visual perceptual abilities, auditory memory, academic achievement, and intelligence measures. The data initially look contradictory; but at least some of this confusion, they point out, apepars to be due to the lack of adequate experimental controls and manipulations. It is clear that meaningful information in this area can be gained only through the careful selection of subjects; the use of proper control populations for comparisons; and systematic, detailed tests of the children's functioning. An example of such gains is provided by one study that attempted to address many of these concerns. These sentiments are also addressed by Dawson, who, in a review of studies with autistic children, provides another opportunity to examine the role of lateralization in relation to language and affective development. Studies of cognitive abilities, handedness, EEG, and speech perception, as well as neuropsychological testing, provide data in support of the notion that autism involves abnormal development of the left hemisphere and overactivation of the right hemisphere. Dawson concludes her chapter by offering a set of four criteria to be used in evaluating the primacy of specific types of brain dysfunction in autism.

Chapter 14 by Netley and Rovet, on X-chromosome abnormalities, and Chapter 17 by Brumback, on childhood depression, address the relationships these authors see existing between these disorders and abnormal forms of lateralization. Both chapters point out the implications of such abnormal patterns not only for cognitive disorders but for social and personality problems as well. Netley and Rovet review the literature concerned with relationships between abnormal numbers of X chromosomes and factors related to cognitive abilities such as verbal and spatial skills, and to personality factors such as aggression, activity, and assertiveness. Central to their focus is the question of the relationship between biology and behavior. In the final chapter in this section, Brumback suggests that biological depressive illness is associated with dysfunctions of the left and right cerebral hemispheres. He goes on to outline how disruptions in factors such as verbal and spatial skills can lead to problems with peer, parent, and teacher interactions, and consequent impairment of normal personality development.

13

Misconceptions and New Conceptions about Early Brain Damage, Functional Asymmetry, and Behavioral Outcome

JACQUELINE LIEDERMAN
Boston University

Although it is well recognized that brain organization varies between individuals, we have only begun to explore whether individuals with atypical brain organization are especially impaired or talented. One kind of variation that has caught the public's attention is the way higher cognitive functions are differentially distributed between the two cerebral hemispheres. In most people, each hemisphere is specialized to play a dominant role within a unique class of functions, and the two hemispheres work in a complementary manner. In individuals with atypical organization, (i.e., those with anomolous or atypical "cerebral dominance") the "wrong" hemisphere may mediate a function or the usual complementarity of the hemispheres may be absent. An individual will be said to have atypical functional asymmetry if a hemisphere is more important as the substrate for a function than it is in the average person. This chapter describes several of the variants of atypical functional asymmetry, some of the ways that these atypicalities arise, and reasons one could expect such a redistribution of function to have cognitive and/or behavioral consequences. Thus, this chapter focuses on whether the way that specialized functions are distributed across the cerebrum is of any consequence to the quality of performance of those functions.

It will be argued that the implications of atypical functional asymmetry depend primarily on the cause of the atypicality. Atypical functional asymmetry will be shown to occur not only as a response to brain damage but also as a normal genetic variant. Next, two basic kinds of atypical functional asymmetry will be described: atypical functional asymmetry due to atypical structural organization of the cerebral cortices, and atypical functional asymmetry *despite* typical cortical structural organization. In the former instance, atypical functional asymmetry may be due to a variety of compensatory changes in the brain subsequent to brain damage. In the latter instance, atypical functional asymmetry may be due to unusual patterns of subcortical–cortical interactions and/or to atypical interhemispheric interactions. An attempt will be made to look for relationships between the patterns of atypical functional asymmetry (as deduced from physiological and behavioral measures of laterality), the mechanisms underlying these patterns (as deduced primarily from neurobiological data from animals), and the consequences of these patterns for behavioral outcome (as indicated by relative strengths and weaknesses in performance).

To avoid defining what is "normal" in terms of functional asymmetry, this chapter will focus instead on what is typical of humans as a group. Thus, the term "typical functional asymmetry" will refer to the modal brain, in which the left hemisphere is more important for the analysis of stimuli as discrete, finely timed events, whereas the right hemisphere is more important for the synthesis of stimuli over space and time into configurational gestalts. Therefore, behaviors such as speech, speech-sound discrimination, praxis, and syntactic comprehension are mediated primarily by the left hemisphere, whereas the perception of three-dimensional space, visuospatial patterns, and musical chords is mediated primarily by the right hemisphere. Dominance for a function does not imply exclusive control of that function (except perhaps for the left hemisphere's control of the production of multiword oral utterances). Instead, a kind of functional asymmetry is assumed in which the two hemispheres work in concert despite their differential aptitude and style of processing.[1]

Discussion of the relationship among early brain damage, functional asymmetry, and behavioral outcome has been obfuscated by two long-standing misconceptions in the literature:

MISCONCEPTION 1: ALL CHILDREN WITH ATYPICAL FUNCTIONAL ASYMMETRY HAVE SUFFERED BRAIN DAMAGE

This assumption is popular among many educators who believe that children with mixed or reversed lateral preferences should be suspected of having suffered brain damage and therefore should be given remedial work (see Chapter 8 by Harris and Chapter 18 by Bryden, this volume). This belief was encouraged by reports that there is an increased incidence of left-handers or individuals with mixed lateral preference within populations suffering from a variety of mental disabilities: mental retardation (Hicks & Barton, 1975; Silva & Satz, 1979), dyslexia (Witelson, 1977), epilepsy (Satz, Yanowitz, & Willmore, 1984), childhood autism (Boucher, 1977), and stuttering (Moore, 1976). In 1973, Bakan, Dibb, and Reed formally proposed that all instances of left-handedness arise from brain damage.

Several kinds of data, however, show that atypical functional asymmetry can occur in individuals who are neurologically intact at birth. For example, Ratcliff, Dila, Taylor, and Milner (1980) studied a series of patients by means of arteriograms and sodium amytal testing. Any patients suspected of perinatal brain damage were excluded from the sample. Yet even within this select group of patients, right-hemispheric or bihemispheric control of speech occurred in 34% of the sample. Although most of Ratcliff *et al.*'s subjects were suspected of being left-handed, others have shown that even some right-handers (crossed dextrals) suffer aphasia subsequent to right-hemisphere strokes (Bromwell, 1899). Taken together, these data indicate that atypical functional asymmetry can occur in both left- and right-handed individuals without a prior history of neurological disorder.

Another way to judge whether atypical functional asymmetry can occur in neurologically intact individuals is to observe the behavior of infants soon after birth (when environmental experience is at a minimum). Although most infants of two right-handed parents prefer to turn rightward at birth, there are children with normal perinatal histories who prefer to turn their heads leftward (Liederman & Coryell, 1981, 1982; Liederman & Kinsbourne, 1980) and rotate their heads further to the left than to the right (Liederman, 1986).

Perhaps most telling is the fact that even within neurologically intact adults, various measures of functional asymmetry are often not well correlated, resulting in the occurrence of so-called mixed laterality. For example, an individual who processes verbal information better when it is presented to the right rather than to the left visual field may not show a corresponding right-ear advantage for dichotic presentations of verbal sounds (Fennell, Bowers, & Satz, 1977) or a right-sided mouth asymmetry during speaking (Graves, 1983). Similarly, an asymmetrical preference for right rather than left ear during monaural stimulation, as indicated by larger auditory brain stem evoked potentials, is correlated with hand preference (Levine, Liederman, & Riley, 1986) but not ear preference during dichotic listening (Levine & McGaffigan, 1983). In addition, the hand, foot, ear, and eye preferences within an individual are not well correlated (Porac & Coren, 1981).

Even more surprising, hand preference per se is not a unitary phenomenon. Healey, Liederman, and Geschwind (1986) and Liederman and Healey (1987) demonstrated that even within "right-handed" individuals, hand preferences for various activities are independent. Certain activities that involve fine motor coordination (such as shaving) are preferentially performed by the right hand, in right-handers. Other manual activities (such as placing a hand down to do a cartwheel, or snapping one's fingers) are less lateralized.

Taken together, these data suggest that: (1) deviations from a typical pattern of asymmetry are not uncommon; (2) no single mechanism accounts for the formation of all asymmetries (see Liederman, 1983, for a more complete discussion) and (3) atypical functional asymmetry need not be a consequence of brain damage.

MISCONCEPTION 2: KNOWLEDGE OF THE LOCUS OF BRAIN DAMAGE IS SUFFICIENT TO PREDICT BEHAVIORAL OUTCOME; BEHAVIORAL LATERALITY DATA PROVIDE NO ADDITIONAL INFORMATION

According to this second perspective, knowing the locus and structural characteristics of the damaged tissue alone would be sufficient to predict the behavioral consequences. Contrary to that view, the point will be made that laterality measures may provide a window through which one can assess how the brain has responded to the damage. From a configural systems perspective, information about the particular location of a lesion would reveal little unless one knew the organizational configuration of the system before and after the lesion occurred. The same lesion will have radically different consequences depending on the organization of the remaining brain. A left-sided lesion will lead to almost irreversible aphasia in most individuals with functional asymmetry typical of right-handers, whereas those individuals with functional asymmetry typical of a left-hander will easily recover from such a lesion (Subirana, 1958). This may have little to do with the amount or kind of tissue damaged in the two cases, and everything to do with the kind of cerebral organization of which the tissue was once a part, or has become a part because of compensatory neural changes.

In addition, the effect of a lesion depends on the developmental stage of the individual at the time of the lesion. The rate and length that neurons will grow new axonal collaterals is greater during early than later development (Gall & Lynch, 1980). In fact, it is probably only in response to very early brain damage that "anomalous" connections are instituted (i.e., synapses are formed between regions that would not be connected in the normative brain).

The other effect of age on recovery of function has to do with the notion that regions become more committed to their primary function, which results in a progressive loss of equipotentiality with development (Bullock, Liederman, & Todorovic, 1987). During early development, the two hemispheres may be relatively competent to assume each other's functions. This is because in infancy the two hemispheres may differ structurally only in terms of the proportion of neurons that are suited to a hemisphere's major function. Thus, within each hemisphere, the majority of neurons may form networks that are well suited for that hemisphere's specialization, whereas a minority population may be suited for the other hemisphere's specialization. Over time, even though the primary specialization of a hemisphere (and therefore the degree of functional asymmetry) may be stable, the degree of residual plasticity may decrease with progressive commitment of tissue to the major function (Bullock, 1986, personal communication; Levy, 1983a).

The importance of age for recovery of function was dramatically demonstrated by Goldman and Galkin (1978), who made frontal lesions in fetal monkeys who were subsequently replaced within the uterus until term. When tested at 1 and 2 years of age, these monkeys were competent at frontal lobe tasks. Histological examination revealed that retrograde degeneration of the dorsomedial thalamus had not occurred, suggesting that the thalamic axons had projected collaterals to structures other than their normal targets. This compensatory sprouting of projecting fibers (discussed later) subserved recovery of frontal lobe functions by permitting nonfrontal cortical areas to receive inputs ordinarily limited to the frontal cortex.

NEW CONCEPTIONS ABOUT THREE KINDS OF BRAIN ORGANIZATION THAT MAY UNDERLIE ATYPICAL LATERALITY: GENERAL ISSUES

There are two basic ways that anomalous cerebral organization can occur: Either the cerebral cortex can be structured in an atypical way, or there can be abnormal activation of normally structured cortical tissue. Abnormal activation of normally structured cortical tissue can occur because of atypical subcortical–cortical interactions or because of atypical interhemispheric interactions (see Table 13-1). The point will be made that despite (or because of) the plasticity of the developing brain, certain variations in cerebral organization are not sufficient to provide an adequate substrate for normal language and cognition.

Brain Organization 1: Atypical Structural Cerebral Organization

When the brain is damaged, functions are sustained by means of the operation of the undamaged residual tissue. In this section, four kinds of compensatory neural changes will be discussed: (1) compensatory unmasking, (2) compensatory sprouting, (3) compensatory hypertrophy, and (4) compensatory maintenance. In the next section, the expected pattern of functional asymmetry and performance associated with each of these compensatory mechanisms will be described.

COMPENSATORY MECHANISMS UNDERLYING FUNCTIONAL PLASTICITY IN RESPONSE TO BRAIN DAMAGE

Compensatory Unmasking. Compensatory unmasking can be defined as a kind of neural change that occurs when the destruction of neurons in one part of the brain releases a secondary part of the brain for subserving that function. In contrast to the other three compensatory mechanisms that affect the rate of growth and/or death of a neuron, compensatory unmasking is passive in that it is the by-product of a shift in the balance of a system due to the loss of a component of that system. Compensatory unmasking can be due to the destruction of either a collection of cell bodies or a fiber tract. An example of compensatory unmasking as a result of the destruction of cell bodies was provided by Sprague (1966), who reported that cats showed unilateral neglect subsequent to a unilateral cortical lesion. Destruction of the superior colliculus on the side opposite to the cortical lesion

Table 13-1. Brain Organizations Underlying Atypical Behavioral Laterality

1. Cerebral *structure* atypically organized with typical activation
2. Atypical *cortical–subcortical reciprocal activation* with typical cerebral structure
3. Atypical *interhemispheric interaction* with typical cerebral structure

restored function (i.e., abolished the unilateral neglect) by restoring the balance of opposing attentional mechanisms.

An example of compensatory unmasking as a result of the destruction of fibers was provided by Wall (1977). Wall argued that most regions receive inputs from a variety of sources, and that competition among inputs renders some of the inputs "silent" in terms of their influence. Damage to one set of inputs, however, changes the balance of inputs to a region, with the result that the previously silent synapses are now in the majority and have a more dominant influence on the function of the receiving area. In this context, it is relevant that most of the regions that seem to take over a function were receiving inputs from a variety of modalities even before the time of insult (see Burnstine, Greenough, & Tees, 1984).

Compensatory Sprouting of Local or Projecting Fibers. Compensatory sprouting of local or projecting fibers can be defined as a kind of neural change that occurs when denervation of a synaptic region (due to damage or underutilization of that region) results in sprouting of axonal collaterals by intact neighboring neurons. This is a basic mechanism, which may also underlie compensatory hypertrophy (to be discussed). According to Ebbesson (1984), the sprouting of collaterals is adaptive in that it usually serves to reinstate a pattern of neural connectivity that is characteristic of the brain either at an earlier stage of development or in an animal lower on the phylogenetic scale. In general, therefore, the sprouted connections establish neural circuits that are more diffuse than the circuits that were disrupted by the original lesion.

Collateral sprouting, however, is not always adaptive. During very early development, sprouted collaterals may occasionally form anomalous connections, permitting synapses between brain regions that are not connected in the normative brain. For example, Schneider (1979) has shown that early lesions to the midbrain tectum of hamsters result in aberrant collateral sprouting, with the result that hamsters turn to the opposite side from where a food pellet is presented.

Compensatory Hypertrophy. Compensatory hypertrophy can be defined as a kind of neural change that occurs when the neural tissue normally associated with an intact region expands its capacity with reference to its usual function in response to a second system's: (1) damage (Goldman-Rakic & Rakic, 1984), (2) underutilization (Cotman & Nieto-Sampedro, 1982), or (3) underdevelopment (suggested by Geschwind & Galaburda, 1987). Compensatory hypertrophy can be due to neural growth (e.g., reactive synaptogenesis) or to lack of death (inhibition of the usual rate of neuronal death and/or collateral retraction). An example of underutilization of one region resulting in compensatory hypertrophy within another is that after young animals have been deprived of vision, there is a gradual increase in auditory cortex dendritic branching and/or the number of dendritic spines (Burnstine, Greenough, & Tees, 1984; Greenough & Green, 1981). More relevant to the current discussion, there may be between-hemisphere compensatory hypertrophy: If left-hemisphere damage occurs early enough, there may be over development of homologous right-hemisphere regions (Geschwind & Galaburda, 1987). Thus, in fetal monkeys, ablation of a cortical region on one side of the brain results in hypertrophy of the homologous area on the opposite side (Goldman-Rakic & Rakic, 1984). (There can also be compensatory hypertrophy of areas adjacent to the lesioned area on the same side.) It is likely that between-hemisphere compensatory hypertrophy has neurochemical implications, because damage to one cerebral hemisphere increases acetylcholine activity in the opposite hemisphere (Kretch, Rosenzweig, & Bennett, 1963).[2]

Compensatory Maintenance. Compensatory maintenance can be defined as a kind of neural change that occurs when early brain damage causes maintenance of a primitive neural feature, which during the normal course of development would otherwise have atrophied. For example, two groups of cats were subjected to hemispherectomy either as kittens or as adult cats (Villablanca, Burgess, & Sonnier, 1984). The young cats had better preservation of sensory and motor abilities than the older cats did, and their brains contained anomalous contralateral fibers from the intact hemisphere to the contralateral thalamus and red nucleus. Villablanca *et al.* (1984) argued that these abnormal projections were probably not formed after the lesion, but were present in the neonatal kitten at the time of ablation. If that were the case, the role of early hemispherectomy would have been to sustain preexisting contralateral pathways, thereby allowing bilateral control by the remaining hemisphere. Villablanca *et al.*'s (1984) hypothesis is reasonable in that it has been shown that some interhemispheric fibers exist transiently and disappear with development (Innocenti, 1981; Ivy, Akers, & Killackey, 1979) (see Table 13-2).

HOW COMPENSATORY NEURAL CHANGES COULD AFFECT FUNCTIONAL ASYMMETRY AND THE QUALITY OF PERFORMANCE

Summary of Popular Predictions. Compensatory unmasking, sprouting, hypertrophy, and maintenance may each be associated with distinct patterns of atypical functional asymmetry and performance. For purposes of illustration, the following discussion will be restricted to the case where compensatory neural changes are triggered by a *focal unilateral left-hemisphere lesion received during infancy.* To simplify the discussion, it is also being assumed that the damaged area cannot subserve its usual function(s) to any extent, and therefore is not contributing noise to the system. The corollaries of each kind of compensatory neural change in terms of functional asymmetry and quality of performance will be described. For a summary, please refer to Table 13-3.

Compensatory changes may involve the undamaged regions of the same (left) hemisphere as was damaged *(within-hemisphere compensatory changes)* and/or regions within the undamaged contralateral (right) hemisphere *(between-hemisphere compensatory changes).* An example of within-hemisphere compensatory changes was provided by Goldman (1971), who claimed that dorsolateral frontal cortex takes over the function of orbitofrontal cortex in response to early lesions in primates. Her evidence was inferential, based on patterns of behavioral recovery. An example of between-hemisphere compensatory change was provided by Levine and Mohr (1979), who reported a series of cases of aphasic patients with

Table 13-2. Kinds of Compensatory Neural Changes Subsequent to Brain Damage

1. *Compensatory unmasking:*
   Release of a secondary system by destruction of the part of the brain that primarily subserved that function.
2. *Compensatory sprouting:*
   Sprouting of axonal collaterals by intact neighboring neurons in response to denervation of a synaptic region (due to damage or underutilization of that region).
3. *Compensatory hypertrophy:*
   Expansion of a region (by means of either collateral sprouting or a reduction of neural death) in response to either (a) damage, (b) underutilization, or (c) underdevelopment of a different neural region.
4. *Compensatory maintenance:*
   Maintenance of a primitive neural feature in response to early brain damage.

Table 13-3. Changes in Behavioral Laterality and Quality of Performance Due to Between-Hemisphere Compensatory Neural Changes

Kind of compensatory neural change	Effect on laterality and quality of performance of "left-hemisphere processes"	Effect on laterality and quality of performance of "right-hemisphere processes"
Between-hemisphere compensatory unmasking and/or sprouting	Reversed functional asymmetry; mild deficits	Normal right-sided advantage; mild deficits
Between-hemisphere compensatory hypertrophy	Reduced left-sided advantage; mild deficits	Exaggerated right-sided advantage; talents
Compensatory maintenance	Lack of left-sided advantage; few if any deficits	Lack of right-sided advantage; few if any deficits

Note: Only the effects of left-hemisphere damage are considered.

a single left-hemisphere stroke who recovered from aphasia until a second stroke in the right-hemisphere reinstituted the aphasia.

All within-hemisphere compensatory changes require that the residual undamaged tissue be the primary substrate for more functions than in the normal course of development. Such "squeezing" of functions within an area may have the following consequences: (1) a reduced degree of functional asymmetry for those left-hemispheric functions; (2) a reduction in the precision with which behaviors corresponding to those left-hemispheric functions are controlled; and (3) no change in the size of the advantage for the functions normally controlled by the undamaged (right) hemisphere. For example, damage to part of Wernicke's area would reduce the size of the left-hemisphere advantage for verbal processing, but it would not affect the size of the right-hemisphere advantage for visuospatial processing. In terms of the quality of performance, some loss of precision or efficiency would be expected. Schneider (1979) reports an example in which squeezing functions within an area reduced the precision of behavior. Partial damage to the superior colliculi of young hamsters resulted in reorganization of the residual superior colliculi and a loss of precision in orientation ability.

Between-hemisphere compensatory changes could result in a number of different patterns of functional asymmetry, depending on the particular compensatory mechanism. For ease of discussion, it is being assumed that between-hemisphere compensatory changes would be restricted to the homologous regions in the hemisphere opposite to the one damaged. (At this time, however, there is no reason to assume that changes need be restricted to homologous regions, especially because many callosal projections are heterotopic rather than homotopic (Selnes, 1974).

Between-hemisphere compensatory unmasking and between-hemisphere compensatory sprouting should have the following consequences in common: First, for the specific case under consideration, where the focal region within the left hemisphere was sufficiently damaged to be rendered nonfunctional, control of the function would be shifted to the opposite hemisphere. Second, for both kinds of compensatory neural change, the behavior may seem recovered, but the pattern of errors may indicate that the unmasked or newly established networks in the opposite hemisphere mediate performance by means of a new set of rules. For example, what have been interpreted as anomalous linguistic strategies have been observed in patients whose left hemispheres have been surgically removed, and who are speaking by means of the isolated right hemispheres (e.g., Dennis, 1980).

The difference between these two compensatory mechanisms is that the compensatory unmasking would result in an *immediate* shift in laterality and an *immediate* onset of behaviors directed toward mediating the required function. (Note that even though the change in laterality would be immediate, there would still be a learning curve as the previously secondary system became more accomplished at the task.) In contrast, in the case of compensatory sprouting, the new collaterals would activate the right hemisphere to a greater extent than it would normally be activated in the undamaged brain. There would be a *gradual* shift in laterality and a *gradual* appearance of new behavioral capacities corresponding to the *growth* of new collaterals and the establishment of new neural networks.

Therefore the predictions for both between-hemisphere compensatory unmasking and sprouting are that one would expect a reversal of functional asymmetry for the function(s) primarily subserved by the damaged side *and* a reduction in the size of the advantage for the function(s) normally controlled by the homologous region of the undamaged hemisphere. Thus, there would be a *right*-hemisphere advantage for verbal processing and a smaller-than-average right-hemisphere advantage for visuospatial processing.

Both of these compensatory neural changes would lead to a reduction in the precision of control of both left- and right-hemisphere functions. The degree of recovery of left hemisphere functions would be inversely proportional to age (because of progressive decreases in equipotentiality), whereas the extent to which right-hemisphere functions would be jeopardized is controversial and will be discussed in a later section concerned with whether functions squeeze each other.

Between-hemisphere compensatory hypertrophy does not seem to occur in response to full-blown lesions of an entire left-hemisphere region. Instead, the known instances are thought to be in response to (1) scattered minor left-hemispheric structural aberrations sustained very early in development, or (2) underdevelopment of regions within the left hemisphere (Geschwind & Galaburda, 1987). In terms of the pattern of functional asymmetry, one would expect a normal or smaller-than-average left-hemisphere advantage for verbal materials, and a larger-than-average right-hemisphere advantage for visuospatial materials. Thus, compensatory hypertrophy should result in a behavioral deficiency corresponding to the specialized function(s) of the lesioned side (e. g., a dyslexia or an aphasia due to an early left-sided lesion), and an extreme talent corresponding to the specialized function(s) of the unlesioned side (i.e., extreme visuospatial skills). Gordon (1980, 1983) has observed that dyslexic patients, as a group, have better-than-average visuospatial talents. Similarly, Geschwind and Galaburda (1987) reviewed a series of cases that they claim fit this description.

Between-hemisphere compensatory maintenance is another neural change that occurs only during very early development. In the cases reported to date, compensatory maintenance has had the effect of making a system more bilateral than it would typically be, in terms of either input to a hemisphere or output from a hemisphere. For example, in the visual system of rats, there is a transient ipsilateral retinotopic projection that is normally only contralaterally organized. Similarly, in the motor system, Kato, Hirano, Katagiri, and Sasaki (1985) observed uncrossed corticospinal fibers in the newborn rat that are totally absent by day 6. After unilateral cortical damage, these ipsilateral fibers may be maintained, explaining why a substantial number of uncrossed corticospinal fibers from the undamaged hemisphere are observed in such animals after they have matured (in rats: Hicks & D'Amato, 1970; in hamsters: Reh & Kalil, 1982).[3]

Thus, compensatory maintenance serves to decrease the extent to which there is functional asymmetry. In terms of performance characteristics, the most obvious consequences would be expected within the motor system. For example, one might predict that there would be some loss of precision due to an increase in spillover movements (Nass, 1985).

Many of the predictions as to the outcomes of compensatory neural changes are based on assumptions that are popular among neuropsychologists. For example, it is generally assumed that the hemisphere that primarily subserves a function is better suited to that function in terms of its structure. This assumption has been less than adequately tested. Similarly, there is the notion that "more is better," that is, that the larger the amount of space available in a hemisphere to subserve a function, the better the function will be executed.

On the basis of these two assumptions, neuropsychologists have made tenuous predictions about the effect of squeezing two functions into one region. They have also talked about asymmetries in the extent to which one hemisphere can serve as the substrate for conducting the functions of the other hemisphere.

Because resolution of these fundamental questions is crucial for the current inquiry, in the next section these questions will be addressed in turn. The discussion will reveal just how far we are from being certain of any of these propositions.

Unresolved Controversies That Jeopardize These Predictions

THE IMPORTANCE OF A PARTICULAR KIND OF CIRCUITRY OR A SPECIFIC AMOUNT OF SPACE FOR ADEQUATE FUNCTION. Two structural differences are usually cited as the basis for functional asymmetry. The appropriately specialized hemisphere is assumed to have better circuitry for a particular function and/or a greater amount of space in the region relevant for that function. Considering how widespread these beliefs are, it is surprising that so little is known about the significance of hemispheric differences in circuitry and space.

Indirect evidence about circuitry differences between the hemispheres has been based on the following reasoning: Since recovery of function after brain damage is limited, the two sides of the brain must not be equipotential for function (Witelson, 1983). The problem with this logic is that a persistent deficit after a unilateral lesion could also be caused by (1) an attempt to use the damaged hemisphere; (2) inhibition from the damaged hemisphere to the nondamaged hemisphere, preventing the latter from taking over the function (Kinsbourne, 1975); or (3) crowding of functions into the undamaged hemisphere. The lack of full recovery does suggest that the hemispheres were initially being deployed differently, but it does not prove that it is because of its cytoarchitectonic structure (i.e., its circuitry) that the contralateral hemisphere does not fully take the function. Observation of hemidecorticate children presents additional inferential obstacles, because some children with only one hemisphere do not show linguistic deficits when compared to age- and IQ-matched controls (Bishop, 1983).

Other indirect evidence suggesting that there are hemispheric differences in cytoarchitecture has come from differential hemispheric rates of clearance of Xenon-133, which is used during cerebral blood flow. The relatively slow clearance rate of the left hemisphere has been interpreted as indicating that the left hemisphere has more gray matter, whereas the right hemisphere has more white matter (Gur *et al.*, 1980). Similarly, Thatcher, Krause, and Hrybyk (1986) have observed a greater amount of EEG coherence between regions in the right as opposed to the left hemisphere, which they interpreted as evidence for more white matter on the right side.

There have been only two cytoarchitectonic studies that compared cortical tissue on the left versus right sides of the brain. Scheibel (1980) examined the dendritic pattern of pyramidal neurons in and around Broca's area. Neurons from the left side of the brain had more higher order dendritic branches than on the right side. According to Scheibel (1980), such branches generally develop late, are small in diameter, have high resistance values, and form Type I (i.e., excitatory) synapses. In contrast, neurons from the right side of the brain had more lower order dendrites than those from the left side. Such branches generally are relatively wide in diameter, have low resistances, and form Type II (i.e., inhibitory) synapses. This could suggest that the right-hemisphere neurons have a branching pattern that permits inhibition to flow freely, whereas left-hemisphere neurons have a pattern that allows widespread activation. It is not immediately obvious how these cytoarchitectonic characteristics map onto the popular notion (Semmes, 1968) that the representation of function is ''focal'' in the left hemisphere and ''diffuse'' in the right hemisphere.

Seldon (1981, 1982) examined left and right cortex in and around the region of Wernicke's area. He concluded that the greater amount and density of the neuropil in the region of Wernicke's area on the left side, and its particular dendritic arrangement, permit greater response specificity as compared to that on the right side. In contrast, the cortical columns on the right side had greater overlap, greater variability of dendritic orientation, and a more diffuse organization than those on the left side. These left–right differences correspond to Semmes's (1968) focal–diffuse dichotomization of hemispheric function.

The results of these studies should be interpreted with caution, because both were somewhat preliminary. Scheibel (1984) examined only six cells per region from eight patients, six of whom were right-handed, and the location of the cells was not verified by histology. In contrast, Seldon (1982) examined 622 neurons and performed extensive histological analysis, but he did not specify the number of subjects or their hand preference and gender. At any rate, conclusions as to global left–right cytoarchitectonic differences should not be based on studies of only Broca's and Wernicke's areas.

There is also only limited support for the phrenological belief that the bigger a region is, the better it functions as a substrate for a behavior. If a larger size were crucial, it would seem odd that the brain would remodel itself by *decreasing* the total number of neurons (Cotman & Nieto-Sampedro, 1982). In addition, hemispheric differences in size are not all easily interpreted. For example, a larger left than right planum temporale is usually associated with a larger left than right angular gyrus region (Eidelberg & Galaburda, 1982). However, the size of Wernicke's area is not correlated with the size of Broca's area (Falzi, Perrone, & Vignolo, 1982).

Similarly, Ratcliff *et al.* (1980) observed that not all patients with a longer left than right Sylvian fissure (as inferred from cerebral angiogram) showed suppression of speech after left-hemisphere injection with sodium amytal. Of 23 right-handed subjects, speech suppression occurred after both left- and right-hemisphere injections in 4 patients and after right-hemisphere injection in 1 patient. In addition, Pieniadz, Naeser, Koff, and Levine (1983) found that right-handed global aphasics recovered from their left-hemisphere stroke more quickly when their right occipital petalia was larger than their left one (an atypical pattern). In their sample, 8 of 14 patients showed that ''atypical'' pattern of cerebral asymmetry. Since these patients had aphasia after a stroke on the left side, and it was the smaller side, we can infer that the side with the smaller occipital petalia was involved with speech processing prior to the insult. Apparently, the larger region is not necessarily the one that will predominate during a behavior.

Perhaps the best demonstration that bigger may not be better was a series of four dyslexic cases who all had symmetrical planum temporale and a greater than usual total amount of tissue in that region (Galaburda, Sherman, Rosen, Aboitiz, & Geschwind, 1985). This may be an instance where the lack of selective cell death, and therefore greater amounts of surviving tissue, is a sign of pathology.

In fact, the usual brain-to-body weight ratio may be a good predictor of ability only when one is making between-species comparisons. Within a species, a relatively small brain may be sufficient for normal species-typical behavior.[4] For example, Lorber and Priestley (1981) have shown that patients who have suffered from hydroencephaly since an early age and who have cortices that are reduced to a fraction of their normal size can still develop language and score within the normal range on IQ tests. Similarly, Chow (1968) has shown that cats could do pattern discrimination when only a small fraction of the optic tract axons were spared, even though acuity was diminished.

Therefore, the relative size of various brain regions may not affect function in the intact brain. It may not matter if the larger of the two hemisphere's regions predominates while executing a function. As will be discussed next, however, after brain damage the size of the intact neural areas may be important, because a small area may be recruited to subserve a greater number of functions than usual.

IS THERE A SQUEEZING OF FUNCTIONS IN RESPONSE TO BRAIN DAMAGE?

Is there a trade-off between language and visuospatial abilities due to a space squeeze? The behavioral outcome after reorganization may depend on whether the damaged area originally subserved language or visuospatial functions. It has been claimed that when the damage occurs early in life, language is spared at the expense of visuospatial abilities. For example, Bullard-Bates and Satz (1983) reported the case of a left-handed woman with a static lesion in the left hemisphere, confirmed by CAT scan. This patient also had atrophy of the right hand and foot, which Satz *et al.* (1984) claimed was a sign that the lesion was sustained around the time of birth. The patient had superior language skills, coupled with a dramatic impairment of visuospatial constructive skills. On the basis of her robust left-ear advantage during dichotic listening, it was suggested that linguistic function had shifted to her undamaged right hemisphere. The authors concluded that linguistic function was given priority over visuospatial function in the right hemisphere, thereby sparing language at the expense of visuospatial ability.

Satz, Orsini, Saslow, and Henry (1985) reviewed 12 cases of left-handers with a history of birth trauma or early brain damage. Seven of these 12 cases had clear evidence of early left-sided brain damage. Nine of the 12 cases lacked left-handed relatives (the other 3 histories were not known). All 12 patients had visuospatial deficits despite their relatively intact language abilities. Similarly, Tizard, Paine, and Crothers (1954) described four cases of right hemiplegia; three were associated with visuospatial deficits. Lansdell (1969) tested 18 epileptics, 15 of whom sustained their lesions prior to age 5. Even though the damage was left-sided, performance was more deficient on the nonverbal than the verbal scale of the Wechsler-Bellevue IQ Test.

Kohn and Dennis (1974) reported four cases of left hemidecortication in which there were verbal rather than visuospatial deficits. This might seem like an exception to this rule of "verbal" sparing. As Satz *et al.* (1985) point out, however, despite the early onset of hemiplegia, surgery was delayed until the age of 10 to 18 years. Thus, language may have been deficient and spatial skills may have been spared because, prior to surgery, language functions were controlled for at least a decade by the damaged left hemisphere.

There is one set of data that suggests that men may be more vulnerable to crowding of function than women. Novelly and Naugle (1986) studied patients who had left-hemispheric epileptogenic focal lesions and whose seizure onset was in childhood. None of the lesions invaded the parietal lobe. The hemisphere dominant for speech was ascertained by means of the sodium amytal procedure. Between-hemisphere compensatory neural changes, as indicated by right-hemisphere speech, was associated with a significantly reduced performance IQ in males ($N = 9$) but not in females ($N = 10$). This could be a by-product of sex differences in the way in which functions are organized within a hemisphere in neurologically intact adults (Kimura & Harshman, 1984). Or it could reflect differences between the sexes in terms of neural plasticity, which could be mediated by differences in hormones.

Do non-brain-damaged left-handers, with bilateral speech representation, suffer from a space squeeze? The nonclinical population that shows the highest incidence of brains with atypical functional asymmetry is that of left-handers. There is agreement that some left-handers have some sort of bilateral representation of speech, although estimates vary between 15% (Rasmussen & Milner, 1977) and 70% (Satz, 1979). On this basis, one would predict a squeeze of right-hemisphere functions. Yet there are virtually no data that show that the average left-hander performs *below the normal range* on any psychometric test (see Briggs, Nebes, & Kinsbourne, 1976, and Hardyck & Petrinovich, 1977 for reviews). As Satz *et al.* (1985) have pointed out, Levy (1974) claimed that a small sample of left-handed college students showed visuospatial deficits, but subsequent studies (e.g., Fennell, Satz, Van den Abell, Bowers, & Thomas, 1978; Newcombe & Ratcliff, 1973) have failed to support that claim. It may be that left-handers with "bilateral" speech nonetheless rely on their left hemisphere for language, thereby leaving the right hemisphere free to subserve the usual right-hemispheric functions.

IS THE RIGHT HEMISPHERE MORE PLASTIC THAN THE LEFT HEMISPHERE? The behavioral outcome of brain damage may also be affected by the relative plasticity of each hemisphere (i.e., how readily one hemisphere can subsume the other hemisphere's function). On the basis of their clinical experience, Geschwind and Galaburda (1985a) suggest that the right hemisphere takes over language more readily than the left hemisphere takes over spatial function(s). According to Goldberg and Costa (1981), the right hemisphere's plasticity is attributable to its greater degree of multimodal organization as compared to the left hemisphere.

If it is true that the right hemisphere shows greater plasticity than the left hemisphere, this runs counter to Goldman's (1971) suggestion that the earlier a region develops, the *earlier* it becomes "committed" to its function(s), and the *less* able it is to serve as a substrate for recovery of function. Most regions of the right hemisphere develop *earlier* than those of the left hemisphere (Best, Chapter 1, this volume; Geschwind & Galaburda, 1987).

The right hemisphere, however, may not be more "plastic" than the left hemisphere, as claimed, but instead may simply be called on more frequently to take over the left hemisphere's function(s) because of the greater vulnerability of the left hemisphere to damage. Liederman (1983) reviewed the literature and concluded that the left hemisphere is more vulnerable to early damage than is the right hemisphere. Recent data support that conclusion. Volpe, Herscovitch, Perlman, and Raichle (1983) used PET scans to study six premature babies who experienced major intraventricular hemorrage with cerebral involvement. Although the sample is very small, it is interesting that all six cases had more marked damage on the left than on the right side. Similarly, of 56 cases of early lesions reported by Hecaen, Perenin, and Jeannerod (1984), 40 were left-sided. Finally, Geschwind and Galaburda (1987) observed that the left hemisphere is more vulnerable to arterovenous malformations and certain kinds of migrational anomalies.

In sum, there are insufficient data to conclude that the right hemisphere takes over function(s) more readily than does the left hemisphere. In fact, there is one piece of data that contradicts this conclusion, and another that is inconclusive. First, Ment *et al.* (1983) studied 11 preterm infants by means of cerebral blood flow. Deviant cerebral blood flow values for the left, but not the right, hemisphere were related to performance on the Bayley Infant Development Scale at age 1 year. Second, Strauss and Verity (1983) examined four patients (aged 12 to 32) with infantile hemiplegia who had undergone hemispherectomy. The repercussions of left versus right hemispherectomy did not differ: In both cases there were residual visuospatial deficits, with sparing of verbal and praxic skills. The reason that these data may be considered inconclusive is that the CAT scans and EEGs at follow-up were abnormal for all four cases, even allowing for the fact that one hemisphere had been surgically removed.

Recapitulation. In summary, the predictions about functional asymmetry and behavioral outcome summarized in Table 13-3 are a snapshot of a moving stream of predictions. They are based on the set of assumptions just described, which, it has been argued, have not been justified by sufficient research. Therefore, Table 13-3 serves as a summary of the current view, but it is not likely to be the final view.

Brain Organizations 2 and 3: Atypical Activation of Otherwise Normally Structured Cerebral Hemispheres

The enormous amount of structural variability in neurologically intact individuals, as well as the amount of variability in functional asymmetry in individuals with typical structural asymmetries, suggests that too much emphasis has been placed on *structural* differences between the hemispheres as the single source of variation responsible for functional asymmetry. Clearly, there must be atypicalities in functional asymmetry that occur *despite* normal structural laterality. As has been pointed out by Kinsbourne (1970) and even more recently by Levy (1983; Levy, Heller, Banich, & Burton, 1983), variations in functional asymmetry may also be due to *differential utilization or activation of various regions of the brain.*

In the next section, two ways that the cerebral hemispheres can be atypically activated so as to influence the ultimate pattern of functional asymmetry will be described. These involve atypical cortical–subcortial interactions and atypical interhemispheric interactions. Together, these mechanisms will define a dynamic process whereby various structural asymmetries of the cortex are differentially activated in different contexts.

BRAIN ORGANIZATION 2: ATYPICAL SUBCORTICAL–CORTICAL INTERACTIONS

A Selective Activation Mechanism That Is Probably Thalamic. Classical activation theory, based on the writings of Moruzzi and Magoun (1949), assumed that the hemispheres could be aroused only to an equal extent. Some modern theorists, such as Friedman and Polson (1981), still make this assumption. However, several sets of data support the notion that there can be regional or hemispheric selectivity in the distribution of arousal. For example, cerebral blood flow studies such as Gur and Reivich's (1980) show that there is asymmetrical blood flow during the performance of verbal versus spatial tasks. Such data demonstrate that the hemispheres are not always activated to the same extent. Similarly, electrophysiological data recorded in infants by Molfese, Freeman, and Palermo (1975) have been interpreted by Kinsbourne (1980) as evidence that speech stimuli can turn on a selector that predominantly activates the left hemisphere. This asymmetrical activation in the newborn does not indicate that the two cortices are differentially analyzing the input. According to Kinsbourne (1980), it merely indicates that on the basis of certain features of the input, a subcortical mechanism differentially activates one hemisphere for processing.

There is also evidence that an individual can consciously decide to activate a hemisphere selectively. A vivid example of this was provided by Gott, Hughes, and Whipple (1984). They reported the case of a neurologically intact woman who could control both the onset and the duration of two different mental states. During the first state, her mentation was dominated by verbal/analytic kinds of processes. During the second state, her mentation was dominated by nonverbal/visuospatial kinds of processes. Hemisphere alpha ratios indicated that the left hemisphere was more active than the right during her left-hemisphere state and that the right hemisphere was more active than the left during her right-hemisphere state. During the EEG recording, the subject was required to do two verbal tasks and two spatial tasks, first while in the left-hemisphere state and then while in the right-hemisphere state. She was able to do the tasks even when required to maintain the "wrong" hemisphere as the most active, but her performance was best when the "correct" hemisphere was the one that she was directed to keep most active.

Asymmetrical activation of the hemispheres is probably mediated by a selector mechanism organized on a thalamic level (Kinsbourne, 1980). Ojemann and Ward (1971) have suggested ventrolateral thalamus; Crosson (1985) has suggested ventroanterior thalamus. A third ventral thalamic nucleus, the reticular nucleus, has been nominated by Scheibel (1980) as the best candidate for the mediator of selective attention.

The reticular nucleus of the thalamus surrounds the lateral and ventral surfaces of the thalamus like a screen (Jones, 1975). The activity of the reticular nucleus of the thalamus is primarily controlled by inputs from two areas. One input consists of incoming stimuli via the brain stem reticular formation; the other input consists of stimuli that have undergone higher order processing via frontal granular and sensorimotor regions of the cortex. The reticular nucleus has no direct output to the cortex. The output of the reticular nucleus is mediated primarily by the other nuclei of the thalamus. As Scheibel (1980) suggests, "the concept emerges of a reticularis complex selectively gating interaction between specific thalamic nuclei and the cerebral cortex under the opposed but complementary control of the brain stem reticular core and the frontal granular cortex."

According to Scheibel, this gate can be extremely selective with reference to stimuli in several modalities, because most of the reticular thalamic nucleus neurons respond to visual, somatic, and auditory stimuli. In addition, the receptive fields of the reticular nucleus are organized in an overlapping fashion, so that a point in space with reference to the body is represented in a multimodal fashion. Therefore, a unit responding to stimulation of the hind limb will usually be maximally sensitive to auditory stimuli originating well to the rear of the organism. These sensory maps also correspond to motor maps in the tectum.

Scheibel has claimed that this nucleus can be selective in terms of the "species" of input. Although it has not been demonstrated, one could conjecture that it could be selective for stimuli that require linguistic or visuospatial processing and could prime one or the other hemisphere to be ready for a certain input (either on the basis of a low-level detector mechanism, or from a downstream signal issuing from frontal cortical areas). Similarly, it could alert a hemisphere to be ready to receive a stimulus on the basis of its afferent input from the brain stem. Thus, as Scheibel suggests, the reticular nucleus of the thalamus may be thought of as a "mosaic of gatelets" that are selective to some specific receptive field or kind of input.

Schlag and Waszak (1970, 1971) have shown that reticularis neurons discharge profusely at times when other thalamic cells are silenced. They interpret these data as indicating that the reticularis neurons impose inhibition on the many neurons of both specific and nonspecific thalamic nuclei to which they project. These data would be consistent with the notion that the reticularis neurons act as a kind of gate.

Atypical Selector Mechanism: Its Effect on Behavioral Laterality and Quality of Performance. Atypical activation of otherwise typically structured cerebral cortex could result in several patterns of atypical functional asymmetry. A faulty selector mechanism could lead to either a *mismatch* between the activation required for a particular input and the specialization of the hemisphere activated, an *imbalance* so that one hemisphere is either tonically or phasically under-activated, or a *cancellation* where the activation pattern by the selector is at odds with the particular pattern of interhemispheric activation. Each of these will be considered in turn.

In a mismatch, the selector could be defective in that the wrong hemisphere is activated. In that case, functional asymmetry would be reversed and performance would be deficient. There have been several demonstrations that the degree of activation of the appropriately specialized hemisphere influences performance. Gur and Reivich (1980) reported that during spatial tasks, when the right hemisphere was more active than the left as indicated by cerebral blood flow, performance was better than when the left hemisphere was more active. Even more compelling was the case study reported by Gott *et al.* (1984). As mentioned previously, their subject was able voluntarily to activate and sustain left-hemisphere activation irrespective of the nature of the task that she was concurrently performing. Which hemisphere was more activated, however, had repercussions on her performance. Her verbal fluency and the number of three-syllable words that she wrote during an essay were significantly greater when her left hemisphere was more activated than her right hemisphere. Conversely, her ability to perform a circle-matching task and other spatial tasks was significantly better when her right hemisphere was more activated than her left. (Oddly enough, hemispheric activation did not affect her performance on the Verbal versus Performance scales of the WAIS.[5]) Nonetheless, her performance was deficient whenever she preferentially activated the "wrong" hemisphere.

An imbalance of activation could produce greater-than-average activation of one hemisphere and relative under-activation of the other hemisphere. This would result in extreme functional asymmetry scores for tasks for which the activated side is specialized, and weak laterality scores for tasks for which the underactivated side is specialized. Moreover, for tasks where both hemispheres must cooperate, there would be a deficient contribution by the relatively underactivated side. A summary of these various outcomes is provided in Table 13-4.

There are some data with dyslexic children that have been related to an imbalance activation deficit. Bakker, Moerland, and Goekoop-Hoefkens (1981) and Bakker and Vinke (1985) have suggested that there are two groups of dyslexic children who differ in terms of which hemisphere is relatively underutilized. L-types show dichotic right ear advantages, make "word-mutilating" reading errors (e.g., omissions and additions of letters), and depend on left-hemisphere reading strategies. P-types do not show dichotic right-ear advantages, make "time-consuming" reading errors (e.g., fragmentations and repetitions of letters), and rely on a right-hemisphere reading strategy. These dyslexic children were given a therapeutic regime consisting of sessions of hemisphere-specific stimulation, directed toward the child's presumably less active hemisphere. In both studies, therapeutic "activation" of an otherwise underutilized hemisphere improved performance for the L but

Table 13-4. Modes of Interhemispheric Activation that Might Affect Behavioral Laterality

1. Interhemispheric shielding
2. Interhemispheric sharing
3. Interhemispheric equilibrium

not the P dyslexics. Unfortunately, the interpretation of the effect is clouded by the fact that the therapy did not consistently induce electroencephalographic changes indicative of greater activation of the underutilized right hemisphere in the L dyslexics.

A relative lack of functional asymmetry would occur if there were strong dissociations between elements of the activation system. This could induce a lack of selective activation: Both hemispheres would be diffusely activated for all tasks, and there would be a lack of behavioral asymmetry. One would expect performance to be degraded for any task requiring focal attention.

A Second Activation Mechanism That Is Probably Neurochemical. A second cortical activation mechanism might involve either tonic or phasic asymmetries in either neurotransmitter levels, turnover, or receptor distribution. For example, Glick, Ross, and Hough (1982) reported that there is a left-sided predominance of dopamine in the striatal area in humans. Oke, Keller, Mefford, and Adams (1978) have shown that in humans, there are greater amounts of norepinephrine in the left than in the right pulvinar nucleus. Similarly, left temporal lobe regions show greater choline–acetyltransferase activity than do corresponding areas of the right hemisphere (Amaducci, Sorbi, Alabanese, & Gainotti, 1981).

The Influence of Tonic and Phasic Neurochemical Asymmetries on Behavioral Outcome. Taken together, these relatively tonic neurochemical asymmetries may set the tone of activation of a region and induce certain low-level behavioral asymmetries. For example, the turning asymmetries that dominate behavior during the first 3 months of an infant's life (Liederman & Kinsbourne, 1980; Turkewitz, 1977) may be attributable in part to a tonically high level of dopamine on the left side. These infant turning biases certainly seem analogous to the circling tendencies of rats with inborn dopaminergic asymmetries (Glick *et al.*, 1982).

Flor-Henry (1979) reviewed data that could be interpreted as indicating the effect of phasic neurochemical asymmetries on functional asymmetry. Some patients with depressive psychosis changed their preferred hand for writing when shifting into depression or into mania.

BRAIN ORGANIZATION 3: ATYPICAL INTERHEMISPHERIC INTERACTION

The third component of an activation model is a mechanism that modifies and equilibrates transmission of activation (or information) between the hemispheres. Three modes of interaction can be suggested: (1) a shielding mode for the insulation of one hemisphere from potentially interfering activity from the other hemisphere; (2) a sharing mode for the interhemispheric exchange of information or the products of processing; and (3) an equilibrium mode for the regulation of activation imbalances (see Table 13-5).

Interhemispheric Shielding Mode: Its Effect on Functional Asymmetry and Quality of Performance. This is a mechanism that permits one hemisphere temporarily to shield itself from receipt of signals from the other hemisphere. Such a mechanism would permit the two hemispheres to serve as relatively insulated work stations for the independent processing of inputs that would otherwise interfere with one another.

There is reason to believe that this shielding capacity, referred to as "hemispheric independence," is not fully developed until late adolescence. This conjecture is based on a series of experiments by Liederman (Liederman & Meehan, 1986; Liederman, Merola, & Hoffman, 1986; Merola & Liederman, 1985, 1986) that show that projecting conflicting tasks to separate hemispheres as opposed to a single hemisphere is beneficial to adults but not to 10-year-old children. By age 18, division of confusing tasks between the hemispheres is beneficial for 92% to 98% of the subjects tested (Liederman & Meehan, 1986; Merola & Liederman 1987). Note that the sharing of information between the hemispheres—as measured, for example, by intermanual transfer of tactile information (Galin, Johnstone, Nakell, & Herron, 1979)—may mature earlier than the ability to shield information from transfer.

Even though the ability to use the two hemispheres independently increases during early adolescence, the extent to which the left hemisphere showed an advantage for verbal processing does not change significantly from early adolescence to adulthood, within the same subjects (Liederman *et al.*, 1986). This suggests that degree of hemispheric shielding does not affect the direction or degree of functional asymmetry. What it does affect is the efficiency with which a hemisphere can work on its portion of the task without interruption by the other hemisphere.

Interestingly, Thatcher, McAlaster, Lester, Horst, and Cantor (1983) reported that one of the best correlates of IQ in adults is a low autocorrelation between left- and right-hemisphere electroencephalographic activity. Similarly, children with high scholastic aptitude scores show significantly more hemispheric shielding than do those with low scores (Merola & Liederman, 1987). These data suggest that there are individual as well as developmental differences in the extent to which the cerebral hemispheres can work independently, and that this may have implications for cognitive ability.

Interhemispheric Sharing Mode: Its Effect on Behavioral Laterality and Quality of Performance. This is a mechanism that permits the products of processing from one hemisphere to be shared with the other hemisphere. It is the opposite of hemispheric shielding, and probably develops before it. A lack of interhemispheric sharing may not affect functional asymmetry, but it certainly will affect cognitive ability. The brain would be equivalent to that of a split-brain; the language capacity of the left hemisphere would be isolated,

Table 13-5. Changes in Behavioral Laterality and Quality of Performance Due to an Atypical Subcortical Activation of the Left Hemisphere

1. *Mismatch:* Normal level of activation of the left hemisphere but at the wrong times
   Decreased left-hemisphere advantage
   Impaired performance

2. Tonic or phasic *overactivation* of the left hemisphere
   Extreme left-hemisphere advantage
   Overreliance on left-hemispheric processing style resulting in *deficits* for "non-left-hemisphere functions"

3. Tonic or phasic *underactivation* of the left hemisphere
   Reduced hemisphere advantage for "left-hemisphere functions"
   Overreliance on right-hemispheric processing style, resulting in *deficits* for "left-hemisphere functions"

except for brain stem connections, from the visuospatial processors of the right hemisphere. The effect on the behavior of the developing child is hard to predict. Callosal agenesis patients do not constitute a good model of deficient hemispheric shielding because of the extreme degree of compensatory hypertrophy that occurs in the anterior commissure (Chiarello, 1980). What would be informative would be a case of a child who underwent split-brain surgery as soon as the corpus callosum became functional (i.e., at approximately age 3). Such a case would presumably involve less compensatory hypertrophy of neighboring structures than would occur in the case of agenesis.

Interhemispheric Equilibrium Mode: Its Effect on Functional Asymmetry and Quality of Performance. This is a mechanism that prevents asymmetrical activation of the hemispheres from being so imbalanced that one hemisphere is virtually shut down. Such an equilibrium function could be provided by the corpus callosum. The callosum, in this context, would serve to keep the less active hemisphere in a moderate state of readiness for subsequent processing. Guiard (1980), Kinsbourne (1970), and Levy (1977) have all pointed to the hemi-inattention of patients whose corpus callosum was severed as a sign that the corpus callosum normally modulates activity levels between the hemispheres. Hemi-inattention refers to the situation in which a person is unaware of stimuli on one side of space. Each of these authors, from somewhat different perspectives, has argued that split-brain subjects ignore information that appears contralateral to the less activated hemisphere, because the corpus callosum is not there to balance the degree of arousal.

Data that are compatible with this interpretation have been provided by Glick, Crane, Jerussi, Fleisher, and Green (1975). They showed that the turning biases of rats (and the striatal dopaminergic asymmetry underlying this behavioral asymmetry) are significantly exaggerated after ventral callosal sections. This suggests that the amount of CNS asymmetry is exaggerated when the modifying influence of the callosum is removed.

SUMMARY OF THE EFFECTS ON BEHAVIOR OF ATYPICAL PATTERNS OF CORTICAL ACTIVATION BY SUBCORTICAL OR CONTRALATERAL CORTICAL REGIONS

In sum, even within brains with typical cerebral cortical asymmetries, functional asymmetry and the quality of performance may be altered by the pattern of subcortical–cortical interactions and/or the pattern of interhemispheric interactions. If the subcortical selector is mismatched to the cortical asymmetries, or the subcortical selector is mismatched with certain tonic or phasic neurochemical asymmetries, functional asymmetries may be reduced or reversed and performance will be impaired. Similarly, depending on the mode of hemispheric interaction, asymmetries may be severely exaggerated and performance may be impaired.

DIRECTIONS FOR FUTURE RESEARCH

The Need for Improved Measures of Functional Asymmetry, and the Mechanisms Underlying It in Humans

It has been shown that variations in the pattern of functional asymmetry within and between individuals are a product of individual differences in (1) structural asymmetries at the level of the cortex and (2) the pattern of activation of the cortex on one side by a contralateral cortical area or a subcortical area. The differential contribution of these various influences can be dissociated only to a limited extent. For example, current methods permit only minimal assessment of the functioning of the thalamic selector mechanism. Early brain stem evoked potentials (in particular, Wave III+) have been shown to be asymmetrical in right- but not left-handed individuals (Levine & McGaffigan, 1983; Levine, Riley, & Liederman, 1988). Changes in Wave III are thought to be affected by activity occurring at the level of the medial nucleus of the trapezoid body (Fullerton & Hosford, 1979). There is little reason to believe that the posited selector mechanism is acting at such a low level. In contrast, one could record middle latency evoked potentials, and an asymmetry at that level might be relevant to thalamic function. Before this can be determined, however, there need to be more clinicoanatomical studies of left versus right middle latency potentials in patients with lateralized thalamic lesions.

In terms of assessment of callosal function, more experiments need to be done using the only methods that are currently available. These include magnetic resonance imagery, measurement of autocorrelations between callosally connected regions during various kinds of behavioral tasks (Thatcher *et al.*, in press), computation of interhemispheric transfer times, and use of strictly behavioral probes like those devised by Merola and Liederman (1985).

Structural atypicalities can best be determined at autopsy, but the functional correlates can only be assessed when the person is alive. For such information in humans, we must wait for the results from the pioneering research by Sandra Witelson, who is administering neuropsychological batteries to terminally ill patients who have agreed to donate their brains for autopsy (cf. Witelson, 1985).

An indirect method of assessing functional organization is to exploit the double-lesion method. This method involves a first lesion that induces an initial set of symptoms, an intermediate period of recovery, and then a second lesion that reverses the recovery. An example is the one previously reviewed in which Levine and Mohr (1979) reported that left-hemisphere strokes induced an aphasia from which patients recovered, but that when these patients suffered a second stroke, this time on the right side, aphasia was reinstated.

The Need for Better Medical Records

Since so much of our understanding of outcome depends on the cause of the lesion and the kind of brain within which the lesion occurred, we need to educate both neurologists and obstetricians to keep more complete medical records. This is required especially for *prenatal* complications given the importance of the timing of the lesion in terms of neural plasticity. Schwartz (1985) has shown that approximately one-third of the medical complications reported by mothers (e.g., extreme vomiting during pregnancy, necessitating hospitalization) do not appear in the hospital medical records. In addition, physicians have not been sensitized to the importance of the hand preference not only of the patient, but also of other family members (Geschwind & Galaburda, 1987).

A Recommendation for a Large-Scale Collaborative Study

Finally, a study needs to be done that would directly answer the question of whether, after brain damage, atypical functional asymmetry is a good or a bad prognostic sign. Research has been reviewed that shows that after early brain damage, several kinds of compensatory neural changes can occur (such as compensatory unmasking, sprouting, hypertrophy, and maintenance). These reorganizations have been shown to affect functional asymmetry and may have either positive or negative implications for the quality of performance. A collaborative project needs to be undertaken that involves a large number of newborn infants with well-defined pre- versus perinatal lesions that are confined to one hemisphere as verified by CAT scan. These children would be recruited from right-handed families without left-handed relatives. When the subjects reached adulthood, they would be divided into two groups: those with and those without atypical functional asymmetry. The basic question would be: Which group shows fewer neuropsychological deficits—those with, or those without, typical functional asymmetry? After that study, a new chapter on the history of the relationship among early brain damage, functional asymmetry and behavioral outcome will be required.

ACKNOWLEDGMENTS

I would like to thank the following students for their helpful comments on earlier versions of this manuscript: Patrick McNamara, Carol Hoffman, Nancy Hutner, and Libby Baker.

NOTES

1. It is interesting to note that Levy and Gur (1980) argue that this kind of "modal" brain organization may be found only within a small portion of the population.

2. This could indicate compensatory hypertrophy, or it could reflect increased activity due to increased functional demand (Kretch *et al.,* 1963), or compensatory unmasking due to release of the contralateral hemisphere from inhibition (Kinsbourne, 1975).

3. It is being suggested here that some ipsilateral fibers are due to compensatory maintenance of a transient pathway. But Kato *et al.* (1985) suggest another possibility, that is, that the transient uncrossed fibers in the newborn serve as a guide for collateral sprouting.

4. There are two additional points. First, the pattern of neuronal connections within a region is more critical than the absolute number and/or size of neurons in that region. Second, size variations *between* species may be more important than size variations *within* a species. The size of the nuclei that control bird song in canaries (Nottebohm, Kasparian, & Pandazis, 1981) and zebra finches and marsh wrens (Nottebohm, 1984) varies directly in proportion to the size of the birds' adult song repertoire (i.e., the number of syllable types produced).

5. This may be because IQ subscales do not provide pure measures of verbal versus visuospatial ability.

REFERENCES

Amaducci, L., Sorbi, A., Alabanese, A., & Gainotti, G. (1981). Choline-acetyl transferase (CHAT) activity differs in right and left human temporal lobes. *Neurology, 31,* 799–805.

Bakan, P., Dibb, G., & Reed, P. (1973). Handedness and birth stress. *Neuropsychologia, 11,* 363–366.

Bakker, D. J., Moerland, R., & Goekoop-Hoefkens, M. (1981). Effects of hemispheric stimulation on the reading performance of dyslexic boys: A pilot study. *Journal of Clinical Neuropsychology, 3,* 155–159.

Bakker, D. J., & Vinke, J. (1985). Effects of hemisphere-specific stimulation on brain activity and reading in dyslexics. *Journal of Clinical and Experimental Neuropsychology, 7*(5), 505–525.

Bishop, D. V. (1983). Linguistic impairment after left hemidecortication for infantile hemiplegia: A reappraisal. *Quarterly Journal of Experimental Psychology: Human Experimental Psychology, 35a*(1), 199–207.

Boucher, J. (1977). Hand preference in autistic children and their parents. *Journal of Autism and Childhood Schizophrenia, 7,* 177–187.

Bromwell, B. (1899). On crossed aphasia. *Lancet, 8,* 1473–1479.
Briggs, G., Nebes, R., & Kinsbourne, M. (1976). Intellectual differences in relation to personal and family handedness. *Quarterly Journal of Experimental Psychology, 28,* 591–601.
Bullard-Bates, P. C., & Satz, P. (1983). A case of the pathological left-hander. *Journal of Clinical Neuropsychology, 5,* 128–129.
Bullock, D., Liederman, J., & Todorovic, D. (1987). Reconciling stable asymmetry with recovery of function: An adaptive systems perspective on functional plasticity. *Child Development, 58,* 689–697.
Burnstein, J. H., Greenough, W. T., & Tees, R. C. (1984). Intermodal compensation following damage or deprivation: A review of behavioral and neural evidence. In C. R. Almli & S. Finger (Eds.), *Early brain damage* (Vol. 1, pp. 3–34.) New York: Academic Press.
Chiarello, C. (1980). A house divided? Cognitive function with callosal agenesis. *Brain and Language, 11,* 128–136.
Chow, K. L. (1968). Visual discriminations after extensive ablation of optic tract and visual cortex. *Brain Research, 9,* 363–366.
Cotman, C. W., & Nieto-Sampedro, M. (1982). Brain function, synapse renewal, and plasticity. *Annual Reviews of Psychology, 33,* 371–401.
Crosson, B. (1985). Subcortical functions in language: A working model. *Brain and Language, 25,* 257–292.
Dennis, M. (1980). Capacity and strategy for syntactic comprehension after left and right hemidecortication. *Brain and Language, 10,* 287–317.
Ebbesson, S. (1984). Evolution and ontogeny of neural circuits. *Behavioral and Brain Sciences, 7,* 321–366.
Eidelberg, D., & Galaburda, A. M. (1982). Symmetry and asymmetry in the human posterior thalamus: I. Cytoarchitectonic analysis in normal persons. *Archives of Neurology, 39,* 325–332.
Falzi, G., Perrone, P., & Vignolo, L. (1982). Right–left asymmetry in anterior speech region. *Archives of Neurology, 39,* 239–240.
Fennell, E., Bowers, D., & Satz, P. (1977). Within-modal and crossed-modal reliabilities of two laterality tests. *Brain and Language, 4,* 63–69.
Fennell, E., Satz, P., Van den Abell, T., Bowers, D., & Thomas, R. (1978). Visuo-spatial competence, handedness, and cerebral dominance. *Brain and Language, 5,* 206–214.
Flor-Henry, P. (1979). Laterality, shifts of cerebral dominance, sinistrality and psychosis. In J. Gruzelier & P. Flor-Henry (Eds.), *Hemisphere asymmetries of function in psychopathology* (pp. 3–18). Elsevier North-Holland.
Friedman, A., & Polson, M. (1981). Hemispheres as independent resource systems: Limited-capacity processing and cerebral specialization. *Journal of Experimental Psychology: Human Perception and Performance, 7*(5), 1031–1058.
Fullerton, B., & Hosford, H. (1979). Effects of midline brain stem lesions on the short-latency auditory evoked responses. *Society of Neuroscience Abstracts, 5,* 20.
Galaburda, A., Sherman, G., Rosen, G., Aboitiz, F., & Geschwind, N. (1985). Developmental dyslexia: Four consecutive patients with cortical anomalies. *Annals of Neurology, 18,* 222–233.
Galin, D., Johnstone, J., Nakell, L., & Herron, J. (1979). Development of the capacity for tactile information transfer between hemispheres in normal children. *Science, 204,* 1330–1332.
Gall, C., & Lynch, G. (1980). The regulation of fiber growth and synaptogenesis in the developing hippocampus. In R. K. Hunt (Ed.) *Neural development: I. Current topics in developmental biology* (Vol. 15, pp. 159–182). New York: Academic Press.
Geschwind, N., & Galaburda, A. M. (1987). *Cerebral lateralization: Biological mechanisms, associations and pathology I.* Cambridge, MA: MIT Press.
Glick, S. D., Crane, A., Jerussi, T., Fleisher, L., & Green, J. (1975). Functional and neurochemical correlate of potentiation of striatal asymmetry by callosal section. *Nature, 254,* 616–617.
Glick, S. D., Ross, D. A., & Hough, L. B. (1982). Lateral asymmetry of neurotransmitters in human brain. *Brain Research, 234,* 52–63.
Goldberg, E., & Costa, L. D. (1981). Hemisphere differences in the acquisition and use of descriptive systems. *Brain and Language, 14,* 144–173.
Goldman, P. S. (1971). Functional development of the prefrontal cortex in early life and the problem of neuronal plasticity. *Experimental Neurology, 32,* 366–387.
Goldman, P. S., & Galkin, T. (1978). Prenatal removal of frontal association cortex in the fetal rhesus monkey: Anatomical and functional consequences in post-natal life. *Brain Research, 152,* 451–485.
Goldman-Rakic, P. S., & Rakic, P. (1984). Experimental modification of gyral patterns. In N. Geschwind & A. M. Galaburda (Eds.), *Cerebral dominance: the biological foundations* (pp. 179–192). Cambridge, MA: Harvard University Press.
Gordon, H. W. (1980). Cognitive asymmetry in dyslexic families. *Neuropsychologia, 18,* 645–656.

Gordon, H. W. (1983). Learning disabled are cognitively right. In M. Kinsbourne (Ed.), *Topics in learning disabilities* (Vol. 3, pp. 29–39). Gaithersburg, MD: Aspen Systems Corporation.

Gott, P. S., Hughes, E. C., & Whipple, K. (1984). Voluntary control of two lateralized conscious states: Validation by electrical and behavioral studies. *Neuropsychologia, 22*(1), 65–72.

Graves, R. (1983). Mouth asymmetry, dichotic ear advantage and tachistoscopic visual field advantage as measures of language lateralization. *Neuropsychologia, 21*(6), 641–649.

Greenough, W. T., & Green, E. J. (1981). Experience and the changing brain. In J. L. McGaugh, J. G. March, & S. B. Kiesler (Eds.), *Aging: Biology and behavior* (pp. 159–200). New York: Academic Press.

Guiard, Y. (1980). Cerebral hemispheres and selective attention. *Acta Psychologica, 46,* 41–61.

Gur, R. C., & Reivich, M. (1980). Cognitive task effects on hemispheric blood flow in humans: evidence for individual differences in hemispheric activation. *Brain and Language, 9,* 78–92.

Gur, R. C., Packer, I., Hungerbuhler, J., Reivich, M., Obrist, W., Amarnek, W. S., & Sackeim, H. A. (1980). Differences in the distribution of gray and white matter in human cerebral hemispheres. *Science, 207,* 1226–1228.

Hardyck, C. & Petrinovich, L. F. (1977). Left-handedness. *Psychological Bulletin, 84,*(3), 385–404.

Healey, J. M., Liederman, J., & Geschwind, N. (1986). Handedness is not a unidimensional trait. *Cortex, 22*(1), 33–53.

Hécaen, H., Perenin, M. T., & Jeannerod, M. (1984). The effects of cortical lesions in children: Language and visual functions. In C. R. Almli & S. Finger (Eds.), *Early brain damage* (Vol. 1, pp. 277–298). New York: Academic Press.

Hicks, R. A., & Barton, A. (1975). A note on left-handedness and severity of mental retardation. *Journal of Genetic Psychology, 127,* 323–324.

Hicks, S. P., & D'amato, C. J. (1970). Motor–sensory and visual behavior after hemispherectomy in newborn and mature rats. *Experimental Neurology, 29,* 416–438.

Innocenti, G. M. (1981). Growth and reshaping of axons in the establishment of visual callosal connections. *Science, 212,* 824–827.

Ivy, G. O., Akers, R. M., & Killackey, H. P. (1979). Differential distribution of callosal projection neurons in the neonatal and adult rat. *Brain Research, 173,* 532–537.

Jones, E. G. (1975). Some aspects of the organization of the thalamic reticular complex. *Journal of Comparative Neurology, 162,* 285–308.

Kato, T., Hirano, A., Katagiri, T., & Sasaki, H. (1985). Transient uncrossed corticospinal fibres in the newborn rat. *Neuropathology and Applied Neurobiology, 11,* 171–178.

Kimura, D., & Harshman, R. (1984). Sex differences in brain organization for verbal and non-verbal function. In G. J. de Vries, J. P. C. De Bruin, H. B. M. Uylings, & M. A. Corner (Eds.), *Progress in brain research* (Vol. 61, pp. 423–439). Amsterdam: Elsevier.

Kinsbourne, M. (1970). The cerebral basis of lateral asymmetries in attention. *Acta Psychologica, 33,* 193–201.

Kinsbourne, M. (1975). Minor hemispheric language and cerebral maturation. In E. H. Lenneberg & E. Lenneberg (Eds.), *Foundations of language development: A multi-disciplinary approach* (Vol. 2). New York: Academic Press.

Kinsbourne, M. (1980). A model for the ontogeny of cerebral organization in non-right-handers. In J. Herron (Ed.), *Neuropsychology of left-handers* (pp. 177–185). New York: Academic Press.

Kohn, B., & Dennis, M. (1974). Selective impairments of visuospatial abilities in infantile hemiplegics after right cerebral decortication. *Neuropsychologia, 12,* 505–512.

Kretch, D., Rosenzweig, M. R., & Bennett, E. L. (1963). Interhemispheric effects of cortical lesions on brain biochemistry. *Science, 32,* 352–353.

Land, P. W., & Lund, R. D. (1979). Development of the rat's uncrossed retinotectal pathway and its relationship to plasticity studies. *Science, 205,* 698–700.

Lansdell, H. (1969). Verbal and nonverbal factors in right-hemisphere speech: Relation to early neurological theory. *Journal of Comparative apd Physiological Psychology, 69,* 734–738.

Levine, D. N., & Mohr, J. P. (1979). Language after bilateral cerebral infarctions: Role of the minor hemisphere. *Neurology, 29,* 927–938.

Levine, R. A., & McGaffigan, P. (1983). Right–left asymmetries in the human brainstem: Auditory evoked potentials. *Electroencephalography and Clinical Neurophysiology, 55,* 532–537.

Levine, R. A., Riley, P. & Liederman, J. (1988). The brainstem auditory evoked potential asymmetry is replicable and reliable. Neuropsychologia, (in press).

Levy, J. (1974). Psychobiological implications of bilateral asymmetry. In S. Dimond & J. Beaumont (Eds.), *Hemispheric function and the human brain* (pp. 121–183). New York: Wiley.

Levy, J. (1977). Manifestations and implications of shifting hemi-inattention in commissurotomy patients. In S. Weinstein & R. P. Friedland (Eds.), *Advances in neurology* (pp. 83–92). New York: Raven Press.

Levy, J. (1983a). Individual differences in cerebral hemisphere asymmetry: Theoretical issues and experimental considerations. In J. B. Hellige (Ed.), *Cerebral hemisphere asymmetry: Method, theory, and application* (pp. 465–497). New York: Praeger Publishers.

Levy, J. (1983b). Is cerebral asymmetry of function a dynamic process? Implications for specifying degree of lateral differentiation. *Neuropsychologia, 21*(1), 3–11.

Levy, J., & Gur, R. C. (1980). Individual differences in psychoneurological organization. In J. Herron (Ed.), *Neuropsychology of left-handedness* (pp. 199–208). New York: Academic Press.

Levy J., Heller, W., Banich, T., & Burton, L. A. (1983). Are variations among right-handed individuals in perceptual asymmetries caused by characteristic arousal differences between hemispheres? *Journal of Experimental Psychology: Human Perception and Performance, 9*(3), 329–358.

Liederman, J. (1983). Mechanisms underlying instability in the development of hand preference. In G. Young, S. J. Segalowitz, C. M. Corter, & S. E. Trehub (Eds.), *Manual specialization and the developing brain* (pp. 71–92). New York: Academic Press.

Liederman, J. (1987). Neonates show an asymmetric degree of head rotation but lack an ATNR asymmetry: Neuropsychological implications. *Developmental Neuropsychology, 3*(2), 101–112.

Liederman, J., & Coryell, J. (1981). How right hand preference may be facilitated by rightward turning during infancy. *Developmental Psychobiology, 14*(5), 439–450.

Liederman, J., & Coryell, J. (1982). The origin of left hand preference: Pathological and non-pathological influences. *Neuropsychologia, 20*(6), 721–725.

Liederman, J., & Healey, (1987). Independent dimensions of hand preference: Reliability of the factor structure and the handedness inventory. *Archives of Clinical Neuropsychology, 1,* 371–386.

Liederman, J., & Kinsbourne, M. (1980). Rightward biases in neonates depends upon parental right handedness. *Neuropsychologia, 18,* 579–584.

Liederman, J., & Meehan, P. (1986). When is between-hemisphere division of inputs advantageous? *Neuropsychologia, 24*(6), 863–874.

Liederman, J., Merola, J., & Hoffman, C. (1986). Longitudinal data indicate that hemispheric independence increases during early adolescence. *Developmental Neuropsychology, 2*(3), 183–201.

Lorber, J., & Priestley, B. C. (1981). Children with large heads: A practical approach to diagnosis in 557 children, with reference to megalencephaly. *Developmental Medicine and Child Neurology, 23,* 494–504.

Ment, L. R., Scott, D. T., Lange, R. C., Ehrenkranz, R. A., Duncan, C. C., & Warshaw, J. B. (1983). Postpartum perfusion of the preterm brain: Relationship to neurodevelopmental outcome. *Child's Brain, 10,* 266–272.

Merola, J. L., & Liederman, J. (1985). Developmental changes in hemispheric independence. *Child Development, 56,* 1184–1194.

Merola, J. L., & Liederman, J. (1987). Developmental versus individual differences in the ability of the hemispheres to operate independently. *International Journal of Neuroscience. 35,* 195–204.

Molfese, D. L., Freeman, R. B., & Palermo, D. S. (1975). The ontogeny of brain lateralization for speech and nonspeech stimuli. *Brain and Language, 2,* 356–368.

Moore, W. H. (1976). Bilateral tachistoscopic word perception of stutterers and normal subjects. *Brain and Language, 3,* 434–442.

Moruzzi, G., & Magoun, H. W. (1949). Brain stem reticular formation and activation of the EEG. *Electroencephalography and Clinical Neurophysiology, 1,* 455–473.

Nass, R. (1985). Mirror movement asymmetries in congenital hemiparesis: The inhibition hypothesis revisited. *Neurology, 35,* 1059–1062.

Newcombe, F., & Ratcliff, G. (1973). Handedness, speech lateralization and ability. *Neuropsychologia, 11,* 399–407.

Nottebohm, F. (1984). Learning, forgetting, and brain repair. In N. Galaburda & A. Galaburda (Eds.), *Cerebral dominance: The biological foundation* (pp. 93–113). Cambridge, MA: Harvard University Press.

Nottebohm, F., Kasparian, S., & Pandazis, C. (1981). Brain space for a learned task. *Brain Research, 213,* 99–109.

Novelly, R., & Naugle, R. (1986). *Acquired right hemisphere speech: Gender specific effects on VIQ vs. PIQ.* Paper presented at the annual meeting of the International Neuropsychological Society, Denver, Colorado.

Ojemann, G. A., & Ward, A. A. (1971). Speech representation in ventrolateral thalamus. *Brain, 94,* 669–680.

Oke, A., Keller, R., Mefford, I., & Adams, R. (1978). Lateralization of norepinephrine in human thalamus. *Science, 200,* 1411–1413.

Pieniadz, J. M., Naeser, M. A., Koff, E., & Levine, H. L. (1983). CT scan cerebral hemispheric asymmetry measurements in stroke cases with global aphasia: Atypical asymmetries associated with improved recovery. *Cortex, 19,* 371–391.

Porac, C., & Coren, S. (1981). *Lateral preferences and human behavior.* New York: Springer-Verlag.

Rasmussen, T., & Milner, B. (1977). The role of early left-brain injury in determining lateralization of cerebral speech functions. *Annals of the New York Academy of Sciences, 299,* 353–369.

Ratcliff, G., Dila, C., Taylor, L., & Milner, B. (1980). The morphological asymmetry of the hemispheres and cerebral dominance: A possible relationship. *Brain and Language, 11,* 87–98.

Reh, T., & Kalil, K. (1982). Functional role of regrowing pyramidal tract fibers. *Journal of Comparative Neurology, 211,* 276–283.

Satz, P. (1979). A test of some models of hemispheric speech organization in the left- and right-handed. *Science, 203,* 1131–1133.

Satz, P., Orsini, D., Saslow, E., & Henry, R. (1985). The pathological left-handedness syndrome. *Brain and Cognition, 4,* 27–46.

Satz, P., Yanowitz, J., & Willmore, J. (1984). Early brain damage and lateral development. In R. Bell, J. Elias, R. Green, & J. Harvey (Eds.), *Interfaces in psychology* (pp. 87–107). Texas: Texas University Press.

Scheibel, A. B. (1980). Anatomical and physiological substrates of arousal: A view from the bridge. Chairman's overview of part II. In J. A. Hobson & M. A. B. Brazier (Eds.), *The reticular formation revisited* (pp. 55–66). New York: Raven Press.

Scheibel, A. B. (1984). A dendritic correlate of human species. In N. Geschwind & A. Galaburda (Eds.), *Cerebral dominance: The biological foundation* (pp. 43–52). Cambridge, MA: Harvard University Press.

Schneider, G. E. (1979). Is it really better to have your brain lesion early? Revision of the Kennard principle. *Neuropsychologia, 17,* 557–584.

Schlag, J., & Waszak, M. (1970). Characteristics of unit responses in nucleus reticularus thalami. *Brain Research, 21,* 286–288.

Schlag, J., & Waszak, M. (1971). Electrophysiological properties of units of the thalamic reticular complex. *Experimental Neurology, 32,* 79–97.

Schwartz, M. (1985). *Perinatal stress factors and laterality: A preliminary report.* Paper presented at the annual meeting of the International Neuropsychological Society, San Diego, California.

Seldon, H. L. (1981). Structure of human auditory cortex: I. Cytoarchitectronics and dendritic distributions. *Brain Research, 229,* 277–294.

Seldon, H. L. (1982). Structure of human auditory cortex: III. Statistical analysis of dendritic trees. *Brain Research, 249,* 211–221.

Selnes, O. A. (1974). The corpus callosum: Some anatomical and functional considerations with special reference to language. *Brain and Language, 1,* 111–139.

Semmes, J. (1968). Hemispheric specialization: A possible clue to mechanism. *Neuropsychologia, 6,* 11–26.

Silva, D. A., & Satz, P. (1979). Pathological left-handedness: Evaluation of a model. *Brain and Language, 7,* 8–16.

Sprague, J. M. (1966). Interaction of cortex and superior colliculus in mediation of visually guided behavior in the cat. *Science, 153,* 1544–1547.

Strauss, E., & Verity, C. (1983). Effects of hemispherectomy in infantile hemiplegics. *Brain and Language, 20,* 1–11.

Subirana, A. (1958). The prognosis in aphasia in relation to cerebral dominance and handedness. *Brain, 81,* 415–425.

Thatcher, R. W., Krause, P. J., & Hrybyk, M. (in press). *Corticocortical associations and EEG coherence: A two compartmental model.*

Thatcher, R. W., McAlaster, R., Lester, M. L., Horst, R. L., & Cantor, D. S. (1983). Hemispheric EEG asymmetries related to cognitive functioning in children. In A. Perecman (Ed.), *Cognitive processing in the right hemisphere* (pp. 125–146). New York: Academic Press.

Tizard, J. P. M., Paine, R. S., & Crothers, B. (1954). Disturbances of sensation in children with hemiplegia. *Journal of the American Medical Association, 155,* 628–632.

Turkewitz, G. (1977). The development of lateral differences in the human infant. In S. Harnad, R. W. Doty, L. Goldstein, J. Jaynes, & G. Krauthamer (Eds.), *Lateralization in the nervous system* (pp. 251–260). New York: Academic Press.

Villablanca, J. R., Burgess, J. W., & Sonnier, B. (1984). Neonatal cerebral hemispherectomy: A model for post lesion reorganization of the brain. In S. Finger and C. R. Almli (Eds.), *The behavioral biology of early brain damage* (Vol. 2, pp. 179–210). New York: Academic Press.

Volpe, J. J., Herscovitch, P., Perlman, J. M., & Raichle, M. E. (1983). Positron emission tomography in the newborn: Extensive impairment of regional cerebral blood flow with intraventricular hemorrhagic intracerebral involvement. *Pediatrics, 72*(5), 589–601.

Wall, P. D. (1977). The presence of ineffective synapses and the circumstances that unmask them. *Philosophical Transactions of the Royal Society, London, Series B, 278,* 361–372.

Witelson, S. F. (1977). Neural and cognitive correlates of developmental dyslexia: Age and sex differences. In C. Shagass, S. Gershon, & A. J. Friedhoff (Eds.), *Psychopathology and brain dysfunction* (pp. 15–49). New York: Raven Press.

Witelson, S. F. (1983). The bumps on the brain: Right–left asymmetry in brain anatomy and function. In S. Segalowitz (Ed.), *Language functions and brain organization* (pp. 117–144). New York: Academic Press.

Witelson, S. F. (1985). The brain connection: The corpus callosum is larger in left-handers. *Science, 221,* 665–668.

14

The Development of Cognition and Personality in X Aneuploids and Other Subject Groups

CHARLES NETLEY
JOANNE ROVET
Hospital for Sick Children, Toronto

This chapter deals with issues formulated on the basis of studies of males and females with abnormal numbers of X chromosomes. These studies have indicated that individuals with such conditions frequently have specific abnormalities in intellectual and personality functioning which appear to be the result of disturbances in neural organization and, in some cases, of hormonal dysfunctioning and environmental adversity. Although much of the data to be presented comes from investigations of the chromosomally abnormal, some have been obtained in studies of other subject groups. Thus, although the initial context concerns the relationships between the X chromosome, brain function, and behavior, more general issues of how biology and behavior interrelate are also discussed. The material and concepts to be described fall into two general classes, the first concerned with cognition and the second with personality. Each is reviewed separately.

COGNITION AND SOME BIOLOGICAL FACTORS

There is now a fairly sizable body of evidence indicating that X aneuploid states, defined by anomalous numbers of X chromosomes, are associated with specific impairments of verbal or spatial ability (Stewart, 1982) In the case of phenotypic females with Turner syndrome (TS) who have one X chromosome rather than the normally occurring two, spatial, but not verbal, ability is depressed when these skills are assessed by either psychometric or experimental procedures (Garron, 1977; Rovet & Netley, 1982; Waber, 1979). Similar studies of males with an extra X 47,XXY karyotype usually have indicated that verbal ability is impaired but spatial ability is not (Netley & Rovet, 1982c; Robinson, Lubs, Nielsen, & Sorensen, 1979); Walzer *et al.*, 1978). Although the evidence is somewhat less consistent, a number of investigators have found that extra X females with a 47,XXX complement also have a specific deficit in language or verbal ability but have relatively normal levels of spatial skills (Pennington, Puck, & Robinson, 1980; Rovet & Netley, 1983; Stewart, Netley, & Park, 1982). Not surprisingly, given their patterns of intellectual functioning, both TS females and extra X males and females frequently have educational difficulties and commonly satisfy the criteria for diagnosis as learning-disabled (Pennington & Smith, 1983).

As we have argued elsewhere (Netley, 1983; Netley & Rovet, 1983) any explanation for the specific intellectual disorders of subjects with X chromosome aneuploid states that is based on gender-specific socialization processes faces difficulties, principally because phenotypic sex is not consistently related to the pattern of cognitive functioning in the various aneuploid conditions (Rovet & Netley, 1981). Thus, among females the occurrence of a verbal or spatial deficit depends on whether there is a supernumerary or a missing X. In addition, socialization theory does not readily explain why extra X males and females are more alike intellectually than are extra-X and missing-X females. Similar difficulties emerge if explanations based on prenatal variations in sex hormones (Hines, 1982; Reinsich, Gandelman, & Spiegel, 1979) are offered because, as with socialization, the hormonal events producing phenotypic sex are inconsistently related to the pattern of cognitive functioning in X aneuploids. Sex specific hormonal functions associated with puberty are also unlikely to be directly responsible for the various patterns of deficit in TS and extra-X individuals since their disorders can be observed well before adolescence (Netley & Rovet, 1982c) and are unchanged by pubertal onset whether occurring naturally or in response to hormonal treatments (Stewart, Bailey, Netley, Rovet, & Park, 1986).

Our own attempts to explain findings in this area were first prompted by the research and formulations of Waber (1976, 1977). Waber advanced the notion that variations in developmental rate around puberty could account for the normally occurring female superiority on verbal tests and the male superiority on spatial tasks (Maccoby & Jacklin, 1974). She examined this issue in studies of slow- and fast-maturing males and females and found that, regardless of sex, slow maturers were more able spatially than verbally, whereas fast maturers tended to show the opposite pattern of skills (Waber, 1976, 1977). She also presented data that suggested that maturation rates influenced hemispheric organization, with slow development being more associated than fast development with a greater left-hemisphere advantage for verbal processing (Waber, 1976, 1977). Subsequent studies have demonstrated that these associations have been difficult to replicate (e.g., Waber, Mann, Merola, & Moylan, 1985).

As we have pointed out previously (Netley & Rovet, 1983), there are a number of intellectual and biological parallels between X aneuploids and early and late maturers. TS females with bone ages advanced relative to stature (Almqvist, Linsten, & Lindvall, 1963) resemble fast maturers in their relatively strong verbal abilities. Extra-X males and females with delayed rates of bone age maturation prior to puberty, on the other hand, resemble slow maturers in their relatively strong nonverbal abilities (Stewart *et al.,* 1979). Moreover, individual differences in bone age maturation and the dermatoglyphic index of prenatal rate of growth resulting from variations in mitotic cell division rates (Mittwoch, 1973; Polani, 1981), total finger ridge count (TFRC), are associated with the degree to which the verbal abilities of extra-X males approximate normal (Netley & Rovet, 1982c). That is, those with higher or more normal TFRCs have verbal abilities higher and, therefore, more normal than do those with lower TFRCs.

Further evidence for similarities between Waber's initial observation with the maturationally atypical and X aneuploids have been provided by studies that have examined hemispheric specialization. Waber (1976, 1977) reported that early maturers failed to show the expected right-ear (left-hemisphere) advantage on a dichotic listening test using verbal stimuli, a finding that has also been shown to characterize 45,X females (Gordon & Galatzer, 1980; Netley, 1977; Netley & Rovet, 1982a; Waber, 1979). Extra-X males, on the other hand, appear to have different anomalies in hemispheric specialization because they have lower than normal degrees of left-hemispheric specialization for language processing and greater than normal degrees of right-hemispheric specialization for nonverbal as well as verbal processing (Netley & Rovet, 1984).

We have reported previously that the index of prenatal growth rate, TFRC, was negatively correlated with half-field and dichhaptic indices of right-hemispheric specialization for nonverbal processing (Netley, 1983). More recently we undertook a more comprehensive investigation of this phenomenon using a six-part battery of left- and right-hemispheric specialization tests. Three of the tests, dichotic listening for CVs and digit series and a half-field letter identification task, were assumed to reflect left-hemispheric specialization for verbal processes. The other three, half field dot estimation, dichotic listening using melodic stimulus pairs, and a dichhaptic recognition task, were assumed to reflect right-hemispheric specialization for nonverbal processes. These tasks were administered to 28 47,XXY males and groups of 79 or 97 chromosomally normal controls (see Netley & Rovet, 1984, for details). The scores of the extra-X males on each test were analyzed in terms of phi coefficients (Kuhn, 1973) and interpreted in terms of deviation scores using the distributions of the phi scores of the controls. Scores for the three verbal tests were then averaged to provide a composite left-hemisphere (LH) score and the three nonverbal tests averaged to provide a composite right-hemisphere (RH) score for each extra-X male. These two indices of hemispheric specialization were then correlated with the TFRCs of the 28 47,XXY males. The only result that was significant was the negative correlation between RH and TFRC of $-.508$ ($p < .01$), which increased to $-.665$ ($p < .01$) when 4 left-handed cases were excluded. No correlations between TFRCs and LH scores were significant.

We have also analyzed the laterality data in a more elaborate way by first factor-analyzing them and then correlating individual factor scores with TFRCs in the 47,XXY sample. The factor analysis resulted in three factors, the first of which reflected right-hemisphere functioning (defined primarily by high loadings on the dichhaptic and half-field dots tasks). The second and third factors were less clear-cut but seemed to reflect left-hemisphere verbal processing; factor 2 loaded highest on dichotic digits and factor 3 on half-field letters. Among the 27 47,XXY boys with complete data, the only significant correlation was between the right-hemisphere factor 1 and TFRC ($r = -.428$, $p < .05$).

These findings are consistent with the concept that slow rates of prenatal growth interfere with the development of hemispheric specialization in 47,XXY males, and raise the possibility that their intellectual deficits are the result of abnormal brain organization. We have examined this possibility by subdividing our extra-X male subjects into four groups on the basis of their composite LH and RH scores averaged across tests of a verbal and nonverbal nature as described earlier. The criteria used for this purpose were as follows: If a boy's RH score was higher than zero (and higher, therefore, than the mean of the normative group of chromosomally normal subjects), he was designated RH high; if not, RH low. If his LH score was less than zero (lower, therefore, than the mean of the chromosomally normal subjects), he was designated LH low; if not, LH high. Of the 29 47,XXY boys with complete data, this procedure resulted in 6 LH low/RH low cases, 15 LH low/RH high cases, 3 LH high/RH low cases, and 5 LH high/RH high cases. An analysis of variance with LH and RH as independent variables and performance IQ as the dependent variable was not significant. However, one that examined verbal IQ was significant and indicated the verbal IQs of RH high subjects were lower than those of the RH low cases ($p = .015$). The data are summarized in Table 14-1.

These findings are consistent with the notion that delays in prenatal growth disturb the development of brain organization in extra-X males, which in turn leads to impairments in verbal intelligence. At one point (Netley & Rovet, 1984) we formulated an explanation for these findings, which borrowed from the concepts advanced by Corballis and Morgan (1978). These authors proposed that in the normal course of development there exists a maturational gradient favoring the more rapid development of the left hemisphere as compared to the right. This, they argued, leads to the establishment of left-hemisphere dominance for language and other complex cognitive operations and, because of left-to-right inhibitory processes, leaves to the right hemisphere only residual perceptual skills. We proposed that

Table 14-1. Means and Standard Deviations of WISC-R Verbal and Performance IQ in 29 47,XXY Boys Classified According to Patterns of Hemispheric Specialization

		LH low RH low	LH low RH high	LH high RH low	LH high RH high
Verbal IQ	Mean	90.50	75.67	102.00	83.60
	S.D.	10.43	15.49	3.46	18.53
Performance IQ	Mean	102.83	96.47	110.00	100.80
	S.D.	12.19	11.46	10.54	18.94

the left-sided advantage would be attenuated in slowly maturing extra-X males and females, with the result that (1) their right hemispheres would assume a greater than normal role in verbal and other forms of higher cognitive activity and (2) the development of left-hemispheric functioning would be inhibited by the right (Netley & Rovet, 1984).

Some recent formulations by Geschwind and his colleagues (Geschwind & Behan, 1982; Geschwind & Galaburda, 1985) have suggested an alternative to this explanation. They advanced the concept that variations in prenatal levels of testosterone (or sensitivity to its effects) influence the development of the two hemispheres and the growth of intellectual skills. According to their hypothesis, a high level of testosterone slows the maturation of the left hemisphere, increasing the likelihood of left-handedness, delayed language, and such clinical conditions as reading or learning disabilities. They also proposed that an elevation in testosterone interferes with the growth of the thymus, thereby disturbing the development of the immune system and increasing the probability of autoimmune disorders among affected individuals. A consequence of this hypothesis is that left-handedness, language disorder, and autoimmune disease should be correlated phenomena, and, indeed, Geschwind and Behan (1982) and Geschwind and Galaburda (1985) do present evidence consistent with such associations.

The hypothesis of Geschwind and his colleagues (Geschwind & Behan, 1982; Geschwind & Galaburda, 1985) is similar to that advanced by ourselves (Netley & Rovet, 1984) in several ways. Like ours, it deals with prenatally occurring processes that influence hemispheric maturation and cognition. They differ, however, on the issue of whether testosterone or growth rate at the cellular level is responsible for disturbances in functional neural development. Although there is insufficient evidence at this time to decide between these proposals, there are a number of findings that argue against the Geschwind view, at least as applied to 47,XXY males. One arises from the observations that although extra-X males are more likely than normal males to be non-right-handed (Netley & Rovet, 1982b; Theilgaard, 1981), language-delayed (Annell, Gustavson, & Tenstam, 1970), and at risk for autoimmune disease (Rhodes, Markham, Maxwell, & Monk-Jones, 1969), there is little reason to believe that they are exposed to higher than normal levels of testosterone during fetal life. The limited evidence suggests just the opposite, in fact, since testosterone levels at birth have been found to be lower than normal in a small 47,XXY sample (Sorensen, Nielsen, Wohlert, Bennett, & Johnsen, 1981). Another difficulty for the proposal of Geschwind and his associates (Geschwind & Behan, 1982; Geschwind & Galaburda, 1985) is presented by some analyses of relations between immunological functioning and cognition in 47,XXY boys conducted by ourselves and Dr. A. Shore of the Department of Pediatrics. at the Hospital for Sick Children, Toronto. Dr. Shore was interested in determining whether immunological functioning was disturbed in these subjects, all of whom were clinically normal. Because a measure of immune responsiveness, the plaque-forming cell (PFC) antibody response, was lower in 22 47,XXY boys than in controls, he con-

Table 14-2. Correlations between TFRCs, LH, and RH in Growth-Delayed Males and Females (data for 47,XXY given for comparison)

	Males	Females	47,XXY
	($N = 26$)	($N = 16$)	($N = 28$)
LH	−.035, NS	.162, NS	.163
RH	.464, $p < .02$	.456, $p < .10$	−.508, $p < .01$

cluded that their immune functioning was abnormal. Although this finding was consistent with the Geschwind proposal, other findings were not. In particular, there were no correlations between PFC and the LH, RH laterality indices or the IQ measures among these extra-X boys, suggesting that their immunological status was unrelated to their hemispheric organization and intellectual functioning.

Collectively, these observations provide some evidence against the testosterone hypothesis of Geschwind, Behan, and Galaburda (Geschwind & Behan, 1982; Geschwind & Galaburda, 1985) in relation to X aneuploids. On the other hand, we have obtained data that tend to support the notion that prenatal growth, as reflected by the TFRC measure rather than testosterone, is important for lateralization and cognitive development in the chromosomally normal. Some come from studies conducted in our laboratory in which we have examined the relationship between LH, RH hemispheric specialization measures (assessed by the same procedures used with our X aneuploid subjects) and TFRCs in children presenting with clinically significant delays in preadolescent growth or sexual maturation. Some results are presented in Table 14-2 and are interesting for two reasons. First, they indicate that prenatal growth rate is related to right-hemispheric functioning in maturationally delayed children, albeit in a way that differs from that seen in extra-X males. Second, since these associations are found in male and female growth-delayed cases who present no signs of autoimmune disorder (as determined by clinical examination in the Hospital Endocrine Clinic), they provide no support for the importance of either sex hormones or immunological disorder in relation to hemispheric specialization.

Additional evidence supporting the importance of prenatal growth rate in relation to hemispheric organization in general is provided by the relationship of TFRCs to handedness in growth-delayed subjects and 47,XXY males. In every case the left-handed subgroups have lower TFRCs than the right-handed majorities (TFRCs in the left- and right-handed groups of growth delayed males, females, and 47,XXY cases are as follows: 113.20 ($N = 5$) versus 154.76 ($N = 21$), $p < .05$; 119.66 ($N = 3$) versus 128.23 ($N = 13$), NS; 84.75 ($N = 4$) versus 110.25 ($N = 24$) NS.)

Although the evidence presented thus far does not support the hypothesis of Geschwind and his associates, we have collected data that are partially consistent with their proposal. These were obtained in studies of male and female patients with the autoimmune conditions of Hashimoto's thyroiditis ($N = 25$; mean age 12.9 years ± 1.7), lupus ($N = 8$; mean age 16.1 years ± 2.9) and juvenile rheumatoid arthritis (JRA) ($N = 15$; mean age 10.0 years ± 3.3). These individuals were examined using the WISC-R, the Wide Range Achievement Test—Revised (WRAT-R), and the laterality battery used with 47,XXY males. In addition, many of their parents completed the Personality Inventory for Children (PIC), thereby providing us with parental perceptions of adjustment, development, and educational progress. The intellectual characteristics of these subjects, divided into male and female subgroups, are summarized in Table 14-3. As Geschwind and his group would predict, the mean verbal IQ (103.6) of these subjects is significantly lower than their performance IQ (112.2, $p = .016$). An effect they presumably would not have predicted,

Table 14-3. Intellectual Test Results of Male and Female Patients with Autoimmune Disorders

		Hashimoto's thyroiditis		Lupus		JRA	
		Male	Female	Male	Female	Male	Female
Verbal IQ	$\bar{x}$	—	104.4	100.0	97.0	103.8	106.2
	S.D.		13.7	14.1	9.2	13.2	11.7
Performance IQ	$\bar{x}$	—	115.3	96.3	111.0	106.7	113.3
	S.D.		15.6	8.0	8.9	10.3	11.6

Note: The female group is composed of 25 Hashimoto's thyroiditis, 5 lupus, and 9 JRA patients. The male group consists of 3 lupus and 6 JRA patients.

however, is the interaction between abilities and sex such that relatively low verbal ability characterizes female but not male patients with autoimmune disorders (the interaction of sex and IQ is significant at the $p = .053$ level). This, of course, suggests that high prenatal testosterone levels are unlikely to be responsible for the relatively low verbal IQs of patients with autoimmune disease since, if this were the case, the male rather than the female subjects would be expected to have verbal deficits.

Given that prenatal exposure to testosterone is improbable as an explanation for these results, what is the explanation? Since our investigations of extra-X males had suggested that the TFRC index of prenatal growth rate was a significant correlate of their cognitive functioning, we examined its relationship to intellectual and educational performance in our female autoimmune patients. Our methodology in these studies was to use multiple regression analyses treating TFRCs and the hemispheric variables, LH and RH, as independent variables and the following as dependent variables: IQs; WRAT-R reading, spelling, and arithmetic standard scores; and the PIC Achievement, Development, and Intellectual Screening scales. In the analyses of the WRAT-R and PIC data, the verbal and performance IQs of the subjects were included as independent variables in order to partial out their contributions to measured and perceived educational and developmental difficulties.

The analysis employing the intellectual data as dependent variables was negative since it revealed no significant association between the verbal and performance IQs of the subjects and their LH, RH scores or their TFRCs. However, a number of significant associations emerged between the independent and dependent variables in the analysis of the WRAT-R and PIC data. These are summarized in Table 14-4. They indicate that TFRC was a significant predictor of measured reading skills and parental perceptions of achievement problems in these girls with autoimmune-related conditions. They indicate, further, that TFRC in combination with the LH, RH hemispheric specialization variables were significant predictors of parent-based reports of intellectual problems. This suggests that prenatal growth rates influence processes associated with the acquisition of reading and also general educational proficiency in females with autoimmune diseases. Although these results are independent of measured intellectual abilities, and therefore unlike those obtained with 47,XXY males, they do suggest that similar processes operate in both types of subjects. In this context, it is interesting that recent evidence obtained in a study of chick embryos has indicated that the growth of the thymus during fetal life is dependent on the maturation of the cephalic neural crest (Bockman & Kirby, 1984). It is conceivable, therefore, that the associations between intellectual, hemispheric, and immunological processes reported by Geschwind, Behan, and Galaburda (Geschwind & Behan, 1982; Geschwind &

Table 14-4. Summary of Significant Multiple Regression Results Obtained in Analyses of Data of Female Patients with Autoimmune Disorders

Independent variable	F	P	Partial r	Changed R^2
		WRAT; Reading Standard Score ($N = 30$)		
1. Verbal IQ	9.04	<.01	.494	.244
2. TFRC	7.43	<.01	.383	.111
		PIC: Achievement Problems ($N = 20$)		
1. TFRC	6.40	<.05	−.512	.262
		PIC: Development Problems ($N = 20$)		
1. TFRC	6.07	<.05	−.502	.252
		PIC: Intelligence		
1. TFRC	4.12	NS	−.431	.186
2. RH	5.79	<.05	.518	.218
3. LH	6.33	<.01	.481	.137

Galaburda, 1985) may depend, not on prenatal hormonal events, but on prenatal neural maturation.

A THEORETICAL PROPOSAL

The relationships between biological and behavioral variables in X aneuploids, growth-disturbed patients, patients with autoimmune disease, and normal males and females are complex and perhaps not interpretable in terms of any single set of principles. As we have seen, the proposals of Geschwind and his colleagues seem inadequate for explaining the variations in cerebral and intellectual functioning in X aneuploids and patients with autoimmune disorders. They also fail to explain (or at least predict) the apparent associations between handedness and TFRCs or the correlations between TFRCs and RH functioning in growth-delayed males and females. The theory of Waber (1976, 1977) does not deal specifically with prenatally occurring events in X aneuploids or other patient groups and so also seems incomplete. Our own proposal, borrowed in part from Corballis and Morgan's concept of a left–right hemispheric developmental gradient, seems satisfactory for extra-X and TS subjects (Netley & Rovet, 1983) but encounters problems (Netley, 1983) when attempting to explain normal sex differences in hemispheric organization and ability. This is so because TFRCs of chromosomally normal females are usually lower than those of males (Penrose, 1967), which would imply that they should be less verbally competent and more hemispherically specialized than males. The available evidence is just the opposite on both points (McGlone, 1980).

The following modification of theory, which incorporates elements of the proposals of Corballis and Morgan (1978) and Geschwind and Galaburda (1985), as well as some of our earlier views, may be more satisfactory. In essence, it postulates a cycle of hemispheric maturation, with first the right hemisphere maturing more rapidly than the left, then the left more rapidly than the right, and finally a state where maturational rate of both are equal. Similar proposals are contained in this book in Chapter 1 by Best and Chapter 4 by Turkewitz. The evidence for the first stage in this cycle has been described by Geschwind and Galaburda (1985), for example, Chi, Dooling, and Gilles (1977) and for the second, that provided by Corballis and Morgan (1978) in their extensive review. The final stage of hemispheric equivalence in growth rates is an inference based on the reasonable assumption that some steady state of balanced maturation is achieved by the two hemispheres. The model also assumes, with Corballis and Morgan (1978), that language is of paramount importance during development and, with a number of others (e.g., Kinsbourne & Hiscock, 1977), that the left hemisphere has a small inherent advantage over the right for this component of cognitive development. It is also assumed, however, that the right hemisphere may, in a stage of accelerated maturation, acquire language functions to some extent as well. It is further postulated that inhibition effects operate between the hemispheres, with the more mature inhibiting the functional development of the less mature. The final assumption made in the model is that the proposed cycle of hemispheric maturational advantage depends on growth rate such that the sequence, if slow, is extended in time and, if fast, is shortened in time.

The consequences and implications of these ideas are as follows: In the case of extra-X males and females with the slowest rates of early growth, the right-hemisphere maturational advantage would be present longer during infancy and childhood. As a result, right-hemisphere cognitive development would be maximized for spatial processes, and even verbal processes would be established to some extent at this site. For these subjects, right-to-left inhibition effects would be strong, and left-to-right inhibition minimal. With faster-growing 47,XXY and 47,XXX cases, the period of right-hemisphere preeminence would be reduced, and left-to-right inhibition increasingly strong. Insofar as this occurs—and this would be a function of growth rate—RH development would fall to more normal levels, and the negative correlation between TFRC and RH functioning would be observed.

Among chromosomally normal males with high rates of growth (Ounsted, 1972), the period of right-hemisphere preeminence would be brief and quickly followed by a left-hemisphere maturational advantage which would tend to resolve into a hemispherically balanced state of equivalent maturation. Among these subjects, language development would be somewhat slowed by right-to-left inhibition. With higher rates of growth (and a lower left-hemisphere maturational advantage and a consequent reduction in left-to-right inhibition) right spatial processes would emerge more successfully. The result would be relatively strong hemispheric specialization and a positive correlation between TFRC and RH correlation such as we found in our study of growth-delayed males.

Chromosomally normal females with lower rates of prenatal growth than males would typically begin language development with left-hemisphere maturation only slightly past the highest level, with left-to-right inhibition strong and right to left inhibition weak. As a result, right-hemisphere processes would develop slowly, thus interfering with the emergence of this aspect of hemispheric specialization. Insofar as the growth rate of females approaches that of males, however, right hemispheric specialization would increase, thereby accounting for the positive correlation between TFRCs and RH in growth-delayed females.

TS females with the highest growth rates would be in the terminal state of hemispheric equivalence, with inhibition effects effectively canceling each other out. Both hemispheres would participate in language development, with a resulting loss of hemispheric specialization and the emergence of spatial skills. The specifics of this proposal are presented in summary form in Figure 14.1.

It is unclear at this point whether observations on individuals with autoimmune disease can be incorporated into this model. They appear to have small but significant deficits in verbal ability and to have somewhat higher TFRCs than normal females (140.2 ± 43.5 versus 127.2 ± 52.5 for 46,XX females) (Penrose, 1967). In these respects they resemble normal males more than normal females. If so, it might be argued that their left-hemisphere maturational advantage corresponds to that of males, meaning that right-to-left inhibition

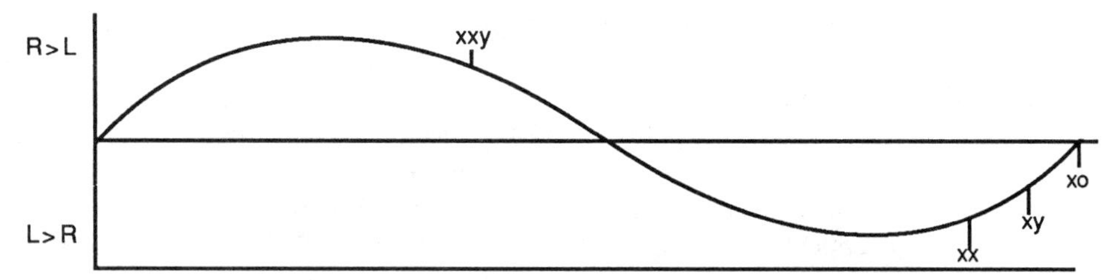

Figure 14-1. Stage of hemispheric maturation in X aneuploid and normal males and females during early cognitive development.

	XXY	XX	XY	XO
Ability pattern	Verbal low, spatial normal	Small verbal over spatial superiority	Small spatial over verbal superiority	Verbal normal, spatial low
Inhibition effects	Strong right-to-left inhibition	Strong left-to-right inhibition	Weak but positive left-to-right inhibition	Nil
Hemispheric specialization	Shifted to right dominance for verbal and nonverbal processing	Lower degrees of RH specialization for spatial processes	Greater specialization than females	Much reduced
TFRC × hemispheric functioning	Negative correlation with RH	Positive correlation with RH	Positive correlation with RH	To be determined

effects are larger than for normal females. More data are required in order to test this possibility.

PERSONALITY AND SOME BIOLOGICAL FACTORS

There are now considerable data that indicate that 47,XXY males frequently show signs of being temperamentally atypical and at risk for maladjustment (Stewart, Netley, & Park, 1982). Some have been obtained in studies of adults (Schiavi, Theilgaard, Owen, & White, 1984), and some from longitudinal examinations of neonatally identified children and adolescents (Bancroft, Axworthy, & Ratcliffe, 1982; Stewart, Bailey, Netley, Rovet, Park, Cripps, & Curtis, 1982; Walzer *et al.*, 1978). Collectively, they indicate that extra-X males are less aggressive, assertive, and active than chromosomally normal males. Although these studies, despite wide differences in methods, have produced findings that are reasonably consistent, they have not explained why these anomalies occur in 47,XXY males. They have, however, provided data that tend to make some of the simpler forms of explanation unlikely. These can be stated as follows:

1. They are due to a disturbance in parenting induced by the knowledge of chromosomal abnormality.
2. They are the response of an affected individual to the intellectual or physical abnormalities sometimes associated with the conditions.
3. Hormonal abnormalities emerging in and after puberty somehow interfere with adjustment.
4. They arise from abnormalities in hormonal processes operating in prenatal life.

The first of these seems unlikely to be correct since parental knowledge of chromosomal state is not a necessary condition for the presence of the temperamental anomalies (Bancroft *et al.,* 1982). The second seems improbable because they can be observed during infancy and in the absence of any clearly defined intellectual or physical disorder (Walzer *et al.,* 1978). Pubertal hormones are also insufficient for much the same reason: The atypical behaviors are apparent before puberty and in the absence of any demonstrable hormonal abnormality (Stewart, Bailey, *et al.,* 1982). The fourth, referring to disturbances in prenatal hormonal events, cannot be ruled out simply because no data that bear on the issue have yet been collected. However, the absence of any clinically evident physical abnormality, which would arise from significant hormonal dysfunction during this time, makes it unlikely.

Our investigations of 47,XXY boys have provided findings that suggest that a complex set of influences may be responsible for their anomalies in temperament and adjustment. In these we have assessed hormonal functioning (testosterone, estradiol, follicle-stimulating hormone or FSH, and luteinizing hormone or LUH); quality of parenting (independently and reliably rated by two investigators); and hemispheric specialization (the previously described LH, RH variables), handedness, IQ, and the TFRC measure. Each of these parameters served as an independent variable in a series of multiple regression analyses. Dependent-variable measures of personality and adjustment were obtained by parental report using the Personality Inventory for Children (PIC) and, somewhat later, the Child Behavior Check List (CBCL).

We analyzed these sets of independent and dependent variables at two points in time, before and during puberty. Before puberty, assessments of hormonal functioning were obtained at a mean age of 10.2 years (S.D. .69) and hemispheric specialization at a mean age of 10.7 years (S.D. 1.08). The dependent variables in this case were derived from the PIC, which was completed by a parent when the boys had an average age of 11.9 years (S.D. 1.38).

The results of these assessments on 23 prepubertal extra-X males are summarized in Table 14-5 and indicate in part what was reported previously. Verbal IQ was relatively low in the extra-X boys, and their LH and RH scores were respectively depressed and elevated. Hormonal functioning was generally within normal prepubertal limits. Parental responses to the PIC indicated the presence of problems in achievement and development and, as we previously reported (Stewart, Bailey, *et al.,* 1982), below-average levels of activity.

The results of the multiple regression analyses of these data are summarized in Table 14-6. Some were as common sense would predict. Verbal IQ, for example, was negatively related to those PIC scales reflecting problems in achievement, development, and the atypical adjustment problems measured by the Delinquency and Psychosis scales. Also as expected, the PIC's Family Relations scale, which reflects difficulties in the domestic environment, was negatively associated with rated quality of parenting. The result of most interest, however, was that the LH variable was negatively related to the PIC Withdrawal scale and positively to its Hyperactivity scale. Since the mean Hyperactivity score and the mean composite LH score of these boys were below average, this suggests that increases in LH (that is, increases to the level of average or higher) lead to higher, more normal levels of activity and reductions in tendencies toward withdrawal behavior among these boys. Stated in another way, these findings indicate that, prior to puberty, the integrity of left-hemispheric functioning in 47,XXY boys is a more powerful predictor of those personality characteristics that distinguish them from chromosomally normal males than any other factor, including quality of parenting and hormone levels.

A similar analysis was conducted using observations collected when the 23 boys were somewhat older and when most were showing signs of puberty. The same independent

Table 14-5. Characteristics of Sample of Prepubescent 47,XXY Boys in Multiple Regression Analyses

	Mean	S.D.
Intelligence		
Verbal IQ	84.65	14.69
Performance IQ	102.78	12.87
Laterality		
RH	.449	.709
LH	−.415	.633
TFRC		
Hormones		
Estradiol	83.96 pmol/L	57.68
Testosterone	.98 nmol/L	1.04
LUH	2.82 IU/L	2.65
FSH	3.21 IU/L	1.52
Personality (from PIC)		
Achievement	56.4*	11.1
Development	55.3*	9.6
Somatic concern	59.1	16.3
Depression	56.6	14.3
Family relations	53.2	10.3
Delinquency	55.7	10.6
Withdrawal	57.2	11.7
Anxiety	53.8	11.5
Psychosis	57.1	13.7
Hyperactivity	44.2*	8.6
Social skills	52.7	10.8
Intellectual screening	60.9*	19.9

*Significantly different from scores of normal boys.

variables were employed in this study, but the dependent variables were those provided by the CBCL, which was completed by parents of the 47,XXY boys when their mean age was 13.5 years (S.D. 1.18). The hormonal and intellectual data were collected as close as possible to each boy's 13th birthday. Hemispheric functioning was assessed using the previously described laterality battery administered at a mean age of 10.9 years

Table 14-6. Stepwise Multiple Regression Analysis Results between Independent and PIC Dependent Variables for 23 Extra-X Males

	Parenting quality	LH	Hand	FSH	VIQ	PIQ
Achievement					−.678	
Development				−.412	−.690	
Somatic complaints						
Depression						
Family relations	−.841					
Delinquency						−.520
Withdrawal		−.427				
Anxious						
Psychosis			−.424		−.462	
Hyperactivity		.561			.488	−.662
Social skills						−.490
Intellectual screening			−.423		−.792	

Note: Only significant associations at the .05 or less level are presented. Values are partial correlations.

Table 14-7. Characteristics of Sample of Pubescent 47,XXY Boys in Multiple Regression Analyses

	Mean	S.D.
Intelligence		
Verbal IQ	86.13	13.84
Performance IQ	101.74	13.40
Laterality		
RH	.342	13.40
LH	−.399	.665
TFRC		
Hormones		
Estradiol	146.26 pmol/L	48.38
Testosterone	5.60 nmol/L	5.08
LUH	9.83 IU/L	10.18
FSH	22.78 IU/L	22.59

(S.D. 1.12). Table 14-7 summarizes the sample's scores on the independent variables. They are similar to those of the younger sample excepting that hormonal activity was now within normal limits for pubertal 47,XXY males. This includes the fact that their FSH levels were higher than values for chromosomally normal pubertal males (Stewart *et al.*, 1986). Table 14-8 summarizes their CBCL results. These provide somewhat stronger, though less specific, evidence for anomalous patterns of adjustment than do the earlier PIC results, since all scales deviate significantly from the test's normative standards.

The results of the multiple regression analysis of these data are presented in Table 14-9. They differ in some respects from those obtained with the prepubertal sample, but in others they are similar. Thus, verbal IQ remained a significant correlate of social and academic performance, and the LH variable significantly related to the relative absence of what the CBCL designates as "uncommunicativeness." However, other associations are clearly different. Quality of parenting emerged as a wide-ranging negative correlate of numbers of scales reflecting the presence of behavior problems. Hormonal functioning,

Table 14-8. Mean Child Behavior Check List Scores for 23 Extra-X Males

	Mean	S.D.
Behavior problems		
Internalizing	60.7	10.2
Externalizing	58.4	9.2
Competence		
Social	43.3	10.0
Activities	40.1	7.8
School	37.6	14.1
Scales		
Somatic complaints	60.7	9.9
Schizoid	59.8	8.6
Uncommunicative	60.6	10.2
Immature	63.2	8.6
Obsessive–compulsive	56.7	8.1
Hostile—withdrawal	61.9	8.7
Delinquent	61.3	7.6
Aggressive	56.6	10.0
Hyperactive	61.6	9.2

Table 14-9. Stepwise Multiple Regression Analysis Results between Independent and Dependent CBCL Variables

	Parenting quality	LH	RH	Testosterone	LUH	Estradiol	VIQ
PIQ							
Behavior problems							
External	−.653		−.469	−.554			
Competence							
Activity						.623	
Social						.716	
School						.679	
Scales							
Somatic complaints							
Schizoid			−.488				
Uncommunicativeness	−.482	−.443	−.505		−.419		
Immature				−.552			
Obsessive–compulsive	−.416			−.480			.440
Hostile—withdrawal	−.416			−.603			
Delinquency	−.728						
Aggressivity	−.572		−.514		−.525		
Hyperactivity	−.550	−.576	−.453	−.480	−.525		

Note: Only significant association at the .05 level or less presented. Values are partial correlations.

testosterone level in particular, was now significantly negatively related to various indices of maladjustment. In addition, the RH variable, previously unrelated to any PIC scale, has become a significant negative correlate of scales reflecting social and behavioral functioning.

A THEORETICAL PROPOSAL

The results obtained in this study suggest that the anomalous personalities and patterns of social relationships of 47,XXY males have their origins in a complex and changing system of environmental and biological events. Prior to puberty, when they are most clearly distinguished by low levels of spontaneous activity, the impact of variations on the adequacy of the environment has little or no effect on this aspect of the behavioral functioning. During this period, aside from their levels of intelligence, only the normality of their left-hemisphere-based processing of verbal information predicts the degree to which they are free from tendencies toward withdrawal and low activity.

The situation after the initiation of puberty appears quite different. During this time, when they appear to present more signs of deviance, the impact of environmental disturbance on adjustment in 47,XXY males is much stronger and more pervasive, as are individual differences in sex hormones, especially levels of testosterone. In addition, in this period right-hemispheric processes also come to be very significant contributors to behavioral adjustment.

Although theorizing about the results of the study is probably premature at this point, a recent paper by Tucker and Williamson (1984) has provided a set of proposals that may be useful in formulating the beginnings of an explanation. They proposed that the two hemispheres make different contributions to features of behavior that fall under the headings of motivational and emotional functioning. In their system they suggest that the left hemisphere has a particular role in mediating tonic activation level, which in turn influences motor functioning and motivationally directed actions. It is conceivable that in prepubertal 47,XXY males, deficits in left-hemispheric functioning are responsible for their lower than expected levels of activity and for their tendencies toward withdrawal. In Tucker and Williamson's system, the right hemisphere's function is different. Its role is to respond flexibly and phasically to environmental change and, further, to mediate emotional (as opposed to motivational) processes. It is possible that as puberty begins, the exaggerated right-hemispheric functioning of 47,XXY males provides greater adaptive capabilities in the face of such stresses as poor parenting and the physical immaturities associated with deficits in testosterone production (Leventhal & Tomarken, 1986). Such a view suggests that the patterns of adjustment and personality style shown by 47,XXY males are the result of complex processes that are biologically and environmentally determined. It suggests, further, that this system is not invariant in time but, as developmental psychopathologists might predict, depends on influences that change as a function of age and stage in development (Sroufe & Rutter, 1984).

At this point it is impossible to know whether the influences of hormones, hemispheric specialization, and family life on social/emotional behaviors in 47,XXY males will remain the same after puberty. It is equally impossible to know whether they or the somewhat different pattern of influences seen in the prepubertal cases are specific to extra-X males or, alternatively, may be generalized to both normal individuals and those with various behavioral or biological abnormalities. However, the issues of hemispheric influences on noncognitive behavior and the developmental course of such interactions seem worthy of investigation in the future.

REFERENCES

Almqvist, S., Linsten, J., & Lindvall, N. (1963). Linear growth, sulfation factor activity and chromosomal constitution in 22 subjects with Turners syndrome. *Acta Endocrinologica, 42,* 168–186.

Annell, A. L., Gustavson, K. H., & Tenstam, J. (1970). Symptomatology in school boys with positive sex chromatin (the Klinefelter syndrome). *Acta Psychiatrica Scandinavica, 46,* 71–80.

Bancroft, J, Axworthy, D. I., & Ratcliffe, S. (1982). The personality and psychosocial development of boys with 47,XXY chromosome constitution. *Journal of Child Psychology and Psychiatry, 23,* 169–180.

Bockman, D., & Kirby, M. (1984). Dependence of thymus development on derivatives of the neural crest. *Science, 223,* 498–500.

Chi, J. G., Dooling, E. C., & Giles, F. H. (1977). Gyral development of the human brain. *Annals of Neurology, 1,* 86–93.

Corballis, M., & Morgan, M. (1978). On the biological basis of human lateralization: I. Evidence for a left–right gradient. *The Behavioural and Brain Sciences, 2,* 261–336.

Garron, D. (1977). Sex linked recessive inheritance of spatial and numerical abilities and Turner's syndrome. *Psychological Review, 77,* 147–152.

Geschwind, N., & Behan, P. (1982). Left-handedness: Association with immune disease, migraine and developmental learning disorder. *Proceedings of the National Academy of Sciences of the USA, 79,* 5097–5100.

Geschwind, N., & Galaburda, A. M. (1985). Cerebral lateralization: Biological mechanisms, associations and pathology: I. A hypothesis and a programme for research. *Archives of Neurology, 42,* 428–459.

Gordon H., & Galatzer, A. (1980). Cerebral organization in patients with gonadol dysgenesis. *Psychoneuroendocrinology, 5,* 235–244.

Hines, M. (1982). Prenatal gonadol hormones and sex differences in human behaviour. *Psychological Bulletin, 92,* 56–80.

Kinsbourne, M., & Hiscock, M. (1977). Does cerebral dominance develop? In S. Segalowitz & F. Gruber (Eds.), *Language development and neurological theory.* New York: Academic Press.

Kuhn, G. M. (1973). The phi-coefficient as an index of ear difference in dichotic listening. *Cortex, 9,* 447–457.

Leventhal, H., & Tomarken, A. J. (1986). Emotion: Today's problems. *Annual Review of Psychology, 37,* 565–610.

Maccoby, E., & Jacklin, C. (1974). *The psychology of sex differences.* Stanford, CA: Stanford University Press.
McGlone, J. (1980). Sex differences in human brain asymmetry: A critical survey. *The Behavioural and Brain Sciences, 3,* 215–263.
Mittwoch, U. (1973). *Genetics of sex differentiation.* New York: Academic Press.
Netley, C. (1977). Dichotic listening of callosal agenesis and Turner's syndrome patients. In S. Segalowtiz & F. Gruber (Eds.), *Language development and neurological theory.* New York: Academic Press.
Netley, C. (1983). Sex chromosome abnormalities and the development of verbal and nonverbal abilities. In C. L. Ludlow & J. A. Cooper (Eds.), *Genetic aspects of speech and language disorders.* New York: Academic Press.
Netley, C., & Rovet, J. (1982a). Atypical hemispheric lateralization in Turner syndrome subjects. *Cortex, 18,* 377–384.
Netley, C., & Rovet, J. (1982b). Handedness in 47,XXY males. *Lancet,* July 31, p. 267.
Netley, C., & Rovet, J. (1982c). Verbal deficits in children with 47,XXY and 47,XXX karyotypes: A descriptive and experimental study. *Brain and Language, 17,* 58–72.
Netley, C., & Rovet, J. (1983). Relationships among brain organization, maturation rate and the development of verbal and nonverbal ability. In S. Segalowitz (Ed.), *Language functions and brain organization.* New York: Academic Press.
Netley, C., & Rovet, J. (1984). Hemispheric lateralization in 47,XXY Klinefelter's syndrome boys. *Brain and Cognition, 3,* 10–18.
Ounsted, M. (1972). Gender and intra-uterine growth: With a note on the use of the sex proband as a research tool. In C. Ounsted & D. C. Taylor (Eds.), *Gender differences: Their ontogeny and significance.* Edinburgh: Churchill Livingstone.
Pennington, B., Puck, M., & Robinson, A. (1980). Language and cognitive development in 47,XXX females followed since birth. *Behaviour Genetics, 10,* 31–41.
Pennington, B., & Smith, S. (1983). Genetic influences on learning disabilities and speech and language disorders. *Child Development, 54,* 369–387.
Penrose, L. (1967). Fingerprint patterns and the sex chromosomes. *Lancet, 1,* 298–300.
Polani, P. E. (1981). Chromosomes and chromosomal mechanisms in the genesis of maldevelopment. In K. Connolly & H. Prechtl (Eds.), *Maturation and development.* Philadelphia: Lippincott.
Reinsich, J., Gandelman, R., & Spiegel, F. (1979). Prenatal influences on cognitive abilities: Data from experimental animals and human genetic and endocrine syndromes. In M. Wittig & A. Petersen (Eds.), *Sex related differences in cognitive functioning.* New York: Academic Press.
Rhodes, K., Markham, R. L., Maxwell, P. M., & Monk-Jones, M. E. (1969). Immunoglobins and the X chromosome. *British Medical Journal, 3,* 439–441.
Robinson, A., Lubs, H., Nielsen, J., & Sorensen, K. (1979). Summary of clinical findings: Profiles of children with 47,XXY, 47,XXX and 47,XYY karyotypes. *Birth Defects: Original Article Series, 15,* 261–266.
Rovet, J., & Netley, C. (1981). Turner syndrome in a pair of dizygotic twins: A single case study. *Behaviour Genetics, 11,* 65–72.
Rovet, J., & Netley, C. (1982). Processing deficits in Turner's syndrome. *Developmental Psychology, 18,* 77–94.
Rovet, J., & Netley, C. (1983). The triple X syndrome in childhood: Recent empirical findings. *Child Development, 54,* 831–845.
Schiavi, R. C., Theilgaard, K., Owen, D. R., & White, D. (1984). Sex chromosome anomalies, hormones and aggressivity. *Archives of General Psychiatry, 41,* 93–99.
Sorensen, K., Nielsen, J., Wohlert, M., Bennett, P., & Johnsen, S. G. (1981). Serum testosterone with karyotype 47,XXY (Klinefelter's syndrome) at birth. *Lancet, 2,* 1112–1113.
Sroufe, L. A., & Rutter, M. (1984). The domain of developmental psychopathology. *Child Development, 55,* 17–29.
Stewart, D. (1982). Children with sex chromosome aneuploidy: Follow-up studies. *Birth Defects: Original Article Series, 18* (Whole Volume).
Stewart D., Netley, C., Bailey, J. D., Haka-Ikse, K., Platt, J., Holland, W., & Cripps, M. (1979). Growth and development of children with X and Y chromosome aneuploidy: A prospective study. *Birth Defects: Original Article Series, 15,* 75–114.
Stewart, D. A., Bailey, J. D., Netley, C., Rovet, J., Park, E., Cripps, M., & Curtiss, J. A. (1982). Growth and development of children with X and Y chromosome aneuploidy from infancy to pubertal stage: The Toronto study. *Birth Defects: Original Article Series, 18,* 99–154.
Stewart, D. A., Netley, C., & Park, E. (1982). Summary of clinical findings with 47,XXY, 47,XYY and 47,XXX karyotypes. *Birth Defects: Original Article Series, 18,* 1–6.

Stewart, D. A., Bailey, J. D., Netley, C., Rovet, J., & Park, E. (1986). Growth and development from early to mid adolescence of children with X and Y chromosome aneuploidy: The Toronto Study. Birth Defects: Original Article Series, 22, 119–182.

Theilgaard, A. (1981). The personalities of XYY and XXY man. In W. Schmid & J. Nielson (Eds.), *Human genetics and behaviour*. Elsevier: North Holland Biomedical.

Tucker, D. M., & Williamson, P. A. (1984). Asymmetric neural control systems in human self regulation. *Psychological Review, 91,* 185–215.

Waber, D. P. (1976). Sex differences in cognition: A function of maturation rate? *Science, 192a,* 572–574.

Waber, D. P. (1977). Sex differences and the rate of physical growth. Developmental Psychology, *13,* 29–38.

Waber, D. P. (1979). Neuropsychological aspects of Turner syndrome. Developmental Medicine and Child Neurology, *21,* 58–70.

Waber, D. P., Mann, M. B., Merola, J., & Moylan, P. M. (1985). Physical maturation rate and cognitive performance in early adolescence: A longitudinal examination. Developmental Psychology, *21,* 666–681.

Walzer, S., Wolff, P. H., Bowman, D., Silbert, A. R., Bashir, A. S., Gerald, P. S., & Richmond, J. B. (1978). A method for the longitudinal study of behavioural development in infants and children: The early development of XXY children. *Journal of Child Psychology and Psychiatry, 19,* 213–229.

15

Cognitive Sequelae of Unilateral Lesions Acquired in Early Childhood

DOROTHY M. ARAM
Rainbow Babies and Childrens Hospital, Cleveland, Ohio

HARRY A. WHITAKER
The Neuropsychiatric Institute, Fargo, North Dakota

One approach to studying early hemispheric specialization for higher cognitive functions has been to study children with known brain lesions. The literature addressing the effect of early brain lesions on children's cognitive development, in general, has involved one of three types of children:

1. Reports of cognitive functioning following lesions acquired after a period of presumably normal language development (the acquired lesions or acquired aphasia in childhood literature)
2. Studies of children with hemiplegia during infancy or early childhood (the infantile or childhood hemiplegia literature)
3. Studies of individuals who have undergone hemispherectomies and therefore continue to function with one remaining hemisphere (the hemidecorticate literature).

Studies documenting the effects of acquired lesions have been reported since the late 1800s, with several relatively well known studies of sizable numbers of children having occurred in the last 40 years, including those of Alajouanine and Lhermitte (1965), Guttmann (1942), Hecaen (1976, 1983), Woods (1980), Woods and Carey (1979), Woods and Teuber (1978).

Reports of cognitive abilities among infantile hemiplegics, especially those addressing the relationship between the side of hemiplegia and language functioning, have appeared since Cotard (1868). Dennis and Whitaker (1977) reviewed a series of 19th- and 20th-century studies relating left and right hemiplegias to impaired language. Several studies have addressed IQ, visual–spatial, motor and language abilities among left and right hemiplegic children (Aicardi, Amsili & Chevrie, 1969; Annett, 1973; Basser, 1962; Byers & McLean, 1962; Hammil & Irwin, 1966; Hood & Perlstein, 1955; Kershner & King, 1974).

Finally, a series of studies with hemidecorticate individuals have documented the differential effect of the remaining right or left hemisphere in subserving a range of cognitive abilities. In the past 10 years, there have been a number of case studies that have provided highly detailed descriptions of language and other aspects of cognition in individuals with a remaining single hemisphere. In addition to several case studies, for example, Day and Ulatowska (1979), probably Maureen Dennis and her colleagues are best known for their work with hemidecorticate patients, (e.g., Dennis, 1980a; Dennis & Kohn, 1975; Dennis, Lovett, & Wiegel-Crump, 1981; Dennis & Whitaker, 1976, 1977; Kohn & Dennis, 1974).

SUBJECT SPECIFICATION AND MEASUREMENT

Limitations in Subject Specifications

In much of this earlier literature, however, several subject and measurement variables have been poorly specified, leaving the interpretation of much of the data highly questionable. Among the important subject variables typically not adequately accounted for have been: (1) specification of lesion unilaterality, including the related issues of how lesion location was determined and the etiology of the lesion; (2) inclusion of patients with seizure disorders; (3) premorbid cognitive and linguistic status of subjects; and (4) failure to use control subjects.

Crucial to inferences made about the relationship between site of lesion and any behavior measured is careful specification of the location of the lesion. Probably the most basic requirement is determining the unilaterality of the given lesion—an important part of the work related to adults with acquired lesions but, in the pre–CT scan era, absent in most of the available work with children. In the majority of studies, the presumed unilaterality of a lesion is based on clinical findings, at times supported by EEG results, angiography, surgical findings, or—in a few instances—autopsy. Some studies, notably Annett (1973) and Dennis and Whitaker (1977), have identified the more involved hemisphere as that contralateral to the hemiplegia or hand with the poorest motor performance. Not until the past four years have studies reported CT scan confirmation of lesion location. CT localization still has some limitations; negative CT findings but positive motor and behavioral findings have been observed by most researchers working with pediatric neurology populations. The recent advent of other forms of imaging, notably Magnetic Resonance Imaging, has permitted identification of some lesions with greater clarity. The only studies that have reported CT scan findings for all children are those of Aram and colleagues (Aram, Rose, Rekate, & Whitaker, 1983; Aram, Ekelman, Rose, & Whitaker, 1985; Aram, Ekelman, & Whitaker, 1986; Aram, Ekelman, & Satz, in press); Ferro and colleagues (Ferro, Martins, Pinto, & Castro-Caldas, 1982; Ferro, Martins, & Tavora, 1984); Rankin, Aram, and Horwitz (1981); Stiles-Davis, Sugarman, and Nass (1985); Vargha-Khadem and colleagues (Vargha-Khadem, Frith, O'Gorman, & Watters, 1983; Vargha-Khadem, O'Gorman, & Watters, 1985); and Visch-Brink and Van de Sandt-Koenderman (1984). Although these recent studies have begun to document side of hemispheric involvement, almost no attempt has been made to specify intrahemispheric localization.

Related to the issue of lesion unilaterality is the fact that most reports have included children for whom bilateral involvement is either stated or presumed, because of the etiology of the lesion. Woods and Teuber (1978) reexamined the incidence of acquired aphasias in childhood after lateralized lesions, and found that, before 1940, the incidence of aphasia following right-hemisphere lesions was one-third. Since the 1940s they found that aphasia occurred in fewer than 10% of right-lesioned patients, and, if known left-handers were excluded, the incidence fell to 5%. They attributed this changing pattern of reported childhood aphasia to the introduction of antibiotics and mass immunizations in the 1940s, thereby checking systemic infections that may well have led to bilateral involvement. Thus, much of the pre-1940 data is suspect for bilateral involvement.

Even in relatively recent studies, patients for whom bilateral involvement may be inferred on the basis of etiology are included. For example, in the often referenced 1976 paper by Hecaen, 16 of the original 26 patients (62%) had incurred lesions following head trauma, a situation likely to produce bilateral damage, although only 3 patients were classified as presenting bilateral involvement. Similarly, in a recent Italian series reported in

1981 by Riva and Cazzaniga of 27 right- and 24 left-lesioned children, 10 had incurred neonatal asphyxia, 5 premature delivery, 3 encephalitis, and 6 arteriovenous malformations where the location and the extensiveness of the bleed were not clearly specified. Even in the otherwise commendable work of Vargha-Khadem and her colleagues, patients with tumors and head trauma were included. The group of children studied by Aram and colleagues appears to be the only group reported for whom all lesions have been secondary to unilateral vascular insults.

A second factor often not specified for subjects is the inclusion of children with seizure disorders. This practice further confounds the unilateral effect of a lesion for at least three reasons:

1. The effect of the epileptiform discharge on behavior, particularly if it spreads bilaterally
2. The effect of anticonvulsants on higher cognitive functions
3. The long-term effect of epileptiform discharges on brain cells.

Almost without exception, studies either make no mention of seizures or include seizure-disordered children. In some—for example, Kiessling, Denckla, & Carlton (1983)—an attempt has been made to include only "well-controlled" patients, yet the past and current seizure history is rarely detailed, and control presumably is established through use of anticonvulsants. In some studies, the inclusion of children with seizure disorders seriously casts suspicion on findings attributed to unilateral lesions. For example, Woods (1980) reported that children with early right-hemisphere lesions are deficient in both Verbal IQ (VIQ) and Performance IQ (PIQ), in comparison to control subjects, whereas children with later-acquired right-hemisphere lesions only are deficient in PIQ. Fifty percent of the early right-lesioned group, however, consisted of children with seizure disorders, in contrast to 15% of the group with later onset of right lesions. The fact that Annett (1973), among others (e.g., Jabbour & Lundevold, 1963; Perlstein & Hood, 1957), have demonstrated a relationship between recurrent fits (epilepsy) and decreased IQ, appears to have gone unnoticed by a number of investigators who continue to include children with seizure disorders, discounting the role of seizures and anticonvulsants in the results they obtain.

A third major limitation in subject specification for the majority of children with unilateral lesions is their premorbid cognitive and linguistic status, which at least in some cases has been suspect. Except in a few recent case studies, (e.g., Ferro *et al.*, 1982, 1984; Pohl, 1979), typically little is known about premorbid status, or what is known often implicates potentially more generalized involvement. Children experiencing neonatal asphyxia or prematurity, for example, are at risk for CNS involvement beyond deficits secondary to acquired unilateral lesions. In rare instances patients with pre- or perinatal complications are excluded, although this is an uncommon occurrence, due at least in part to the rarity of children with unilateral lesions. Although documentation of prior status, including intellectual abilities, hand preference, and the like, can be more readily established for children sustaining lesions at older ages, this important information is often neglected.

Finally, studies are quite inconsistent in comparing results with lesioned children to control populations. What variables to control for or what constitutes an appropriate comparison group may be highly debatable, yet it is doubtful that "standardized" normative data suffice, given the multitude of factors known to influence higher cognitive functioning. As Milner has commented (1973, pp. 115–116, following Woods & Teuber): "In trying to draw valid conclusions from unavoidably small numbers of cases of spontaneously occurring unilateral cerebral injury, almost everything hinges on the choice of appropriate control subjects."

Several of the more recent studies have used comparison subjects, some chosen to reflect a particular stage of development (e.g., Stiles-Davis, Sugarman, & Nass, 1985); others to represent grade-level performance, (e.g., Woods & Carey, 1979) or chronological comparisons (Kershner & King, 1974). Vargha-Khadem *et al.* (1985) selected control subjects matched by age and Full Range IQ to lesioned subjects. One might question the rationale of matching by IQ, which appears to be an effect of the lesion rather than a variable to be controlled. Several studies have used sibling controls (Kiessling *et al.*, 1983; Riva & Cazzaniga, 1981; Woods, 1980; Woods & Teuber, 1978), although because of age differences this introduces the problem of comparing performance on age-dependent tasks. Nonetheless, several of the childhood lesion studies have used control subjects despite the serious question of what constitutes an appropriate control for a unilaterally brain-lesioned child.

Limitations in Systematic Measurement

Except for the hemidecorticate studies and a few case studies, no study of children with acquired lesions or early-onset hemiplegia reported systematic measures other than intelligence test results, until the past 10 years. The majority of the earlier studies relied on clinical impressions of cognitive abilities. Reliance on clinical impressions introduces questions of the reliability of the judgment made and the criteria for language loss and language recovery. For example, Woods and Teuber (1978) reported that no patient under 8 years of age when the lesions occurred was still clinically aphasic when examined neurologically at the time of their follow-up study. Yet when Woods and Carey (1979) used objective measures of language ability, including picture naming and various syntactic tasks, they found that if the lesion both occurred after 1 year of age and caused a language deficit, aphasic deficits were still present at the time of testing. The contrast between the Woods and Teuber (1978) and the Woods and Carey (1979) studies, based largely on the same subject population but using clinical impression in the former and objective measures in the latter, suggest that clinical impression may not be a reliable indicator of language status.

A final limitation concerns the lack of uniformity in follow-up testing. Most studies have reported findings at one point in time, usually several years post–lesion onset. A few have followed children over a period of years, although the follow-up schedule for each child often was variable or not documented. With some notable exceptions, few studies have reported findings as a function of time since lesion onset.

Failure to follow children with acquired lesions over time creates at least two important limitations: (1) the recovery and development process cannot be charted; and (2) unless testing is undertaken well beyond what is considered the period of normal language development, any differences may represent a delay, presumably necessitated by hemispheric reorganization for language, rather than a permanent deficit.

REVIEW OF RECENT STUDIES

With these subject and measurement constraints as background, the following reviews what little is known about higher cognitive functions in children with unilateral lesions, drawing principally from work that has appeared within the past 7 years. The intent here is to understand the consequences of lesions acquired early in life for later cognitive development. To understand the relationship between the site of hemispheric involvement and later abilities, a clear picture of the lesion and of cognitive performance is needed. Although the hemidecorticate studies have been exemplary in specifying anatomical involvement and cognitive tasks, they are not included in the following review for two reasons: (1) most hemidecorticate patients have a history of long-standing seizure disorders and anticonvulsant therapy; and (2) there is an important theoretical difference between functioning with one remaining hemisphere and functioning with two hemispheres, one of which is damaged.

Ideally, a review such as this would include only studies that: (1) involve children with clearly specified lesion sites, known premorbid status, and no seizures; (2) select normal control children on the basis of a range of variables known to influence language performance, such as sex, age, social class, and similar medical histories exclusive of neurological involvement; (3) use objective measures of the aspects of cognitive development under study; and (4) follow the children over time to determine whether the lags in performance represent delayed or deficient development. These ideal studies, however, are not available. Therefore, in this review, studies that meet two principal criteria have been included: (1) report of objective assessment of some aspect of higher cognitive functions for children with unilateral lesions, and (2) lesion specification for the majority of subjects. As will be seen, the second criterion, a clear unilateral lesion, is less than perfectly met in most instances. In fact, if all studies that include some children with known bilateral involvement or with lesions secondary to trauma, tumors, and other conditions that implicate bilateral involvement were eliminated, only a few case studies and some of the studies reported by Aram and colleagues would remain.

Source of Data

CASE STUDIES

The case studies that provide both objective data and a clearly specified unilateral lesion are those listed in Table 15-1. The earliest are Yeni-Komshian (1977), where 1 of 4 subjects sustained a unilateral left frontoparietal lesion at 11 years of age, and Pohl (1979), reporting a 6-year-old left-lesioned boy. In 1980 Maureen Dennis described the ability of a 9-year-old girl, 3 months post onset of a left temporoparietal infarct, to retell the story of Little Red Riding Hood. The girl's expressive syntax, communicative intent as revealed in the propositions in the story, and ability to judge the grammaticality of her own utterances were described. Ferro, Martins, and colleagues have reported three studies, one addressing visual neglect in three children sustaining right lesions at 5, 6, and 9 years of age (Ferro, Martins, & Tavora, 1984); a second documenting aphasia following a right striatoinsular infarction at 6 years of age in a left-handed girl (Ferro, Martins, Pinto, & Castro-Caldas, 1982); and a third study reporting crossed aphasia in a 15-year-old boy with a right-hemisphere tumor (Martins, Ferro, & Trindade, 1984). Aram, Rose, Rekate, and Whitaker (1983) compared a 7-year-old girl with an acquired lesion in the area of the head of the caudate and the anterior limb of the internal capsule who presented language loss but no dysarthria, to that of an 11-year-old girl with a more posterior subcortical lesion for whom language remained normal, but a mild dysarthria presented. Finally, Visch-Brink and Van de Sandt-Koenderman (1984) discussed paraphasia in several children with acquired aphasia, all but one of whom had bilateral involvement, the exception being an 11-year-old boy with a unilateral left-hemisphere lesion.

Table 15-1. Case Studies Reviewed

Investigators	Subjects	Focus	Findings
Yeni-Komshian, 1977	11-year-old: L-frontoparietal	Dichotic listening	Strong LEA (left-ear advantage) and REA, persisting to follow-up at 14 months
Pohl, 1979	6-year-old: L lesioned	Dichotic listening	Strong LEA and REA extinction persisting to follow-up at 13 months. REA extinction not related to stimulus length or training.
Dennis, 1980b	9-year-old: L-temporoparietal	Communicative intent; expression; comprehension; reading	Comprehension, expression, and communicative intent all ↓ at 3-month follow-up; dissociation between auditory and reading comprehension, the latter being relatively preserved.
Ferro, Martins, Pinto, & Castro-Caldas, 1982	6-year-old: R-striatoinsular infarct	Subcortical effects	Acute nonfluent aphasia, LEA extinction, visual neglect, and ↓ word and sentence repetition. Two weeks post onset, aphasia cleared, but articulation, reading, and handwriting difficulties persisted.
Aram, Rose, Rekate, Whitaker, 1983	7- and 11-year-olds: L-subcortical	Subcortical effects	Lesion in the putamen, anterior limb of internal capsule and head of caudate resulted in ↓ comprehension and nonfluent aphasia but no dysarthria; lesion in globus pallidus, posterior limb of internal capsule and body of caudate was related to dysarthria but no language loss.
Ferro, Martins, & Tavora, 1984	5-, 6-, and 9-year-olds: R-lesioned	Visual neglect	Visual neglect demonstrated acutely with complete recovery within 1 month post lesion onset.
Martins, Ferro, & Trindade, 1984	15-year-old: R-lesioned	Crossed aphasia	Fluent aphasia, reading, writing, and visual–spatial disturbance occurred secondary to right occipitotemporal tumor; 1 month post surgery, a severe global aphasia was associated with rostral extension of the tumor.
Visch-Brink & Van De Sandt-Koenderman, 1984	Case 1: 11-year-old: L-lesioned	Paraphasias	Five months post onset, difficulties persisted in spoken syntax, oral reading, and repetition of words and sentences. Neologisms and literal and verbal paraphasias present on naming tasks.

GROUP STUDIES

The studies reporting on groups of children with acquired lesions for whom specific objective findings are reported, including lesion specification, are listed in Table 15-2. Woods and Carey (1979) reported what appears to be the first large-scale study of specific behavioral data beyond IQ test results, providing information pertinent to naming, syntax, and spelling for 27 patients with left-hemisphere lesions. The following year, Woods (1980) published an extensive comparison of the effects of early and late left and right lesions on Verbal and Performance IQ. Both studies used control subjects for comparison, the 1979 study using 48 normal 5th-, 7th-, 9th-, and 11th-graders and the 1980 study making use of 37 closest-in-age siblings. Unfortunately, unilaterality of lesions for both studies was based on clinical neurological findings inconsistently supported by surgery, angiography, brain scans, and EEG. Five of 50 (10%) in the 1980 study were documented to present mild bilateral deficits, and 11 of 50 (20%+) had histories of severe and/or prolonged seizures. Riva and Cazzaniga (1981) also examined the effects of left and right lesions sustained before or after 1 year of age on IQ, comparing the findings to sibling and cousin controls. Pneumoencephalograms, arteriograms, and CTs were used to identify lesion location; still, 10 of 51 subjects (20%) had suffered neonatal asphyxia, and 5 were the product of premature delivery. Rankin, Aram, and Horwitz (1981) described the language of 3 left-hemiplegic and 3 right-hemiplegic 6- to 8-year-olds. Despite CT scan confirmation of pre- or perinatally sustained unilateral lesions, here, too, one left-lesioned child should not have been included because of having contracted meningitis at 5 years of age. Kiessling, Denckla, and Carlton (1983) studied 8 right- and 8 left-hemiplegic children, comparing their performance to siblings on a range of higher cognitive tasks including syntax, visual–spatial skills, and academic achievement. Although the study provided relatively rich data, unilaterality of the lesions was determined on the basis of performance on the Annett pegboard and results of clinical neurological examination, with 9 of the 16 subjects demonstrating some degree of bilateral involvement.

Vargha-Khadem and colleagues (1983, 1985) have presented two highly detailed studies, one addressing aspects of language and memory and the other academic achievement in large groups of left- and right-lesioned subjects. CT scans were used to identify lesions in all subjects, although patients with tumors and those with lesions secondary to trauma were included. Nonetheless, their studies provide what appears to be the most extensive data available on large numbers of brain-lesioned children.

Recently, Stiles-Davis, Sugarman, and Nass (1985) presented a detailed experimental study of the development of spatial and class relations in 4 left-lesioned and 4 right-lesioned 2½- to 3½-year-old children, comparing these children's performance to groups of stage-graded normally developing children. All lesioned children were hemiparetic, with no contralateral findings indicated on the basis of the clinical neurological examination. CT scan data was available for all children, although for 3 of 8 children, CT scans were normal despite the presence of positive clinical findings.

Finally, Aram *et al.* (1985, 1986) reported two studies of 8 left-lesioned and 8 right-lesioned children with several additional studies in progress comparing the lesioned children's performance to that of carefully matched controls on a range of IQ and language measures. Although these studies are not without their faults, they have been particularly stringent in including only children with unilateral lesions while excluding subjects with any evidence of bilateral involvement, seizures, or questionable premorbid status.

The findings of these various case and group studies will be summarized next, beginning with an abbreviated summary of the work of other investigators, followed by a somewhat more detailed report of the findings thus far from our group. Information will be

Table 15-2. Group Studies Reviewed

Investigators	N	Lesion side	Focus	Findings
Woods & Carey, 1979	27	Left[a]	Naming, syntax, spelling, rhyming	Children with lesion onset after 1 year of age were poorer than controls on syntax, naming, and spelling tests; those with lesions before 1 year were deficient in spelling only.
Woods, 1980	27 23	Left[a] Right	Age, IQ	Lesion laterality / Lesion onset: <1 year / >1 year Left: ↓ VIQ, PIQ / ↓ VIQ, PIQ Right: ↓ VIQ, PIQ / ↓ PIQ
Riva & Cazzaniga, 1981	27 24	Right[a] Left	Lesion $\leqslant$ 1 year effect on IQ	Lesion laterality / Lesion onset: <1 year / >1 year Left: ↓ VIQ, PIQ / ↓ VIQ, PIQ Right: ↓ PIQ / ↓ PIQ
Rankin, Aram, & Horwitz, 1981	3 3	Left[a] Right	Syntax, lexicon, articulation	Left-lesioned children were inferior on tasks of speech production, vocabulary comprehension, and syntactic comprehension and production.
Kiessling, Denckla, & Carlton, 1983	8 8	Right[a] Left	Motor function, syntax, memory, academic achievement	Left-lesioned children were significantly poorer than rights or controls on syntactic awareness and sentence repetition. Both lefts and rights were poorer than controls on short-term memory, digit repetition, and confrontation naming. Left-hand impairment related to arithmetic computation.

Vargha-Khadem, Frith, O'Gorman, & Watters, 1983	24 22	Left[a] Right	Age of lesion onset and effect on reading, spelling, arithmetic, and paired associate learning	All lesioned groups ↓ in comparison to normals in reading and spelling, although more pronounced among left lesions, especially acquired postnatally. Mental arithmetic and digit span did not discriminate among groups. Left-lesioned significantly impaired in paired associate learning.
Nass, Sadler, & Sidtis, 1984	8 4	Left[a] Right	Dichotic speech, syllable, and pitch discrimination	Congenital left- and right-hemisphere damage associated with poorer performance on dichotic tests contralateral to damaged hemisphere. In contrast to findings with adults, pitch discrimination ↓ in left-lesioned children and speech discrimination ↓ in right-lesioned children.
Vargha-Khadem, O'Gorman, & Watters, 1985	28 25	Left[a] Right	Age at lesion onset, severity, IQ, language, and motor performance	Language deficits occurred in all left-lesioned groups but were most pronounced when onset was after 5 years of age. Left- and right-lesioned children, grouped by age of lesion onset, were not significantly different in IQ. Postnatally acquired left lesions result in lower VIQ, and postnatal right lesions result in lower PIQ.
Stiles-Davis, Sugarman, & Nass, 1985	4 4	Right[a] Left	Spatial and class relations	Early right lesions resulted in spatial deficits exemplified by the failure to generate next-to relations.
Aram, Ekelman, Rose, & Whitaker, 1985	8 8	Left Right	IQ, syntax, lexicon	IQ scores in right- and left-lesioned children were not reliably indicative of lesion laterality; lexical comprehension and production were reduced in both right- and left-lesioned children; syntactic production was reduced in lefts but not rights.
Aram, Ekelman, & Whitaker, 1986	8 8	Left Right	Spoken syntax	Left-lesioned children ↓ on multiple measures of simple and complex sentence structure.

[a]Denotes some question of bilateral involvement.

reviewed by cognitive area, first addressing results of central auditory testing, then visual–perceptual skills, followed by performance on various areas of academic achievement—reading, written language, spelling, and mathematics. Finally, IQ and language abilities will be discussed, with the latter discussion focusing on the work we have been doing.

Cognitive Areas Reviewed

CENTRAL AUDITORY PROCESSING

The case studies of Yeni-Komshian (1977) and Pohl (1979) specifically addressed dichotic listening for left-hemisphere-lesioned subjects. Yeni Komshian's 11-year-old incurred a massive lesion to the left frontoparietal area, requiring that the left middle cerebral artery (LMCA) be ligated above the level of the Circle of Willis. Pohl's 6-year-old suffered occlusion of the LMCA following a diphtheria-tetanus revaccination. Both patients presented pronounced and persistent aphasic symptoms. They were retested over time on the dichotic measures until 1 year post lesion onset. Both children exhibited a pronounced left-ear advantage persisting through the year's follow-up, coupled with extinction of the right-ear response under dichotic conditions. Pohl demonstrated that the right-ear extinction was independent of stimulus length and not modifiable through verbal training. Both investigators interpreted their findings as showing a transfer in hemispheric dominance of speech for these subjects with massive left-hemisphere lesions. In contrast, Yeni-Komshian's bilaterally involved children initially demonstrated a marked REA, with an inability to process competing stimuli, but then improved in processing dichotic stimuli corresponding to improvement in language functioning. As well, Ferro *et al.* (1984), in their study of visual neglect, reported initial left-ear extinction in a 6-year-old with a right striatoinsular infarction, which returned to normal in 2 weeks, along with a second patient with a massive right fibroplastic meningioma where the left-ear extinction persisted after 1 month.

Nass, Sadler, and Sidtis (1984) compared the performance on dichotic listening tests of 8 children with congenital left-hemisphere damage and 4 with congenital right-hemisphere damage to that of adults with unilateral hemisphere lesions. Similar to adults, both left- and right-hemisphere-damaged children were poorer in the ear contralateral to the damaged hemisphere. However, the pattern of deficits among the children was opposite from that of the adults: The congenital left-hemisphere-damaged group was poorer in pitch discrimination than either the right-damaged or the control group, and the congenital right-hemisphere group was significantly worse in syllable discrimination than either the left-damaged or the control group. The investigators attributed these unexpected findings to the crowding hypothesis (Woods & Teuber, 1973; see also Liederman, Chapter 13, this volume).

VISUAL PERCEPTUAL ABILITIES

Several investigators have reported findings pertinent to visual–perceptual abilities of brain-lesioned children based on performance on a range of IQ or related tasks. For example, Kiessling *et al.* (1983) reported that results on the Raven's Progressive Matrices did not correlate significantly with side of lesion as determined by hand performance on the Annett pegboard; it must be kept in mind, however, that over half of their subjects had bilateral involvement. Nonetheless, these results are in agreement with Hecaen and Albert (1978) and with observations in our own laboratory that demonstrate no side of lesion effect of the Raven's, suggesting that Raven's scores may be affected by damage to either hemisphere or, conversely, completed satisfactorily by either a verbal–logical or visual–spatial strategy.

Among the studies of children with well-demarcated unilateral lesions only Ferro *et al.* (1984) and Stiles-Davis *et al.* (1985) specifically have addressed visual–perceptual abilities. The absence of visual neglect among children with brain lesions is noted by many investigators and is consistent with our own observations, except in the acute period. Ferro *et al.* (1984) presented findings for three right-lesioned subjects who initially presented symptoms of visual neglect on a visual constructional task, the Benton visual retention task, a letter cancellation, and a line bisection task. All subjects' performance returned to normal within 1 month of lesion onset, leading these investigators to suggest that the rarity of visual neglect in children may stem from lack of right-hemisphere dominance for attention, creating a situation in which either hemisphere could activate attention bilaterally. Except as can be extrapolated from performance on other tasks, no studies with unilaterally lesioned children have attempted to study visual attention in any detail.

Stiles-Davis *et al.* (1985) studied the process of development of spatial and class relationships for 4 left- and 4 right-lesioned children, longitudinally from 2 to 2½ to 3 to 3½ years of age, and compared these children's performance to that of 32 normally developing children. The investigators used a series of manipulative classification tasks that had been previously demonstrated to show a systematic relationship to age among normally developing children. The children were encouraged to group objects by varying the composition of the sets of toys provided. They were provided with toys that could encourage either spatial or class grouping, such as yellow or green rings and yellow or green columns. They also had tasks in which stickers affixed to the bottom of certain toys could prompt a child to shift focus from the spatial grouping of objects to a sequential, item-by-item search for the objects with stickers on them. The results of the study showed that the right-lesioned children failed to generate *next-to* relations (i.e., placing one object next to another) with the same frequency as normal or left-hemisphere-damaged children, although they did demonstrate *in* and *on* relations (i.e., containing an object within another) with normal frequency. They also demonstrated that the right-lesioned children were developing normally in their conceptualization of class relations when they did not have to construct certain spatial forms. The importance of this study is that it documents, for the first time, an early spatial deficit in young right-hemisphere-lesioned children, demonstrating that lateralization of some spatial functions would appear to be present very early in life.

AUDITORY MEMORY

Several investigators have reported results of digit repetition tasks, usually from an IQ measure, although the results are contradictory. Kiessling *et al.* (1983) report that digit repetition tends to be lower in both left- and right-lesioned subjects than for matched controls, but not significantly so, while Rudel and Denckla (1974) suggest that backward repetition is lower in right-lesioned than in left-lesioned children; and Vargha-Khadem *et al.* (1983) reported that digit repetition tasks did not differentiate between right- or left-lesioned groups and controls matched for age and IQ. It appears that only Vargha-Khadem *et al.* (1983) thus far have reported data for memory tasks other than digit repetition. Her group administered a paired associates learning task from the Wechsler Memory Scales. On this task the left-lesioned patients performed significantly poorer than the rights or controls, leading these investigators to suggest that some learning ability may be irrevocably impaired for children with left lesions.

ACADEMIC ACHIEVEMENT

Probably the most outstanding sequelae of unilateral lesions in children commented on in the older literature has been the academic difficulties that occur even in the face of what was thought to be complete recovery of language functions. Hecaen (1976, 1983), who provided no information about the measured used or specific findings, reports that while reading disorders are frequent in the acute period (said to be 40% in the left-lesioned subjects), they are of no localizing value and they disappear rapidly and completely. In contrast, Alajouanaine and Lhermitte (1965), studying 32 left-lesioned children, reported that 18 of the 32 had difficulty understanding written language and that for half of these (9), reading was totally lost. None of the 32 followed normal progress at school, and only 2 were said to have a satisfactory social evolution. Kiessling *et al.* (1983) and Vargha-Khadem *et al.* (1983) appear to be the first to report specific reading measures and results with groups of left- or right-lesioned children (both studies, however, included children with some degree of bilateral involvement). Kiessling *et al.* (1983) presented the WRAT reading recognition words, and Vargha-Khadem *et al.* (1983) presented a series of reading measures including word recognition, reading speed, and comprehension. Both groups of investigators found that although there was a tendency for both left- and right-lesioned groups to perform lower than controls, left-lesioned groups performed significantly lower than right-lesioned children or controls, with the greatest reading deficits presented by left-lesioned subjects who had postnatally acquired lesions.

Although the limited evidence suggests a greater deficit in reading recognition, and probably in comprehension, among left-lesioned than among right-lesioned children, this is most probably only a very limited part of the story. For example, Dennis (1980b), in a case study of a 9-year-old studied 3 months after the onset of a left temporoparietal infarction, demonstrated a dissociation between age-appropriate reading comprehension and a significant auditory comprehension deficit.

Likewise, although most reports suggest that written language deficits may be the most common and persistent of the higher cognitive sequelae of the left-brain-lesioned children, (e.g., Alajounaine & Lhermitte, 1965; Hecaen, 1976, 1983), this need not necessarily be true, as demonstrated by Dennis's 9-year-old, for whom written language at 2 weeks post onset was better preserved than oral language.

Woods and Carey (1979) appear to be the first to provide systematic spelling data for children with unilateral lesions. These investigators found that their left-lesioned subjects, regardless of age of lesion onset, had significantly poorer performance than control subjects. Further, all lesioned subjects, irrespective of whether or not they initially were aphasic following lesion onset, had greater difficulty spelling than did controls when studied many years after lesion onset. Vargha-Khadem *et al.* reported that all left-lesioned subjects performed marginally worse than right-lesioned or control subjects, with significant deficits apparent for left-lesioned subjects incurring postnatal lesions. All left-lesioned subjects had greater difficulty with low-frequency than with high-frequency words. These investigators also report qualitative data relative to the morphophonemic and impaired phonemic structure in the errors of the left-lesioned patients.

The very limited data reported for mathematical abilities is contradictory. Hecaen (1983) suggests that acalculia is the only major neuropsychological deficit associated with impaired language in left-lesioned children, whereas Kiessling *et al.* (1983) report that math achievement as measured by the WRAT arithmetic subtest is correlated significantly with left-hand function (i.e., lack of right-hemisphere impairment). On the other hand, Vargha-Khadem *et al.* (1983) report that the WISC mental arithmetic subtest does not discriminate among left-lesioned, right-lesioned, and control groups. Clearly, much remains to be learned about all aspects of academic achievement as it relates not only to lesion lateralization, but also to lesion location within a hemisphere.

INTELLIGENCE

The IQ scores of brain-lesioned children have been by far the most extensively reported measure, but they are probably the most questionable data, given that even many of the best available group studies are confounded by inclusion of patients with probable bilateral involvement and patients with seizure disorders. Rather than attempting to disentangle the morass in this literature, we selectively illustrate some major points. Exemplary of even recent studies reporting IQ scores are those of Woods (1980) and Riva and Cazzaniga (1981), who report contradictory findings. For patients sustaining left and right lesions prior to or after 1 year of age, Woods (1980) reported that lesions sustained before 1 year of age to either the right or left hemisphere impaired both VIQ and PIQ below the mean for normal controls. In contrast, after 1 year of age, the effect depended on side of lesion; that is, left lesions impaired both Verbal and Performance IQs, but right lesions impaired PIQ alone. Riva and Cazzaniga (1986) reported that age of lesion onset made no difference and that, regardless of age, early and late right-hemisphere lesions lowered only Performance scores, whereas left-hemisphere lesions lowered both Verbal and Performance scores. The problem in attempting to resolve these contradictory findings is that both investigators included seizure-disordered patients and other patients with etiologies suggestive of bilateral involvement.

Annett (1973) addressed some of these variables related to IQ differences in an extensive study of left and right hemiplegic children with particular reference to familial history of sinistrality and motor performance of both hands. Earlier reports of Full Scale IQs for right and left hemiplegic children suggested that the mean Full Scale IQs for right and left hemiplegic children are really very close, although the right hemiplegics (i.e., left-lesioned children) perform slightly less well than do the left hemiplegics.

Annett (1973) also examined several variables related to Full Scale IQ in her group and reported:

1. No evidence of selective impairment associated with side of hemiplegia
2. A significant inverse correlation between physical disability and IQ, in part at least secondary to limitations in motor manipulation and most probably due to greater incidence of bilateral involvement
3. A marked drop in IQ, especially Performance IQ, when the nonhemiplegic hand was impaired (evidence of bilateral involvement)
4. Association between low IQ and recurrent epilepsy
5. An interaction between age, etiology, and IQ, with hemiplegia sustained early during the postnatal period being associated with the lowest IQs.

The conclusion is that it is essentially impossible to reconcile differences among the reports of IQ and lesions when all these variables are present. Furthermore, it will probably be more productive to look at lesioned children's performance on specific linguistic, spatial–perceptual, memory, and other neuropsychological tasks than to dwell on results of more global IQ measures.

Authors' Work in Progress

Considering our own work, we will review our findings relative to language abilities, especially syntax. Our work is a longitudinal study of children with unilateral brain lesions, initially focusing on syntax but more recently becoming broader in scope. In the first phase of the study we studied only children with congenital heart disorders who had incurred a unilateral infarction secondary to cardiac catheterization or surgery. Currently we have expanded the study to include a broader group of children with unilateral lesions, so that we now have a group of 22 left-lesioned children and 15 right-lesioned children. Because the work with this larger group is currently in progress, here we will report data only from the original 8 left- and 8 right-lesioned children.

Subjects were identified from a review of approximately 1,400 charts of children 10 years or younger who underwent a cardiac catheterization at Rainbow Babies and Childrens Hospital in Cleveland, Ohio, within the 5 years preceding the onset of the study (1976–1981). The chart review served two main purposes: (1) to identify all children who experienced neurological complications suggestive of unilateral lesions following cardiac catheterization or subsequent surgery, and (2) to obtain identifying data for the noncomplicated cardiac patients that would serve as a means for selecting control subjects. From this chart review, 51 living children with neurological complications following catheterization or subsequent surgery were identified. Of these 51 children, all but 16 were excluded for the following reasons: 7 for preexisting abnormal neurological, genetic, or developmental problems; 22 because of clinical and/or CT-scan evidence of bilateral hemisphere involvement; 4 because of the nonavailability of technically acceptable CT scans; 2 because of a questionable relationship between unilateral symptoms and catheterization or surgery.

The 16 children retained in the study all had available: (1) clinical neurological examinations indicating unilateral findings alone; (2) CT scan confirmation of the unilateral nature of their acquired lesions; (3) evidence of normal neurological, genetic, and developmental status prior to the lesion onset; and (4) parental consent to participate in the longitudinal study. Particular care was given to excluding patients with bilateral involvement, including seizure disorders. It should be noted that for one of these children, RS3, an EEG was taken after the initial studies were completed, revealed spike activity in the left as well as the right temporal lobe and therefore he has been excluded from further studies. Although the exclusion criteria reduced the number of children available for study, those retained comprise a rigorously selected group with respect to the unilaterality of their lesions.

All subjects were children with congenital heart disorders; therefore, controls were selected from the 1,400 charts of cardiac patients reviewed. Controls were chosen on the basis of chronological age, sex, and race. An attempt was also made to match by severity of heart disorder, degree of cyanosis present, number of hospitalizations required, and socioeconomic status, although it was not possible to control these variables as rigorously as age, sex, and race. No subject or control was from a bilingual home, although one right and one left subject–control pair were raised in homes where Black English is spoken. Further, children were not selected as controls and were excluded as subjects if there was evidence in the chart of preexisting neurological, genetic, or developmental disorders, or pre- or perinatal complications beyond the congenital heart disorder.

Table 15-3 summarizes age at lesion onset, age at testing, and neurological findings for the lesioned subjects. Of particular importance to the present study was the fact that at initial testing, all but two subject–control pairs were 5 years of age or younger (left subject–control pairs 7 and 8), with over half of the children 3 years of age or younger. Consequently, only two subject–control pairs could be assessed for academic achievement, since the remaining children were younger than school age. Six of the 8 left-lesioned subjects incurred lesions during the first 6 months of life, and 4 of the 8 right subjects did so during the first year. Thus, the majority of subjects acquired lesions very early in life,

Table 15-3. Neurological Status for Subjects with Left and Right Lesions

Subject	Age at onset (yr.–mo.)	Age at exam (yr.)	Hemiparesis[a]				Spasticity[a]		Relative hyper-reflexia[a]		Hand preference	Days post onset	CT scan findings	
			Side	Face	Arm	Leg	Arm	Leg	Arm	Leg			Hemi-sphere involved	Lesion location[b]
Left lesions														
LS1	5	2.00	R	3	3	2	2	0	2	2	L	2	L	Pre- and retrorolandic with basal ganglia
LS2	6	3.13	R	0	2	1	1	0	2	1	L	40	L	Small pre- and retrorolandic without basal ganglia
LS3	2	3.08	R	0	2	0	1	1	2	1	L	4	L	Extensive pre- and retrorolandic without basal ganglia
LS4	4	3.92	R	0	2	1	1	0	2	1	L	2	L	Extensive pre- and retrorolandic without basal ganglia
LS5	1	4.30	0	0	0	0	0	0	0	0	L	2	L	Retrorolandic without basal ganglia
LS6	3	5.37	R	0	1	0	0	1	0	0	R	417	L	Small pre- and retrorolandic without basal ganglia
LS7	2–0	6.16	R	1	2	0	2	0	1	0	L	2	L	Retrorolandic without basal ganglia
LS8	6–2	8.15	R	1	3	2	2	1	3	2	L	738	L	Pre- and retrorolandic with basal ganglia
Right lesions														
RS1	2	1.67	L	0	2	0	N	N	0	0	R	179	R	Small pre- and retrorolandic without basal ganglia
RS2	1–5	2.52	L	1	1	0	1	0	0	0	R	3	R	Prerolandic without basal ganglia
RS3	4	2.68	L	1	3	1	2	1	2	0	R	2	R	Extensive pre- and retrorolandic without basal ganglia
RS4	9	3.19	L	1	1	0	0	0	1	0	R	1	R	Prerolandic without basal ganglia
RS5	3–1	4.37	L	1	1	2	1	2	2	2	R	11	R	Prerolandic without basal ganglia
RS6	2–9	5.05	L	0	1	2	1	2	0	2	R	431	R	Subcortical with basal ganglia
RS7	2–4	5.59	L	1	2	1	0	0	1	2	R	278	R	Atypical: Increased sulci in distribution of right middle cerebral artery
RS8	7	5.82	0	0	0	0	0	0	0	0	R	3	R	Prerolandic without basal ganglia

[a] 0 = none detectable; 1 = mild; 2 = moderate; 3 = severe; N = missing data.
[b] Using Brunner's classification (1981).

resulting in little variability among subjects in age at lesion onset. All subjects were neurologically stable, with one or more years elapsing between onset of lesion and testing. All subjects and their controls were seen for initial testing during the fall of 1982 and winter of 1983. The testing consisted of: (1) clinical neurological examination by a pediatric neurologist, who also coded all CT-scan findings; and (2) language, cognitive, and academic testing.

At the time of initial testing, the 8 left- and 8 right-hemisphere-lesioned children and their matched controls were between 18 months and 8 years of age. Both left- and right-lesioned subjects were found to have lower IQ scores than their controls, yet most functioned within the normal range or higher. For children old enough to obtain comparative Verbal and Performance IQ estimates, discrepancies between Verbal and Performance scores did not distinguish between right- and left-lesioned subjects.

Language testing revealed that lexical comprehension and production were impaired in both subject groups when compared to their matched controls, yet appeared to be more impaired in right-lesioned subjects than in lefts. These findings, however, were somewhat equivocal and at least in part appear to reflect the relatively gross measures used to estimate lexical comprehension (Peabody Picture Vocabulary Test) and lexical production (Expressive One-Word Picture Vocabulary Test). Syntactic expression, on the other hand, was markedly deficient for left-lesioned subjects, despite the fact that left-lesioned subjects had slightly higher intelligence scores than did right subjects. Syntactic comprehension did not reveal definitive differences between left and right subjects and their controls, although this may in part be a function of the children's young age and their inability to perform more sensitive tasks of syntactic comprehension. For example, although the Token Test for Children was administered to all children 3 years and older, 8 children could not complete the test, because of failure to indicate color and shape reliably.

Spontaneously elicited spoken language samples were analyzed from each subject and control child. Comparisons were made between subjects and their controls and between left and right subject–control difference scores on a series of measures of overall sentence accuracy and simple and complex sentence structures. Results summarizing these findings are presented in Table 15-4. Significant results emerged for the majority of syntactic measures for left subject–control groups; in contrast, right subject–control groups differed on few syntactic measures. Left subjects, when compared to their controls, (1) produced shorter mean length of utterances (MLUs); (2) had lower overall DSS scores; (3) had a lower percentage of total sentences correct; (4) attempted more simple sentences and produced a greater number of simple sentences in error; (5) produced a fewer number of main verbs, interrogative reversals, and wh-questions, with their productions being developmentally less mature; (6) produced fewer grammatical marker attempts per sentence and a greater number of grammatical marker errors; (8) produced fewer sentences containing conjunctions or embeddings and produced a greater percentage of complex sentences in error; and (9) produced fewer embedded clause types and produced more errors in sentences containing embedded clauses.

Right subjects, when compared with their controls, (1) produced shorter MLUs; (2) had a greater number of simple sentence constructions in error; (3) produced fewer main verbs, although developmental level was comparable; (4) produced developmentally less mature negative forms; and (5) produced more grammatical marker errors, although the number of grammatical marker attempts per sentence was comparable.

When comparing left and right subjects in terms of subject–control difference scores, difficulties in syntactic production emerged that differentiated these two groups. Differences between subject and control MLUs were greater for lefts than for rights. Left subjects

Table 15-4. Summary of Syntactic Findings

	Left subjects/ left controls[a]	Right subjects/ right controls[a]	Left subject/control differences/ right subject/control differences[b]
Overall sentences			
MLU	*	*	*
DSS	*	NS	NS
% total sentences correct	*	*	NS
Simple sentences			
% attempted	*	NS	NS
% correct	*	*	NS
DSS			
Pronouns			
Mean	NS	NS	NS
Total	NS	NS	NS
Main verb			
Mean	*	NS	NS
Total	*	*	NS
Interrogative reversals			
Mean	*	NS	NS
Total	*	NS	*
Wh-questions			
Mean	*	NS	*
Total	*	NS	NS
Negatives			
Mean	*	*	NS
Total	NS	NS	NS
GMN	*	NS	NS
GME	*	*	NS
Complex sentences			
% attempted	*	NS	*
% correct	*	NS	*
Embedding			
Number	*	NS	*
% correct	*	NS	*
Conjunctions			
Number	NS	NS	NS
% corrrect	NS	NS	NS

* = Significant at or beyond the .05 level.
NS = Not significant.
[a] = Randomized Test for Matched Pairs.
[b] = Mann Whitney U Test.

also produced fewer wh-questions and interrogative reversals than did right subjects, with developmental levels of production being lower for left than right subjects for wh-questions. Lefts produced significantly fewer complex sentences and had a greater percentage of complex sentences in error than rights. Lefts produced significantly fewer embedded clause types than rights and produced a greater percentage of errors in sentences containing an embedded clause.

This study demonstrated that for virtually all measures of spoken syntax, left subjects performed less well than did their matched controls. Although they attempted to use a greater percentage of simple sentences than did their controls, this simply reflects the fact that, being developmentally less able than their controls, they were using proportionately fewer complex sentences. On several measures of simple sentence structures, right subjects, compared to their controls, also were less competent. Although right subjects typically attempted to use as many structures as did their controls, they made more errors, especially in simple sentences and in use of grammatic markers. Their ability to handle complex sentences, including embeddings and conjunctions, however, was comparable to their controls.

SUMMARY

One approach to the question of an asymmetrical hemispheric contribution to cognitive development is to assess functional impairments following early brain damage. Until fairly recently, however, much of the literature on the cognitive sequelae of early lesions to one or the other hemisphere has suffered from a variety of shortcomings, making it difficult to draw clear conclusions. Most of the published studies are confounded by the inclusion of subjects with bilateral involvement and/or seizure disorders; many fail to report systematic measures of the function being studied; many do not provide suitable long-term follow-up data, making it difficult to distinguish between delayed development and permanent impairment; and most have failed to provide appropriate control subjects. Focusing on more recent research, which avoids some, if not all, of these problems, it is reasonable to conclude that early left- and early right-hemisphere lesions are not comparable in their cognitive sequelae.

It is reasonable to conclude that early right-hemisphere lesions may produce some spatial deficits, such as in grouping, but tests like the Raven's Progressive Matrices seem to be equally affected (or not affected, as the case may be) by early lesions on either side. Not surprisingly, auditory processing is compromised in the ear contralateral to the side of lesion; however, results of auditory immediate memory studies (digit span) do not suggest a lateralized effect. Auditory verbal memory (paired associate learning) is affected by early left-hemisphere lesions. Reading and spelling are more likely to be impaired by early left-hemisphere lesions than by right. Some language measures, such as lexical comprehension and production, are equally affected by early lesions on either side; other language measures, such as syntactic production, are markedly asymmetrically affected (early left-hemisphere lesions). Subjects with early left lesions produced syntactically simpler output (fewer complex sentences) that exhibited many more syntactic errors, than those produced by their controls and by early right-lesioned subjects.

Asymmetrical functions of the hemispheres in the adult are no longer debatable, but one may still ask whether this known brain asymmetry is present early in development or acquired later. The evidence reviewed in this chapter clearly implies that functional asymmetries are present from the earliest measureable point in time. This evidence also suggests that there likely are permanent residua from early brain damage; recovery is probably not complete. However, a proper long-term follow-up study, into adult age, has not yet been done; thus the delay hypothesis must remain an option. There remains much to be done in studying the differential cognitive and linguistic capacities of the left and right hemispheres. Investigating the consequences of unilateral brain lesions in children is one of the most appropriate methods for studying this question. It can proceed meaningfully only if subjects are carefully selected and compared to proper controls with a set of systematic and explicit functional measures.

ACKNOWLEDGMENT

Preparation of this chapter was supported in part by National Institute of Health Grant #NS17366 to the first author (D.M.A.).

REFERENCES

Aicardi, J., Amsili, J., & Chevrie, J. J. (1969). Acute hemiplegia in infancy and childhood. *Developmental Medicine and Child Neurology, 11,* 162–173.

Alajouanine, T., & Lhermitte, F. (1965). Acquired aphasia in children. *Brain, 88,* 653–662.

Annett, M. (1973). Laterality of childhood hemiplegia and the growth of speech and intelligence. *Cortex, 9,* 4–33.

Aram, D. M., Ekelman, B. L., Rose, D. F., & Whitaker, H. A. (1985). Verbal and cognitive sequelae following unilateral lesions acquired in early childhood. *Journal of Clinical and Experimental Neuropsychology, 7,* 55–78.

Aram, D. M., Ekelman, B. L., & Satz, P. (1986). Trophic changes following early unilateral lesions. *Developmental Medicine and Child Neurology, 28,* 165–170.

Aram, D. M., Ekelman, B. L., & Whitaker, H. A. (1986). Spoken syntax in children with acquired hemisphere lesions. *Brain and Language, 27,* 75–100.

Aram, D. M., Rose, D. F., Rekate, H. L., & Whitaker, H. A. (1983). Acquired capsular/striatal aphasia in childhood. *Archives of Neurology, 40,* 614–617.

Basser, L. S. (1962). Hemiplegia of early onset and the faculty of speech with special reference to the effects of hemispherectomy, *Brain, 85,* 427–460.

Byers, R. K., & McLean, W. T. (1962). Etiology and course of certain hemiplegias with aphasia in childhood. *Pediatrics, 29,* 376–383.

Cotard, J. (1868). Etude sur l'atrophie cérébrale. Thèse pour le doctorat en Medecine. Paris: A. Parent.

Cooper, J. A. (1982). *Residual impairments in children with a history of acquired aphasia.* Unpublished doctoral dissertation, University of Washington, Seattle.

Day, P. S., & Ulatowska, H. K. (1979). Perceptual, cognitive, and linguistic development after early hemispherectomy: Two case studies. *Brain and Language, 7,* 17–33.

Dennis, M. (1980a). Capacity and strategy for syntactic comprehension after left or right hemidecortication. *Brain and Language, 10,* 287–307.

Dennis, M. (1980b). Strokes in childhood: Communicative intent, expression and comprehension after left hemisphere arteriopathy in a right-handed nine-year-old. In R. W. Rieber (Ed.), *Language development and aphasia in children* (pp. 45–67). New York: Academic Press.

Dennis, M., & Kohn, B. (1975). Comprehension of syntax in infantile hemiplegics after cerebral hemidecortication: Left hemisphere superiority. *Brain and Language, 2,* 472–482.

Dennis, M., Lovett, M., & Wiegel-Crump, C. A. (1981). Written language acquisition after left or right hemidecortication in infancy. *Brain and Language, 12,* 54–91.

Dennis, M., & Whitaker, H. A. (1976). Language acquisition following hemidecortication: Linguistic superiority of the left over the right hemisphere. *Brain and Language, 3,* 404–433.

Dennis, M., & Whitaker, H. A. (1977). Hemispheric equipotentiality and language acquisition. In S. J. Segalowitz & F. A. Gruber (Eds.), *Language development and neurological theory* (pp. 93–106). New York: Academic Press.

Ferro, J. M., Martins, I. P., Pinto, F., & Castro-Caldas, A. (1982). Aphasia following right striato-insular infarction in a left-handed child: A clinico-radiological study. *Developmental Medicine and Child Neurology, 24,* 173–182.

Ferro, J. M., Martins, I. P., & Tavora, L. (1984). Neglect in children. *Annals of Neurology, 15,* 281–284.

Guttmann, E. (1942). Aphasia in children. *Brain, 65,* 205–219.

Hammil, D., & Irwin, O. C. (1966). IQ differences of right and left spastic hemiplegic children. *Perceptual Motor Skills, 22,* 193–194.

Hécaen, H. (1976). Acquired aphasia in children and the ontogenesis of hemispheric functional specialization. *Brain and Language, 3,* 114–134.

Hécaen, H. (1983). Acquired aphasia in children: Revisited. *Neuropsychologia, 21,* 581–587.

Hécaen, H., & Albert, M. L. (1978). *Human neuropsychology.* New York: Wiley.

Hood, P. N., & Perlstein, M. A. (1955). Infantile spastic hemiplegia: II. Laterality of involvement. *American Journal of Physical Medicine, 34,* 457–466.

Jabbour, J. T., & Lundervold, A. (1963). Hemiplegia: A clinical and electro-encephalographic study in childhood. *Developmental Medicine and Child Neurology, 5,* 24–31.

Kershner, J. R., & King, A. J. (1974). *Perceptual and Motor Skills, 39,* 1283–1289.

Kiessling, L. S., Denckla, M. B., & Carlton, M. (1983). Evidence for differential hemispheric function in children with hemiplegic cerebral palsy. *Developmental Medicine and Child Neurology, 25,* 727–734.

Kohn, B., & Dennis, M. (1974). Selective impairments of visuo-spatial abilities in infantile hemiplegics after right cerebral hemidecortication. *Neuropsychologia, 12,* 505–512.

Martins, I. P., Ferro, J. M., & Trindade, A. (1984, June). *Acquired crossed aphasia in a child.* Paper presented at the meeting of the International Neuropsychology Society, Aachem, Germany.

Milner, B. (1973). Discussion of "Early onset of complimentary specialization of cerebral hemispheres in man." *Transactions of American Neurological Association, 98,* 115–117.

Nass, R. D., Sadler, A. E., & Sidtis, J. J. (1984). Differential effects of congenital right and left hemisphere injury on dichotic tests of specialized auditory function. *Annals of Neurology, 16,* 388.

Oelschlaeger, M. L., & Scarborough, J. (1976). Traumatic aphasia in children: A case study. *Journal of Communication Disorders, 9,* 281–288.

Perlstein, M. A., & Hood, P. N. (1957). Infantile spastic hemiplegia: Intelligence and age of walking and talking. *American Journal of Mental Deficiency, 61,* 534–542.

Pohl, P. (1979). Dichotic listening in a child recovering from acquired aphasia. *Brain and Language, 8,* 372–379.

Rankin, J. M., Aram, D. M., & Horwitz, S. J. (1981). Language ability in right and left hemiplegic children. *Brain and Language, 12,* 292–306.

Riva, D., & Cazzaniga, L. (1986). Late effects of unilateral brain lesions before and after the first year of age. *Neuropsychologia, 24,* 423–428.

Rudel, G. R., & Denckla, M. B. (1974). Relation of forward and backward digit span to neurological impairment in children with learning disabilities. *Neuropsychologia, 12,* 109–118.

Stiles-Davis, J., Sugarman, S., & Nass, R. (1985). The development of spatial and class relations in four young children with right cerebral hemisphere damage: Evidence for an early spatial–constructive deficit. *Brain and Cognition, 4,* 388–412.

Vargha-Khadem, F., Frith, U., O'Gorman, A. M., & Watters, G. V. (1983, June). *Learning disabilities in children with unilateral brain damage.* Paper presented at the meeting of the International Neuropsychological Society, Lisbon, Portugal.

Vargha-Khadem, F., O'Gorman, A. M., & Watters, G. V. (1985). Aphasia and handedness in relation to hemispheric side, age at injury and severity of cerebral lesion during childhood. *Brain, 108,* 677–696.

Visch-Brink, E. G., & Van de Sandt-Koenderman, N. (1984). The occurrence of paraphasias in the spontaneous speech of children with an acquired aphasia. *Brain and Language, 23,* 258–271.

Woods, B. T. (1980). The restricted effects of right-hemisphere lesions after age one: Wechsler test data. *Neuropsychologia, 18,* 65–70.

Woods, B. T., & Carey, S. (1979). Language deficits after apparent clinical recovery from childhood aphasia. *Annals of Neurology, 6,* 405–409.

Woods, B. T., & Teuber, H. L. (1973). Early onset of complementary specialization of cerebral hemispheres in man. *Transactions of American Neurological Association, 98,* 113–117.

Woods, B. T., & Teuber, H. L. (1978). Changing patterns of childhood aphasia. *Annals of Neurology, 3,* 273–280.

Yeni-Komshian, G. H. (1977, April). *Speech perception in brain injured children.* Paper presented at the Conference on the Biological Bases of Delayed Language Development, New York.

16

Cerebral Lateralization in Autism: Clues to Its Role in Language and Affective Development

GERALDINE DAWSON
University of Washington

It is well recognized by now that the syndrome of early infantile autism, described by Kanner in 1943, is a severe and chronic developmental disability of neurological origin. Autism affects several basic areas of functioning, including language comprehension and expression, and social and affective behavior. Autistic symptoms include social aloofness or indifference, severe receptive and expressive language impairments, stereotyped mannerisms and ritualistic traits, and onset before 30 months (Rutter, 1978). Developmental outcome in autism varies widely. Fifty percent of autistic individuals remain mute their entire lives, but approximately 25% eventually are able to master the formal aspects of language expression, although their social usage remains awkward (Baltaxe & Simmons, 1975; Fish, Shapiro, & Campbell, 1966; Rutter, 1974; Simmons & Baltaxe, 1975; Wolff & Chess, 1965). There is less variability in outcome in the social realm. Some remain aloof and uninterested in social relationships, whereas the better adapted individuals may desire social relationships but are at a loss in knowing how to form and sustain them. There are few, if any, instances of marriage by autistic individuals, although approximately 25% are self-sufficient and have normal intelligence (DeMyer *et al.*, 1974). It is not known whether the persistence of social disabilities in autism reflects their primacy in the disorder, or the lack of adequate therapies in this realm. Given that, until recently, therapies with autistic children have tended to focus on language rather than social behavior, the latter explanation is plausible.

The etiological basis of autism is also varied. Autism has been associated with prenatal risk factors (Gillberg & Gillberg, 1983; Knobloch & Pasamanick, 1975; Lobascher, Kingerlee, & Gubbay, 1970) and genetic background (Folstein & Rutter, 1977). Autism and autistic-like behavior have been associated with central nervous system (CNS) viral infection (Chess, 1971), neonatal conditions such as retrolental fibroplasia (Keeler, 1958), tuberous sclerosis (Lotter, 1974), congenital syphilis (Rutter, Greenfield, & Lockyer, 1967), infantile seizures (Creak, 1963; Kolvin, Ounsted, & Roth, 1971; Taft & Cohen, 1971), metabolic disturbances (Knobloch & Pasamanick, 1975), and widespread neurolipidosis (Creak, 1963). Similarly, there is significant variability across autistic individuals in neurological findings, which include neurological soft signs, abnormal electroencephalograms (EEGs), atypical cerebral lateralization, and seizures (e.g., Creak & Pampiglione, 1969; Dawson, Finley, Phillips, & Galpert, 1986; Gubbay, Lobascher, & Kingerlee, 1970; Kolvin *et al.*, 1971; Rutter, Greenfeld, & Lockyer, 1967; Small, 1975).

The focus of this chapter is on studies of cerebral lateralization in autism. Several questions regarding the specific role of abnormal hemispheric functioning in autism will be raised. To what extent are the impairments of autistic children related to abnormal hemispheric functioning? What are possible reasons for the relatively high frequency of abnormal cerebral lateralization in autistic populations? What implications does information about cerebral lateralization have for clinical intervention with autistic children? In addition, a number of interpretive problems found in studies of cerebral lateralization with autistic individuals will be described, and some suggestions for alleviating them will be offered.

HEMISPHERE FUNCTIONING IN AUTISM: A REVIEW OF THE EVIDENCE

Behavioral Profile

Although significant variability in the cognitive and language skills of autistic persons exists, one commonly found profile is adequate to superior right-hemisphere skills, such as visuospatial abilities, along with impoverished left-hemisphere skills, including language, gestural communication, and other symbolic abilities (Dawson, 1983; Hoffman & Prior, 1982; Lockyer & Rutter, 1970). To illustrate, in Figure 16-1, the mean subtest scores from the Block Design, Object Assembly, Verbal Comprehension, and Vocabulary subtests from the Wechsler Scale are shown for four groups: (1) 10 autistic individuals of varying IQ; (2) a subgroup of 7 autistic individuals with IQ below 70; (3) 10 mentally retarded individuals (matched to Group 1 on IQ, chronological age, and handedness); and 10 persons with verifiable bilateral or diffuse brain damage (matched to Group 1 on chronological age). This discrepancy in skill level across domains also has been found in a number of studies of the sensorimotor skills of young autistic children (Dawson & Adams, 1983; Riquet, Taylor, Benaroya, & Klein, 1981; Sigman & Ungerer, 1984). For example, in one study by Dawson and Adams (1984), it was found that most preschool-age autistic children had adequate object permanence ability (a skill requiring visuospatial memory) but were severely deficient in language and gestural imitation ability. Thus, autistic persons may have adequate visuospatial skills, but, at least during the first several years of life, language, gestural communication, and social abilities are universally impaired.

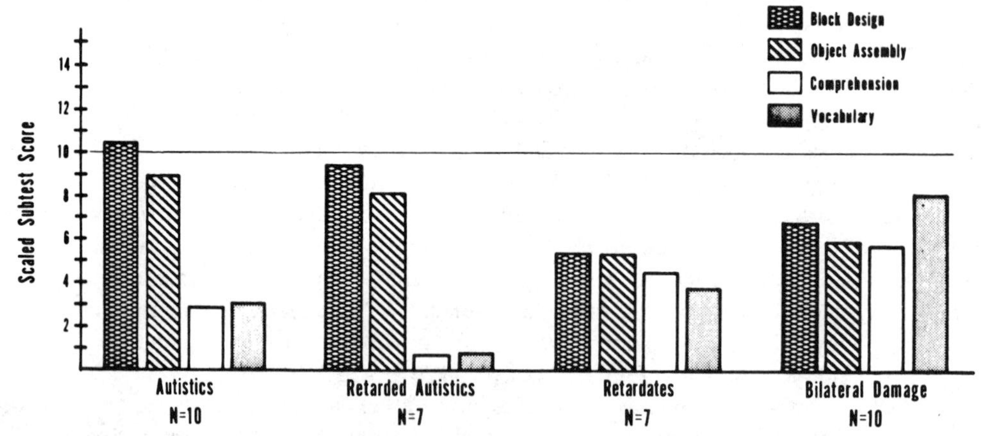

Figure 16-1. Mean scaled scores for selected spatial (Block Design and Object Assembly) and verbal (Comprehension and Vocabulary) subtests from the Wechsler Intelligence Scales. Reprinted by permission from "Lateralized Brain Dysfunction in Autism: Evidence from the Halstead-Reitan Neuropsychological Battery" by G. Dawson, 1983, *Journal of Autism and Developmental Disorders, 13,* pp. 269–286.

At least two studies have systematically assessed left- and right-hemisphere-related skills in autistic individuals. Dawson (1983) administered part of the Halstead-Reitan Neuropsychological Battery to a group of 10 autistic subjects and compared their performance to age-, handedness-, and IQ-matched mentally retarded subjects, as well as to age-matched patients with demonstrable diffuse or bilateral brain damage. Based on tests that measured perceptual and sensorimotor functioning on the right and left sides of the body, it was found that the autistic group exhibited significantly greater left- than right-hemisphere dysfunction. Moreover, autistic subjects showed significantly greater left-hemisphere impairment than did mentally retarded individuals. Mentally retarded subjects showed a more even pattern of hemisphere impairment, whereas the patients with bilateral damage showed a slight elevation in right-hemisphere impairment. An examination of individual autistic subjects' protocols revealed that 5 subjects exhibited primarily left-hemisphere (right-sided) dysfunction, 4 exhibited significant bilateral involvement, and 1 showed mild and primarily right-hemisphere impairment. Based on the subjects' Verbal IQ scores on the Wechsler Intelligence Scale, it was found that language ability was significantly related to degree of left- but not of right-hemisphere impairment. Performance IQ was not related to left-hemisphere impairment.

Hoffman and Prior (1982) administered a neuropsychological battery that included tasks that measured either left- or right-hemisphere functions to 10 autistic individuals. It was found that the autistic group performed significantly worse than chronological age (CA)–matched, but not mental age (MA)–matched, control subjects on "left-hemisphere" tasks, which typically involved either verbal or nonverbal sequential processing. In contrast to MA-matched control subjects, however, autistic subjects performed at chronological age level on "right-hemisphere" tasks, which involved visuospatial processing.

Handedness

Several studies have found an increased incidence of non-right-handedness among autistic individuals. In a study comparing young autistic and normal subjects, Colby and Parkinson (1977) found that 65% of the autistic group was non-right-handed (compared to 12% of the normal CA-matched group). They did not differentiate between left-handed and mixed-handed children. Barry and James (1978) did not find significant differences in the distributions of handedness (right-, left-, and mixed-) among autistic, normal CA-matched, and mentally retarded IQ-matched groups. They noted, however, that the autistic group, as a whole, showed significantly more variability in degree of hand dominance compared to mentally retarded and normal groups. In addition, they found some evidence for a developmental trend toward greater dominance with age in the autistic group. This developmental trend was not found in two other studies (Boucher, 1977; Tsai, 1983).

Boucher found no difference in the distributions of handedness of autistic and language-matched normal subjects. When older autistic subjects were analyzed separately, slightly higher frequencies of left-handedness (9% versus 2%) and mixed-handedness (39% versus 32%) were found in the autistic group. Boucher concluded from this that non-right-handedness is a persistent characteristic of the autistic population. Unfortunately, the small number of subjects in this study prevents any firm conclusion. In a sample of 70 autistic persons of a wide age range (2 to 13 years), Tsai found little evidence of a relationship between age and hand dominance. He reported that a high percentage of subjects exhibited mixed hand dominance—54%, as compared with Annett's (1967) finding of 37% in a sample of 5- to 15-year-old normal children. Also, subjects with mixed-handedness tended to be the most developmentally impaired.

Fein, Humes, Kaplan, Lucci, and Waterhouse (1984) evaluated 75 children who fell in the broad category of Pervasive Developmental Disorders, as well as children with childhood schizophrenia. These authors also found that mixed dominance was associated with lower functioning, but not with age. Thirty percent of their sample exhibited mixed dominance; 13% and 36% exhibited left- and right-handedness, respectively. The percentage of non-right-handedness in this sample is slightly lower than that found in others (Soper & Satz, 1984; Tsai, 1983). Perhaps this is because of the heterogeneity of their sample, which was not restricted to autistic children.

Based on a sample of 51 autistic children, Soper and Satz (1984) reported that 40% were right-handed, 20% were left-handed, and 40% showed "ambiguous" handedness (defined as inconsistent hand usage on the same task). The existence of a substantial group of ambiguous-handed subjects required a revision of Satz's original model of pathological left-handedness to include this third anomalous group (see Satz, 1972, 1973, for a description of his statistical model for determining locus of brain dysfunction from handedness patterns). Based on this revision, they demonstrated that, given that a person is both autistic and left-handed, the probability that the *primary* lesion is in the left hemisphere is very high (.95). Furthermore, they argue that the probability that cases of left-handedness and ambiguous handedness are pathological (i.e., have suffered early brain damage) is also high (.83) and virtually certain for ambiguous handedness. According to their model, there is good reason to believe that autism is associated in many cases with bilateral dysfunction, but that in approximately 20% of cases, the primary lesion is in the left hemisphere.

In summary, there is substantial variability in the handedness patterns of autistic individuals. In fact, some autistic persons may show a type of handedness pattern rarely shown in the normal population, that is, ambiguous handedness. Most studies have found that the distribution of handedness patterns for autistic persons differs from that of the normal population; higher frequencies of non-right-handedness are reported for the autistic population. The question of whether handedness pattern is associated with level of impairment and/or locus of brain dysfunction in autism deserves further study.

As in the normal population, the relationship between hand dominance and speech lateralization in the autistic population does not appear to be strong. In two studies that directly measured both hand dominance and hemispheric activation during speech, no relationship between handedness and speech lateralization was found (Dawson, Finley, Phillips, & Galpert, 1986; Dawson, Warrenburg, & Fuller, 1982).

Neuroanatomical Studies

Several studies using CT scans or pneumoencephalograms with autistic children have been reported. The first of these was carried out by Hauser, DeLong, and Rosman (1975). Using pneumoencephalograms, they found pathological enlargement of the left temporal horn in 15 of 18 cases. Some cases were found to have enlargement of both temporal horns, or mild variable enlargement of the lateral ventricles, especially the left. In contrast, Caparulo *et al.* (1981) were unable to find a definite pattern of focal abnormalities. Only 2 of the 22 autistic children in their study showed clearly abnormal CT scans, and these involved increased ventricular size.

Several studies have measured neuroanatomical asymmetries, in addition to evaluating gross structural features. In the first of such studies, Hier, LeMay, and Rosenberger (1979) found that 57% of autistic subjects showed reversed asymmetry in the parietooccipital region (i.e., right wider than left). This was in contrast to comparison groups of mentally retarded subjects and miscellaneous neurological patients in which approximately a quarter showed reversals. Gillberg and Svendsen (1983) found that right occipital enlargement was only marginally more common in autistic subjects than in normal subjects. However, they found that in 10 of their 27 autistic cases, the left frontal horns of the ventricular system was significantly wider than in normal subjects. Similarly, Damasio, Mawrer, Damasio, and Chui (1980) found that only 18% of autistic subjects showed greater right than left width in the occipital region, but that an additional 35% lacked asymmetry in this region. Tsai, Jacoby, and Stewart (1983) also found that autistic children often failed to show clear asymmetry in the parietooccipital and frontal lobes. Although none of the aforementioned studies found gross structural abnormalities to be common among autistic persons, mild but variable enlargement of the ventricles was often reported.

Although CT scanning methods have detected only subtle cortical abnormalities in autistic individuals, recent studies using magnetic resonance imaging techniques suggest that many autistic individuals may have significant subcortical abnormalities. Specifically, Courchesne (in press) found evidence of hypoplasia of vermal lobules VI and VII of the cerebellum in 14 out of 18 autistic subjects examined. These results suggest that, if structural abnormalities are to be implicated in autism, they are likely to be subcortical in nature. The influence of such early subcortical abnormalities on cortical development has yet to be determined.

In summary, the available evidence suggests that only a small percentage of autistic individuals have obvious structural cortical abnormalities. A somewhat higher than expected percentage of autistic persons, however, appear either to have reversed neuroanatomical asymmetry from normal persons or to be lacking in asymmetry. As Geschwind and Galaburda (1985a) have pointed out, it is difficult to make inferences about either the locus of brain damage or functional representation from neuroanatomical asymmetries in developmentally disabled or brain-damaged populations. There is evidence from animal studies that early damage may lead to enlargement of the homologous area on the side opposite the lesion, as well as the *areas adjacent to the lesion* (Goldman, 1978). This enlargement may result from the death of fewer neurons and perhaps larger size of neurons in the intact regions because neurons in the damaged area are no longer competing for synaptic connections. If so, studies of neuroanatomical asymmetries in abnormal populations are not likely to report consistent findings given the likely variability in the effects of early damage on the development of neuroanatomical structure.

Functional Lateralization for Speech and Other Stimuli

Measures of handedness and neuroanatomical asymmetries, though valuable markers of abnormal brain organization and development, will not necessarily be strongly correlated with patterns of functional usage of the hemispheres during language, cognitive, or affective processing. In this section, studies that directly measured speech lateralization in autistic individuals will be reviewed.

DICHOTIC LISTENING

Ear preference tasks have been used in five studies with autistic children. In the first of these, Blackstock (1978) simply observed which ear autistic children preferred for listening to music and verbal passages. Given a choice, autistic children tended to prefer their left ear for both types of stimuli, whereas normal children listened to musical passages more often with the left but to verbal passages with the right ear. A more sophisticated approach was used by Prior and Bradshaw (1979). They presented 19 autistic children and 19 primary school–age normal children with a traditional dichotic listening task that used words for stimuli. The normal group showed the expected right-ear advantage (REA). In contrast, the autistic group showed greater variability with only 5 of the 19 autistic children exhibiting a REA. Seven showed a left-ear advantage (LEA), and 7 showed no preference. Lateralized autistic subjects were more likely to have had speech before 5 years of age, as indicated by their medical histories. Wetherby, Koegel, and Mendel (1981) reported similar findings. When words were used as stimuli in a dichotic listening task with 6 autistic individuals of a wide age range, 3 subjects exhibited a REA, 2 showed a LEA, and 1 showed no preference. Interestingly, 1 subject, who was followed longitudinally, showed a decrease in degree of LEA as his language abilities increased. Hoffman and Prior (1982) also administered a dichotic listening task to 10 autistic individuals who, as a group, were found to exhibit a significant LEA. However, normal controls also showed a LEA, which compromises these results. Individual data were not reported. Finally, Arnold and Schwartz (1983) used a variation on the traditional dichotic listening task with 8 autistic children. In this task, CV sounds were presented dichotically with a separation of 50 milliseconds, and children were asked to "Point to the ear you heard the sound in first." Seven of the 8 autistic children pointed more often to their right ear. It is difficult to judge how the unusual presentation of stimuli and more complex verbal instructions may have influenced results.

In summary, to date, there have been five studies using ear preference with autistic children. Of these, four studies reported that a substantial number of autistic subjects showed either a LEA or no ear preference. Unfortunately, the strength of these findings is diminished by the small number of subjects in one study and by the failure of the normal control group to show a REA in another study. There was some evidence that degree or direction of lateralization may be associated with language abilities in autistic children. This possibility will be explored more fully in subsequent sections of this chapter. A summary of the studies using ear preference with autistic children is provided in Table 16-1.

ELECTROPHYSIOLOGICAL STUDIES

A variety of electrophysiological techniques have been used to measure hemispheric activity in autistic persons. In the first of these, Small (1975) recorded resting EEG data obtained from 7 autistic children and age- and sex-matched normal controls. EEG activity was recorded from right and left occipital regions. Based on measures of integrated EEG activity, normal children showed significantly higher values on the left side than on the right, whereas the autistic children showed no difference in hemispheric activity. In this same report, Small also examined the relationship between focal EEG abnormalities and behavioral characteristics in a heterogeneous group of children, which included 147 autistic children, 50 mentally retarded children, and 37 children with various psychiatric disorders. Two-thirds of the autistic group showed abnormal EEGs. Based on the total sample, significant correlations were found between generalized, anterior, and/or left-sided abnormalities and lower IQ scores and ratings of speech development. There were no significant associations with right-sided abnormalities. Tanguay (1976) recorded auditory evoked potentials from a group of ten 2- to 5-year-old autistic children and normal controls during sleep. Normal subjects showed hemispheric asymmetry in their evoked potentials during REM (rapid eye movement) sleep, whereas autistic subjects showed no such differences.

In a more recent study by Ogawa and his colleagues (Ogawa *et al.*, 1982), 21 2- to 8-year-old autistic children and 28 CA-matched normal children were studied. During click stimulation, 42% of the normal subjects showed significant hemispheric differences in cu-

Table 16-1. Dichotic Listening Studies of Individuals with Autism

Reference	N	CA	Mean IQ	Diagnosis	Method	Results
Blackstock, 1978	11	$\overline{X}=0.3$ yr	Not given	Autistic (Rutter's criteria)	Speakers placed to right and left of Ss. S had to put ear to speaker to hear stimuli. Stimuli: 3 musical passages, 3 verbal passages	Autistic Ss, as a group, listened to both musical and verbal passages with L ear. Normal Ss listened to musical passages with L ear, verbal passages with R ear.
	7	$\overline{X}=5.4$ yr	Not given	Normal		
Prior & Bradshaw, 1979	19	8–13 yr	PPVT: 68 MA: 3–14 yr	Autistic (Prior's criteria)	Dichotic listening: Words	Normal: Significant group REA Autistic: 5 REA 7 LEA 7 no EA Lateralized autistic Ss more likely to have had speech before 5 years of age.
	19	Primary-school age	PPVT MA: 8 yr	Normal		
Wetherby, Koegel, & Mendel, 1981	6	8–24 yr	Not given	Autistic (NSAC criteria)	Dichotic listening: Words Two language tests (TACL and PPVT)	3 REA 2 LEA 1 no EA One S followed longitudinally; As language improved, LEA decreased.
Hoffman & Prior, 1982	10	$\overline{X}=11$ yr (7–14 yr)	87 (76–109)	Autistic (Rutter's criteria)	Dichotic listening: Words	Both autistic and MA control group showed LEA. CA control group showed REA.
	10	Matched on CA	100 (85–112)	Normal		
	10	Matched on MA (8–10 yr)	107 (97–120)	Normal		
Arnold & Schwartz, 1983	8	6–14 yr	PPVT: 6 yr (3–12 yr)	Autistic (Rimland's Checklist)	Dichotic listening: CVs, presented dichotically with separation of 50 msec. Response: "Point to ear you heard the sound in first."	Autistic: 7 REA 1 LEA Aphasic: 1 REA 6 LEA Normal: 6 REA 0 LEA
	8	7–11 yr	PPVT: 5 yr (3–7 yr)	Aphasic "varied in symptoms" MLU: $X=2.5$		
	8	6–13 yr	Not given	Normal		

mulative EEG activity, whereas no autistic children did so. During flash stimulation, however, 28% of the autistic children showed significant occipital hemispheric differences (compared with 64% of normal children). These results suggest that, for 28% of the autistic children in this sample, abnormal brain functioning was more pronounced for auditory than for visual stimuli.

The first study to use electrophysiological techniques to assess hemispheric activation during language and cognitive processing in autistic individuals was carried out by Dawson, Warrenburg, and Fuller (1982). Measures of right- and left-hemisphere alpha power (8–13 Hz) were used to infer underlying cortical activation. This technique makes use of the well-known finding that alpha attenuation is associated with active information processing. Thus, differential right- and left-hemisphere alpha attenuation can be used as a measure of hemispheric asymmetry during cognitive processing. We measured alpha from right and left parietal lobes during two language tasks, two visuospatial tasks, and a baseline period. Ten autistic individuals ranging from 8 to 34 years of age were tested. Normal subjects were matched for chronological age, sex, handedness, and familial handedness pattern. Results were analyzed in terms of ratios of right- to left-hemisphere alpha; higher ratios indicated relatively greater left-hemisphere activation, lower ratios indicated relatively greater right-hemisphere activation. Normal subjects showed the expected pattern of greater left-hemisphere dominance during speech as compared to spatial tasks. Autistic subjects' pattern of hemispheric asymmetry did not differ significantly from that of normal subjects during spatial tasks. However, they showed significantly greater right-hemisphere dominance during the language tasks than did normal subjects. These data are illustrated in Figure 16-2. Note the high degree of right-hemisphere dominance during the verbal memory task for the autistic subjects. The two groups' patterns were not significantly different from each other during the baseline period. Examination of individual results showed that 7 of the 10 autistic subjects showed greater right-hemisphere dominance (i.e., lower right/left hemisphere alpha ratios) during the language tasks than during the visuospatial tasks.

The alpha-blocking method was also used with this sample of autistic subjects to assess cerebral activation during a series of four motor imitation tasks (two oral static postures, two oral sequential movements, two manual static postures, and two manual sequential movements) (Dawson, Warrenburg, & Fuller, 1983). The tasks were designed such that subjects could not use visual feedback to make accurate imitations of the experimenter but, rather, were required to rely on an internal body representation. Normal subjects exhibited a left-hemisphere dominant pattern of hemispheric activation during all four motor imitation tasks (Dawson, Warrenburg, & Fuller, 1985). Autistic subjects showed greater right-hemisphere activation, in general, than normal subjects on all four tasks. A right-dominant pattern was particularly evident on the oral imitation tasks. In addition, older autistic subjects showed more normal (i.e., more left-dominant) patterns than did younger subjects. No such developmental trend was found in normal subjects.

We (Dawson, Finley, Phillips, & Galpert, 1986) recently completed a study of hemispheric asymmetries using auditory speech-evoked potentials. There were several aims of this study. First, we expanded the ability range and size of the sample in order to assess how representative our findings were of the general autistic population. Second, we chose a technique for measuring lateralization that required no verbal response and minimal attentional capabilities on the part of subjects. The technique had been used to demonstrate hemispheric asymmetries in young infants (Molfese, Freeman, & Palermo, 1975). Finally, we wanted to explore systematically the relationship between patterns of hemispheric acti-

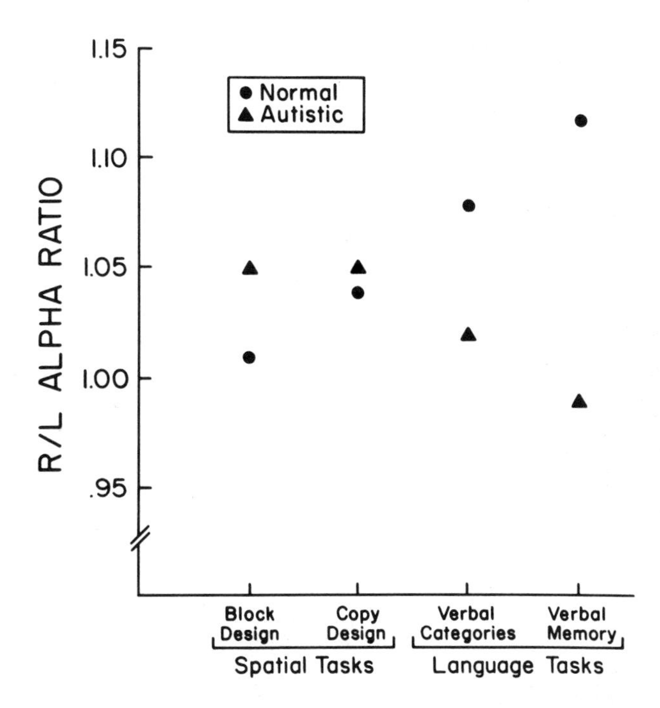

Figure 16-2. Mean R/L alpha ratios obtained during spatial and verbal tasks for autistic and normal control groups. Reprinted by permission from "Cerebral Lateralization in Individuals Diagnosed as Autistic in Early Childhood" by G. Dawson, S. Warrenburg, and P. Fuller, 1982, *Brain and Language, 15,* pp. 353–368.

vation during speech processing and various language abilities of autistic children. In this regard, three alternative hypotheses were tested:

1. Given the evidence from both neuropsychological testing and measures of cerebral dominance that there may exist two subgroups in the autistic population—one with primarily left-sided brain dysfunction and one with bilateral dysfunction—it is possible that the variability in language acquisition may be explained in terms of the compensatory capabilities of the right hemisphere for left-hemisphere dysfunction. That is, individuals with unilateral dysfunction may be superior in language to those with bilateral dysfunction because of the right hemisphere's compensatory capability. If this were true, one would expect that superior language abilities would be found in those autistic individuals who showed *right*-hemisphere dominance for speech.

2. Alternatively, regardless of the possibility of subgroups in autism, such a compensatory mechanism as outlined in hypothesis 1 may not occur in developmentally disabled populations. If so, superior language abilities instead may be directly related to the left hemisphere's capability for language. In this case, superior language should be found in individuals with *left*-hemisphere dominance for speech.

3. Fein *et al.* (1984) have recently argued that autistic children's failure to develop clearly lateralized function is better characterized as an absence or reduction of cerebral dominance for all stimuli. They further suggested that this reduction in cerebral asymmetry reflects a general developmental lag or retardation and not selective left-hemisphere dys-

function. According to this hypothesis, one would predict that poorer language abilities would be associated with a *reduction* or *absence* of cerebral asymmetry for speech.

Seventeen autistic children ranging from 16 to 18 years of age and 17 normal chronological age–matched children were tested. IQ scores for autistic children ranged from 53 to 91. Measures of hemispheric asymmetry were differences in the averaged cortical evoked responses taken from right- and left-hemisphere temporoparietal scalp locations to a linguistic stimulus (''da''). Autistic subjects were administered a comprehensive battery of language tests, which included measures of articulation, syntax, receptive and expressive vocabulary, and verbal comprehension, as well as two measures of visuospatial ability (Block Design and Object Assembly subtests from the Wechsler Intelligence Scale).

Normal subjects showed consistent hemispheric asymmetries in the early components of the evoked response, including the amplitude and latency of N1, and the amplitude of P2 (see Figure 16-3). The autistic and normal groups differed significantly on measures of the direction of hemispheric asymmetry (right minus left differences for N1 amplitude and for N1 latency). Based on the group-averaged evoked potentials, the autistic subjects appeared to show little asymmetry, as can be seen in Figure 16-3. Examination of individual

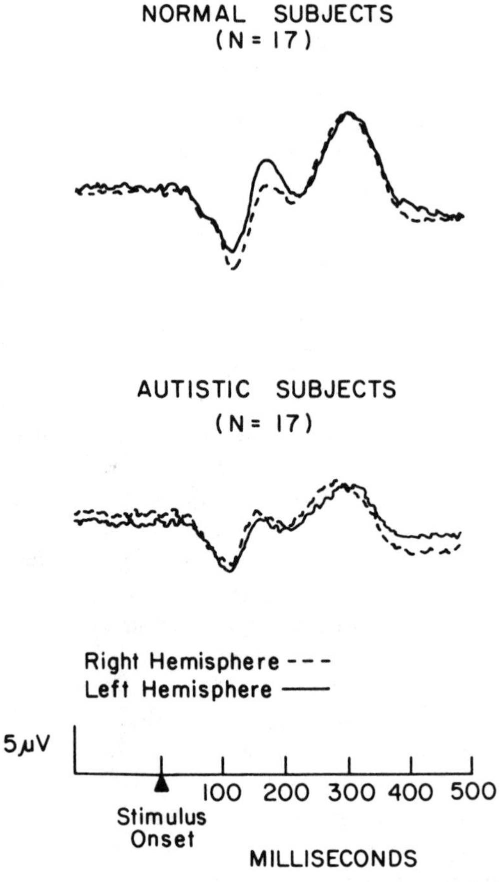

Figure 16-3. The left- and right-hemisphere averaged speech evoked potentials for autistic and normal groups ($N = 17$, each group). (Polarity: Positive is up.) Reprinted by permission from ''Hemispheric Specialization and the Language Abilities of Autistic Children'' by G. Dawson, C. Finley, S. Phillips, and L. Galpert, 1986, *Child Development, 57,* 1440–1453.

Table 16-2. Hemispheric Asymmetries in the Averaged Evoked Responses to Speech

Measure	Absolute degree of asymmetry	Left minus right hemisphere: Entire group	Subjects with reversed asymmetry	Subjects with normal asymmetry
N1 amplitudes				
Autistic *N*	17	17	10	7
Mean	4.34	−1.83	−5.23	3.05
S.D.	4.89	6.36	5.84	3.04
Normal *N*	17	17	5	12
Mean	2.73	2.10	−1.09	3.24
S.D.	2.51	3.09	1.03	2.65
N1 latencies				
Autistic *N*	1	17	11	6
Mean	7.49	2.60	9.53	−6.93
S.D.	6.76	9.91	7.96	3.83
Normal *N*	17	17	6	11
Mean	11.09	−3.29	5.63	−14.06
S.D.	10.93	10.50	2.28	12.68

responses, however, revealed that this was due to the averaging of subjects who showed a reversed direction with those who showed a normal direction of asymmetry. This is supported by data displayed in Table 16-2. Here it is evident that subjects with a reversed direction of asymmetry actually showed greater than normal degrees of asymmetry—more so than either normal subjects or autistic subjects with normal lateralization (−5.23 microvolts versus 3.05 and 3.24 microvolts, respectively). Note also the difference in degree of asymmetry shown between autistic and normal subjects, who exhibited a reversed direction (−5.23 microvolts versus −1.09). Normal subjects with reversed asymmetry showed the least degree of asymmetry, whereas the opposite was true for autistic subjects.

N1 latencies for the right and left hemispheres for normal and autistic subjects are shown in Figure 16-4. Interestingly, normal and autistic subjects' left-hemisphere re-

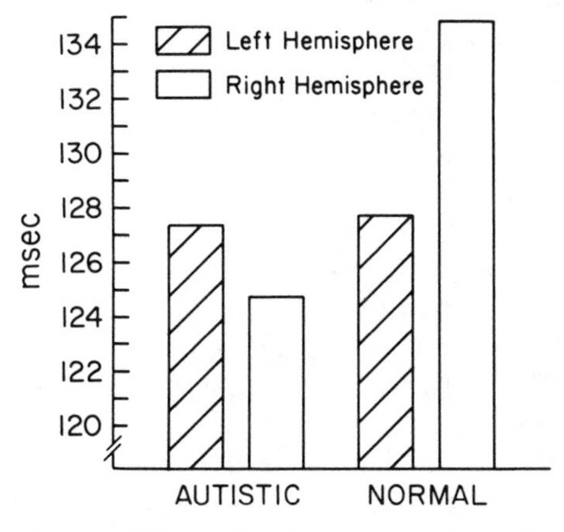

Figure 16.4. Mean N1 latencies in milliseconds of the averaged speech evoked potentials for autistic and normal control groups ($N = 17$, each group). Reprinted by permission from "Hemispheric Specialization and the Language Abilities of Autistic Children" by G. Dawson, C. Finley, S. Phillips, and L. Galpert, 1986, *Child Development, 57,* 1440–1453.

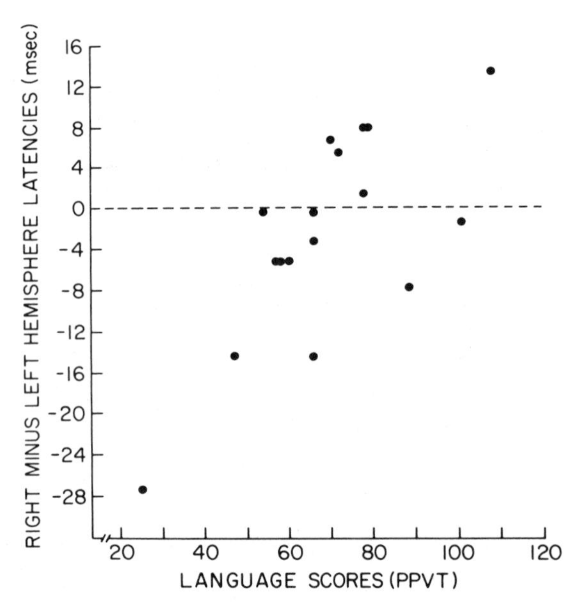

Figure 16-5. Scatter plot displaying individual autistic subjects' scores on the Peabody Picture Vocabulary Test and patterns of hemispheric asymmetry, as measured by right-minus left-hemisphere N1 latencies of the averaged speech evoked potential. Negative latency differences indicate reversed hemispheric asymmetry from normal. Reprinted by permission from "Hemispheric Specialization and the Language Abilities of Autistic Children" by G. Dawson, C. Finley, S. Phillips, and L. Galpert, 1986, *Child Development, 57,* 1440–1453.

sponses did not significantly differ. Rather, it was the right-hemisphere response that significantly differed between autistic and normal subjects.

Correlations between right- minus left-hemisphere asymmetry (based on either N1 amplitude or N1 latency differences) and language abilities indicated that superior language abilities, in almost all measures of language, were associated with a normal (left-dominant) direction of cerebral asymmetry for speech. Poorer language abilities were found in those subjects with both a reversed direction of asymmetry and greater degrees of asymmetry. This relationship is illustrated in Figure 16-5, which is a scatter plot displaying individual autistic subjects' scores on the Peabody Picture Vocabulary Test and patterns of hemispheric asymmetry, as measured by right- minus left-hemisphere N1 latencies. For many of the language abilities, including articulation, receptive and expressive syntactical skills, receptive and expressive vocabulary, and verbal comprehension ability, significant correlations with direction of asymmetry remained after age was partialed out.

Correlations between language abilities and N1 amplitudes carried out separately for each hemisphere yielded interesting results. Language abilities were associated with right-hemisphere amplitudes but were not related to left-hemisphere amplitudes. These correlations are shown in Table 16-3. These data suggest the possibility that deficient language in autism is associated with overactivation of the right hemisphere, which in turn may reflect inadequate left-hemisphere inhibitory mechanisms.

Visuospatial skills were also correlated with direction of hemispheric asymmetry for speech, but only for the N1 latency measure. Improved visuospatial performance was associated with a normal direction of hemispheric asymmetry for speech.

Correlations between chronological age and degree or direction of hemispheric asymmetry were not found for normal subjects. However, age-related changes in hemispheric

Table 16-3. Correlations between N1 Amplitude of the Averaged Evoked Response to the Linguistic Stimulus and Language Abilities for Each Hemisphere

	Hemisphere			
	Right		Left	
Language ability	*r*	*p*	*r*	*p*
Arizona Articulation Test	.43	.08	.01	N.S.
Peabody Picture Vocabulary	.61	.01	.16	N.S.
Northwestern Syntax				
Screening test: Receptive	.46	.05	.19	N.S.
Expressive	.43	.08	.06	N.S.
Wechsler subtests: Vocabulary	.60	.01	.08	N.S.
Comprehension	.61	.01	.21	N.S.
Mean Length of Utterance	.52	.03	.00	N.S.
Length Complexity Index	.55	.03	.12	N.S.

asymmetry were found for autistic subjects. With increasing chronological age, subjects were more likely to exhibit left-hemisphere dominance, for speech. This finding is consistent with previous research showing older autistic subjects to be more likely to show left-hemisphere dominance for motor imitation (Dawson, Warrenburg, & Fuller, 1983).

Returning to the original hypotheses of this study, outlined previously, our results support hypothesis 2. These data suggest that inferior language ability in autism is associated with a greater degree of hemispheric asymmetry favoring the right hemisphere. These results are not consistent with hypothesis 1, which predicted that right-hemisphere speech would be associated with improved language, nor with hypothesis 3, which predicted that inferior language ability would be associated with normal but reduced cerebral asymmetry.

Based on these results, the following two possibilities regarding the relationship between language ability and cerebral lateralization in autism are suggested. First, it is possible that the variability in patterns of hemispheric activation found in autistic populations reflects meaningful subgroups based on underlying neuropathology. According to this idea, one subgroup of autistic individuals with severe left-hemisphere dysfunction relies on the right hemisphere's inadequate language-processing capabilities, which results in both poor language and visuospatial abilities and a highly right-dominant pattern of speech lateralization. It is assumed that a right-hemisphere compensatory mechanism such as has been documented in cases of early left-hemisphere brain trauma is lacking. A second subgroup of autistic individuals suffers from a lesser degree of left-hemisphere dysfunction such that left-hemisphere speech processing is possible and language skills are improved. A third subgroup is also likely. These austistic individuals may show significant bilateral involvement, which may preclude language acquisition altogether. These individuals most likely would be mute (and therefore were not included in the study described earlier) and perhaps would fail to show right- or left-hemisphere lateralization for speech.

A second possibility is that the variability in patterns of cerebral asymmetry for speech in autism may reflect developmental changes in hemispheric processing of language. According to this interpretation, early left-hemisphere dysfunction may lead to an overreliance on the right hemisphere. Given that the autistic child is deprived of social and prelinguistic stimulation early in life by virtue of his or her inability to make sense of and respond to such stimulation, left-hemisphere dysfunction would be exacerbated by the lack of postnatal stimulation. Furthermore, the ability of the autistic child to engage in various object-related activities such as puzzles would only serve to enhance asymmetrical development of the hemispheres favoring the right hemisphere. Thus, by the time the autistic child does begin to use language to communicate (typically around 5 years of age), the child may tend to rely on right-hemisphere strategies to do so, given that these strategies are more mature and functional. As the child develops more communicative language, however, the left hemisphere may begin to take over, given its inherent predisposition for the processing of speech stimuli (see Molfese & Betz, Chapter 6, this volume).

SUMMARY AND DISCUSSION

Taken together, data from the several studies just reviewed indicate that many autistic individuals exhibit an abnormal pattern of hemispheric activation suggestive of left-hemisphere dysfunction. All six electrophysiological studies found significant differences in pattern of hemispheric activity between autistic and comparison groups. In all but two studies, auditory stimuli were used. In the two studies that examined cerebral specialization for visual stimuli, autistic subjects were more likely to show a normal pattern of hemispheric activity. A summary of the electrophysiological studies reviewed is presented in Table 16-4.

The specific role of abnormal hemispheric functioning in autism is unknown, but several hypotheses will be discussed. It is very likely that differences in the degree, nature, and origin of hemispheric dysfunction exist across autistic individuals and that these differences partially account for the variability in patterns of hemispheric activity found in the autistic population. This variability has led some authors to minimize the potential contribution of hemispheric dysfunction to autism (Fein *et al.*, 1984). However, it is quite likely that this variability may be related to severity of behavioral symptoms and developmental outcome. In this light, the variability in the degree and type of dysfunction may allow us to draw more direct conclusions about specific relationships between underlying neural pathology and the behavioral symptoms of autism. Additionally, the variability may reflect developmental influences. It is quite possible that developmental changes in patterns of hemispheric processing occur in individuals who have sensory or perceptual deficits from an early age.

THE ROLE OF ABNORMAL HEMISPHERIC FUNCTIONING IN AUTISM

Left Hemisphere Hypothesis

Several authors (Dawson, 1983; Dawson, Warrenburg, & Fuller, 1982, 1983; Geschwind & Galaburda, 1985a, 1985b, 1985c; Prior & Bradshaw, 1979) have proposed that left-hemisphere pathology plays a central role in autistic symptomatology. It is generally recognized that the underlying cause of left-hemisphere dysfunction likely will vary across individuals given the heterogeneous etiological findings and other accompanying types of brain dysfunction. Cortical dysfunction may be secondary to brain-stem abnormalities (Dawson & Lewy, in press). According to the left-hemisphere hypothesis, however, cortical dysfunction in autism is not diffuse; left-hemisphere functions are more impaired than are right-hemisphere functions.

Even if this hypothesis is correct, it remains unclear whether the abnormal left-hemisphere development arises because of prenatal or postnatal influences. Most likely, the timing of the deleterious influences varies across individuals. One strong proponent of the existence of prenatal influences on cerebral lateralization is Geschwind, who wrote exten-

Table 16-4. Electrophysiological Studies of Lateralization in Individuals with Autism

Reference	*N*	CA	Mean IQ	Diagnosis	Method	Results
Small, 1975	7	Not given	Not given	Autistic (criteria not reported)	Resting EEG recorded from right and left occipital regions	Normal Ss showed higher mean integrated voltage values from LH than from RH. Autistic Ss showed no hemispheric asymmetry.
Tanguay, 1976	10	2–5 yr	Not given	Autistic (DSM-III criteria)	Auditory evoked potentials taken during sleep	Normal Ss showed larger RH than LH potentials during REM. Autistic Ss showed no significant hemispheric differences.
	10	4–5 yr	Not given	Normal		
Ogawa, Sugiyama, Ishiwa, Suzuki, Ishihara, & Sato, 1982	21	2–8 yr	Not given	Autistic (Kranner's criteria), R-handed	EEG activity recorded during click and flash stimulation	During click stimulation, 42% of normal Ss showed significant hemispheric asymmetry, no autistic Ss did so. During flash stimulation, 64% of normal Ss showed hemispheric asymmetry, 28% of autistic Ss did so.
	28	2–8 yr	Not given	Normal R-handed		
Dawson, Warrenburg, & Fuller, 1982	10	9–34 yr	FSIQ: 69 (40–113)	Autistic (Rutter's criteria)	RH and LH parietal alpha taken during 4 cognitive tasks: 2 verbal, 2 spatial	Autistic and normal Ss did not differ during spatial tasks; autistic Ss showed greated RH activation during verbal tasks than normal Ss. 7/10 autistic Ss showed RH dominance during verbal tasks. For autistic Ss only, greater asymmetry related to increases in IQ and age.
	10	9–34 yr	Not given	Normal matched on gender, CA, handedness.		
Dawson, Warrenburg, & Fuller, 1983	10	9–34 yr	FSIQ: 69 (40–113)	Autistic (Rutter's criteria)	RH and LH parietal alpha taken during 4 motor imitation tasks: 2 manual, 2 oral	Autistic Ss showed greated RH activity than normal Ss, particularly during oral imitation. Older autistic Ss more likely to exhibit normal patterns of asymmetry.
	10	9–34 yr	Not given	Normal matched on gender, CA, handedness.		
Dawson, Finley, Phillips, & Galpert, 1986	17	6–18 yr	71 (53–91)	Autistic (CARS score, DSM-III criteria)	RH and LH cortical auditory evoked potentials to linguistic stimulus. Battery of language tests.	11/17 autistic Ss showed RH dominance for speech. RH dominance associated with poorer language abilities and greater degree of asymmetry. Older Ss more likely to show normal direction of asymmetry.
	17	6–18 yr	PPVT: 125	Normal, matched on gender and CA.		

sively on this subject before his death in 1985. Geschwind and Galaburda (1985a) proposed that a wide range of learning disabilities, including dyslexia, dysphasia, stuttering, and autism, are related to abnormal cerebral dominance for language caused by intrauterine hormonal influences. They argue that, given evidence suggesting that the right hemisphere develops earlier than the left (Taylor, 1969), harmful influences that occur during fetal and early postnatal life are more likely to affect the development of the left hemisphere, which is at risk over a longer period of time. Furthermore, it is suggested that a delay of left cortical development results in more successful competition by right-hemisphere neurons for available synapses and thus leads to diminished rates of neuronal death in the right hemisphere. This is offered as a possible explanation for the enhanced right-hemisphere skills found in some language-impaired individuals. To summarize, this view suggests prenatal influences that permanently alter the neural organization of the brain in such a way that the left hemisphere is no longer preferred for linguistic processing.

Our data presented above suggest an alternative possibility. Recall the developmental interpretation offered—that is, that changes in pattern of hemispheric activation (toward normal left-hemisphere dominance for language) occur as the child develops communicative speech. Such a notion suggests that, in autism, the basic neural organization, in terms of innate language representation, is not different from that of normal individuals—but that the development and functional use of the left hemisphere is severely delayed and results in an early functional preference for right-hemisphere processing strategies. This is not to say that the postnatal influences of inadequate linguistic and social stimulation will not have an effect on neural development, but it is proposed that these effects are of a lesser degree than that proposed in Geschwind's model, and are likely to have their greatest impact on those parts of the brain that develop most rapidly during the postnatal period, such as the frontal cortex. This hypothesis cannot be tested directly without a longitudinal study of hemispheric functioning in autistic individuals.

If, at least in some cases, postnatal influences of the processing deficits, themselves, are having a significant effect in distorting development, then the question arises of which symptoms of autism are the result of the primary dysfunction, and which are the result of these secondary influences of processing deficits on subsequent development. It is possible that some of the behavioral characteristics of autistic children are a function of secondary influences (see Dawson, 1987, for an elaboration of this argument). If this is the case, early intervention aimed at stimulating left-hemisphere development may alleviate some of these secondary symptoms (see Harris, Chapter 12, this volume).[1]

Influences of Subcortical Dysfunction on Hemispheric Functioning

Ornitz (1983, 1985) and Tanguay (Tanguay, Edwards, Buchwald, Schwafel, & Allen, 1982) have stressed the role of subcortical dysfunction in autism. Ornitz emphasizes the disturbances in sensory modulation and motility displayed by some young autistic children—for example, hand flapping and the absence of response to sounds. These behaviors have been found in about 70% of young autistic children. Because the disturbances in sensory modulation occur early, and because of their potential impact on sensory processing in all realms of development, Ornitz has argued that they may have explanatory value with respect to the total behavioral syndrome.

The evidence for brain stem dysfunction in autistic children comes from several sources. Several studies of auditory brain stem evoked responses (ABER) have found subgroups of autistic children to show significant, though variable, abnormalities in the latencies of various peaks (e.g., Fein, Skoff, & Mirsky, 1981; Gillberg, Rosenhall, & Johansson, 1983; Tanguay *et al.*, 1982). Some studies, however, have not found such evidence of brain stem abnormalities (Courchesne, Courchesne, Hicks, & Lincoln, 1985; Rumsey, 1984). Some authors have argued that, since these particular brain stem abnormalities only show up in a subgroup of children, the primacy of brain stem dysfunction in autism cannot be supported. However, Ornitz has cogently countered that the ABER reflects only a subset of neurons within the brain stem. He has suggested that problems in sensory modulation reflect more widespread interconnecting neuronal systems within the reticular formation, involving a system dysfunction rather than pathological changes in a specific group of neurons. Thus, Ornitz has argued that the abnormal ABERs may represent a subgroup of autistic children whose brain stem abnormalities happen also to involve the auditory pathways tapped by the ABER. In support of this, he has pointed out that the percentage of children showing abnormal ABERs is the same as that found to have frank neurological signs. According to Ornitz, the more relevant data on the brain stem hypothesis are measures that reflect reticular formation processes. He and his colleagues (e.g., Ornitz, 1978, 1985; Ornitz, Brown, Mason, & Putnam, 1974; Ornitz, Forsythe, & de la Pena, 1973), as well as other investigators (Piggott, Purcell, Cummings, & Caldwell, 1976) have reported studies that demonstrate abnormalities in the vestibular responses of autistic children.

To explain the findings of abnormal hemispheric activation in autistic individuals, several authors (Dawson & Lewy, in press; Ornitz, 1983, 1985; Tanguay *et al.*, 1982) have discussed the possible influences of subcortical dysfunction on the developing cortex. From this perspective, the symptoms of autism are explained in terms of dysfunction of brain stem systems *and* further distortion of cortical systems that are influenced by the brainstem and its dysfunction. As Ornitz himself has pointed out, however, the developmental influences between subcortical and cortical structures are likely to be reciprocal. Supporting this is Anthony and Graham's (1983) finding that, in young infants, cortical attentional processes can modify the blink reflex, which is organized at the brain stem level. Thus, we are left with a chicken and egg dilemma—which came first and is primary, subcortical or cortical dysfunction?

Some authors supporting the sensory modulation or attentional hypothesis (Fein *et al.*, 1984; Ornitz, 1983) have argued that the processing impairment in autism is of a global and pervasive nature, affecting all realms of cognitive and social development. Consistent with this view, these authors have maintained that autistic individuals more often show *reduced* rather than *reversed* hemispheric asymmetry for *both verbal and visual processing*. However, much of the data on hemispheric activation in autism do not fit this interpretation. As reported above (Dawson, Finley, Phillips, & Galpert, 1986), we found that the more severely affected autistic individuals showed a reversed direction, as well as a *greater degree* of hemispheric asymmetry to speech stimuli compared to normal subjects. Moreover, studies have found that the left hemisphere is more likely to be affected than the right. In our study of alpha blocking during verbal and visuospatial processing (Dawson, Warrenburg, & Fuller, 1982), it was found that the autistic group's pattern of hemispheric activation did not differ from that of normal subjects during the baseline period and visuospatial tasks. Right-hemisphere dominance for language processing cannot be reasonably conceived of as developmental delay in an otherwise normally developing process, since even young infants have been found to exhibit left-hemisphere dominance for speech using similar measures of hemispheric processing (Molfese *et al.*, 1975). Thus, the brain stem hypothesis must account for the fact that, in at least some autistic individuals, the left hemisphere appears to be more severely affected. One possible explanation is that the left hemisphere is more vulnerable to the influence of subcortical dysfunction because of its later development relative to the right hemisphere. However, this asymmetrical influence would have to be of such a degree that, in some autistic individuals, some right-hemisphere functions are not only spared but actually develop to a degree that is superior to normal.

THE ROLE OF ABNORMAL HEMISPHERIC FUNCTIONING IN THE AFFECTIVE AND SOCIAL DEFICITS OF AUTISTIC CHILDREN

Most of the studies of hemispheric lateralization in developmentally disabled children have examined speech lateralization. In order to have a more complete picture of the functional abnormalities associated with these disorders, however, it is important that future studies incorporate stimuli other than speech. A theory that postulates a selective rather than global deficit in brain functioning, such as has been offered in this chapter, must demonstrate normal brain functioning as well as abnormal. A step in this direction was made in our study that used measures of hemispheric activation during both language and visuospatial processing with autistic and normal children and adults (Dawson, Warrenburg, & Fuller, 1982).

If we are to address the question of the nature of brain dysfunction in autism, the affective and social deficits must be accounted for, since it is this realm that differentiates autism from many other developmental disabilities (Bartak, Rutter, & Cox, 1975; DeMyer *et al.*, 1972). During the past two decades, most neuropsychological and behavioral studies of autistic children have focused on cognition and language, to the exclusion of affect and social behavior. Recently investigators have redirected their focus such that the social and affective impairments are now considered important areas of investigation. Given the recency of this shift in focus, there exist few data that characterize the autistic child's social and affective impairments, as well as few data that address neurological bases. For example, it is still a matter of debate whether the autistic child's manner of social interaction is one of active withdrawal or of passivity and lack of interest. Answers to this kind of question bear directly on models of the neurological basis of autism. Thus, the ideas presented below regarding the possible neurological basis of the affective and social deficits in autism will necessarily be speculative, and will most certainly be revised as more data are available.

Motor Imitation

The influence of the autistic child's impairment in motor imitation on early social development has been discussed by the present author in other articles (Dawson & Adams, 1984; Dawson & Galpert, 1986; Dawson, Warrenburg, & Fuller, 1983). There is ample evidence to suggest that motor imitation is a left-hemisphere-mediated function from both brain-damaged (DeRenzi, Pieczuro, & Vignolo, 1966; Duffy, Duffy, & Pearson, 1975; Kimura & Archibald, 1974; Mateer & Kimura, 1977) and normal (Dawson, Warrenburg, & Fuller, 1985) populations. That the autistic child's motor imitation impairment may be a significant part of his or her social impairment is suggested for several reasons. First, a deficiency in motor imitation differentiates autistic children from children with other related developmental disabilities who do not specifically show social problems (i.e., mentally retarded and dysphasic children) (Bartak *et al.*, 1975; DeMyer *et al.*, 1972). Second, in early life, a failure to imitate the actions and facial expressions of others is a universal characteristic of autistic children. There is evidence that indicates that this failure is not motivational in nature (Dawson & Adams, 1984). Third, the degree of motor imitation deficit exhibited by an autistic child has been found to correlate with his or her degree of social impairment (Dawson & Adams, 1984; Wing, 1981). Finally, research on normal early development suggests that motor imitation is one of the earliest and most important forms of social interaction between parents and infants (Meltzoff & Moore, 1977; Papousek & Papousek, 1977; Trevarthen, 1977; Uzgiris, 1981). In our study of alpha asymmetry during a series of motor imitation tasks (Dawson, Warrenburg, & Fuller, 1983), it was found that, in contrast to normal control subjects, autistic individuals are not demonstrating the normal, left-hemisphere-dominant pattern during motor imitation. This provides one link between abnormal left-hemisphere functioning and the social impairments of autistic persons.

Affective Expression and Perception

It is well known that autistic individuals have difficulty comprehending affective expressions and have impoverished expression of affect. In fact, even quite high functioning adult autistic persons, with normal intellectual ability, continue to suffer in this regard (Rutter, 1983). Thus, studies of the neuropsychology of affect, like those reported in Chapter 7 of this volume by Davidson, are quite relevant to understanding autism. Fox and Davidson's (1984) developmental model, in particular, may be of heuristic value in beginning to explore the possible neurological basis of the affective impairments in autism. Based on studies of brain-damaged persons, as well as normal adults and infants, these authors and others have proposed that left-hemisphere-mediated emotions are those involved in social approach, and that those mediated by the right hemisphere are characterized by withdrawal. Studies by Davidson and his colleagues (Davidson & Fox, 1982; Davidson, Schwartz, Saron, Bennet, & Goleman, 1979) suggest that the hemispheric asymmetries for affect are particularly evident in the frontal cortex. According to Fox and Davidson's developmental model, in the early months of life, because of the lack of fully developed interhemispheric connections, basic emotions like pleasure and distress are thought to be unilaterally mediated. As the corpus callosum becomes more functional, however, certain emotions presumed to involve interhemispheric integration become possible. Fox and Davidson have further suggested that interhemispheric integration may also allow for the inhibition of particular right-hemisphere emotions, such as distress, via the left hemisphere. Based on this model, a testable hypothesis is that the autistic person's failure to approach others socially, as well as their inability to inhibit certain negative reactions, such as distress, may be reflective of inadequate left frontal lobe functioning. Moreover, given that the frontal cortex is a later-developing structure, one would expect that the deprivation of social stimulation experienced by the autistic child as a result of processing deficits would have a significant impact on frontal lobe development. To date, there exist no studies of hemispheric activation during affective processing in autistic persons. This would seem a fruitful direction to pursue in the future. Given that the social and affective impairments persist throughout the autistic person's lifetime, even when their linguistic and cognitive abilities have reached normal levels, it is possible that, in higher-functioning autistic persons, one would find abnormal hemispheric activation during affective processing, concurrent with normal activation during language processing. To test this, it would be important to sample several brain loci, including temporal (at which asymmetries for linguistic stimuli would be most evident) and frontal (at which asymmetries for affective stimuli would most likely exist).

SUMMARY AND CONCLUSIONS

In this chapter, I have reviewed several types of evidence that suggest that autism involves abnormal functioning of the left hemisphere. This evidence is based on studies of cognitive abilities, handedness, clinical EEGs, neuropsychological testing, and measures of hemispheric activity during speech and other stimuli.The specific role of left-hemisphere dysfunction in autism is still unknown. Data presented in the present chapter support a strong relationship between the direction of hemispheric activity during speech and the severity of language impairment in autism. Autistic persons with more adequate language skills have been found to be more likely to show the normal left-dominant pattern of hemispheric asymmetry for speech; those with more impaired language were more likely to show both a greater degree of asymmetry and right-hemisphere dominance for speech. Whether there actually occurs a shift in hemispheric processing of speech as the autistic child develops language is a question that can be answered directly only with a longitudinal study of hemispheric processing of speech in autistic individuals. Our data suggest that, at least in early development, autism can be associated with an overactivation of the right hemisphere. It is possible that this overactivation is caused by the lack of adequate inhibitory left-hemisphere mechanisms.

Several hypotheses regarding the role of abnormal hemispheric functioning in autism were discussed. These hypotheses emphasize the left-hemisphere-related functions of motor imitation, language, and symbol formation as being central to autism. The role of brain stem dysfunction and its effect on hemispheric development also were discussed. It was suggested that abnormal hemispheric functioning may be secondary to the ontogenetic influences of brain stem dysfunction.

Finally, a number of testable hypotheses regarding the possible role of inadequate left-hemisphere development in the affective and social impairments of autistic persons were offered. In particular, it was speculated that, given the left hemisphere's involvement in those emotions associated with social approach, overactivation of the right hemisphere in autistic persons may result in a failure to have interest in and approach others, and lead to the withdrawal from others that is often described in autistic children.

To conclude, I offer a set of criteria for evaluating the primacy of specific types of brain dysfunction in autism. These criteria are as follows:

1. *Universality:* The specific type of brain dysfunction must be shown to exist in all autistic individuals. An important qualification of this criterion, however, is that the specific type of dysfunction need only be present at an early point in development and, with improvements in functioning, may no longer be apparent in mature, higher functioning individuals. Therefore, in order to evaluate universality properly, the investigator must include younger, more impaired children and interpret data from a developmental (at least cross-sectional, if not longitudinal) perspective using concurrent measures of developmental level. Any study that simply averages behavioral and neurophysiological data across subjects who vary in developmental level cannot present an accurate picture of the nature of autism.

2. *Exclusivity:* The specific type of brain dysfunction must be shown to exist exclusively in autistic individuals. A qualification of this criterion is that exclusivity will not be found when comparisons are being made between clinical populations that *share a diagnostic symptom.* For example, given that dysphasic and autistic individuals share the symptom of deficient language comprehension and expression, and given that this symptom is considered a defining characteristic of both disorders, neurological measures that specifi-

cally pertain to this symptom (e.g., hemispheric lateralization for speech), should show similar findings for both groups. In order to evaluate exclusivity, studies must include relevant comparison groups, such as normal, developmental age–matched controls and mentally retarded and dysphasic comparison groups.

3. *Symptom relevance or validity:* It should be demonstrated that the severity of the specific type of brain dysfunction under study correlates with at least one of the cardinal symptoms of autism (e.g., language and/or social abilities). Furthermore, the logical, functional relationship between the neurological correlate and the behavior of interest must be established (for example, the relationship between left-hemisphere dysfunction and social withdrawal).

4. *Deviant, rather than delayed, functioning:* Given that many autistic persons are also mentally retarded, it is possible that a neurological finding may reflect the overlay of developmental delay rather than autism. Thus, most investigators tend to give more weight to findings that indicate deviant, rather than simply delayed, functioning. In order to evaluate this criterion, studies should incorporate both developmental age–matched normal control subjects and a mentally retarded comparison group. One point of interpretation should be made, however. It is possible that autism involves the asymmetrical development of functions that, in themselves, are following a normal, albeit delayed, developmental path. If this is correct, it is the asymmetry in development across functions, rather than the functions themselves, that is deviant. Thus, if only one aspect of functioning is studied, it may be found that this function is following a delayed, rather than deviant, pattern. At the same time, this delay in a specific function, relative to other functions, may cause an overall distortion in development that is itself deviant in nature. In order to address this issue, whether one is studying brain functioning, behavior, or their relationship, it is necessary to look at *patterns* of functioning across several domains and to assess the relative development of those domains.

The study of the neurological basis of autism is still in its infancy. Given the rarity of the syndrome and the great difficulty in identifying and testing autistic persons, progress in this field of study may be greatly accelerated by collaboration between investigators using identical diagnostic criteria and experimental designs. Interdisciplinary collaboration also will continue to be extremely important in making strides in understanding the complex nature of brain–behavior relationships in autism.

ACKNOWLEDGMENT

Preparation of this chapter was supported by NIMH grant MH36612 awarded to Geraldine Dawson.

NOTE

1. We have been investigating intervention techniques for facilitating social and communicative development in young autistic children, which, in fact, may facilitate left-hemisphere functioning. One such technique involves imitating the actions of the autistic child, including toy play, facial expressions, and vocalizations. In two studies (Dawson & Adams, 1984; Tiegerman & Primavera, 1984), it was found that simultaneous imitation of autistic children's actions led to significant increases in a variety of social behaviors, including eye contact and vocalizations.

REFERENCES

Annett, M. (1967). The binomial distribution of right, mixed, and left handedness. *Quarterly Journal of Experimental Psychology, 19,* 327–333.

Anthony, B. J., & Graham, F. K. (1983). Evidence for sensory-selective set in young infants. *Science, 220,* 742–743.

Arnold, G., & Schwartz, S. (1983). Hemispheric lateralization of language in autistic and aphasic children. *Journal of Autism and Developmental Disorders, 13,* 129–139.

Baltaxe, C. A., & Simmons, J. Q. (1975). Language in childhood psychosis: A review. *Journal of Speech and Hearing Sciences, 30,* 439–458.

Barry, R. J., & James, A. L. (1978). Handedness in autistics, retardates, and normals of a wide age range. *Journal of Autism and Childhood Schizophrenia, 8*(3), 315–323.

Bartak, L., Rutter, M., & Cox, A. (1975). A comparative study of infantile autism and specific developmental receptive language disorder: I. The children. *British Journal of Psychiatry, 126,* 127–145.

Blackstock, E. G. (1978). Cerebral asymmetry and the development of early infantile autism. *Journal of Autism and Childhood Schizophrenia, 8,* 339–353.

Boucher, J. (1977). Hand preference in autistic children and their parents. *Journal of Autism and Childhood Schizophrenia, 7*(2), 177–187.

Caparulo, B. K., Cohen, D. J., Rothman, S. L., Young, J. G., Katz, J. D., Shaywitz, S. E., & Bennett, B. A. (1981). Computed tomographic brain scanning in children with developmental neuropsychiatric disorders. *Journal of the American Academy of Child Psychiatry, 20,* 338–357.

Chess, S. (1971). Autism in children with congenital rubella. *Journal of Autism and Childhood Schizophrenia, 1,* 33–47.

Colby, K. M., & Parkinson, C. (1977). Handedness in autistic children. *Journal of Autism and Childhood Schizophrenia, 7,* 3–9.

Courchesne, E. (in press). Neuroanatomical systems involved in infantile autism: The implications of cerebellar abnormalities. In G. Dawson (Ed.), *Autism: New perspectives on diagnosis, nature, and treatment.* New York: Guilford Press.

Courchesne, E., Courchesne, R. Y., Hicks, G., & Lincoln, A. J. (1985). Functioning of brainstem auditory pathway in nonretarded autistic individuals. *Electroencephalography and Clinical Neurophysiology, 61,* 491–501.

Creak, M. (1963). Schizophrenic syndrome in childhood: Progress report of a working party. *Cerebral Palsy Bulletin, 3,* 501–503.

Creak, M., & Pampiglione, G. (1969). Clinical and EEG studies on a group of 35 psychotic children. *Developmental Medicine and Child Neurology, 11,* 218–227.

Damasio, H., Maurer, R. B., Damasio, A. R., & Chui, H. C. (1980). Computerized tomographic scan findings in patients with autistic behavior. *Archives of Neurology, 37,* 504–510.

Davidson, R. J., & Fox, N. A. (1982). Asymmetrical brain activity discriminates between positive and negative affective stimuli in human infants. *Science, 21,* 1235–1237.

Davidson, R. J., Schwartz, G. E., Saron, C., Bennet, J., & Goleman, D. J. (1979). Frontal versus parietal EEG asymmetry during positive and negative affect. *Psychophysiology, 16,* 202–203.

Dawson, G. (1983). Lateralized brain dysfunction in autism: Evidence from the Halstead-Reitan Neuropsychological Battery. *Journal of Autism and Developmental Disorders, 13,* 269–286.

Dawson, G. D. (1987). The role of abnormal hemispheric specialization in autism. In E. Schopler & G. Mesibov (Eds.), *Neurobiological issues in autism* (pp. 213–227). New York: Plenum.

Dawson, G., & Adams, A. (1984). Imitation and social responsiveness in autistic children. *Journal of Abnormal Child Psychology, 12,* 209–225.

Dawson, G., Finley, C., Phillips, S., & Galpert, L. (1986). Hemispheric specialization and the language abilities of autistic children. *Child Development, 57,* 1440–1453.

Dawson, G., & Galpert, L. (1986). A developmental model for facilitating the social behavior of autistic children. In E. Schopler & G. Mesibov (Eds.), *Social problems in autism* (pp. 237–260). New York: Plenum.

Dawson, G., & Lewy, A. (in press). Subcortical influences on higher cortical functions in autism: Role of attentional mechanisms. In G. Dawson (Ed.), *Autism: New perspectives on diagnosis, nature and treatment.* New York: Guilford.

Dawson, G., Warrenburg, S., & Fuller, P. (1982). Cerebral lateralization in individuals diagnosed as autistic in early childhood. *Brain and Language, 15,* 353–366.

Dawson, G., Warrenburg, S., & Fuller, P. (1983). Hemisphere functioning and motor imitation in autistic persons. *Brain and Cognition, 2,* 346–354.

Dawson, G., Warrenburg, S., & Fuller, P. (1985). Left hemisphere specialization for facial and manual imitation. *Psychophysiology, 22,* 237–245.

DeMyer, M. K., Alpern, G. D., Barton, S., DeMyer, W. E., Churchill, D. W., Hingtgen, J. N., Bryson, C. Q., Pontius, W., & Kimberlin, G. (1972). Imitation in autistic, early schizophrenic, and nonpsychotic subnormal children. *Journal of Autism and Childhood Schizophrenia, 2,* 264–287.

DeMyer, M. K., Barton, S., Alpern, G. D., Kimberlin, C., Allen, J., Yang, E., & Steele, R. (1974). The measured intelligence of autistic children: A follow-up study. *Journal of Autism and Childhood Schizophrenia, 4.* 42–60.

DeRenzi, E., Pieczuro, A., & Vignolo, L. A. (1966). Oral apraxia and aphasia. *Cortex, 2,* 50–73.

Duffy, R., Duffy, J., & Pearson, K. (1975). Pantomime recognition in aphasics. *Journal of Speech and Hearing Research, 18,* 115–132.

Fein, D., Humes, M., Kaplan, E., Lucci, D., & Waterhouse, L. (1984). The question of left hemisphere dysfunction in autism. *Psychological Bulletin, 95,* 258–281.

Fein, D., Skoff, B., & Minsky, A. F. (1981). Clinical correlates of brain dysfunction in autistic children. *Journal of Autism and Developmental Disorders, 11,* 303–315.

Folstein, S., & Rutter, M. (1977). Genetic influences and infantile autism. *Nature, 265,* 726–728.

Fish, B., Shapiro, T., & Campbell, M. (1966). Long-term prognosis and the response of schizophrenic children to drug therapy: A controlled study of trifluoperazine. *American Journal of Psychiatry, 123,* 32–39.

Fox, N. A., & Davidson, R. J. (1984). Hemispheric substrates of affect: A developmental model. In N. A. Fox & R. J. Davidson (Eds.), *The psychobiology of affective development* (pp. 353–381). Hillsdale, NJ: Erlbaum.

Geschwind, N., & Galaburda, A. M. (1985a). Cerebral lateralization: Biological mechanisms, association, and pathology: I. A hypothesis and a program for research. *Archives of Neurology, 42,* 428–459.

Geschwind, N., & Galaburda, A. M. (1985b). Cerebral lateralization: Biological mechanisms, association, and pathology: II. A hypothesis and a program for research. *Archives of Neurology, 42,* 521–552.

Geschwind, N., & Galaburda, A. M. (1985c). Cerebral lateralization: Biological mechanisms, associations, and pathology: III. A hypothesis and a program for research. *Archives of Neurology, 42,* 634–654.

Gillberg, C., & Gillberg, I. C. (1983). Infantile autism: A total population study of reduced optimality in the pre-, peri-, and neonatal period. *Journal of Autism and Developmental Disorders, 13*(2), 153–166.

Gillberg, C., Rosenhall, U., & Johansson, E. (1983). Auditory brainstem responses in childhood psychosis. *Journal of Autism and Developmental Disorders, 13,* 181–195.

Gillberg, C., & Svendsen, P. (1983). Childhood psychosis and computed tomographic brain scan findings. *Journal of Autism and Developmental Disorders, 13,* 19–32.

Goldman, P. S. (1978). Neuronal plasticity in primate telencephalon: Anomalous projections induced by prenatal removal of frontal cortex. *Science, 202,* 768–770.

Gubbay, S. S., Lobascher, M., & Kingerlee, P. (1970). A neurological appraisal of autistic children: Results of a Western Australian survey. *Developmental Medicine and Child Neurology, 12,* 422–429.

Hauser, S. L., DeLong, G. R., & Rosman, N. P. (1975). Pneumographic findings in the infantile autism syndrome: A correlation with temporal lobe disease. *Brain, 98,* 667–688.

Hier, D. B., LeMay, M., & Rosenberger, P. B. (1979). Autism and unfavorable left–right asymmetries of the brain. *Journal of Autism and Developmental Disorders, 9,* 153–159.

Hoffman, W. L., & Prior, M. R. (1982). Neuropsychological dimensions of autism in children: A test of the hemispheric dysfunction hypothesis. *Journal of Clinical Psychology, 4,* 27–41.

Kanner, L. (1943). Autistic disturbances of affective contact. *Nervous Child, 2,* 217–250.

Keeler, W. R. (1958). Autistic patterns and defective communication in blind children with retrolental fibroplasia. In P. H. Hock & J. Zubin (Eds.), *Psychopathology of communication.* New York: Grune and Stratton.

Kimura, D., & Archibald, Y. (1974). Motor functions of the left hemisphere. *Brain, 97,* 337–350.

Knobloch, H., & Pasamanick, B. (1975). Some etiological and prognostic factors in early infantile autism and psychosis. *Pediatrcis, 55,* 182–191.

Kolvin, I., Ounsted, C., & Roth, A. (1971). Studies in childhood psychosis: V. Cerebral dysfunction and childhood psychoses. *British Journal of Psychiatry, 118,* 407–414.

Lobascher, M. E., Kingerlee, P. E., & Gubbay, S. D. (1970). Childhood autism: Aetiological factors in 25 cases. *British Journal of Psychiatry, 117,* 525–529.

Lockyer, L., & Rutter, M. (1970). A five-to-fifteen year study of infantile psychosis: IV. Patterns of cognitive ability. *British Journal of Social and Clinical Psychology, 9,* 152–163.

Lotter, V. (1974). Factors related to outcome in autistic children. *Journal of Autism and Childhood Schizophrenia, 4,* 263–277.

Mateer, C., & Kimura, D. (1977). Impairment of nonverbal oral movement in aphasia. *Brain and Language, 4,* 262–272.

Meltzoff, H., & Moore, M. K. (1977). Imitation of facial and manual gestures by human neonates. *Science, 198,* 75–78.

Molfese, D. L., Freeman, R. B., & Palmero, D. S. (1975). The ontogeny of brain lateralization for speech and non-speech stimuli. *Brain and Language, 2,* 356–368.

Ogawa, T., Sugiyama, A., Ishiwa, S., Suzuki, M., Ishihara, T., & Sato, K. (1982). Ontogenic development of EEG-asymmetry in early infantile autism. *Brain and Development, 4,* 439–449.

Ornitz, E. M. (1978). Neurophysiologic studies. In M. Rutter & E. Schopler (Eds.), *Autism: A reappraisal of concepts and treatment* (pp. 243–250). New York: Plenum.

Ornitz, E. M. (1983). Neuroanatomical basis of early infantile autism. *International Journal of Neuroscience, 19,* 85–124.

Ornitz, E. M. (1985). Neurophysiology of infantile autism. *Journal of the American Academy of Child Psychiatry, 24*(3), 251–262.

Ornitz, E. M., Brown, M. B., Mason, A., & Putnam, N. H. (1974). Effect of visual input on vestibular nystagmus in autistic children. *Archives of General Psychiatry, 31,* 369–375.

Ornitz, E. M., Forsythe, A. B., & de la Pena, A. (1973). Effect of vestibular and auditory stimulation on the REMs and REM sleep in autistic children. *Archives of General Psychiatry, 29,* 786–791.

Papousek, H., & Papousek, M. (1977). Mothering and cognitive headstart: Psychobiological considerations. In H. R. Schaffer (Ed.), *Studies in mother–infant interaction* (pp. 63–85). New York: Plenum.

Piggott, L., Purcell, G., Cummings, G., & Caldwell, D. (1976). Vestibular dysfunction in emotionally disturbed children. *Biological Psychiatry, 11,* 719–729.

Prior, M. R., & Bradshaw, J. L. (1979). Hemisphere functions in autistic children. *Cortex, 15,* 73–81.

Riquet, C., Taylor, N., Benaroya, S., & Klein, L. (1981). Symbolic play in autistic, Down's, and normal children of equivalent mental age. *Journal of Autism and Developmental Disorders, 11,* 439–448.

Rumsey, J. (1984). Auditory brainstem responses in pervasive developmental disorders. *Biological Psychiatry, 19,* 1403–1418.

Rutter, M. (1974). The development of infantile autism. *Psychological Medicine, 4,* 147–163.

Rutter, M. (1978). Diagnosis and definition. In M. Rutter & E. Schopler (Eds.), *Autism: A reappraisal of concepts and treatment* (pp. 1–25). New York: Plenum.

Rutter, M. (1983). Cognitive deficits in the pathogenisis of autism. *Journal of Child Psychology and Psychiatry, 24,* 513–531.

Rutter, M., Greenfield, D., & Lockyer, L. (1967). A five to fifteen year follow-up study of infantile psychosis: II. Social and behavioral outcome. *British Journal of Psychiatry, 113,* 1183–1199.

Satz, P. (1972). Pathological left-handedness: An explanatory model. *Cortex, 8,* 121–137.

Satz, P. (1973). Lefthandedness and early brain insult: An explanation. *Neuropsychologia, 11,* 115–117.

Sigman, M., & Ungerer, J. (1984). Cognitive and language skills in autistic, mentally retarded, and normal children. *Developmental Psychology, 20,* 293–302.

Simmons, J. Q., & Baltaxe, C. (1975). Language patterns of adolescent autistics. *Journal of Autism and Childhood Schizophrenia, 5,* 333–351.

Small, J. G. (1975). EEG and neurophysiological studies of early infantile autism. *Biological Psychiatry, 10,* 385–389.

Soper, H. V., & Satz, P. (1984). Pathological left-handedness and ambiguous handedness: A new explanatory model. *Neuropsychologia, 22,* 511–515.

Taft, L., & Cohen, H. J. (1971). Hypoarrhythmia and infantile autism: A clinical report. *Journal of Autism and Childhood Schizophrenia, 1,* 327–336.

Tanguay, P. E. (1976). Clinical and electrophysiological research. In E. R. Ritvo (Ed.), *Autism: Diagnosis, current research and management.* New York: Spectrum Publications.

Tanguay, P. E., Edwards, R. M., Buchwald, J., Schwafel, J., & Allen, V. (1982). Auditory brainstem evoked responses in autistic children. *Archives of General Psychiatry, 39,* 174–180.

Taylor, D. C. (1969). Differential rates of cerebral maturation between sexes and between hemispheres: Evidence from epilepsy. *The Lancet,* 140–142.

Tiegerman, E., & Primavera, L. (1984). Imitating the autistic child: Facilitating communicative gaze behavior. *Journal of Autism and Developmental disorders, 14,* 27–28.

Trevarthen, C. (1977). Descriptive analysis of infant communicative behavior. In H. R. Schaffer (Ed.), *Studies in mother–infant interaction* (pp. 227–270). New York: Academic Press.

Tsai, L. Y. (1983). The relationship of handedness to the cognitive, language, and visuo-spatial skills of autistic patients. *British Journal of Psychiatry, 142,* 156–162.

Tsai, L. Y., Jacoby, C. G., & Stewart, M. A. (1983). Morphological cerebral asymmetries in autistic children. *Biological Psychiatry, 18,* 317–327.

Uzgiris, I. C. (1981). Experience in the social context. In R. L. Schiefelbusch & D. D. Bricker (Eds.), *Early language: Acquisition and interaction* (pp. 139–168). Baltimore, MD: University Park Press.

Wing, L. (1981). Language, social and cognitive impairments in autism and severe mental retardation. *Journal of Autism and Developmental Disorders, 11,* 31–44.

Wolff, S., & Chess, S. (1965). An analysis of the language of fourteen schizophrenic children. *Journal of Child Psychology and Psychiatry, 6,* 29–41.

Wetherby, A. M., Koegel, R. L., & Mendel, M. (1981). Central auditory neurons system dysfunction in echolalic autistic individuals. *Journal of Speech and Hearing Research, 24,* 420–429.

17

Childhood Depression and Medically Treatable Learning Disability

ROGER A. BRUMBACK
University of Oklahoma College of Medicine

Although it has been firmly established that disturbances in specific sensorimotor, intellectual, and cognitive functions result from focal structural abnormalities in the cerebral hemispheres (Broca, 1861; Geschwind, 1965; Luria, 1966; Mesulam, 1985), little interest has been generated in the concept that similar neurological and neuropsychological changes occur secondary to nonstructural abnormalities of the cerebral hemispheres. Focal paralysis (Meyer & Portnoy, 1959) and aphasia (Gascon, Victor, & Lombroso, 1973; Landau & Kleffner, 1957) have been reported to follow the electrophysiological disturbance of epilepsy in which no structural brain abnormality can be detected. The intravenous administration of dimethyltryptamine (a potent serotonin antagonist) to normal volunteers has been reported to produce transient left extensor plantar response (Babinski reflex) and left-sided hyperreflexia (Sai-Halasz, Brunecker, & Szara, 1958). The metabolic disturbances of systemic hypoglycemia, electrolyte derangement, and hyperpyrexia have all been reported to produce focal neurological and/or neuropsychological signs of cerebral dysfunction, which disappear with correction of the metabolic problem (Meyer & Portnoy, 1959; Montgomery & Pinner, 1964). Evidence is mounting that biological depressive illness, which is a metabolic derangement affecting specific brain neurotransmitters, is also associated with specific neurological and neuropsychological signs suggesting focal cerebral dysfunction.

BIOLOGICAL DEPRESSIVE DISORDER

Depression was recognized as a specific illness under the name *melancholia* as long ago as the 4th century B.C., and Aretaeus of Cappadocia provided a description of the disorder in the 2nd century A.D. that is still accurate today (Brumback, 1985a; Jelliffe, 1931):

> Those affected with melancholia are not everyone of them affected according to one particular form; they are either suspicious of poisoning or flee to the desert from misanthropy or turn suspicious or construct a hatred of life . . . the patients are dull or stern, dejected or unreasonably torpid without any manifest cause . . . they also become peevish, dispirited, sleepless, and start up from a disturbed sleep. Unreasonable fear also seizes them . . . they become thin by their agitation and loss of refreshing sleep . . . at a more advanced stage, they complain of a thousand futilities and desire to die.

Throughout the centuries vivid descriptions of depressive symptomatology have been provided in the writings and paintings of poets, authors, and artists who either suffered from depressive illness or witnessed others with depression. However, there was little medical or scientific understanding of depression as a biological disorder (Robertson, 1979) until the development in recent years of validated diagnostic criteria for differentiating biological depression from other psychiatric disorders or from ordinary sadness and grief (American Psychiatric Association Task Force on Nomenclature, 1980; Feighner *et al.*, 1972; Spitzer, Endicott, & Robins, 1978).

Despite this current acceptance by the medical community of the biological nature of depressive illness in adults, there has been considerable reluctance to acknowledge biological depression in children, and most mental health professionals have tended to deny its existence. Meanwhile, the findings that significant learning disturbances occur in normally intelligent children without visual or hearing impairments, and that these learning difficulties are frequently associated with behavioral problems such as hyperactivity, somatization, hyperreactivity, sadness, withdrawal, hostility, anger, lying, stealing, fire setting, and aggressiveness, has been widely recognized. Although the biological nature of the learning disturbances has gained support from the recent postmortem findings of focal anatomical abnormalities of the cerebral cortex of dyslexic patients (Galaburda & Kemper, 1979; Galaburda, Sherman, Rosen, Aboitiz, & Geschwind, 1985; Geschwind & Galaburda, 1985; Kemper, 1984), the associated behavioral symptoms have often been attributed to the child's chronic frustrations in dealing with difficult schoolwork and with problematic family and peer social relationships. Accordingly, behavioral disturbances would be expected to be worsened by situations that stress the child's specific cognitive disability, whereas behavioral problems should not be encountered if the learning disabilities involve skills not ordinarily stressed in school or social situations (Geschwind, 1984; Grossman, 1977). However, treatment programs (including counseling) directed at reducing perceived stresses have achieved only limited success in relieving behavioral symptomatology. The only generally accepted "biological" behavior problem has been the syndrome of hyperactivity, which has been treated with stimulant medication in almost epidemic proportions (Barkley, 1981). Yet, such stimulant pharmacotherapy has not seemed to alter the long-term poor prognosis for many affected children (Blouin, Bornstein, & Trites, 1978; Huessy & Cohen, 1976; Riddle & Rapoport, 1976). Fortunately, a few dissenting voices suggested that a specific medically treatable biological affective illness (similar to that in adults) did occur in children and was a major cause of childhood behavior problems and learning difficulties (Connell, 1972; Frommer, 1967; Ling, Oftendal, & Weinberg, 1970; Polvan & Cebiroglu, 1972). Beginning in 1973, Weinberg and colleagues developed criteria (Table 17-1) for the diagnosis of depression in childhood (Brumback, 1976; Brumback, Dietz-Schmidt, & Weinberg, 1977; Brumback & Weinberg, 1977a; Weinberg & Brumback, 1976; Weinberg & McLean, 1986; Weinberg, Rutman, Sullivan, Penick, & Dietz, 1973). Subsequent investigators using these and comparable criteria have validated the occurrence of biological depressive illness in childhood (Cantwell & Carlson, 1983; Carlson & Cantwell, 1979; Hodges & Siegel, 1985; Offord & Joffe, 1985; Poznanski, Mokros, Grossman, & Freeman, 1985); however, these strict diagnostic criteria, though resulting in reproducible categorization in various investigative studies, have proved somewhat restrictive for the clinical purpose of recognizing medically treatable depression in individual patients. Clinically, depressive illness is more readily diagnosed on the basis of: (1) the presence of a constellation of depressive symptoms (from Table 17-2) that resolve with appropriate antidepressant therapy, and (2) a positive family history, since there appears to be a multifactorial genetic basis for depressive disorder, and children from families with other depressed members are at high risk for developing depression.

The reported frequency of childhood depression (Table 17-3) has varied widely in different studies (Earls, 1984; Kashani *et al.*, 1981; Offord & Joffe, 1985). Surveys of hospitalized children or children referred for evaluation of behavior problems have shown

Table 17-1. Weinberg Criteria for Childhood Depression

A. Presence of both major symptoms I and II and two or more of the remaining eight major symptoms (III–X):
- I. Dysphoric mood (melancholy)
  - a. Statements or appearance of sadness, loneliness, unhappiness, hopelessness, and/or pessimism
  - b. Mood swings, moodiness
  - c. Irritable, easily annoyed
  - d. Hypersensitive, cries easily
  - e. Negative, difficult to please
- II. Self-deprecatory ideation
  - a. Feeling of being worthless, useless, dumb, stupid, ugly, guilty (negative self-concept)
  - b. Beliefs of persecution
  - c. Death wishes
  - d. Desire to run away or leave home
  - e. Suicidal thoughts
  - f. Suicidal attempts
- III. Aggressive behavior (agitation)
  - a. Difficult to get along with
  - b. Quarrelsome
  - c. Disrespectful of authority
  - d. Belligerent, hostile, agitated
  - e. Excessive fighting or sudden anger
- IV. Sleep disturbance
  - a. Initial insomnia
  - b. Restless sleep
  - c. Terminal insomnia
  - d. Difficulty awakening in morning
- V. Change in school performance
  - a. Frequent complaints from teachers regarding daydreaming, poor concentration, poor memory
  - b. Loss of usual work effort in school subjects
  - c. Loss of usual interest in nonacademic school activities
- VI. Diminished socialization
  - a. Decreased group participation
  - b. Less friendly, less outgoing
  - c. Socially withdrawing
  - d. Loss of usual social interests
- VII. Change in attitude toward school
  - a. Does not enjoy school activities
  - b. Does not want or refuses to attend school
- VIII. Somatic complaints
  - a. Nonmigraine headaches
  - b. Abdominal pain
  - c. Muscle aches or pains
  - d. Other somatic concerns or complaints
- IX. Loss of usual energy
  - a. Loss of usual personal interests or pursuits other than school (e.g., hobbies)
  - b. Decreased energy; mental and/or physical fatigue
- X. Unusual change in appetite and/or weight
  - a. Anorexia or polyphagia
  - b. Unusual weight change in past 4 months

B. Each major symptom must be a *discrete change* in the child's usual behavior and must be present for longer than 1 month. A symptom is considered positive when at least one of the characteristic behaviors listed for the category is present.

Source: Adapted from Weinberg *et al.* (1973), Brumback *et al.* (1977), and Weinberg & McLean (1986).

a much higher frequency of depression (approximately 60%), than have the population studies that suggest a frequency of 1% to 2% (Kashani *et al.*, 1983; Kashani & Simonds, 1979; Staton & Brumback, 1981). This latter frequency for depression in the pediatric population is what would be expected (Staton & Brumback, 1981) if the frequency in children is similar to the reported frequency of depression in adults (Clayton, 1981). One possible explanation for a discrepancy in the frequency of depression reported by different

Table 17-2. Symptomatology of Depressive Illness

Physiological	Psychological

Sleep disturbance
  Delayed insomnia
  Frequent awakening
Somatic complaints
  Headaches
  Abdominal pain
  Dizziness
  Vague aches and pains
  Blurred vision
Alimentary tract disturbance
  Eating disorder (increase in or loss of appetite)
  Constipation
Weight change (loss or gain)
Fatigue
Psychomotor disturbance
  Increased body activity (agitation or hyperactivity) or decreased body activity (retardation)
  Increased or decreased mental activity (including impaired concentration and confusion)
Nonreactivity to surrounding events (including inconsolability or nonreactivity to cheering efforts)
Diurnal variation in mood and symptoms (usually worse in the morning)
	Dysphoric mood, unhappiness, sadness, crying spells
	Cognitive negatives
	  Negative feelings about self (low self-esteem, self-deprecation)
	  Negative feelings about relationships or friendships (or paranoia)
	  Negative feelings about the future (pessimism, hopelessness)
	Irritability, anger, poor frustration tolerance, temper outbursts
	Social withdrawal
	Guilt
	Loss of interest or pleasure in usual activities (including loss of interest in school)
	Preoccupation with death and/or suicidal thoughts, threats, or attempts

Table 17-3. Frequency of Childhood Depression in Various Studies

Population evaluated	Frequency of depression	Investigators
Psychiatric inpatients	59%	Petti, 1978
Educational diagnostic center outpatients	58%	Weinberg *et al.*, 1973; Brumback *et al.*, 1977
Family psychiatric unit patients	54%	Colbert *et al.*, 1982
Psychiatric inpatients	53%	McConville *et al.*, 1973
Neurological inpatients	40%	Ling *et al.*, 1970
Parochial school (7th & 8th grades)	33%	Albert & Beck, 1975
Children in residential nurseries	25%	Meierhofer, 1972
Psychiatric inpatients	23%	Pearce, 1977
Child psychiatry outpatient clinic	20%	Feinstein *et al.*, 1984
Elementary school (3rd to 6th grades)	15%	Leon *et al.*, 1980
School psychiatric center patients	13.7%	Bauersfeld, 1972
Military dependents' pediatric outpatient clinic	4%	Cantwell, 1974
General population (randomly selected)	1.9%	Kashani & Simonds, 1979
Nine-year-old children from general population	1.8%	Kashani *et al.*, 1983
Pediatric inpatients	1.8%	Nissen, 1971
School district elementary-age population	1.1%	Staton & Brumback, 1981
Psychiatric clinic patients	0.8%	Cebiroglu *et al.*, 1972
General population	0.14%	Rutter, Graham, & Yule, 1970

investigators is the problem of proper diagnostic assessment of the behaviorally disturbed child. There is a widely accepted notion that children are not able to report their own feelings, emotions, behavior, personal relationships, and problems in psychosocial functioning (Aylward, 1985). This has been shown to be incorrect by studies (Herjanic, Herjanic, Brown, & Wheatt, 1975; Rutter & Graham, 1968) consistently demonstrating that children are reliable reporters (although children are often unable to provide a free-association description of their symptomatology). However, the erroneous assumption has prevented many physicians and mental health professionals from eliciting symptomatology necessary for the diagnosis of childhood depression. Many examiners:

1. Fail to obtain symptom descriptions through directed questioning in a semistructured interview.
2. Use words that have a variety of meanings (such as the word ''depressed'') or use abstract language beyond the child's level of understanding (for example, asking a grade school child about ''inappropriate guilt'').
3. Fail to ask the same question with different wordings to confirm that the child understands and is giving internally consistent responses.
4. Assume that the grade school child has a clear concept of time relationships (rather than relating time to events such as ''since the first day of school'').
5. Dismiss the child's report of emotionally threatening (to the interviewer) symptomatology such as suicidal ideation and sexual activity (Puig-Antich, 1984; Puig-Antich, Chambers, & Tabrizi, 1983).

SYMPTOMATOLOGY OF DEPRESSION IN CHILDREN

The symptomatology associated with depression can generally be divided into two categories: *psychological* (behavioral) and *physiological* (vegetative) symptoms (Table 17-2). Dysphoric mood is the psychological symptom usually considered most characteristic of depression, although the negative thoughts and ideas (''cognitive negatives'') may be more evident. These cognitive negatives consist of: (1) negative thoughts about self (self-depreciation, negative self-concept, or low self-esteem); (2) negative ideas about friendships and other relationships; and (3) negative feelings about the future (hopelessness). The depressed child's self-deprecatory thoughts and statements of being stupid, dumb, ugly, worthless, or useless, and his or her statements of ''I can't do it,'' ''I'm not good enough,'' ''I don't want to,'' can be very irritating to parents and teachers. The depressed child who already feels undesirably ugly may make little effort to dress well or maintain good personal hygiene. Although depressed boys often have a disheveled look, such an appearance does not necessarily mean the boy is depressed; on the other hand, such a look in a young girl is strongly suggestive of depression. A negative attitude toward relationships usually creates interpersonal difficulties, and the depressed child may perceive any restrictions (such as a reasonable bedtime) or punishment as evidence of the parents' hatred of him or her. A mother may find it very hard to hug and comfort a depressed child who says to her, ''You don't love me,'' or, ''You like [sister or brother] better than you like me.'' Depressed children often do not express their feelings of hopelessness and negative ideas about the future; in depressed adults, however, the degree of hopelessness correlates with the risk of suicide (Beck, 1973), and it is possible that a similar correlation exists in depressed children.

About one-third of depressed children will become preoccupied with death and dying

(Brumback *et al.*, 1977; Pearce, 1981). The depressed child may be upset about the past death of a relative or express a desire to be with a dead relative or friend. Somewhat less than 10% of depressed children will have suicidal thoughts, but about half of these will develop a suicide plan or attempt suicide (Brumback *et al.*, 1977). About 15% of depressed children (many of those who also have suicidal thoughts) will have a desire or attempt to run away from home. Depressive illness is a prime consideration in children who attempt suicide or are runaways.

Irritability, anger, and low frustration tolerance are present in about 60% of depressed children (Brumback *et al.*, 1977) and may lead to frequent fights with peers and friends. The depressed child may become enthralled with violence in television programs or movies and develop a fascination with armaments and/or martial arts techniques. Temper tantrums occur in about 40% of depressed children, and willful destructiveness occurs in about one-quarter (Brumback *et al.*, 1977). In contrast, apathy is a major symptom in the nearly 40% of depressed children who do not become irritable or angry. The apathetic depressed child, who seems unfazed by serious problems and unaffected by punishment, is sometimes likened to a "zombie."

Social withdrawal is prominent in about two-thirds of children with depressive illness (Brumback *et al.*, 1977). A depressed child stops playing with other children, a depressed adolescent girl may lose the normal flirtatious interest in boys, and a depressed adolescent boy may avoid girls. The depressed child loses interest in school and other activities. School phobia developing in a child who has generally enjoyed (or at least tolerated) school is strongly suggestive of depression (Agras, 1959; Gittleman-Klein & Klein, 1971). Instead of completely avoiding school, some depressed children may quit clubs and activities; stop doing homework or other assignments; and make irreversible decisions such as giving away, selling, or destroying favorite possessions.

The biological (or physiological or vegetative) symptoms of depression often bring the depressed child to medical attention. The most common of these, disturbed sleep, is clinically apparent in 80% to 90% of depressed children (Brumback *et al.*, 1977). The most characteristic sleep problem is awakening early in the morning and being unable to fall back to sleep (delayed or terminal insomnia). Usually parents are not immediately aware of this problem, but may become suspicious if they happen to awaken while the child is awake or if they find lights or television turned on in the morning. Careful questioning of the depressed child may reveal that he or she awakens frequently during the night and each time has difficulty getting back to sleep. Occasionally, the depressed child may have difficulty falling asleep upon initially going to bed (initial insomnia), but more commonly the depressed child falls asleep without problem. A small number of depressed children (about 5%) will be excessively sleepy and have difficulty awakening in the morning.

Somatic complaints, present in over one-half of all depressed children (Brumback *et al.*, 1977; Kuperman & Stewart, 1979), may be the most prominent presenting symptom, with headache, which may or may not have a migrainous quality (Ling *et al.*, 1970), being the most common. Sometimes the headache may be associated with photophobia, nausea, vomiting, autonomic changes, unsteadiness, and lethargy. Too often, because depressive illness is not considered among the diagnostic possibilities, unnecessary neurodiagnostic tests have been performed to evaluate a headache in a depressed child. Performance of an electroencephalogram (EEG) to evaluate the headache has not infrequently led to the incorrect diagnosis of seizure disorder. Nonspecific and/or epileptiform electroencephalographic abnormalities occur frequently in behaviorally disturbed children without clinical seizure disorder (Klinkerfuss, Lange, Weinberg, & O'Leary, 1965) and cannot be used as the basis for diagnosing epilepsy or beginning anticonvulsant therapy. Abdominal pains ("stomach aches") are also common in depressed children; these pains may occur independently or may be associated with headaches or with constipation. Muscle and joint aches and pains, dizziness, ringing in the ears, blurred vision, and chest pains are other less frequent somatic symptoms.

Disturbances in eating habits, which occur in about one-third of depressed children (Brumback *et al.*, 1977; Pearce, 1981), may be either a reduction or an increase in appetite and may be associated with changes in weight. One of the causes of severe anorexia in children and adolescents is depressive illness, which must be excluded before the diagnosis of the idiopathic disorder anorexia nervosa is made. Constipation is relatively common in depressed children, and a small number (less then 5%) may have encopresis (fecal soiling and/or having stools in underclothes). Enuresis or bed wetting may occur in 20% or more of depressed children (Brumback *et al.*, 1977; Kuperman & Stewart, 1979), often as secondary enuresis (bed wetting that begins after the child has been toilet trained without nighttime accidents) rather than primary enuresis (the child has never had a sustained period of being dry at night).

A change in psychomotor activity level (either an increase or decrease) and a reduction in motor proficiency is present in nearly all depressed children (Brumback *et al.*, 1977; Humphries, Gruber, Hall, & Kryscio, 1985). In a retarded depression there is a decrease in body (motor) activity (hypoactivity). The parent may feel it necessary continually to urge the child to "Hurry up!" or "Move!" Teachers become upset because the child does not complete tasks at the same rate as other children in the classroom. An associated slowing of mental activities may be evident as impaired concentration or confusion, and the child may "always be two steps behind" in understanding directions.

From 40% to 60% of depressed children will have an increase in mental and motor activity level during the depressive illness (Brumback *et al.*, 1977; Brumback & Weinberg, 1977b; Staton & Brumback, 1981). The hyperactive motor behavior is usually nonproductive or non–goal directed (for example, pacing back and forth, repeatedly standing up and sitting down in a chair, fidgeting, or tapping the hands or fingers), and the increased mental activity level may make the child hyperalert to extraneous stimuli and readily distractible (short attention span). Accident proneness may follow upon both the excessive activity and the easy distractibility, and the child may act impulsively. This same constellation of disruptive symptoms has assumed the status of a specific disease entity under a variety of names, including developmental hyperactivity, minimal brain dysfunction (MBD), hyperkinetic syndrome, and recently "attention deficit disorder" (American Psychiatric Association, 1980; Clemmens & Kenny, 1972; Satterfield, Cantwell, & Satterfield, 1974; Stewart, 1970; Stewart, Pitts, Craig, & Dieruf, 1966), in part because of the observation by Bradley in 1937 that treatment with the stimulant drug Benzedrine (racemic amphetamine) produced an almost miraculous reduction in hyperactive symptoms. Subsequently, dextroamphetamine (the more potent amphetamine isomer), methylphenidate, and pemoline proved equally effective. Unfortunately, since many clinicians considered this hyperactive symptom complex to be the only "biological" behavioral disorder in children (that biological nature having been "proved" by the evidence of symptomatic improvement from stimulant pharmacotherapy), children with almost any possibly biological behavioral problems (regardless of the exact symptomatology) were pigeonholed into the diagnostic category of hyperactivity. Moodiness, sadness, and other depressive symptoms commonly identified in hyperactive children (Bohline, 1985) have usually been explained as the consequence of deprivation in infancy, parental rejection, difficulty controlling aggression, and/or an inward conflict over the increased activity level (Zrull, McDermott, & Poznan-

Table 17-4. Hyperactivity and Depression in 223 Consecutive Children Referred for Educational Evaluation

	Hyperactive ($n = 117$)	Not hyperactive ($n = 106$)
Depressed ($n = 136$)	86	50
Not depressed ($n = 87$)	31	56
$\chi^2 = 15.1$; $p < .0001$		

Source: Adapted from Brumback & Weinberg (1977b).

ski, 1970). Yet, despite the unquestioned reduction in hyperactivity produced by stimulant drugs, definite evidence that the child's academic abilities improve has been lacking (Gadow, 1983; Ottenbacher & Cooper, 1983; Whalen & Henker, 1976). Some investigators have found that stimulant medications improve vigilance and reduce activity levels as much in normal volunteers as in hyperactive children (Gadow, 1983; Klorman *et al.*, 1984; Rapoport, Buchsbaum, Weingartner, Zahn, & Ludlow, 1980; Rapport, Murphy, & Bailey, 1982) and have even suggested that learning may deteriorate with stimulant drug treatment (Wetzel, Squire, & Janowsky, 1981). In addition, some children react adversely to stimulant drugs with increasing withdrawal, sadness, and crying. Of all children with excessive psychomotor activity, about three-quarters will have a depressive illness; the other one-quarter of hyperactive children will have some other cause of the hyperactivity (Brumback & Weinberg, 1977b) (Table 17-4). For the latter group, in which the hyperactivity may have no readily apparent explanation (and, therefore, may be idiopathic), use of the term "attention deficit disorder" (American Psychiatric Association, 1980), which merely describes the symptoms, is probably appropriate. Often, this latter group of children with "idiopathic hyperactivity" has a history of excessive motor activity dating back to the child's early infancy (for example, scooting all around the crib in the first weeks of life; an occasional multiparous mother will describe the child as having been hyperactive *in utero* compared to her other pregnancies). In contrast, the hyperactivity in depressed children usually does not appear until after other symptoms of depressive illness become apparent, and remission of the depression ameliorates the hyperactivity (Brumback *et al.*, 1977). Since stimulant drugs have antidepressant properties and have been used successfully in the short-term treatment of depressive episodes (Kiloh, Neilson, & Andrews, 1974; Otow, 1980; Post, Kotin, & Goodwin, 1974; Rudolf, 1956), improvement of hyperactive symptoms with stimulant medication does not prove that hyperactivity is a distinct syndrome. The frequently reported success of antidepressant pharmacotherapy in the treatment of children presenting with hyperactive behavior (Garfinkel, Wender, Sloman, & O'Neill, 1983; Huessy & Wright, 1970; Werry, Aman, & Diamond, 1980), lends support to the suggestion that depressive illness may be an underlying contributing factor in most hyperactive children (Brumback & Staton, 1982a, 1982b). The hyperactive children who apparently have a poor long-term prognosis (Blouin *et al.*, 1978; Huessy & Cohen, 1976; Riddle & Rapoport, 1976) seem to be those with depression, in whom the depressive illness is neither recognized nor properly treated (Brumback & Weinberg, 1977b).

Depressive illness is usually associated with a diurnal variation in symptomatology. The dysphoric mood and other depressive symptoms are generally worse in the morning and tend to improve over the course of the day. Parents may note that the depressed child is a "real bear to get along with" in the morning, but that he or she is more reasonable after school or in the evening.

REPRESENTATIVE BIOLOGICAL CORRELATES OF DEPRESSION

The physiological (biological or vegetative) symptoms of depression (Table 17-2) suggest that depression is more than just a mood change; it involves a profound effect on multiple brain and body systems. The reports of disturbed sleep have neurophysiological correlates in the abnormal polysomnographic patterns recorded in depressed patients (Post & Ballenger, 1984). The normal adult all-night polysomnographic recording reveals a short period of wakefulness after turning out the light, followed by onset of 70 to 100 minutes of non–rapid eye movement (non-REM) sleep before the first rapid eye movement (REM) sleep period begins. The most clearly reproducible characteristic of the sleep pattern in depressed adults is the short REM latency, which is the unusually early onset of the first REM sleep period in relation to the onset of sleep (Taub, 1984; Vogel, Vogel, & McAbee, 1980). Unfortunately, because of the marked age-related maturational variations in the normal polysomnographic sleep pattern in children, it has not yet been possible to confirm a short REM latency in depressed children (Puig-Antich *et al.*, 1982; Puig-Antich, Goetz *et al.*, 1983). Other neurophysiological abnormalities reportedly associated with depressive episodes include an alteration in the frequency and power spectrum of the right-hemisphere activity in quantitatively analyzed electroencephalographic recordings (Abrams & Taylor, 1979; Flor-Henry, 1976, 1983; Marin & Tucker, 1981; Rochford, Weinapple, & Goldstein, 1981; Tucker, 1981; Tucker, Stenslie, Roth, & Shearer, 1981), reduced cerebral blood flow to the posterior right cerebral hemisphere (Uytdenhoef *et al.*, 1983), and poorer performance of the right hemisphere to dichotic listening tests (Yozawitz *et al.*, 1979).

Abnormal growth hormone secretion and changes in the normal circadian fluctuations of hypothalamic–pituitary–adrenal secretion have been found in depressive illness, suggesting a depression-induced dysfunction of the hypothalamic regulatory centers (Post & Ballenger, 1984). Normally, serum cortisol and adrenocorticotrophic hormone (ACTH) levels fluctuate over the 24 hours of a day, with the highest levels recorded in the morning and the lowest levels in the evening. In the normal diurnal cycle (11:00 P.M. bedtime, 7:00 A.M. arousal), cortisol secretion is virtually absent between 8:00 P.M. and 2:00 A.M. and is maximal at approximately 9:00 A.M. In the dexamethasone suppression test (DST), administration of a single oral dose of dexamethasone (1.0 mg in adults or 0.5 mg in children) at 11:00 P.M. will normally almost completely suppress serum cortisol values below 6 micrograms/dl for 24 hours. Most depressed individuals secrete cortisol at night and have an abnormal response to the DST, but the frequency of this abnormal response has been variable in different studies. Most do not suppress the morning cortisol secretion, and many of those who do suppress the morning secretion escape with a rise of serum cortisol before the full 24 hours has elapsed (Carroll, Curtis, & Mendels, 1976a, 1976b; Carroll *et al.*, 1981). Unfortunately, the frequency of positivity on the DST has varied widely in different studies (Emslie, Weinberg, Rush, Weissenburger, & Parkin-Feigenbaum, 1987; Geller, Rogol, & Knitter, 1983; Poznanski, Carroll, Banegas, Cook, & Grossman, 1982; Puig-Antich, Chambers, Halpern, Hanlon, & Sachar, 1979), and its usefulness as a reliable diagnostic test of childhood depression has not yet been established. However, in those individuals with an abnormal DST, normalization of the cortisol responses parallels clinical improvement and a persistently abnormal test despite apparent clinical recovery indicates incomplete remission and probable early relapse.

Normally, basal growth hormone secretion is low, but during the insulin tolerance test, growth hormone secretion is markedly enhanced by the insulin-induced hypoglycemia (blood sugar values 50% below normal). Up to 70% of depressed children hyposecrete growth hormone in response to insulin-induced hypoglycemia (Puig-Antich *et al.*, 1984a, 1984b, 1984c, 1984d). Similar hyposecretion of growth hormone has been described in psychosocial dwarfism (the condition of short stature, sleeplessness, and behavioral disturbance that occurs in young children in environments of social deprivation and which some investigators have suggested is a psychodynamic model of depression); however, the hyposecretion of growth hormone (as well as the sleep and behavioral disturbances) normalize quickly (often within 24 hours) when the deprived child is placed in a caring environment, even a hospital (Guilhaume, Benoit, Gourmelen, & Richardet, 1982; Powell, Brazel, & Blizzard, 1967; Powell, Hopwood, & Barratt, 1973). In contrast, children with a history of a depressive episode (and hyposecretion of growth hormone in response to hypoglycemia) still have hyposecretion of growth hormone many months after complete remission of the depression. In addition, children who are currently depressed or have a history of a recent depressive illness have excessive secretion of growth hormone during delta (slow wave) sleep.

DEPRESSION, NEUROLOGICAL FUNCTION, AND NEUROPSYCHOLOGICAL (COGNITIVE) FUNCTION

Depressive illness adversely affects both cognitive and sensorimotor functioning of the brain, an observation first reported by Bruce (1895), who described the case of a 47-year-old Welsh sailor with recurrent manic-depressive illness, who in his depressive state was completely left-handed, remained relatively immobile, appeared confused, and spoke incoherently in and understood only Welsh. When this patient cycled into a manic state, he was restless, had a mischievous sense of humor, spoke and understood both English and Welsh fluently, was completely right-handed, and produced mirror writing with his left hand. Subsequently, Robinson (1976) reported the somewhat similar case of a 45-year-old manic-depressive right-handed man who had a postoperative Broca-type (nonfluent, expressive) aphasia and right hemiparesis, despite the otherwise successful total excision of a left cerebral convexity meningioma several years previously. This patient's speech and right-sided movement became normal during a manic episode, but the aphasia and hemiparesis returned after drug-induced remission of the mania. Freeman, Galaburda, Cabal, and Geschwind (1985) described a depressed 62-year-old woman whose reduced left-arm swing in walking, left central facial weakness, and marked right gaze preference (head and eyes strongly deviated to the right) resolved after electroconvulsive therapy (ECT)–induced remission of the depressive episode. Cutler, Post, Rey, and Bunney (1981) reported two manic-depressive patients whose persistent tardive oral-buccal-lingual dyskinesias secondary to long-term neuroleptic treatment disappeared during manic episodes and were apparent only during depressive episodes.

Goldstein, Filskov, Weaver, and Ives (1977) and Kronfol, Hamsher, Digre, and Waziri (1978) independently showed that depressed patients had low Wechsler Adult Intelligence Scale (WAIS) Performance IQ scores, but normal WAIS Verbal IQ and Full Scale IQ scores. Flor-Henry (1976, 1983) reported that WAIS Block Design and Object Assembly subtest scores were particularly low in depressed patients. Depressed college students showed significant deficits on paired easy associates, digit symbol, writing speed, and Neckar Cube reversals tests when compared with age-matched nondepressed controls (Berndt & Berndt, 1980). Hemsi, Whitehead, and Post (1968) found that depressed patients improved on Digit Copying and Synonym Learning tests after ECT-induced remission of depression. In a detailed study of 152 depressed individuals, Strömgren (1977) reported a significant correlation between the severity of depression and the degree of memory disturbance on the Wechsler Memory Scale (WMS), and Breslow, Kocsis, and Belkin (1980) confirmed that depressed patients show significant deficits in all three memory subfunctions of the WMS. This depression-associated memory disturbance resolved after ECT-induced (Strömgren, 1977) or imipramine-induced (Glass *et al.*, 1978) remission of the depressive episode. Savard, Rey, and Post (1980) noted significantly more errors on the Halstead-Reitan Categories Test in depressed patients compared to control subjects, and that the high error scores improved toward normal after remission of the depression. More recently, Fromm and Schopflocher (1984) demonstrated neuropsychological findings consistent with right-cerebral-hemisphere dysfunction in depressed middle-aged and elderly adults; appropriate antidepressant treatment improved these neuropsychological deficits, and the most improvement occurred in those functions with the greatest deficit. It has also been suggested that the deterioration in neuropsychological test performance that seems to predict impending death in elderly individuals may be a symptom of depression (Brumback, 1985b).

The study by Weinberg *et al.* (1973) initially delineating diagnostic criteria for childhood depression (conducted at an educational diagnostic center to which children with learning problems were referred by their schoolteachers) used "change in school performance" as one of the criterion symptoms (see Table 17-1). Although the depressed child's poor school performance may be explained in part by poor concentration and a lack of interest in the schoolwork, a change in cognitive (neuropsychological) function also plays a major role. As early as 1965, Rapoport found that imipramine treatment specifically improved handwriting, reading, and arithmetic skills according to both school reports and psychological test findings in a group of 41 depressed, learning-disabled children and adolescents. Warneke (1975) described a 14-year-old manic-depressive boy who had a severe learning disability, with a Wechsler Intelligence Scale for Children (WISC) Verbal IQ of 92 and Performance IQ of 69 during a depressive episode. Following ECT-induced remission of depression, this child's learning disability resolved in association with a dramatic improvement of neuropsychological test scores (posttreatment WISC Verbal IQ of 94 and Performance IQ of 93). Coll & Bland (1979) reported a medication-responsive 14½-year-old manic-depressive boy with pretreatment Wechsler Intelligence Scale for Children, Revised Edition (WISC-R) Verbal IQ of 111, Performance IQ of 91, and Full Scale IQ of 101. Yepes, Balka, Winsberg, and Bialer (1977) found that those aggressive, hyperactive children with symptomatology suggestive of depression, whose behavior improved following amitriptyline pharmacotherapy, also showed improvement on various neuropsychological measures, including the Continuous Performance Test (Rosvold, Mirsky, Sarason, Bransome, & Beck, 1956), the Matching Familiar Figures test, and a short-term memory test. Kaslow, Tanenbaum, Abramson, Peterson, & Seligman (1983), in a study of depressed and nondepressed 4th- and 5th-grade children with normal Peabody Picture Vocabularly Test scores, found that the depressed children (based on their scores on the Children's Depression Inventory [Kovacs, 1981]) were significantly ($p<.001$) slower than nondepressed children in completing a WISC-R–like block designs task and in solving an anagrams task. Mullins, Siegel, and Hodges (1985) also reported that depressed children of this same age showed poorer performance on an anagrams task than did nondepressed children. In another comparison of cognitive problem solving by depressed and nondepressed elementary school children, the depressed children significantly ($p<.01$) made more errors, were less efficient, and had longer response latencies than the nondepressed children on the Matching Familiar Figures test (Schwartz, Friedman, Lindsay, & Narrol, 1982).

At the University of North Dakota School of Medicine Childhood Depression and Hyperactivity Clinic, we studied the possible relationships between depressive illness, specific neurological signs, and learning disturbances, after the chance observation of two depressed, learning-disabled children who had neurological signs of left hemiparesis (including pronation drift of the outstretched left arm, hyperactive left-sided tendon reflexes, and left extensor plantar response) in whom treatment with a tricyclic antidepressant to ameliorate the depression resulted in complete disappearance of the neurological signs (Staton, Wilson, & Brumback, 1981). In one of these children, the left hemiparesis reappeared after medication withdrawal resulted in recurrence of the depression, but the neurological signs again resolved after reinstitution of antidepressant medication produced another remission of the depression. We subsequently noted other depressed children with neurological disturbances (including stuttering and multiple tics) that resolved with remission of the depressive episode (Brumback & Staton, 1981). By utilizing a simplified screening examination for lateralized sensorimotor neurological abnormality (Table 17-5; Figures 17-1 through 17-5); in conjunction with neuropsychological evaluation, we found specific neurological, cognitive, and behavioral symptom patterns associated with depression. Depressed children frequently showed the same mixed lateral preference ("mixed dominance") that has been reported in many other studies of individuals with a variety of behavior and learning problems (Critchley & Critchley, 1978; Geschwind & Behan, 1982; Geschwind & Galaburda, 1984, 1985). Over 75% of our depressed children, however, showed specific postural, movement, and reflex asymmetries involving the left side of the body (examples shown in Figure 17-6), which, in conjunction with neuropsychological asymmetries, provided evidence of the hemisyndrome of dysfunction of the right cerebral hemisphere.

Table 17-5. Simplified Examination for Lateralized Sensorimotor Neurological Abnormality

Part One (Figure 17-1)		
I. Lateral preference (dominance)		
Motor		
A. Hand preference		
Throwing ball	L______	R______
Writing	L______	R______
B. Foot preference		
Kicking ball	L______	R______
Hopping on "best" foot	L______	R______
Sensory		
C. Eye preference		
Looking through a tube or telescope	L______	R______
D. Ear preference		
Listening to telephone	L______	R______
Part Two (Figures 17-2 and 17-3)		
II. Posture with arms extended		
A. Feet together, pronated arms extended in front (palms toward floor)		
0 = no spooning + = spooning	L______	R______
B. Feet together, supinated arms extended in front (palms toward ceiling)		
0 = no pronation or drift		
+ = pronation and/or downward or outward drift	L______	R______
III. Walking (spontaneous and "stressed") 10 to 20 paces and return		
A. Spontaneous walking		
Legs	L______	R______
Arms	L______	R______

B. Walking on tiptoes
Legs L_____ R_____
Arms L_____ R_____
C. Walking on heels
Legs L_____ R_____
Arms L_____ R_____
D. Walking on lateral surfaces (outsides) of feet
Legs L_____ R_____
Arms L_____ R_____
Scoring:
Legs: 0 = normal ability to walk
+ = circumduction of leg (and stiff knee) or inability to stay on tiptoes, heel, or side of foot
Arms: 0 = normal arm swing (palms toward thigh)
+ = no arm swing, or arm held stiffly, or arm postured (elbow flexion, or fisted thumb, or wrist flexion)

IV. Skipping (10 skips forward and return)
0 = skips normally
+ = repeated hops with same leg forward or occasional alternating hops _____

Part Three (Figures 17-4 and 17-5)

V. Tendon reflexes
A. Biceps L_____ R_____
B. Knee L_____ R_____
Scoring:
0 = both sides equal
+ = unequal reflexes (more active side abnormal)

VI. Leg position (lying flat on back, head straight, arms at side, eyes closed, legs spread slightly apart and relaxed)
0 = foot pointing upward (nearly vertical)
+ = leg markedly externally rotated with foot pointing outward (nearly horizontal) L_____ R_____

VII. Plantar response
0 = normal flexion (curling) of toes
+ = no movement or extension of big toe L_____ R_____

DEPRESSION AND THE HEMISYNDROMES OF CEREBRAL HEMISPHERIC DYSFUNCTION

Although learning disabilities affect at least 5% and possibly as many as 30% of school-age children (Cantwell & Forness, 1982; Dworkin, 1985; Feagans, 1983; Kirk & Elkins, 1975; Lerner, 1976; Meier, 1971) most current classification schemes categorize ("split") learning disabilities into so many different specific subtypes (some subtypes so specific as to apply only to a vanishingly few individuals) that correlations with other disorders have been difficult, if not impossible (Boder, 1973; Culbertson & Ferry, 1982; Denckla, 1973; Harris, 1982; Levine, Brooks, & Shonkoff, 1980; Levine, Oberklaid, & Meltzer, 1981; Mattis, French, & Rapin, 1973; Rapin, 1982; Resnick, Allen, & Rapin, 1984; Watson, Watson, & Fredd, 1982). However, by utilizing an admittedly simplistic classification scheme that relates specific behavioral, developmental, academic, neurological, and neuropsychological characteristics to cerebral hemispheric dysfunction, it has been possible to recognize

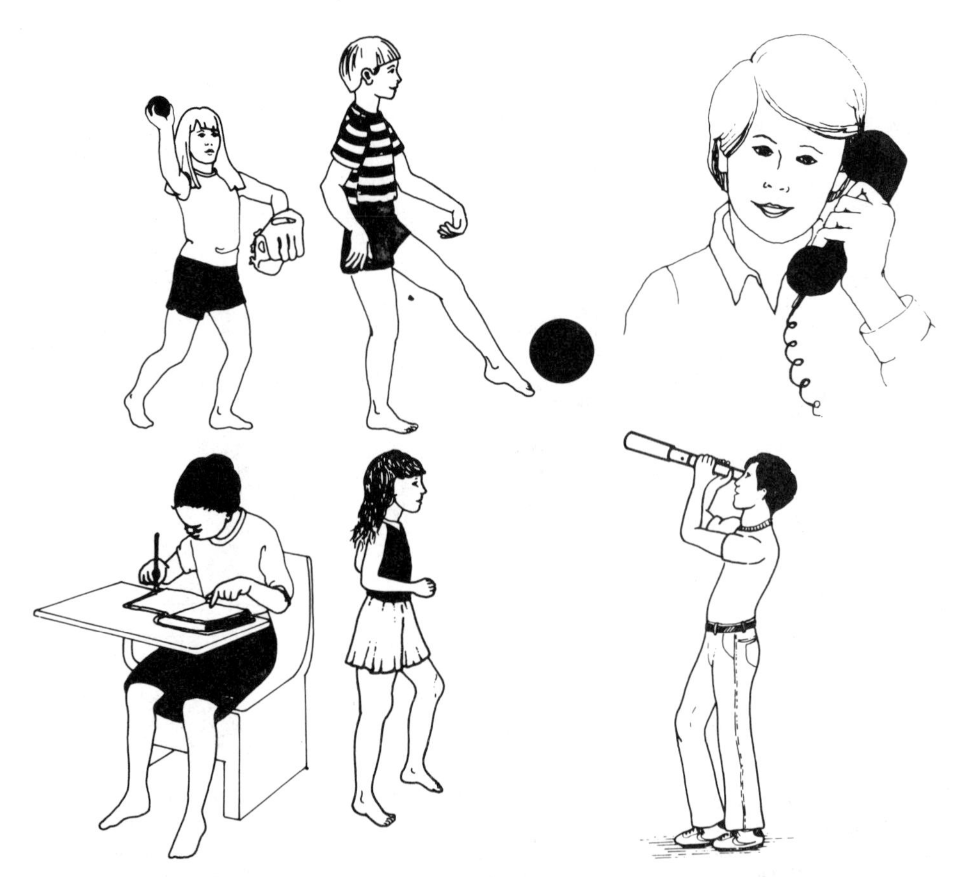

Figure 17-1. Lateral preference (dominance or lateral superiority) is assessed by observing which hand the child uses to throw a ball, which hand is used to write, which foot is used to kick a ball, which foot remains on the ground when the child is asked to stand and hop on one foot, which eye is used to look through a tube or telescope, and which ear is used to listen to a telephone.

two major hemisyndromes (right-cerebral-hemispheric dysfunction and left-cerebral-hemispheric dysfunction) in learning-disabled and behaviorally disturbed children (Table 17-6 and 17-7) and to relate these to childhood depressive illness (Brumback & Staton, 1983). Although lateralized abnormalities on detailed neurological and neuropsychological assessment can provide substantial evidence for lateralized cerebral dysfunction, such evaluations are time consuming, expensive, frequently unavailable, and subject to the problems of obtaining the child's cooperation. Wechsler intelligence test results showing a marked difference between the Verbal IQ score (a measure of left-hemisphere function) and the Performance IQ score (a measure of right-hemisphere function) are suggestive of lateralized cerebral hemispheric dysfunction, with Performance IQ deficit (Verbal IQ score higher than Performance IQ score) implying right-cerebral-hemisphere dysfunction and Verbal IQ deficit suggesting left cerebral dysfunction. However, the statistical significance reported for the size of the WISC-R Verbal–Performance IQ discrepancy of at least 9 IQ points ($p<.15$), 12 IQ points ($p<.05$), or 15 IQ points ($p<.01$) translates only into the degree of confi-

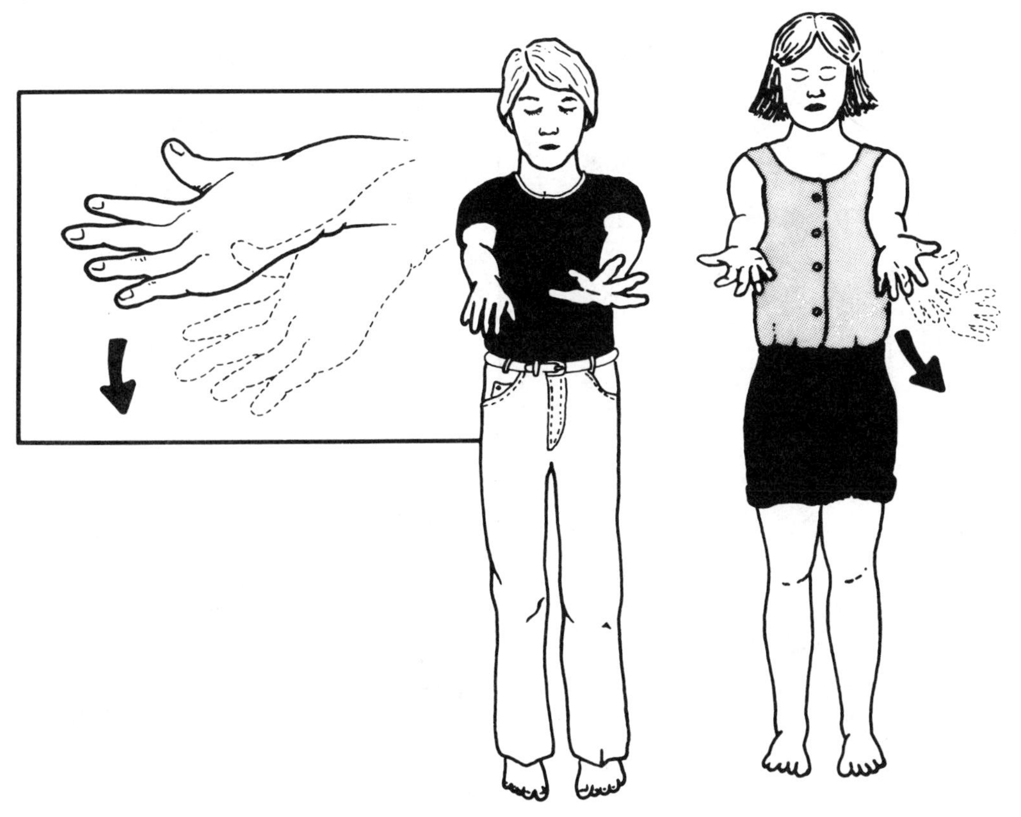

Figure 17-2. The child is told to stand with eyes closed and arms outstretched in front with palms facing the floor or facing the ceiling. Normally the arms will be symmetrically positioned and the hands will be flat. Starting in a symmetrical position with the palms facing the floor, the abnormal posturing will be evident as one hand (in this example, the left hand) bending at the wrist toward the floor (see insert) and the fingers extending backwards to make the top surface of the hand concave (like the end of a spoon, hence the term ''spooning''). When the child stands with the palms of the hands facing upward, one hand may slowly turn over (pronate) and drift outward and/or downward.

dence that the Verbal IQ and Performance IQ scores are actually different (Wechsler, 1974). The average Verbal–Performance IQ discrepancy (regardless of direction) of the normal children used in the standardization of the WISC-R was 9.7 (S.D. = 7.6) IQ points, and 50% of normal children had a discrepancy of at least 9 points, 33% had a discrepancy of at least 12 points, and 25% had a discrepancy of at least 15 points (Kaufman, 1976, 1979; Kaufman, Long, & O'Neal, 1986). Thus, while large Verbal–Performance IQ discrepancies suggest lateralized cerebral dysfunction, the finding of discrepancy alone cannot be used to make a diagnosis. The finding of lateralized sensorimotor neurological abnormalities, however, is a definite indication of lateralized cerebral dysfunction and, in combination with a detailed history of the symptoms associated with each hemisyndrome and the presence of a WISC-R Verbal–Performance IQ discrepancy, can be used to establish the diagnosis of the specific hemisyndrome of lateralized cerebral dysfunction. The most common hemisyndrome (occurring in about one-half to two-thirds of children with

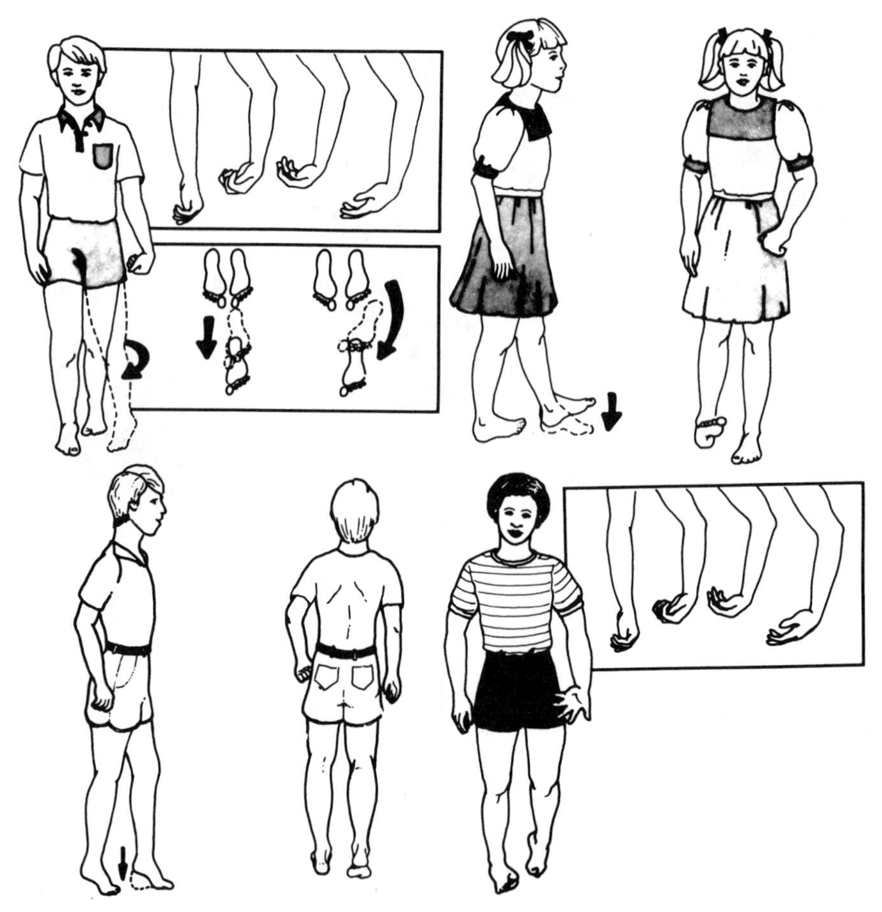

Figure 17-3. The child is observed walking 10 to 20 paces forward and returning during ordinary walking and "stressed" walking. In ordinary walking, the legs move smoothly forward and the arms (with the palms directed toward the thighs) swing an equal distance back and forth. Abnormality is apparent as one leg moving stiffly or swinging outward as shown on the left side of the subject pictured (inset shows the normal pattern of foot movement in the left panel and an abnormal pattern of foot movement in the right panel). There may also be reduced arm swing and/or abnormal arm postures such as those shown in the left arm of the pictured subject or in the inset. Stressed walking consists of walking successively on tiptoes, heels, and outsides (lateral surfaces) of the feet (feet inverted), while the observer notes any asymmetric abilities to remain on the heels, tiptoes, or outsides of the feet, or any abnormal posturing of one hand or arm during the walking tasks, which may be most evident when the child walks on the outsides of the feet.

learning and behavior disturbances) appears to be that of right cerebral dysfunction (Brumback, 1979; Brumback, Jackoway, & Weinberg, 1980, unpublished observations from the Pattonville Study; see Table 17-8), while only about 10% of behaviorally disturbed or learning-disabled children have the hemisyndrome of left cerebral dysfunction; an additional one-quarter to one-third will have a syndrome of bihemispheric dysfunction (a combination of features of both the right cerebral dysfunction hemisyndrome and the left cerebral dysfunction hemisyndrome).

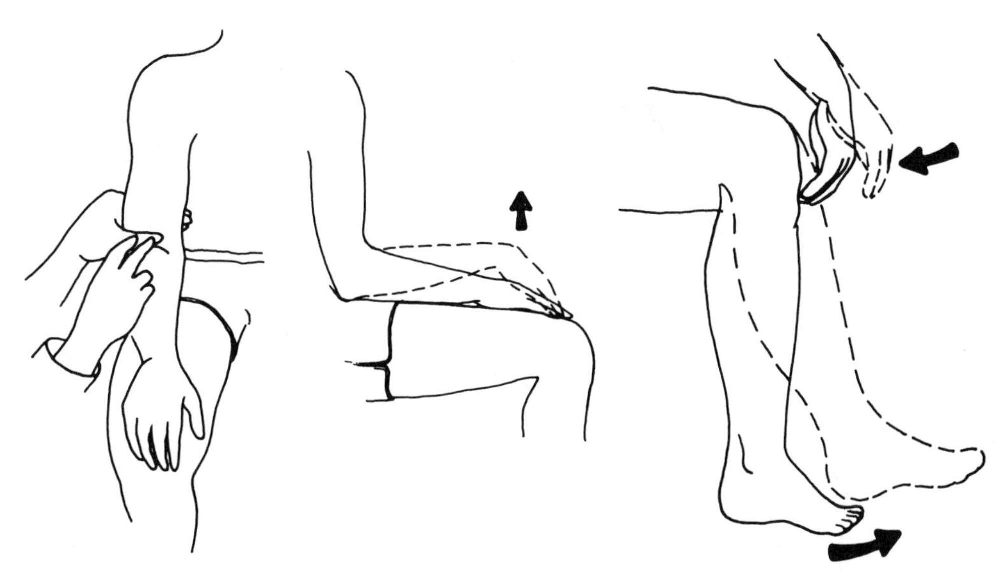

FIgure 17-4. Testing of tendon reflexes requires the use of the fingertips of one hand as a percussion instrument (hammer), which in testing children is less threatening and just as effective as use of a reflex hammer. The examiner strikes a sharp blow with the finger tips over the tendon, causing a reflex contraction of the muscle and a visible twitch or jump at the joint. To test the biceps reflex the child must be in a sitting position with the arms comfortably resting on the thighs, and the examiner gently places a hand around the child's elbow with the thumb on the child's biceps tendon in the elbow crease. Sharply striking the thumb with the other hand causes a quick reflex contraction of the biceps muscle that can be felt by as a movement of the biceps tendon and seen as a slight flexion of the child's arm at the elbow. To test the knee reflex, the child should be sitting high enough that the legs dangle freely, and the examiner sharply strikes with four fingers the slight hollow containing the broad tendon just below the kneecap; reflex contraction of the upper thigh muscle will cause the lower leg to swing forward slightly. The more active side is abnormal when the reflex is asymmetrical.

Hemisyndrome of Right Cerebral Dysfunction

Depression is most commonly associated with the hemisyndrome of right cerebral hemispheric dysfunction (which has also been known by a variety of names, including ''clumsy child'' syndrome, visual-motor disability, developmental apraxia, the developmental Gerstmann syndrome, and developmental dyscalculia). The impaired spatial skills (spatial orientation, spatial imagery, and spatial ordering) of the child with right-cerebral-hemispheric dysfunction interfere with many play activities such as puzzles, coloring books, constructional toys, and ball games. The child may have difficulty correctly handling and using common objects (e.g., properly holding a baseball bat, properly gripping and using a pen or a knife and fork, or properly opening and closing a screw-top jar lid). The child will have difficulty with the figure–ground discrimination required by ''find the hidden object'' picture games. Visuospatial confusion may impair recognition of visual images (such as faces) or the proper matching of names and faces, and the child's inability to recognize acquaintances, particularly from among a group of people, makes peers think the child is ''unfriendly'' or ''stuck-up.'' Judging size, distance, or weight relationships is

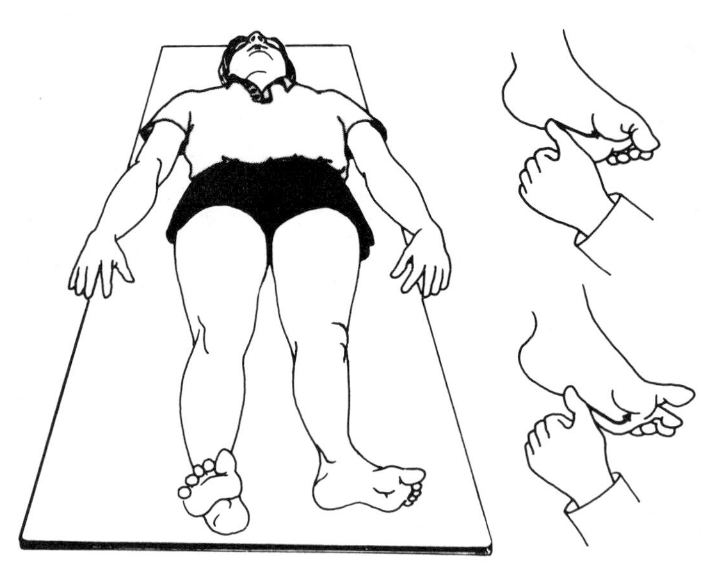

Figure 17-5. The child's leg position at rest is evaluated by having the child lie flat with the head straight, arms at sides, eyes closed, and legs spread slightly apart and relaxed. The legs ordinarily should be relatively symmetrical (usually the toes are directed slightly outward, but occasionally they may be straight or turned slightly inward); marked external rotation of one leg (foot and leg rotated outward) compared to the other leg is abnormal. The plantar reflex (the most sensitive indicator of lateralized cerebral hemispheric dysfunction) can then be performed with the child in the lying position, although ticklishness of the bottom of the foot in some children may preclude its performance. The plantar reflex is elicited by lightly scratching with the thumbnail in one continuous motion along the bottom outside (lateral side) of the foot beginning at the heel, going up to the ball of the foot, continuing across the ball of the foot, and ending just before the base of the big toe. Normally, all the toes will curl (flex). An abnormal response (an extensor plantar response) is for the big toe or all the toes to fail to curl or for the big toe or all the toes to move upward or backward (extend). If the whole foot withdraws because the child is too ticklish, the test cannot be interpreted.

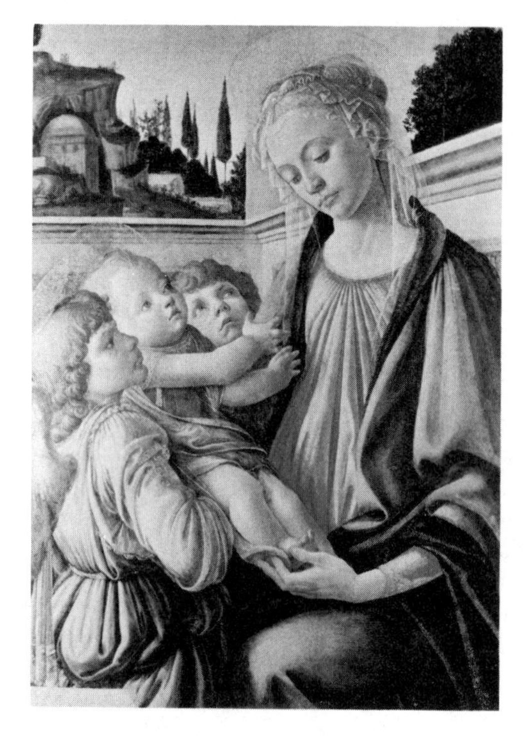

(b) The ease with which neurological signs such as the plantar reflex can be elicited and observed is evidenced in this 15th-century painting, *Madonna and Child with Angels* by Sandro Boticelli, in which the mother's stimulation of the outside of the infant's foot produces the extensor plantar response.

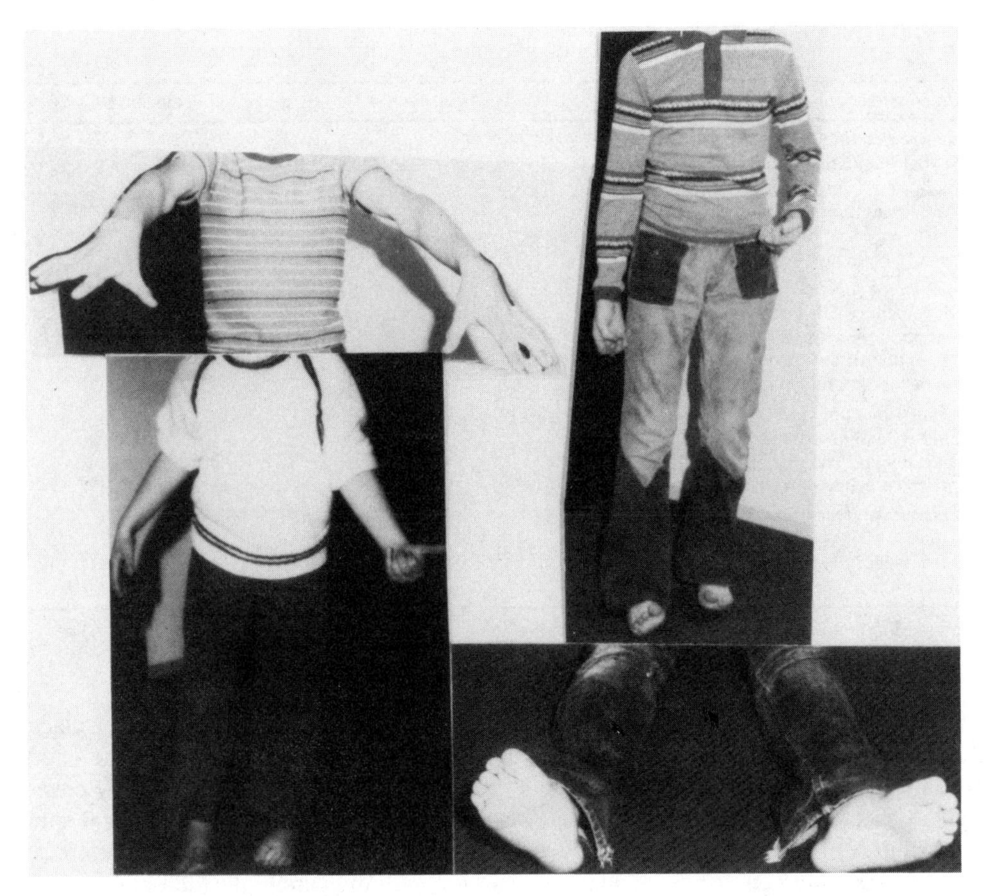

Figure 17-6. Examples of abnormalities involving the left side of the body (suggesting right cerebral hemisphere dysfunction) noted on the sensorimotor neurological examination in four children with depression: wrist drop and spooning of left hand; abnormal posturing of the left arm during stressed walking; outward rotation of the left leg in the lying position.

difficult for children with right cerebral dysfunction. Persistent confusion of directionality (confusion of right versus left is abnormal beyond 7 years of age) and difficulties with body orientation may lead to problems with dressing. The child performs poorly on spatially oriented school skills such as telling time (using a dial or analogue clock), cutting with scissors, sewing, art, and penmanship and other paper-and-pencil tasks. Paperwork is usually messy, with irregular size and shape of letters, figures, symbols, and geometric forms; irregular pressure and frequent erasures; and written lines that are poorly spaced, crowded, and variable in size.

The child persistently reverses letters or numbers (strephosymbolia). Such reversals usually involve symbols that are similar except for their horizontal (left-to-right) orientation (such as the letters *b* and *d*), although some more severely affected children may also have reversals of symbols that differ in vertical (up-and-down) orientation (such as the letters *b* and *p*). Normally, some children reverse the vertical orientation of symbols until 4½ to 5 years of age and the right–left orientation of symbols until the end of first grade (about 6½ to 7 years), but persistent reversal of letters and numbers beyond these ages is abnormal. Although the letter reversals interfere with reading (for instance, the word *big* may be confused with *dig, pig,* or *dip*), the child also has difficulty reading because of an inability

Table 17-6. Laterality of Cerebral Hemispheric Functions

Right cerebral hemisphere	Left cerebral hemisphere
Cognitive function:	*Cognitive function:*
Spatial orientation, imagery, ordering	Language skills (comprehension and expression of oral and written language)
Right–left discrimination	*Sensorimotor function:*
Timing and time perception	Movement of right body
Music appreciation (appreciating pitch and tonality of sound)	Sensation of right body
Sensorimotor function:	Perception of right visual field
Movement of left body	Appreciation of sound from right ear
Sensation of left body	
Perception of left visual field	
Appreciation of sound from left ear	
Emotional function:	
Prosody and emotional gesturing	
Empathy and comprehension of emotionality	
Affective behavior	
Attentional/vigilance function:	
Arousal	
Attentiveness	
Activation	

Source: Modified from Brumback & Staton (1983).

to maintain proper orientation on the printed page. The child will lose his or her place on the line or page; the longer the reading passage, the greater the problem. Some children will attempt to compensate by marking the place on the page with a finger or by covering (with a sheet of paper) all the text except the line being read. Arithmetic problem solving that requires maintenance of the relative position of the digits (such as vertical columns for addition and subtraction or diagonal columns for multidigit multiplication and long division) is characteristically poor for the same reason.

Because of problems conceptualizing "the whole as a series of interconnected parts," the child has great difficulty completing large or multistep tasks or performing assignments with a series of directions. Instead of correctly attributing the difficulties to an inability to perform required multistep tasks, teachers may consider the child to be inattentive or noncompliant because of the "forgotten" assignments or homework. Family members may describe the child as "forgetful," "obstinate" ("he can do it, but he won't"), "disorganized," "always losing his place," "can't keep on track," and needing constant prodding and supervision. Sloppiness may result from difficulties in independently completing the multiple steps required in dressing (for example, putting shoes on before socks instead of after socks, zipping the fly on a pair of pants, buttoning all the buttons on a shirt) and in proper personal hygiene. This sloppiness, sometimes mistakenly considered willful, may result in teasing and interfere with school, peer, and family relationships. The ability to work independently deteriorates along with skill and accuracy in task performance as the length of time necessary for completion of the task increases. The child may be unable to provide an orderly recounting of events or stories (e.g., telling a joke without mixing the punch line and the story) and unable to judge the proper temporal sequence of events (e.g., the concepts of "before" and "after"). Difficulty with processing multiple items may also appear in language skills. In reciting overlearned series (such as the alphabet, numbers from 1 to 20, days of the week, months of the year, and seasons of the year) the child will misorder, repeat, and omit items. Similar errors result in misspelling and occasional misspeaking of multisyllabic (and some smaller) words (for example, *tevelision* for *television,*

Table 17-7. Neurobehavioral Symptomatology Associated with Right Cerebral Hemispheric and Left Cerebral Hemispheric Hemisyndromes (Learning Disabilities)

Right cerebral dysfunction	Left cerebral dysfunction
Toddler: Marked clumsiness and delayed acquisition of motor skills	*Toddler:* Silent, quiet Difficulty understanding when spoken to Little response to instructions or direct questions Delayed speech Poor articulation
Preschool: Avoids playing with puzzles, constructional toys, and coloring books Clumsy play where spatial skills are important (such as ball games) Difficulty with dressing, organizing bedroom, and following instructions	*Preschool:* Delayed *naming* of colors, geometric shapes, numbers, letters Substitution of action words (verbs) for nouns in speech
School age: Loses place on page when reading (may mark place by pointing at each word) Difficulty organizing arithmetic problems Poor handwriting and disorganized, messy paperwork Difficulty judging size, distance, weight Difficulty telling time Inattentive and easily distracted	*School age:* Difficulty reading and word substitutions Difficulty understanding math concepts (symbols) Difficulty spelling Unable to skip
Neurological signs: Abnormal left arm and/or leg postures and reflexes	*Neurological signs:* Abnormal right arm and/or leg postures and reflexes

Source: Modified from Brumback & Staton (1983).

refriteragor for *refrigerator, wnt* for *went, saw* for *was*) (Figure 17-7). The child also will have difficulties solving mathematical equations because of an inability to follow the proper sequence of the various algebraic operations.

An additional factor that adversely affects the child's ability to complete multistep tasks is the dysfunction of the right cerebral hemisphere's attentional/vigilance systems (Heilman & Van Den Abell, 1980; Mesulam, 1981), resulting in relative inattentiveness, easy distractibility by all types of minor environmental stimuli, and motor hyperactivity. It

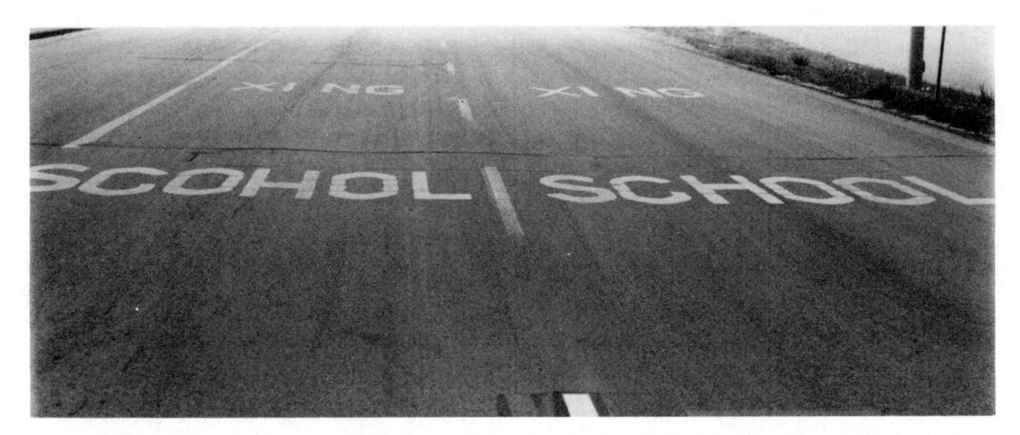

Figure 17-7. Road sign demonstrating the graphic misordering of right cerebral hemispheric dysfunction.

Table 17-8. Relationship of the Symptom of Hyperactivity to Lateralized Cerebral Hemispheric Dysfunction in a Group of 100 Consecutive Children Referred for Evaluation of School Difficulties

	Hyperactive ($N=45$)	Not hyperactive ($N=55$)
Right cerebral dysfunction ($N=57$)	25	32
Left cerebral dysfunction ($N=8$)	0	8
Bihemispheric dysfunction ($N=22$)	13	9
No learning disability ($N=13$)	7	6

Source: Unpublished data from the Pattonville Study of a group of consecutive children referred for evaluation of school learning or behavioral problems to the Educational Diagnostic Center of the Pattonville (St. Louis County, Missouri) School District (Brumback, Jackoway, & Weinberg, 1980).

Note: $p=0.03$ using χ^2 analysis of all groups or using Fisher's exact test (Armitage, 1971) for differences between left and right cerebral dysfunction groups.

is of interest that symptomatology of hyperactivity is notably absent in children with learning disability due to left cerebral dysfunction (see Table 17-8).

Probably the most significant problems for the child with right-cerebral-hemispheric dysfunction are: (1) difficulty in expressing appropriate nonverbal social cues (including happiness or anger) and in responding correctly to those cues expressed by others, and (2) difficulty in expressing and understanding the prosodic portions of language (the emotional and tonal inflections of speech). Inappropriate facial expressions make it difficult for the child to interact with parents and teachers as well as with peers. The child may appear "uninterested" or have an emotional facial expression that is unsuitable for the situation. The child may be considered socially inept because of incorrect and sometimes crude manners. The child will also have difficulty comprehending others' emotional reactions to his or her behavior. Although the child may have relatively good language skills (if left cerebral function is intact), the child's speech will be monotonous and lack emotional changes in pitch and tone or will have improperly placed inflections and inconsistent emotional tones. Since most educational programs emphasize language, symbolic concepts, and verbal skills, however, children with even relatively severe right cerebral dysfunction often have fewer school difficulties than do children with left cerebral dysfunction. In addition, the unkempt appearance, clumsiness, and difficulty with paper-and-pencil tasks of children (especially boys) with right cerebral dysfunction are usually accepted without much concern. Nevertheless, any failures in academic or peer group situations may impair normal personality development (Thompson, 1985).

Hemisyndrome of Left Cerebral Dysfunction

The left-cerebral-hemisphere dysfunction hemisyndrome involves varying degrees of disturbed language function and is much less commonly associated with depression. More severely affected children may present with "delayed" development of language (little speech production and/or poor articulation) in comparison to older siblings or to playmates of the same age, and may be described as "quiet" or "shy," with a poor general vocabulary and a relative lack of spoken language (dysphasia). Poor articulation of spoken words may be evident, but many times the parents can understand and communicate with the child, even though the language is not understandable to an outsider. Sometimes the child will be described as "immature" because the speech is more like that of a much younger child. The preschool child with left cerebral dysfunction will have delay in the normal development (Weinberg, 1982) of the symbolic language milestones of naming colors (3–4½ years), geometric shapes (3½–6 years), numbers (4½–6 years), and letters (5–6½ years). The child will be unable to "find" the correct word or words to describe objects, places, persons, and experiences, and will use descriptive circumlocution (e.g., "the thing you eat on" for *table*), identify an object by its association (e.g., *bed* for *blanket*), and substitute action words (verbs) for nouns (e.g., *throw* for *ball*). Often the child substitutes words that sound similar or can be used in a similar context, but sometimes the words do not relate to the context. For example, a parent asks, "What do you want for lunch?" the child who actually desires a hot dog might respond, "I want a hamburger" (substituting another food item) or "I want a cat" (substituting *cat* for "hot *dog*"). Similar sounding words (e.g., *ball* and *bell*) are easily confused. Speech may consist of only short sentences or incomplete phrases. Frequent speech hesitation (occurring either in initial word sounds or in the middle of words) may be mistaken for stuttering. Parents sometimes state that the child "just can't seem to tell us what he wants" or that "it's like the words are right on the tip of her tongue, but she just can't get them out." If the child is placed in a stressful situation, the substitutions, word-finding difficulties, and hesitations become especially prominent. Difficulties with receptive language may be evident as an apparent lack of understanding when spoken to or given instructions by parents and as a failure to respond to direct questioning or to directions. Instructions often need to be repeated (parents may complain that the child is always asking "What?"). Jokes and riddles that amuse peers may not be understood, although children with left cerebral dysfunction usually enjoy slapstick and visual comedy more than their peers do.

The degree of reading difficulty (dyslexia) experienced by the school-age child with left cerebral dysfunction varies, with some children having only a delay in the rate of acquisition of reading skills such that they can read, but not at expected grade level. The child has as much difficulty reading single words as reading sentences or paragraphs, but can easily follow line by line along the page without losing the place. The severity of the left cerebral dysfunction will determine whether the child is able to master the various stages of the educational process in learning to read, beginning with one-syllable written words in 1st and 2nd grade, followed by compound words (such as homework) in 3rd grade, and progressing to literacy in 4th grade by mastery of the word attack skills necessary for reading polysyllabic words. Reading difficulties of the child with left cerebral dysfunction will often be readily apparent if the child is asked to read aloud a grade-appropriate paragraph (such as in Table 17-9). Although poor word attack skills prevent the child from reading or comprehending many of the words in a written passage, some paragraphs may be understood from other context; the story line of more complicated passages, however, will usually not be understandable. During oral reading the child substitutes familiar words for unfamiliar words, sometimes making the sentence meaningless (e.g., "Tom likes art the fancy red tags," instead of "Tom laughs at the funny blue toys"). In speaking as well as in spelling tasks, the child makes phonemic and graphemic omissions or substitutions (e.g., saying and spelling "elant" for "elephant," "pay" for "pray," "whent" for "went," or "oures" for "hours"). The child will also have difficulty understanding operational concepts and symbols in mathematics (e.g., $2+6$ [2 plus 6] misinterpreted as 2×6 [2 multiplied by 6], resulting in an incorrect answer). Although the graphic aspects of writing may be normal (particularly if right cerebral function is intact), the same substitutions and grammatical and word usage problems that are evident in the child's speech will also be apparent in writing.

Table 17-9. Typical Reading Paragraphs for Grades 1 through 6 Used in Assessment of Left Cerebral Dysfunction

Grade 1

I saw a big tree.
The tree is green.
The girl has a red ball.
Father works on a farm.
Mother and Father go to the store.

Grade 2

Ann and her mother walk to the store.
Mother put the money into her pocket.
Ann plays with her new toy.
Father does hard work on the farm.
Father will eat a big dinner.

Grade 3

Tom and Kathy walk to the same red school.
They both saw the big bird in art class.
Kathy is almost ready to go to the store.
Tom should wait for Kathy in front of the house.
Tom laughs at the funny blue toys.
Kathy likes to help her mother do housework and cook dinner.

Grade 4

Father builds automobiles at his business. His favorite automobile has a shallow red back seat and a deep front seat. The top of the automobile is rough. Father puts white paint on the outside. Mother works at the toy store. She prepares special dolls which look like prisoners. Certain dolls wear goggles. She builds wonderful doll cottages. Ed and Sally study at school. Mother assists Ed with his important school work.

Grade 5

Bill and Peggy study astronomy in school. They learn about the sun, the stars, and the planets. The teacher told them a curious story about a famous scholar who studied the equator of the earth. They were astonished to learn about the inventors who forged the trail of human knowledge. Bill attends a biology class and learns about many different animals. Bill recognized a picture of crocodiles and lizards which the teacher showed to the students. Peggy learns about healthy eating habits in her cooking class. The class is growing tomato plants. Jane made marmalade to take home for her parents.

Grade 6

The summer camping trip to a legendary mining town will be exciting for Paul and Joan. Father is preparing his children for healthy outdoor living. Since camping can be treacherous, Father is carefully supervising all the preparations. Paul and Joan will each pack a burlap knapsack with the necessary camp supplies. Mother constructed a specialized apparatus to hold their immense tent. It is absolutely essential for Joan to receive swimming instruction before the trip. Paul has persuaded his father to visit a cave that bears once used for hibernation.

If right cerebral function is intact, the speech of the child with left cerebral dysfunction (even though sparse or inadequately articulated) will contain a normal (or even increased) amount of emotional tone and pitch. The child uses the marked variation in vocal emotion to compensate for the lack of linguistic output. Children with the most severe degree of left cerebral dysfunction have little expression or comprehension of spoken or written language and frequently rely on nonverbal means of expression such as pointing or using ''autistic'' arm or body movements. When constructional and organizational abilities of the right hemisphere are preserved, some children with moderately severe left cerebral dysfunction may manifest meticulous ordering of the environment and repetitive constructional activities that appear ritualistic. An interesting additional finding in children with left cerebral dysfunction is that they are generally unable to skip properly (skipping, which involves moving forward with alternating hops, can normally be performed by children over 6 years of age).

Children who have only subtle left cerebral dysfunction may still be handicapped in social relationships with more verbal peers and family members. The impaired oral and written communications skills result in a degree of social isolation that prevents the child from expressing concerns and feelings. Even excellent right-hemisphere drawing and constructional skills may not be enough to compensate for a poverty of language skills. Maladaptive acting-out behaviors further interfere with social attachments. Sexual promiscuity in teenage girls with left cerebral dysfunction may be an attempt to compensate for an inability to verbalize feelings of attachment. Aggressive acting out (more commonly observed in boys) may be another maladaptive behavior of the left-cerebral-hemisphere-impaired child who has limited ability to express (verbally) feelings of frustration, anger, and unhappiness. It is probable that lifelong personality disorders, not affective illness, may be the result of the persistent maladaptation in the child with left cerebral dysfunction. Cantwell and Baker (1977, 1980) have reported psychiatric disorders in a high proportion of children with language impairment, and Rutter, Graham, and Yule (1970) found that one-third of the children in the Isle of Wight survey with some degree of left-cerebral-hemispheric dysfunction (specific reading retardation) had diagnosable conduct disorder.

Antidepressant Therapy and Cerebral Dysfunction in Children

Tricyclic antidepressant administration to depressed children with the hemisyndrome of right-cerebral-hemispheric dysfunction results in a dramatic improvement not only in the depression, but also in the symptomatology of the right cerebral dysfunction (Brumback, Staton, & Wilson, 1980; Staton *et al.*, 1981). In a group of 11 depressed children administered neuropsychological test batteries both prior to and 3 to 6 months after instituting tricyclic antidepressant therapy, significant ($p < .05$) improvements occurred in the WISC-R Performance IQ (average 16-point increase); the WISC-R Similarities, Comprehension, Block Design, and Coding subtest scores (average 3- to 4-point increase); the Illinois Test of Psycholinguistic Abilities (ITPA) Visual Reception subtest score (average 8-point increase); the Halstead Categories Test error score; and the Matching Familiar Figures response latencies and error rates (Staton *et al.*, 1981). A larger study of 75 depressed, learning-disabled children (55 males, 20 females) demonstrated that tricyclic antidepressant–induced remission of depression resulted in significant ($p < .02$), though slightly smaller, average improvements in the WISC-R Verbal IQ and Performance IQ (average 8-point increase); WISC-R Similarities, Picture Completion, Picture Arrangement, and Block Design subtest scores (average 1- to 2-point increase); ITPA Visual Reception and Auditory Association subtest scores; Beery-Buktenica Visual–Motor Integration (VMI) score; Halstead Categories Test error score; Trail-making Test B score; Matching Familiar Figures error score; and Stroop-like attention test battery time and error scores (Wilson & Staton, 1984).

Examples of the marked improvements in neuropsychological test function and in ordinary paper-and-pencil tasks (such as draw-a-person, draw-a-clock, and handwriting) that can occur with remission of depression are shown in Table 17-10 and Figure 17-8. Six of the seven cases in Table 17-10 were normally intelligent children with learning disabilities associated with a depressive episode. However, Case #6 was a child diagnosed by the school as mildly mentally retarded (Grossman, 1983) and initially referred for evaluation of hyperactivity. After a careful examination revealed symptomatology of depression, tricyclic antidepressant treatment of his depressive illness also improved his level of intellectual and psychosocial functioning to the low normal or borderline range. Improvement in neuropsychological function with remission of depression is not simply a practice effect, since retesting of unmedicated control children (without depression) has shown no such improvement in test scores over the same time interval (Wilson & Staton, 1984). In addi-

Table 17-10. Examples of Neuropsychological Test Results Associated with Treatment of Depression in Children

	Case #1			Case #2			Case #3		
Measures	Pre	Post	Change	Pre	Post	Change	Pre	Post	Change
Age (yr)	10 0/12	10 3/12		11 9/12	12 2/12		13 6/12	13 11/12	
WISC-R									
Information	11	12	+1	15	14	−1	10	11	+1
Similarities	10	9	−1	16	18	+2	13	11	−2
Arithmetic	15	14	−1	10	10	0	11	11	0
Vocabulary	11	10	−1	13	13	0	14	16	+2
Comprehension	9	8	−1	13	18	+5	11	15	+4
Digit Span	12	10	−2	11	9	−2	10	8	−2
Picture Completion	9	9	0	13	15	+2	5	15	+10
Picture Arrangement	9	10	+1	11	13	+2	6	9	+3
Block Design	8	13	+4	13	15	+2	11	11	0
Object Assembly	12	9	−3	12	14	+2	12	12	0
Coding	5	12	+7	7	11	+4	8	12	+4
Verbal IQ	107	103	−4	120	128	+8	111	117	+6
Performance IQ	90	104	+14	108	126	+18	88	112	+24
Full Scale IQ	99	103	+4	117	130	+13	100	117	+17
WRAT									
Reading	110	110	0	108	103	−5	106	110	+4
Spelling	112	121	+9	108	104	−4	97	98	+1
Arithmetic	85	88	+3	79	85	+6	85	91	+6
ITPA									
Auditory Reception	27	38	+11	—	—	—	—	—	—
Visual Reception	35	37	+2	—	—	—	—	—	—
Auditory Association	42	46	+4	—	—	—	—	—	—
Visual Association	28	44	+16	—	—	—	—	—	—
Porteus Mazes	123	118	−5	131	135	+4	—	—	—
Halstead Categories	0.28	0.08	−0.20	0.33	0.14	−0.19	0.32	0.12	−0.20
Trail Making Test R	11	18	+7	22	18	−4	—	—	—
Trail Making Test B	38	34	−4	46	31	−15	—	—	—
CDI	14	4	−10	27	4	−23	9	3	−6

Note: Pre = Scores prior to treatment of depressive episode; Post = Scores during tricyclic antidepressant-induced remission of depression; WISC-R = Wechsler Intelligence Scale for Children, Revised Edition; WRAT = Wide Range Achievement Test; ITPA = Illinois Test of Psycholinguistic Abilities; CDI = Children's Depression Inventory (Kovacs, 1981)

tion, test improvements are not a nonspecific effect of tricyclic antidepressants, since normal young adult college student volunteers given these same medications show either no change or a slight deterioration in neuropsychological test performance (Ross, Smallberg, & Weingartner, 1984).

In a monumental study of over 150 depressed children, Ossofsky (1974) correlated pretreatment WISC IQ scores with the response to antidepressant (imipramine) treatment. All of the one-sixth of her population of depressed children with a Performance IQ deficit (Performance IQ less than Verbal IQ) had complete remission of the depression with imipramine therapy. Of the two-thirds of depressed children who had essentially equal WISC Performance and Verbal IQ scores, only 50% experienced a remission of depression following antidepressant treatment. The other one-sixth of this population of depressed children had a pretreatment Verbal IQ deficit (WISC Verbal IQ less than Performance IQ), and none of them experienced remission of the depression with pharmacotherapy. We observed a differential improvement of neuropsychological deficits (Table 17-11) with res-

Case #4			Case #5			Case #6			Case #7		
Pre	Post	Change	Pre	Post	Change	Pre	Post	Change	Pre	Post	Change
9 2/12	9 7/12		7 1/12	7 4/12		7 6/12	7 10/12		12 3/12	12 10/12	
12	12	0	13	16	+3	5	5	0	11	13	+2
9	10	+1	15	16	+1	3	3	0	10	16	+6
10	6	−4	12	16	+4	3	5	+2	10	14	+4
10	10	0	18	19	+1	6	3	−3	9	13	+4
8	8	0	14	19	+5	3	5	+2	10	13	+3
6	5	−1	10	11	+1	2	1	−1	7	11	+4
15	14	−1	13	14	+1	3	8	+5	13	15	+2
10	13	+3	16	15	−1	3	8	+5	12	18	+6
12	13	+1	8	11	+3	3	4	+1	12	17	+5
11	16	+5	8	14	+6	10	12	+2	9	16	+7
8	11	+3	7	9	+2	5	3	−2	8	15	+7
98	95	−3	127	146	+19	64	65	+1	100	123	+23
108	124	+16	102	118	+16	67	80	+13	105	143	+38
102	109	+7	118	137	+19	62	70	+8	102	138	+36
100	101	+1	108	122	+14	69	77	+8	110	112	+2
100	100	0	106	121	+15	65	69	+4	103	114	+11
90	97	+7	108	109	+1	65	84	+19	88	99	+11
30	30	0	43	46	+3	22	25	+3	—	—	—
39	43	+4	50	51	+1	22	25	+3	—	—	—
40	38	−2	53	55	+2	10	8	−2	—	—	—
27	31	+4	42	46	+4	7	28	+21	—	—	—
112	127	+15	—	—	—	62	60	−2	127	127	0
0.27	0.30	−0.03	0.30	0.30	0	0.54	0.54	0	0.35	0.35	0
16	14	−2	23	27	+4	—	—	—	17	14	−3
60	39	−21	120	87	−33	—	—	—	32	23	−8
18	6	−12	—	—	—	—	—	—	37	2	−35

olution of depression in children who were grouped on the basis of a WISC-R Verbal IQ/ Performance IQ discrepancy, using a 10 IQ point difference between Verbal IQ and Performance IQ as the cutoff for grouping (Brumback, 1985c; Wilson, Staton, & Brumback, 1982). Following antidepressant treatment, depressed children with an initial Performance IQ deficit showed moderate to marked neuropsychological improvements in alertness, visual sequencing, visual perception, long-term visual retention, perceptual organization, and auditory information processing, as well as significant improvement in all depressive symptoms and depression rating scales. In contrast, the depressed children with an initial Verbal IQ deficit, following treatment, had only slight to moderate neuropsychological improvements in verbal comprehension, reading achievement, practical reasoning, and visual–motor coordination, and had minimal change in depressive symptoms (improving only on the "appearance" items of the self-esteem rating scale). These findings raise the possibility of two distinct types of depression: (1) a depressive illness, associated with right-cerebral-hemisphere deficits, that responds to antidepressant therapy that also improves the associated right cerebral dysfunction; and (2) a depressive disorder without evidence of right-hemisphere deficit, which is poorly responsive or unresponsive to conventional antidepressant treatment. This formulation is consistent with the suggestions (Ross, 1984; Ross & Rush,

this IS ME
one year Ago
In the apartment
I have Lived
For one
Me
Me

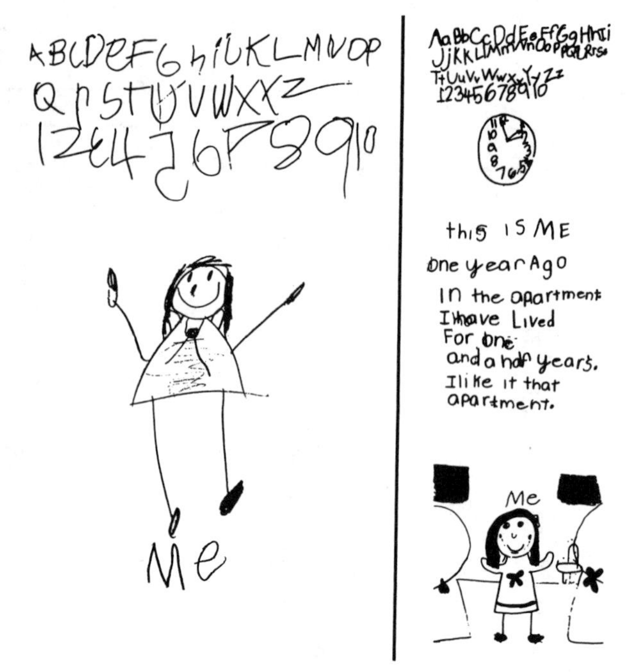

Figure 17-8. Improvement of graphic abilities of children treated for depression: (a) 7-year-old girl. *Left:* Pretreatment (WISC-R Performance IQ 102). *Right:* 3 months later during tricyclic antidepressant–induced remission of depression (WISC-R Performance IQ 118). Reproduced by permission from "Right Cerebral Hemisphere Dysfunction" by R. A. Brumback, R. D. Staton, and H. Wilson, 1984, *Archives of Neurology, 41,* pp. 248–250.

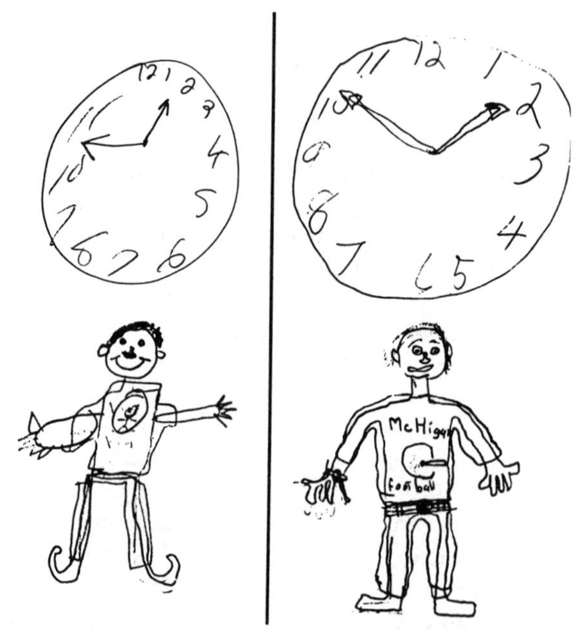

(b) 12-year-old boy. *Left:* Pretreatment (WISC-R Performance IQ 95) *Right:* 5 months later during tricyclic antidepressant–induced remission of depression (WISC-R Performance IQ 112).

Mom is in bean.
Once day a boy was watching
TV and he a puppet reading
and he said the wordes that
he did. He got done and
the show was done and
a book and tried to read it
then he new how to
read.

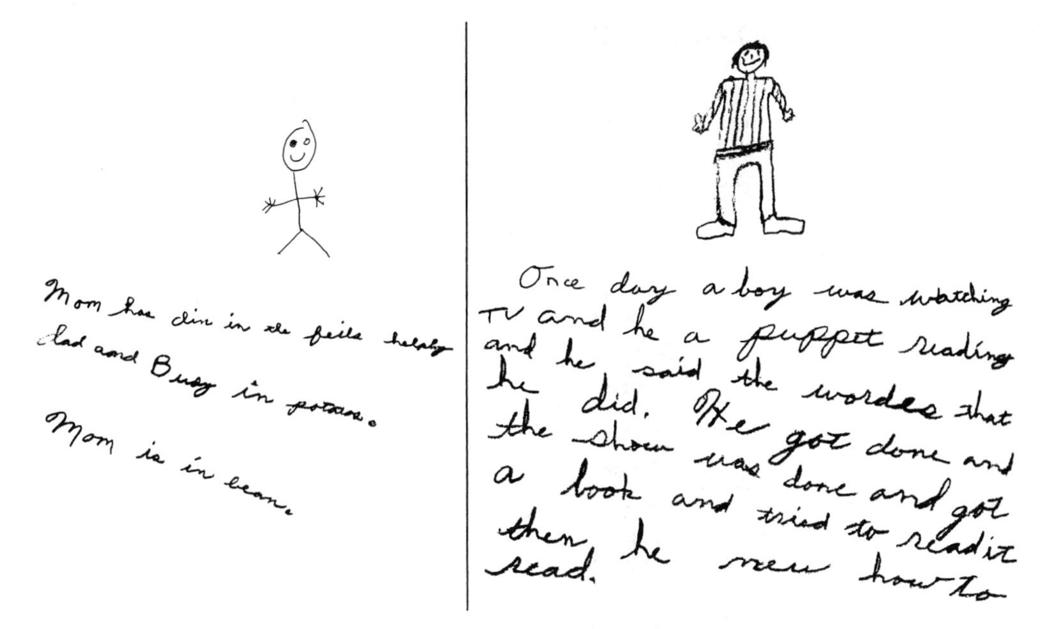

(c) 9-year-old boy (neuropsychological profile of this child shown in Table 10, Case 4). *Left:* Pretreatment. *Right;* Follow-up during tricyclic antidepressant–induced remission of depression.

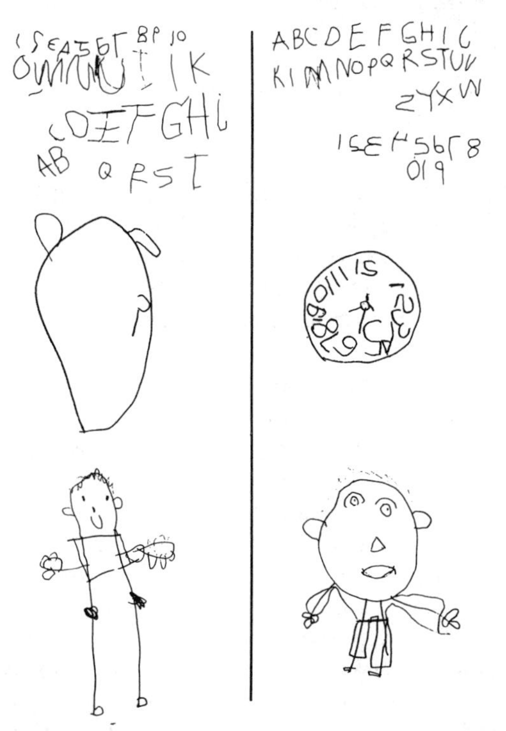

(d) 7-year-old boy (neuropsychological profile of this child shown in Table 17-10, Case 5). *Left:* Pretreatment. *Right:* Follow-up during tricyclic antidepressant–induced remission of depression. Reproduced by permission from "Learning Disability and Childhood Depression" by R. A. Brumback and R. D. Staton, 1983, *American Journal of Orthopsychiatry, 53,* pp. 269–281.

Table 17-11. Neuropsychological Tests[a] Showing Significant[b] Differential Improvement Following Resolution of Depression in Children Grouped According to WISC Verbal IQ/ Performance IQ Discrepancy

Performance IQ deficit[c] (N = 18)	Verbal IQ deficit[d] (N = 18)
WISC-R[e]	WISC-R[e]
Vocabulary	Vocabulary
Picture Completion	Comprehension
Block Design	Verbal IQ
Coding	WRAT
Performance IQ	Reading
ITPA	VMI
Auditory Association	
Halstead Categories	

[a]WISC-R = Wechsler Intelligence Scale for Children, Revised Edition; ITPA = Illinois Test of Psycholinguistic Abilities; WRAT = Wide Range Achievement Test; VMI = Beery-Buktenica Visual Motor Integration Test.

[b]Analysis of variance $p < .05$.

[c]Performance IQ Deficit = Verbal IQ score more than 10 points higher than Performance IQ score.

[d]Verbal IQ Deficit = Performance IQ score more than 10 points higher than Verbal IQ score.

[e]Average WISC-R IQ improvement of 15 points and average WISC-R subtest score improvement of 3 points.

1981) of distinctive right-cerebral-hemisphere and left-cerebral-hemisphere depressions, in which the right-hemisphere depression is associated with more ''endogenous'' or biological symptoms and responds to pharmacotherapy, whereas the left-hemisphere depression is characterized by negative depressive thoughts and ideas and, though poorly responsive to pharmacotherapy, may respond to forms of psychotherapy such as the cognitive therapy of Beck (1976).

Several investigators, after finding no significant differences between mean Wechsler Verbal and Performance IQs in groups of depressed and control nondepressed children (Kashani *et al.*, 1983; Stevenson & Romney, 1984), have recently denied the existence of any depression-associated change in neuropsychological function. To buttress this argument, Stevenson & Romney (1984) cited our earlier study (Brumback, Jackoway, & Weinberg, 1980), in which we also reported no significant differences in the mean Wechsler Performance and Verbal IQs of 100 consecutive children (62% with depression) referred for evaluation of school problems. However, reassessment of our data (Table 17-12) showed that a significant number of the depressed children (but not the nondepressed children) had a Performance IQ 15 points or more lower than the Verbal IQ (Brumback, 1985c), supporting our current thesis that a major *subgroup* of depressed individuals has right-cerebral-hemisphere dysfunction (suggested by the Performance IQ deficit). Averaging IQ scores from large populations of depressed children generally will blur subgroup differences (as in the original analysis of our data). However, Kron *et al.* (1982), evaluating children (some of whom were clinically depressed at the time of the study) of parents who had

Table 17-12. Number of Children with Wechsler[a] Performance IQ or Verbal IQ Deficits[b]

		Performance IQ deficit		No deficit		Verbal IQ deficit	
	N	*n*	%	*n*	%	*n*	%
Depressed	61	21	34	23	38	17	28
Nondepressed	36	5	14	24	67	7	19

Whole table: $\chi^2 = 8.1, p < .01$
Performance deficit versus other groups: $\chi^2 = 3.9, p < .05$

Source: Adapted from Brumback (1985c).

Note: Mean Verbal/Performance IQ discrepancies (regardless of direction):
Depressed 13.2 ± 8.1
Nondepressed 10.8 ± 8.2

[a]Wechsler Intelligence Scale for Children (WISC) or Wechsler Preschool and Primary Scale of Intelligence (WPPSI).

[b]Performance IQ Deficit = Verbal IQ at least 15 points higher than Performance IQ; Verbal IQ Deficit = Performance IQ at least 15 points higher than Verbal IQ; No Deficit = 14 or less point difference between Verbal and Performance IQ.

required hospitalization for treatment of affective disorders, found that: (1) the study children had a mean WISC-R Performance IQ that was 8.4 IQ points lower than that of controls; (2) 39% of the study children had a Performance IQ deficit, compared to only 11% of the controls; and (3) the average Performance IQ deficit was 8.2 IQ points in the study children, compared to only 1.9 IQ points for the control children. In addition, it is possible that depressed children with no evidence of a Verbal–Performance IQ discrepancy during the depressive episode may actually have experienced a depression-associated lowering of their pre-illness Performance IQ, which would only become apparent by retesting after remission of the depressive episode (see Table 17-10, case #4).

It is of interest that neurological signs of right cerebral dysfunction, along with neurophysiological and neuroendocrine abnormalities similar to those identified in depression, have been observed in patients presenting with either obsessive–compulsive disorder or anorexia nervosa, and that clinical improvement follows antidepressant pharmacotherapy (Behar *et al.*, 1984; Maxwell, Tucker, & Townes, 1984; Murphy, Siever, & Insel, 1985). This suggests that these two conditions may be variant forms of depressive illness and that learning-disabled children with either disorder might also experience amelioration of the learning problem after appropriate antidepressant treatment.

NEUROBIOLOGY OF DEPRESSION

Current research indicates that affective illness (depression and mania) results from an episodic disturbance of CNS aminergic neurotransmission by the indolamine serotonin (5-hydroxytryptamine) and/or the catecholamine norepinephrine, which are major modulators of cerebral neuronal activity (Coppen & Wood, 1982; Post & Ballenger, 1984). The norepinephrine-containing neurons are located primarily in the pontine locus ceruleus, and the serotonin-containing neurons are located in the brain stem raphé nuclei. Large numbers of axons originating from these aminergic neurons widely distribute the serotonin and norepinephrine throughout the brain. Although current evidence indicates that the neurons are symmetrically arranged in the brain stem, their axonal projections to the cerebrum and diencephalon appear to be asymmetrical (Robinson, Kubos, Starr, Rao, & Price, 1984). In animal studies, injury to the left cerebral hemisphere produces no change in brain norepinephrine concentrations, whereas damage in the right cerebral hemisphere produces a profound bilateral reduction in cerebral catecholamine levels (Robinson & Coyle, 1980). The only human study to date has shown higher concentrations of norepinephrine in the right thalamic somatosensory relay nuclei (ventralis posterolateralis and ventralis posteromedialis) and in the left pulvinar (Oke, Keller, Mefford, & Adams, 1978).

The change in biogenic amine neurotransmission occurring during depressive and manic episodes profoundly alters the function of nonamine neuronal systems throughout the brain, resulting in the variety of observed clinical symptoms. We have suggested (Brumback & Staton, 1983; Staton *et al.,* 1981) that the depression-associated decrease in cerebral biogenic amine neurotransmission modifies nonamine cerebral systems, worsening cerebral cognitive and sensorimotor functioning (see Figure 17-9). The evidence suggests that right-cerebral-hemispheric and frontal lobe functioning are more adversely affected by depression than are left-hemispheric functions, and this effect may be apparent as a learning disorder. Since metabolic derangements (such as hypoglycemia, hypoxia, and electrolyte disturbances) can reversibly unmask subclinical deficits associated with previous CNS injury (Meyer & Portnoy, 1958), we have suggested that the depression-related reduction in biogenic amine facilitation of nonamine cortical systems may similarly make ordinarily

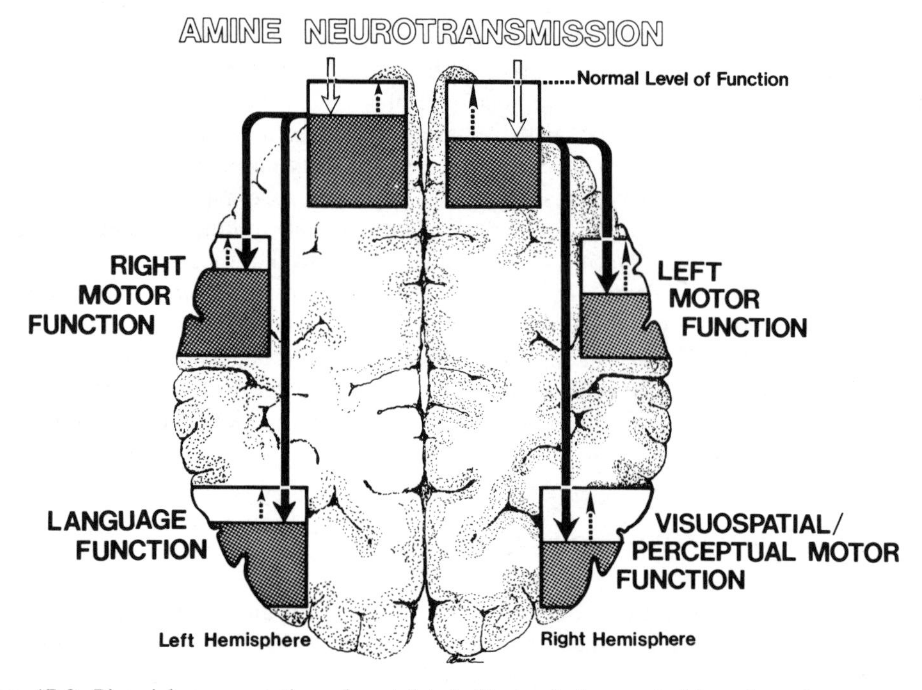

Figure 17-9. Pictorial representation of postulated effects of changes in biogenic amine neurotransmission on cortical function. Reduction (as occurs during a depressive episode) in the cerebral biogenic amine neurotransmission (greater reduction on the right side than on the left side) would decrease the level of functioning of cortical motor, visuospatial–perceptual motor, and language abilities (thick arrows). Conversely, increased amine neurotransmission (as following tricyclic antidepressant–induced remission of depression) would increase the level of crotical functioning (thin arrows). Reproduced by permission from "Cognitive Improvement Associated with Tricyclic Antidepressant Treatment of Childhood Major Depressive Illness" by R. D. Staton, H. Wilson, and R. A. Brumback, 1981, *Perceptual and Motor Skills, 53,* pp. 219–234.

asymptomatic subtle cerebral abnormalities clinically apparent. Thus, otherwise subclinical dysfunction of either cerebral hemisphere would become clinically evident as a learning disability during a depressive episode. Remission of depression corrects the deficient biogenic amine neurotransmission, resolving the learning disability.

Pharmacotherapy for depression is aimed at improving biogenic amine neurotransmission (Richardson & Richelson, 1984; Rosenbaum, Maruta, & Richelson, 1979). The monoamine oxidase (MAO) inhibitors (such as phenelzine and pargyline) prevent the MAO-mediated oxidative deamination (and, therefore, inactivation) of neurotransmitter. Tricyclic antidepressants (such as imipramine and amitriptyline) block the reuptake pump of the presynaptic neuron, preventing removal (inactivation) of the neurotransmitter. Stimulants (such as dextroamphetamine) have a combination of effects, directly stimulating the postsynaptic neuron, enhancing the release of transmitter by the presynaptic neuron, inhibiting MAO, and blocking the reuptake pump of the presynaptic neuron. Because of potentially severe changes in blood pressure, MAO inhibitors are used infrequently, and even though stimulants may produce a relatively rapid antidepressant effect, clinical improvement is usually short-lived and may be followed by a more profound depression. Tricyclic antidepressants are currently the most commonly used drugs for treating depression, but there remains a strong undercurrent of fear among physicians concerning the use of antidepressant medication in children because of the cardiotoxicity noted with massive overdoses (Goldberg, Capone, & Hunt, 1985; Hayes, Panitch, & Barker, 1975; Winsberg, Goldstein, Yepes, & Perel, 1975). However, all medications can be toxic or fatal in overdoses (Editor, *BMJ*, 1979), and even critics of antidepressant usage in children freely prescribe for behaviorally disturbed children medications that may produce serious side effects at therapeutic doses (Gilman, Goodman, Rall, & Murad, 1985), such as stimulants (addictive potential) and neuroleptics (permanent dyskinesias [Gualtieri, Barnhill, McGimsey, & Schell, 1980; Gualtieri, Quade, Hicks, Mayo, & Schroeder, 1984; Staton & Brumback, 1980], hepatotoxicity, and retinotoxicity). In addition, a large experience by us and by others using *therapeutic doses* of antidepressants in children has not revealed any cardiotoxicity or serious toxic side effects, and there is no reason to avoid the use of antidepressants in the treatment of childhood depression.

Different antidepressant drugs have various effects on the presumed aminergic neurotransmitter abnormality of depression, and preliminary studies suggest that there may be a differential response of the cerebral hemispheric dysfunction to different psychotherapeutic drugs (Brumback, Staton, & Wilson, 1984b; Staton, Wilson, & Brumback, 1982). In one study, a greater number of neuropsychological test measures improved following amitriptyline-induced remission compared to imipramine-induced remission of depression (Table 17-13). A manic-depressive child with neurological and neuropsychological signs of right-cerebral-hemispheric dysfunction showed neuropsychological improvement and disappearance of the neurological signs after amitriptyline-induced remission of depression; when he was switched to lithium carbonate pharmacotherapy, however, the behavioral and neurological remission continued, but there was a deterioration of right-hemispheric neuropsychological performance (Table 17-14). Ternes, Woody, and Livingston (1987) described an 11-year-old boy with right cerebral hemisphere dysfunction, depression, and frequent right temporal spikes on his electroencephalogram, who had remission of his depressive symptoms and significant improvement in right hemisphere neuropsychological function following treatment with carbamazepine. These findings suggest that studies of the effect of psychotherapeutic drugs on neurological and neuropsychological function in larger numbers of depressed individuals may identify the differential influence of the various neuroaminergic systems on cerebral function. It may also be possible to develop drug regimens that specifically improve different aspects of cerebral hemispheric function.

Table 17-13. Neuropsychological Test Scores Showing Significant[a] Differential Improvement Following Antidepressant-Induced Remission of Childhood Depressive Episodes

Amitriptyline-induced remission ($n=32$)	Imipramine-induced remission ($n=13$)
WISC-R[b]	WISC-R[b]
Comprehension	Picture Arrangement
Picture Completion	Coding
Object Assembly	ITPA
Performance IQ	Visual Reception
ITPA	Halstead Categories
Visual Association	Porteus Mazes
Halstead Categories	
Trail Making Test B	

Source: Adapted from Staton *et al.* (1982).

[a]Significant improvements (analysis of variance $p<.05$) from pretreatment scores to scores achieved 3 to 6 months later following pharmacotherapy-induced remission of depression.

[b]Average WISC-R IQ improvement of 15 points and average WISC-R subtest score improvement of 3 points.

EVALUATION AND TREATMENT IMPLICATIONS

Epidemiological studies have reported that 5% of all office visits to pediatricians are for behavior or learning problems at school or at home (Anders, 1977). It is imperative that such difficulties not simply be attributed to conduct disorder, attentional disorder, some other behavioral disturbance, or environmental factors without ascertaining the possibility of a biological depressive illness (Brumback & Staton, 1983; Brumback, Staton, & Wilson, 1984a, 1984b; Brumback, Wilson, & Staton, 1984). Although the exact incidence is unknown, depressive symptomatology has been frequently observed in learning-disabled children (Murray & Little, 1981). Weinberg *et al.* (1973) reported 58% and Colberg, Newman, Ney, and Young (1982) reported that 54% of children referred for evaluation of school difficulties or learning disabilities had diagnosable depressive illness when criteria symptoms were actively sought. Weintraub and Mesulam (1983) found that depression was the disabling symptomatology in a group of 14 adolescents and young adults with right-hemisphere-type learning disability. The high incidence of poor social adjustment in long-term follow-up studies of depressed children (Eastgate & Gilmour, 1984; Poznanski, 1981; Poznanski, Krahenbuhl, & Zrull, 1976), seems to relate to the inadequacy of the pharmacotherapy necessary to sustain long-lasting remission of the depression. An intermittent dysfunction (related to inadequate antidepressant therapy) of the right-cerebral-hemisphere ability to understand prosody, emotional gesturing, and other social cues makes it difficult for the child to develop appropriate interpersonal skills, causing failure in most social situations, while other cognitive difficulties complicate academic performance. Repeated school failure and chronic social ineptitude do not permit the child to develop the skills necessary for successful independent living in society. If symptoms of depression are found, it is imperative that the learning-disabled or behaviorally disturbed child receive adequate antidepressant therapy to ensure complete long-term remission of the depression. In addition, learning-disabled children even without apparent diagnosable depressive illness (especially those who have evidence of right-cerebral-hemispheric dysfunction) should prob-

Table 17-14. Right Cerebral Hemispheric Neurologic and Neuropsychological Test[a] Results during Amitriptyline and Lithium Carbonate Treatment of a 10-Year-Old Boy with Manic-Depressive Illness

	Pretreatment	Amitriptyline treatment	Lithium treatment
WISC-R			
Picture Completion	12	14	15
Picture Arrangement	11	15	13
Block Design	10	14	11
Object Assembly	11	13	12
Coding	8	11	4
Performance IQ	102	124	106
WRAT			
Arithmetic	96	135	91
ITPA			
Visual Reception	30	46	36
Visual Association	32	44	28
Left sensorimotor neurological signs	Present	Absent	Absent

Source: Adapted from Brumback *et al.* (1984b).

[a] WISC-R = Wechsler Intelligence Scale for Children, Revised Edition; WRAT = Wide Range Achievement Test; ITPA = Illinois Test of Psycholinguistic Abilities.

ably also be considered for a trial of antidepressant therapy, since recognition of the depressive nature of symptoms may not be possible until treatment-induced improvement has occurred and depression-associated learning disability has resolved. Improvement in academic performance associated with improved neuropsychological functioning after treatment-induced remission of a depressive episode can be dramatic, with disappearance of apparent learning disability. Poor educational achievement associated with chronic learning difficulties ultimately affects adult social functioning, and untreated or improperly treated chronic depression may result in the development of later personality disturbances. Therefore, before attributing school problems in children to untreatable conditions, depressive disorder must be excluded. Appropriate antidepressant therapy should be provided to all children with evidence of depression.

ACKNOWLEDGMENT

The author wishes to acknowledge encouragement by the late Dr. Norman Geschwind to pursue the study of neurological changes associated with depression. Special thanks to Brenda Robinson and Barbara E. Venerus for preparing the drawings of the sensorimotor examination. Mary H. Brumback provided helpful suggestions regarding this chapter.

REFERENCES

Abrams, R., & Taylor, M. A. (1979). Differential EEG patterns in affective disorder and schizophrenia. *Archives of General Psychiatry, 36,* 1355–1358.

Agras, S. (1959). The relationship of school phobia to childhood depression. *American Journal of Psychiatry, 116,* 533–536.

Albert, N., & Beck, A. T. (1975). Incidence of depression in early adolescence: A preliminary study. *Journal of Youth and Adolescence, 4,* 301–307.

American Psychiatric Association Task Force on Nomenclature. (1980). *Diagnostic and statistical manual of mental disorders* (3rd ed.). (DSM-III). Washington, DC: Author.

Anders, T. F. (1977). Child psychiatry and pediatrics: the state of the relationship. *Pediatrics, 60,* 616–620.

Armitage, P. (1971). *Statistical methods in medical research.* Oxford: Blackwell Scientific Publications.

Aylward, G. P. (1985). Understanding and treatment of childhood depression. *Journal of Pediatrics, 107,* 1–9.

Barkley, R. A. (1981). *Hyperactive children: A handbook for diagnosis and treatment.* New York: Guilford Press.

Bauersfeld, K. H. (1972). Diagnose und Behandlung depressiver Krankheitszustände in einer schulpsychiatrischen Beratungsstelle. In A.-L. Annell (Ed.), *Depressive states in childhood and adolescence: Proceedings of the 4th Union of European Psychiatrists Congress* (pp. 281–285). Stockholm: Almqvist & Wiksell.

Beck, A. T. (1973). *The diagnosis and management of depression.* Philadelphia: University of Pennsylvania Press.

Beck, A. T. (1976). *Cognitive therapy and the emotional disorders.* New York: International Universities Press.

Behar, D., Rapoport, J. L., Berg, C. J., Denckla, M. B., Mann, L., Cox, C., Fedio, P., Zahn, T., & Wolfman, M. G. (1984). Computerized tomography and neuropsychological test measures in adolescents with obsessive–compulsive disorder. *American Journal of Psychiatry, 141,* 363–369.

Berndt, D. J., & Berndt, S. M. (1980). Relationship of mild depression to psychological deficit in college students. *Journal of Clinical Psychology, 36,* 868–874.

Blouin, A. G. A., Bornstein, R. A., & Trites, R. L. (1978). Teenage alcohol use among hyperactive children: A five-year follow-up study. *Journal of Pediatric Psychology, 4,* 188–194.

Boder, E. (1973). Developmental dyslexia: A diagnostic approach based on three atypical reading–spelling patterns. *Developmental Medicine and Child Neurology, 15,* 663–687.

Bohline, D. S. (1985). Intellectual and affective characteristics of attention deficit disordered children. *Journal of Learning Disabilities, 10,* 604–608.

Bradley, C. (1937). The behavior of children receiving Benzedrine. *American Journal of Psychiatry, 94,* 577–585.

Breslow, R., Kocsis, J., & Belkin, B. (1980). Memory deficits in depression: Evidence utilizing the Wechsler Memory Scale. *Perceptual and Motor Skills, 51,* 541–542.

Broca, P. (1861). Remarques sur le siège de la faculté du langage articulé, suivies d'une observation d'aphémie. *Bulletin de Société Anatomique Paris* (2nd series), *6,* 332–333, 343–357.

Bruce, L. C. (1895). Notes of a case of dual brain action. *Brain, 18,* 54–65.

Brumback, R. A. (1976). Depressive disorder in childhood. *American Journal of Psychiatry, 133,* 455.

Brumback, R. A. (1979). Use of operational criteria in an office practice for diagnosis of children referred for evaluation of learning or behavioral disorders. *Perceptual and Motor Skills, 49,* 299–311.

Brumback, R. A. (1985a). Neurology of depression. *Neurology and Neurosurgery Update Series, 7*(6), 1–8.

Brumback, R. A. (1985b). "Terminal drop" as a sign of depression in elderly individuals: an hypothesis. *Psychological Reports, 57,* 84–86.

Brumback, R. A. (1985c). Wechsler performance IQ deficit in depression in children. *Perceptual and Motor Skills, 61,* 331–335.

Brumback, R. A., Dietz-Schmidt, S. G., & Weinberg, W. A. (1977). Depression in children referred to an educational diagnostic center: Diagnosis and treatment and analysis of criteria and literature review. *Diseases of the Nervous System, 38,* 529–535.

Brumback, R. A., Jackoway, M. K., & Weinberg, W. A. (1980). Relation of intelligence to childhood depression in children referred to an educational diagnostic center. *Perceptual and Motor Skills, 50,* 11–17.

Brumback, R. A., & Staton, R. D. (1981). Depression-induced neurologic dysfunction. *New England Journal of Medicine, 305,* 642.

Brumback, R. A., & Staton, R. D. (1982a). Right hemisphere involvement in learning disability, attention deficit disorder, and childhood major depressive disorder. *Medical Hypotheses, 8,* 505–514.

Brumback, R. A., & Staton, R. D. (1982b). An hypothesis regarding the commonality of right hemisphere involvement in learning disability, attentional disorder, and childhood major depressive disorder. *Perceptual and Motor Skills, 55,* 1091–1097.

Brumback, R. A., & Staton, R. D. (1983). Learning disability and childhood depression. *American Journal of Orthopsychiatry, 53,* 269–281.

Brumback, R. A., Staton, R. D., & Wilson, H. (1980). Neuropsychological study of children during and after remission of endogenous depressive episodes. *Perceptual and Motor Skills, 50,* 1163–1167.

Brumback, R. A., Staton, R. D., & Wilson, H. (1984a). Psychopharmacology in children. *New England Journal of Medicine, 311,* 473–474.

Brumback, R. A., Staton, R. D., & Wilson, H. (1984b). Right cerebral hemisphere dysfunction. *Archives of Neurology, 41,* 248–250.

Brumback, R. A., & Weinberg, W. A. (1977a). Childhood depression: An explanation of a behavioral disorder of children. *Perceptual and Motor Skills, 44,* 911–916.

Brumback, R. A., & Weinberg, W. A. (1977b). Relationship of hyperactivity and depression in children. *Perceptual and Motor Skills, 45,* 247–251.

Brumback, R. A., Wilson, H., & Staton, R. D. (1984). Behavioral problems in children taking theophylline. *Lancet, 1,* 958.

Cantwell, D. (1974). Prevalence of psychiatric disorder in a pediatric clinic for military dependent children. *Journal of Pediatrics, 85,* 711–714.

Cantwell, D., & Baker, L. (1977). Psychiatric disorder in children with speech and language retardation. *Archives of General Psychiatry, 34,* 583–591.

Cantwell, D., & Baker, L. (1980). Academic failures in children with communication disorders. *Journal of the American Academy of Child Psychiatry, 19,* 579–591.

Cantwell, D., & Carlson, G. A. (Eds.). (1983). *Affective disorders in childhood and adolescence: An update.* New York: SP Medical and Scientific Books.

Cantwell, D., & Forness, S. R. (1982). Learning disorders. *Journal of the American Academy of Child Psychiatry, 21,* 417–419.

Carlson, G. A., & Cantwell, D. P. (1979). A survey of depressive symptoms in a child and adolescent psychiatric population: Interview data. *Journal of the American Academy of Child Psychiatry, 18,* 587–599.

Carroll, B. J., Curtis, G. C., & Mendels, J. (1976a). Neuroendocrine regulation in depression: I. Limbic system–adrenocortical dysfunctions. *Archives of General Psychiatry, 33,* 1039–1044.

Carroll, B. J., Curtis, G. C., & Mendels, J. (1976b). Neuroendocrine regulation in depression: II. Discrimination of depressed from nondepressed patients. *Archives of General Psychiatry, 33,* 1051–1058.

Carroll, B. J., Feinberg, M., Greden, J. F., Tarika, J., Albala, A. A., Haskett, R. F., James, N. McI., Kronfol, Z., Lohr, N., Steiner, M., de Vigne, J. P., & Young, E. (1981). A specific laboratory test for the diagnosis of melancholia. *Archives of General Psychiatry, 38,* 15–22.

Cebiroglu, R., Sümer, E., & Polvan, Ö. (1972). Etiology and pathogensis of depression in Turkish children. In A-L. Annell (Ed.), *Depressive states in childhood and adolescence: Proceedings of the 4th Union of European Psychiatrists Congress* (pp. 133–136). Stockholm: Almqvist & Wiksell.

Clayton, P. J. (1981). The epidemiology of bipolar affective disorder. *Comprehensive Psychiatry, 22,* 31–43.

Clemmens, R. L., & Kenny, T. J. (1972). Clinical correlates of learning disabilities, minimal brain dysfunction and hyperactivity. *Clinical Pediatrics, 11,* 311–313.

Colbert, P., Newman, B., Ney, P., & Young, J. (1982). Learning disabilities as a symptom of depression in children. *Journal of Learning Disabilities, 15,* 333–336.

Coll, P. G., & Bland, R. (1979). Manic depressive illness in adolescence and childhood: Review and case report. *Canadian Journal of Psychiatry, 24,* 255–263.

Connell, H. M. (1972). Depression in childhood. *Child Psychiatry and Human Development, 4,* 71–85.

Coppen, A., & Wood, K. (1982). 5-Hydroxytryptamine in the pathogenesis of affective disorders. In B. T. Ho, J. C. Schoolar, & E. Usdin (Eds.), *Serotonin in biological psychiatry.* Advances in Biochemical Psychopharmacology. (Vol. 34, pp. 249–258). New York: Raven Press.

Critchley, M., & Critchley, E. A. (1978). *Dyslexia defined.* Springfield, IL: Thomas.

Culbertson, J. L., & Ferry, P. C. (1982). Learning disabilities. *Pediatric Clinics of North America, 29,* 121–135.

Cutler, N. R., Post, R. M., Rey, A. C., & Bunney, W. E., Jr. (1981). Depression-dependent dyskinesias in two cases of manic-depressive illness. *New England Journal of Medicine, 304,* 1088–1089.

Denckla, M. (1973). Research needs in learning disabilities, a neurologist's point of view. *Journal of Learning Disabilities, 6,* 441–450.

Dworkin, P. H. (1985). *Learning and behavior problems of school children.* Philadelphia: Saunders.

Earls, F. (1984). The epidemiology of depression in children and adolescents. *Pediatric Annals, 13,* 23–31.

Eastgate, J., & Gilmour, L. (1984). Long-term outcome of depressed children: A follow-up study. *Developmental Medicine and Child Neurology, 26,* 68–72.

Editor, *BMJ.* (1979). Manic states in affective disorders of childhood and adolescence. *British Medical Journal, 1,* 684–685.

Emslie, G. J., Weinberg, W. A., Rush, A. J., Weissenburger, J., & Parkin-Feigenbaum, L. (1987). Depression and dexamethasone suppression testing in children and adolescents. *Journal of Child Neurology, 2,* 31–37.

Feagans, L. (1983). A current view of learning disabilities. *Journal of Pediatrics, 102,* 487–493.

Feighner, J. P., Robins, E., Guze, S. B., Woodruff, R. A., Winokur, G., & Munoz, R. (1972). Diagnostic criteria for use in psychiatric research. *Archives of General Psychiatry, 26,* 57–63.

Feinstein, C., Blouin, A. G., Egan, J., & Conners, C. K. (1984). Depressive symptomatology in a child psychiatric outpatient population: Correlations with diagnosis. *Comprehensive Psychiatry, 25,* 379–391.

Flor-Henry, P. (1976). Lateralized temporal–limbic dysfunction and psychopathology. *Annals of the New York Academy of Sciences, 280,* 777–795.

Flor-Henry, P. (1983). *Cerebral basis of psychopathology.* Littleton, MA: John Wright–PSG.

Freeman, R., Galaburda, A. M., Cabal, R. D., & Geschwind, N. (1985). The neurology of depression: Cognitive and behavioral deficits with focal findings in depression and resolution after electroconvulsive therapy. *Archives of Neurology, 42,* 289–291.

Fromm, D., & Schopflocher, D. (1984). Neuropsychological test performance in depressed patients before and after drug therapy. *Biological Psychiatry, 19,* 55–72.

Frommer, E. A. (1967). Treatment of childhood depression with antidepressant drugs. *British Medical Journal, 1,* 729–732.

Gadow, K. D. (1983). Effects of stimulant drugs on academic performance in hyperactive and learning disabled children. *Journal of Learning Disabilities, 16,* 290–299.

Galaburda, A. M., & Kemper, T. L. (1979). Cytoarchitectonic abnormalities in developmental dyslexia: A case study. *Annals of Neurology, 6,* 94–100.

Galaburda, A. M., Sherman, G. F., Rosen, G. D., Aboitiz, F., & Geschwind, N. (1985). Developmental dyslexia: Four consecutive patients with cortical anomalies. *Annals of Neurology, 18,* 222–233.

Garfinkel, B. D., Wender, P. H., Sloman, L., & O'Neill, I. (1983). Tricyclic antidepressant and methylphenidate treatment of attention deficit disorder in children. *Journal of the American Academy of Child Psychiatry, 22,* 343–348.

Gascon, G., Victor, D., & Lombroso, C. T. (1973). Language disorder, convulsive disorder, and electroencephalographic abnormalities. *Archives of Neurology, 28,* 156–162.

Geller, B., Rogol, A. D., & Knitter, E. F. (1983). Preliminary data on the dexamethasone suppression test in children with major depressive disorder. *American Journal of Psychiatry, 140,* 620–622.

Geschwind, N. (1965). Disconnexion syndromes in animals and man. *Brain, 88,* 237–294.

Geschwind, N. (1984). The brain of a learning-disabled individual. *Annals of Dyslexia, 34,* 319–327.

Geschwind, N., & Behan, P. O. (1982). Left-handedness: Association with immune disease, migraine, and developmental learning disorder. *Proceedings of the National Academy of Science (USA), 79,* 5097–5100.

Geschwind, N., & Galaburda, A. (1984). *Cerebral dominance: The biological foundations.* Cambridge, MA: Harvard University Press.

Geschwind, N., & Galaburda, A. M. (1985). Cerebral lateralization: Biologic mechanisms, associations, and pathology. *Archives of Neurology, 42,* 428–459, 521–552, 634–654.

Gilman, A. G., Goodman, L. S., Rall, T. W., & Murad, F. (Eds.). (1985). *Goodman and Gilman's The pharmacological basis of therapeutics* (7th ed.) New York: Macmillan.

Gittleman-Klein, R., & Klein, D. F. (1971). Controlled imipramine treatment of school phobia. *Archives of General Psychiatry, 25,* 204–207.

Glass, R. M., Uhlenhuth, E. H., Weinreb, H., *et al.* (1978). Imipramine-reversible cognitive deficit in outpatient depressives. *Psychopharmacology Bulletin, 14*(2), 10–12.

Goldberg, R. J., Capone, R. J., & Hunt, J. D. (1985). Cardiac complications following tricyclic antidepressant overdose: Issues for monitoring policy. *Journal of the American Medical Association, 254,* 1772–1775.

Goldstein, S. G., Filskov, S. B., Weaver, L. A., & Ives, J. O. (1977). Neuropsychological effects of electroconvulsive therapy. *Journal of Clinical Psychology, 37,* 187–197.

Grossman, H. J. (1977). Psychiatric examination and MBD. In J. G. Millichap (Ed.), *Learning disabilities and related disorders: Facts and current issues* (pp. 51–54). Chicago: Yearbook Medical Publishers.

Grossman, H. J. (Ed.). (1983). *Classification in mental retardation.* Washington, DC: American Association on Mental Deficiency.

Gualtieri, C. T., Barhnill, J., McGimsey, J., & Schell, D. (1980). Tardive dyskinesia and other movement disorders in children treated with psychotropic drugs. *Journal of the American Academy of Child Psychiatry, 19,* 491–510.

Gualtieri, C. T., Quade, D., Hicks, R. E., Mayo, J. P., & Schroeder, S. R. (1984). Tardive dyskinesia and other clinical consequences of neuroleptic treatment in children and adolescents. *American Journal of Psychiatry, 141,* 20–23.

Guilhaume, A., Benoit, O., Gourmelen, M., & Richardet, J. M. (1982). Relationship between sleep stage IV deficit and reversible HGH deficiency in psychosocial dwarfism. *Pediatric Research, 16,* 299–303.

Harris, A. J. (1982). How many kinds of reading disability are there? *Journal of Learning Disabilities, 15,* 456–460.

Hayes, T., Panitch, M., & Barker, E. (1975). Imipramine dosage in children: A comment on "Imipramine and electrocardiographic abnormalities in hyperactive children." *American Journal of Psychiatry, 132,* 546–547.

Heilman, K. M., & Van Den Abell, T. (1980). Right hemisphere dominance for attention: The mechanism underlying hemispheric asymmetries of inattention (neglect). *Neurology, 30,* 327–330.

Hemsi, L. K., Whitehead, A., & Post, F. (1968). Cognitive functioning and cerebral arousal in elderly depressives and dements. *Journal of Psychosomatic Research 12,* 145–156.

Herjanic, B., Herjanic, M., Brown, F., & Wheatt, T. (1975). Are children reliable reporters? *Journal of Abnormal Child Psychology, 3,* 41–48.

Hodges, K. K., & Siegel, L. J. (1985). Depression in children and adolescents. In E. E. Beckham & W. R. Leber (Eds.), *Handbook of depression: Treatment, assessment, and research* (pp. 517–555). Homewood, IL: Dorsey Press.

Huessy, H. R., & Cohen, A. H. (1976). Hyperkinetic behaviors and learning disabilities followed over seven years. *Pediatrics, 57,* 4–10.

Huessy, H. R., & Wright, A. L. (1970). The use of imipramine in children's behavior disorders. *Acta Paedopsychiatrica, 37,* 194–199.

Humphries, L., Gruber, J., Hall, J., & Kryscio, R. (1985). Motor proficiency in depressed adolescent inpatients: Biochemical and clinical diagnostic correlates. *Developmental and Behavioral Pediatrics, 6,* 259–262.

Jelliffe, S. E. (1931). Some historical phases of the manic-depressive synthesis. *Series of Research Publications—Association for Research in Nervous and Mental Disease, 11,* 3–47.

Kashani, J. H., Husain, A., Shekim, W. O., Hodges, K. K., Cytryn, L., & McKnew, D. H. (1981). Current perspectives on childhood depression: An overview. *American Journal of Psychiatry, 138,* 143–153.

Kashani, J. H., McGee, R. O., Clarkson, S. E., Anderson, J. C., Walton, L. A., Williams, S., Silva, P. A., Robins, A. J., Cytryn, L., & McKnew, D. H. (1983). Depression in a sample of 9-year-old children: Prevalence and associated characteristics. *Archives of General Psychiatry, 40,* 1217–1223.

Kashani, J., & Simonds, J. F. (1979). The incidence of depression in children. *American Journal of Psychiatry, 136,* 1203–1205.

Kaslow, N. J., Tanenbaum, R. L., Abramson, L. Y., Peterson, C., & Seligman, M. E. P. (1983). Problem-solving deficits and depressive symptoms among children. *Journal of Abnormal Child Psychology, 11,* 497–502.

Kaufman, A. S. (1976). Verbal–Performance IQ discrepancies on the WISC-R. *Journal of Consulting and Clinical Psychology, 44,* 739–744.

Kaufman, A. S. (1979) *Intelligent testing with the WISC-R.* New York: Wiley.

Kaufman, A. S., Long, S. W., & O'Neal, M. R. (1986). Topical review of the WISC-R for pediatric neuroclinicians. *Journal of Child Neurology, 1,* 89–98.

Kemper, T. L. (1984). Asymmetrical lesions in dyslexia. In N. Geschwind & A. Galaburda (Eds.), *Cerebral dominance: The biological foundations* (pp. 75–89). Cambridge, MA: Harvard University Press.

Kiloh, L. G., Neilson, M., & Andrews, G. (1974). Response of depressed patients to methylamphetamine. *British Journal of Psychiatry, 125,* 496–499.

Kirk, S. A., & Elkins, J. (1975). Characteristics of children enrolled in the child service demonstration centers. *Journal of Learning Disabilities, 8,* 630–637.

Klinkerfuss, G. H., Lange, P. H., Weinberg, W. A., & O'Leary, J. L. (1965). Electroencephalographic abnormalities of children with hyperkinetic behavior. *Neurology, 15,* 833–891.

Klorman, R., Bauer, L. O., Coons, H. W., Lewis, J. L., Peloquin, L. J., Perlmutter, R. A., Ryan, R. M., Salzman, L. F., & Strauss, J. (1984). Enhancing effects of methylphenidate on young adults' congitive processes. *Psychopharmacology Bulletin, 20,* 3–9.

Kovacs, M. (1981). Rating scale to assess depression in school-aged children. *Acta Paedopsychiatrica, 46,* 303–315.

Kron, L., Decina, P., Kestenbaum, C. J., Farber, S., Gargan, M., & Fieve, R. (1982). The offspring of bipolar manic-depressives: Clinical features. *Adolescent Psychiatry, 10,* 273–298.

Kronfol, Z., Hamsher, K. deS., Digre, K., & Waziri, R. (1978). Depression and hemispheric functions: Changes associated with unilateral ECT. *British Journal of Psychiatry, 32,* 560–567.

Kuperman, S., & Stewart, M. (1979). The diagnosis of depression in children. *Journal of Affective Disorders, 1,* 213–217.

Landau, W., & Kleffner, F. (1957). Syndrome of acquired aphasia with convulsive disorder in children. *Neurology, 7,* 523–530.

Leon, G. R., Kendall, P. C., & Garber, J. (1980). Depression in children: Parent, teacher and child perspectives. *Journal of Abnormal Child Psychology, 8,* 221–235.

Lerner, J. W. (1976). *Children with learning disabilities.* Boston: Houghton Mifflin.

Levine, M. D., Brooks, R., & Shonkoff, J. P. (1980). *A pediatric approach to learning disabilities.* New York: Wiley.

Levine, M., Oberklaid, F., & Meltzer, L. (1981). Developmental-output failure: A study of low productivity in school-aged children. *Pediatrics, 67,* 18–25.

Ling, W., Oftendal, G., & Weinberg, W. A. (1970). Depressive illness in children presenting as severe headache. *American Journal of Diseases of Children, 120,* 122–124.

Luria, A. R. (1966). *Higher cortical functions in man.* New York: Basic Books.

Marin, R. S., & Tucker, G. J. (1981). Psychopathology and hemispheric dysfunction: A review. *Journal of Nervous and Mental Disease, 169,* 546–557.

Mattis, S., French, J. H., & Rapin, I. (1973). Dyslexia in children: Three independent neuropsychological syndromes. *Developmental Medicine and Child Neurology, 17,* 150–163.

Maxwell, J. K., Tucker, D. M., & Townes, B. D. (1984). Asymmetric cognitive function in anorexia nervosa. *International Journal of Neuroscience, 24,* 37–44.

McConville, B. J., Boag, L. C., & Purohit, A. P. (1973). Three types of childhood depression. *Canadian Psychiatric Association Journal, 18,* 133–138.

Meier, J. H. (1971). Prevalence and characteristics of learning disabilities found in second grade children. *Journal of Learning Disabilities, 4,* 1–16.

Meierhofer, M. (1972). Depressive Verstimmungen im frühen Kindesalter. In A.-L. Annell (Ed.), *Depressive states in childhood and adolescence: Proceedings of the 4th Union of European Psychiatrists Congress* (pp. 159–162). Stockholm: Almqvist & Wiksell.

Mesulam, M-M. (1981). A cortical network for directed attention and unilateral neglect. *Annals of Neurology, 10,* 309–325.

Mesulam, M-M. (1985). *Principles of behavioral neurology.* Philadelphia: Davis.

Meyer, J. S., & Portnoy, H. D. (1958). Localized cerebral hypoglycemia simulating stroke. *Neurology, 8,* 601–614.

Meyer, J. S., & Portnoy, H. D. (1959). Post-epileptic paralysis. *Brain, 82,* 162–185.

Montgomery, B. M., & Pinner, C. A. (1964). Transient hypoglycemic hemiplegia. *Archives of Internal Medicine, 114,* 680–684.

Mullins, L. J., Siegel, L. J., & Hodges, K. (1985). Cognitive problem-solving and life event correlates of depressive symptoms in children. *Journal of Abnormal Child Psychology, 13,* 305–314.

Murphy, D. L., Siever, L. J., & Insel, T. R. (1985). Therapeutic responses to tricyclic antidepressants and related drugs in non-affective disorder patient populations. *Progress in Neuro-Psychopharmacology and Biological Psychiatry, 9,* 3–13.

Murray, M. E., & Little, M. (1981). Depression in learning disabled children. *Journal of Psychiatric Treatment and Evaluation, 3,* 193–196.

Nissen, G. (1971). *Depressive syndrome in Kindesund Jugendalter.* Berlin: Springer-Verlag.

Offord, D. R., & Joffe, R. T. (1985). Childhood depression. In W. G. Dewhurst & G. B. Baker (Ed.), *Pharmacotherapy of affective disorders: Theory and practice* (pp. 531–583). New York: New York University Press.

Oke, A., Keller, R., Mefford, I., & Adams, R. N. (1978). Lateralization of norepinephrine in human thalamus. *Science, 200,* 1411–1413.

Ossofsky, H. J. (1974). Endogenous depression in infancy and childhood. *Comprehensive Psychiatry, 15,* 19–25.

Ostow, M. (1980). Treating depression with amphetamines. *American Journal of Psychiatry, 137,* 382–383.

Ottenbacher, K. J., & Cooper, H. M. (1983). Drug treatment of hyperactivity in children. *Developmental Medicine and Child Neurology, 25,* 358–366.

Petti, T. A. (1978). Depression in hospitalized child psychiatry patients: Approaches to measuring depression. *Journal of the American Academy of Child Psychiatry, 17,* 49–59.

Pearce, J. (1977). Depressive disorder in childhood. *Journal of Child Psychology and Psychiatry, 18,* 79–82.

Pearce, J. B. (1981). Drug treatment of depression in children. *Acta Paedopsychiatrica, 46,* 317–328.

Polvan, Ö., & Cebiroglu, R. (1972). Treatment with psychopharmacologic agents in childhood depressions. In A.-L. Annell (Ed.), *Depressive states in childhood and adolescence: Proceedings of the 4th Union of European Psychiatrists Congress* (pp. 467–472.). Stockholm: Almqvist & Wiksell.

Post, R. M., & Ballenger, J. C. (Eds.). (1984). *Neurobiology of mood disorders.* Frontiers of Clinical Neuroscience (Vol. 1). Baltimore: Williams and Wilkins.

Post, R. M., Kotin, J., & Goodwin, F. K. (1974). The effects of cocaine on depressed patients. *American Journal of Psychiatry, 131,* 511–517.

Powell, G. F., Brasel, J. A., & Blizzard, R. M. (1967). Emotional deprivation and growth retardation simulating idiopathic hypopituitarism: I. Clinical evaluation of the syndrome. *New England Journal of Medicine, 276,* 1271–1278.

Powell, G. F., Hopwood, N. J., & Barratt, E. S. (1973). Growth hormone studies before and during catch up growth in a child with emotional deprivation and short stature. *Journal of Clinical Endocrinology, 37,* 674–679.

Poznanski, E., Krahenbuhl, V., & Zrull, J. P. (1976). Childhood depression: A longitudinal perspective. *Journal of the American Academy of Child Psyychiatry, 15,* 491–501.

Poznanski, E., Mokros, H. B., Grossman, J., & Freeman, L. N. (1985). Diagnostic criteria in childhood depression. *American Journal of Psychiatry, 142,* 1168–1173.

Poznanski, E. O. (1981). Childhood depression: The outcome. *Acta Paedopsychiatrica, 46,* 297–304.

Poznanski, E. O., Carroll, B. J., Banegas, M. C., Cook, S. C., & Grossman, J. A. (1982). The dexamethasone suppression test in prepubertal depressed children. *American Journal of Psychiatry, 139,* 321–324.

Puig-Antich, J. (1984). Clinical and treatment aspects of depression in childhood and adolescence. *Pediatric Annals, 13*(1), 37–45.

Puig-Antich, J., Chambers, W., Halpern, F., Hanlon, C., & Sachar, E. J. (1979). Cortisol hypersecretion in prepubertal depressive illness: A preliminary report. *Psychoneuroendocrinology, 4,* 191–197.

Puig-Antich, J., Chambers, W. J., & Tabrizi, M. A. (1983). The clinical assessment of current depressive episodes in children and adolescents: Interviews with parents and children. In D. P. Cantwell & G. A. Carlson (Eds.), *Affective disorders in childhood and adolescence* (pp. 157–179). New York: Spectrum.

Puig-Antich, J., Goetz, R., Davies, M., Fein, M., Hanlon, C., Chambers, W. J., Tabrizi, M. A., Sachar, E. J., & Weitzman, E. D. (1984a). Growth hormone secretion in prepubertal children with major depression: II. Sleep-related plasma concentrations during a depressive episode. *Archives of General Psychiatry, 41,* 463–466.

Puig-Antich, J., Goetz, R., Hanlon, C., Davies, M., Thompson, J., Chambers, W. J., Tabrizi, M. A., & Weitzman, E. D. (1982). Sleep architecture and REM sleep measures in prepubertal children with major depression: A controlled study. *Archives of General Psychiatry, 39,* 932–939.

Puig-Antich, J., Goetz, R., Hanlon, C., Tabrizi, M. A., Davies, M., & Weitzman, E. D. (1983). Sleep architecture and REM sleep measures in prepubertal major depressives: Studies during recovery from the depressive episode in a drug-free state. *Archives of General Psychiatry, 40,* 187–192.

Puig-Antich, J., Goetz, R., Davies, M., Tabrizi, M. A., Novacenko, H., Hanlon, C., Sachar, E. J., & Weitzman, E. D. (1984a). Growth hormone secretion in prepubertal children with major depression: IV. Sleep-related plasma concentrations in a drug-free, fully recovered clinical state. *Archives of General Psychiatry, 41,* 479–483.

Puig-Antich, J., Novacenko, H., Davies, M., Chambers, W. J., Tabrizi, M. A., Krawiec, V., Ambrosini, P. J., & Sachar, E. J. (1984b). Growth hormone secretion in prepubertal children with major depression: I. Final report on response to insulin-induced hypoglycemia during a depressive episode. *Archives of General Psychiatry, 41,* 455–460.

Puig-Antich, J., Novacenko, H., Davies, M., Tabrizi, M. A., Ambrosini, P., Goetz, R., Bianca, J., Goetz, D., & Sachar, E. J. (1984c). Growth hormone secretion in prepubertal children with major depression: III. Response to insulin-induced hypoglycemia after recovery from a depressive episode and in a drug-free state. *Archives of General Psychiatry, 41,* 471–475.

Rapin, I. (1982). *Children with brain dysfunction: Neurology, cognition, language, and behavior.* New York: Raven Press.

Rapoport, J. (1965). Childhood behavior and learning problems treated with imipramine. *International Journal of Neuropsychiatry, 1,* 635–642.

Rapoport, J. L., Buchsbaum, M., Weingartner, H., Zahn, T. P., & Ludlow, C. (1980). Dextroamphetamine: Cognitive and behavioral effects in normal and hyperactive boys and normal men. *Archives of General Psychiatry, 37,* 933–943.

Rapport, M. D., Murphy, H. A., & Bailey, J. S. (1982). The effects of a response cost treatment tactic on hyperactive children. *Journal of School Psychology, 18,* 98–111.

Resnick, T. J., Allen, D. A., & Rapin, I. (1984). Disorders of language development: Diagnosis and intervention. *Pediatrics in Review, 6,* 85–92.

Richardson, J. W., & Richelson, E. (1984). Antidepressants: A clinical update for medical practitioners. *Mayo Clinic Proceedings, 59,* 330–337.

Riddle, D., & Rapoport, J. L. (1976). A two-year follow-up of 78 hyperactive boys: Classroom behavior and peer acceptance. *Journal of Nervous and Mental Disease, 162,* 126–134.

Robertson, B. M. (1979). The psychoanalytic theory of depression: I. The major contributors. *Canadian Journal of Psychiatry, 24,* 341–352.

Robinson, B. W. (1976). Limbic influences on human speech. *Annals of the New York Academy of Science, 280,* 761–771.

Robinson, R. G., & Coyle, J. T. (1980). The differential effect of right versus left hemispheric cerebral infarction on catecholamines and behavior in the rat. *Brain Research, 188,* 63–78.

Robinson, R. G., Kubos, K. L., Starr, L. B., Rao, K., & Price, T. R. (1984). Mood disorders in stroke patients: Importance of location of lesion. *Brain, 107,* 81–93.

Rochford, J. M., Weinapple, M., & Goldstein, L. (1981). The quantitative hemispheric EEG in adolescent psychiatric patients with depressive or paranoid symptomatology. *Biological Psychiatry, 16,* 47–54.

Ross, E. D. (1984). Right hemisphere's role in language, affective behavior and emotion. *Trends in Neurosciences, 7,* 342–346.

Ross, E. D., & Rush, A. J. (1981). Diagnosis and neuroanatomical correlates of depression in brain-damaged patients: Implications for a neurology of depression. *Archives of General Psychiatry, 38,* 1344–1354.

Ross, R. J., Smallberg, S., & Weingartner, H. (1984). The effects of desmethylimipramine on cognitive function in healthy subjects. *Psychiatry Research, 12,* 89–97.

Rosenbaum, A. H., Maruta, T., & Richelson, E. (1979). 1. Drugs that alter mood: I. Tricyclic agents and monoamine oxidase inhibitors. *Mayo Clinic Proceedings, 54,* 335–344.

Rosvold, H. E., Mirsky, A. F., Sarason, I., Bransome, E. D., Jr., & Beck, L. H. (1956). A continuous performance test of brain damage. *Journal of Consulting Psychology, 20,* 343–350.

Rudolf, G. deM. (1956). The treatment of depression with methylamphetamine. *Journal of Mental Science, 102,* 358–363.

Rutter, M., Graham, P., & Yule, W. (1970). *A neuropsychiatric study in childhood.* Clinics in Developmental Medicine, No. 35–36. London: Spastics Society with Heinemann Medical.

Rutter, M., & Graham, P. (1968). The reliability and validity of the psychiatric assessment of the child: I. Interview with the child. *British Journal of Psychiatry, 114,* 563–579.

Rutter, M., Tizard, J., & Whitmore, K. (1970). *Education, health and behavior.* London: Longman.

Sai-Halâsz, A., Brunecker, G., & Szâra, S. (1958). Dimethyltryptamin: Ein neues Psychoticum. *Psychiatria et Neurologia (Basel), 135,* 285–301.

Satterfield, J. H., Cantwell, D. P., & Satterfield, B. T. (1974). Pathophysiology of the hyperactive child syndrome. *Archives of General Psychiatry, 31,* 839–844.

Savard, R. J., Rey, A. C., & Post, R. M. (1980). Halstead-Reitan category test in bipolar and unipolar affective disorders: Relationship to age and phase of illness. *Journal of Nervous and Mental Disease, 168,* 297–304.

Schwartz, M., Friedman, R., Lindsay, P., & Narrol, H. (1982). The relationship between conceptual tempo and depression in children. *Journal of Consulting and Clinical Psychology, 50,* 488–490.

Spitzer, R. L., Endicott, J., & Robins. E. (1978). *Research diagnostic criteria (RDC) for a selected group of functional disorders.* (3rd ed.). New York: Biometrics Research, New York State Psychiatric Institute.

Staton, R. D., & Brumback, R. A. (1980). Neuroleptic-induced reinnervation sprouting in the central nervous system (a model for the development of tardive dyskinesia and supersensitivity psychosis). *Journal of Clinical Psychiatry, 41,* 427–428.

Staton, R. D., & Brumback, R. A. (1981). Non-specificity of motor hyperactivity as a diagnostic criterion. *Perceptual and Motor Skills, 52,* 219–234.

Staton, R. D., Wilson, H., & Brumback, R. A. (1981). Cognitive improvement associated with tricyclic antidepressant treatment of childhood major depressive illness. *Perceptual and Motor Skills, 53,* 219–234.

Staton, R. D., Wilson, H., & Brumback, R. A. (1982). *Differential effects of amitriptyline versus imipramine upon childhood psychological functioning.* Program of the 29th Annual Meeting of the American Academy of Child Psychiatry, Washington, D.C.

Stevenson, D. T., & Romney, D. M. (1984). Depression in learning disabled children. *Journal of Learning Disability, 17,* 579–582.

Stewart, M. A. (1970). Hyperactive children. *Scientific American, 222*(4), 94–98.

Stewart, M. A., Pitts, F. N., Craig, A. C., & Dieruf, W. (1966). The hyperactive child syndrome. *American Journal of Orthopsychiatry, 36,* 861–867.

Strömgren, L. S. (1977). The influence of depression on memory. *Acta Psychiatrica Scandinavica, 56,* 109–128.

Taub, J. M. (1984). Individual variations in the sleep of depression. *International Journal of Neuroscience, 23,* 269–280.

Ternes, J., Woody, R., & Livingston, R. (1987). A child with right hemisphere deficit syndrome responsive to carbamazepine treatment. *Journal of the American Academy of Child and Adolescent Psychiatry, 26,* 586–588.

Thompson, O. W. (1985). The nonverbal dilemma. *Journal of Learning Disabilities, 18,* 400–402.

Tucker, D. M. (1981). Lateral brain function, emotion, and conceptualization. *Psychological Bulletin, 89,* 19–46.

Tucker, D. M., Stenslie, C. E., Roth, R. S., & Shearer, S. L. (1981). Right frontal lobe activation and right hemisphere performance: Decrement during a depressed mood. *Archives of General Psychiatry, 38,* 169–174.

Uytdenhoef, P., Portelange, P., Jacquy, J., Charles, G., Linkowski, P., & Mendlewicz, J. (1983). Regional cerebral blood flow and lateralized hemispheric dysfunction in depression. *British Journal of Psychiatry, 143,* 128–132.

Vogel, G. W., Vogel, F., & McAbee, R. S. (1980). Improvement of depression by REM sleep deprivation: New findings and a theory. *Archives of General Psychiatry, 37,* 247–253.

Warneke, L. (1975). A case of manic-depressive illness in childhood. *Canadian Psychiatric Association Journal, 20,* 195–200.

Watson, B. U., Watson, C. S., & Fredd, R. (1982). Follow-up studies of specific reading disability. *Journal of the American Academy of Child Psychiatry, 21,* 376–382.

Wechsler, D. (1974). *Manual for the Wechsler Intelligence Scale for Children—Revised.* New York: Psychological Corporation.

Weinberg, W. A. (1982). Delayed symbol language skills and their relationship to school performance: diagnosis and management. In K. F. Swaiman & F. S. Wright (Eds.) *The practice of pediatric neurology* (pp. 1098–1120). St. Louis: Mosby.

Weinberg, W. A., & Brumback, R. A. (1976). Mania in childhood: Case studies and literature review. *American Journal of Diseases of Children, 130,* 380–385.

Weinberg, W. A., & McLean, A. (1986). A diagnostic approach to developmental specific learning disorders. *Journal of Child Neurology, 1,* 158–172.

Weinberg, W. A., Rutman, J., Sullivan, L., Penick, E. C., & Dietz, S. G. (1973). Depression in children referred to an educational diagnostic center: Diagnosis and treatment. *Journal of Pediatrics, 83,* 1065–1072.

Weintraub, S., & Mesulam, M.-M. (1983). Developmental learning disabilities of the right hemisphere: Emotional, interpersonal, and cognitive components. *Archives of Neurology, 40,* 463–468.

Werry, J. S., Aman, M. G., & Diamond, E. (1980). Imipramine and methylphenidate in hyperactive children. *Journal of Child Psychology and Psychiatry, 21,* 27–35.

Wetzel, C. D., Squire, L. R., & Janowsky, D. S. (1981). Methylphenidate impairs learning and memory in normal adults. *Behavioral and Neural Biology, 31,* 413–424.

Whalen, C. K., & Henker, B. (1976). Psychostimulants and children, a review and analysis. *Psychological Bulletin, 83,* 1113–1130.

Wilson, H., & Staton, R. D. (1984). Neuropsychological changes in children associated with tricyclic antidepressant therapy. *International Journal of Neuroscience, 24,* 307–312.

Wilson, H., Staton, R. D., & Brumback, R. A. (1982). *Antidepressant treatment responses of children with right hemisphere cognitive deficits.* Program of the 29th annual meeting of the American Academy of Child Psychiatry, Washington, D.C.

Winsberg, B., Goldstein, S., Yepes, L., & Perel, J. (1975). Imipramine and electrocardiographic abnormalities in hyperactive children. *American Journal of Psychiatry, 132,* 542–545.

Yepes, L. E., Balka, E. B., Winsberg, B. G., & Bialer, I. (1977). Amitriptyline and methylphenidate treatment of behaviorally disturbed children. *Journal of Child Psychology and Psychiatry, 18,* 39–52.

Yozawitz, A., Bruder, G., Sutton, S., Sharpe, L., Gurland, B., Fleiss, J., & Costa, L. (1979). Dichotic perception: Evidence for right hemisphere dysfunction in affective psychosis. *British Journal of Psychiatry, 135,* 224–237.

Zrull, J. P., McDermott, J. F., & Poznanski, E. (1970). Hyperkinetic syndrome: The role of depression. *Child Psychiatry and Human Development, 1,* 33–40.

PART FIVE

Lateralization in Learning-Disabled Children

The notion that unilateral dysfunction is at the basis of learning disability stretches back at least 50 years, to the period when Orton (1937) elaborated his model of reading disability. Numerous attempts have been made to draw analogies between acquired dysphasia and developmental dysphasia (Ellis, 1984) and between language breakdown and language acquisition (Caramazza & Zurif, 1978). The logic of this model is straightforward. Since the brain requires certain areas intact to function properly, as evidenced by the deficit in language or cognition when damage occurs to them, developmental dysfunction of these areas may be the source of developmental disability of the associated function. Chapter 16 by Dawson in the previous section is an illustration of where the data seem to uphold this logic. Recent elaborations of models of acquired dyslexia (e.g., Benson, 1985; Ellis, 1984) has strengthened the plausibility of the argument by their very specificity.

The weakness in the logic, however, stems from the nature of problematic development. The child can develop symptoms that look somewhat like those of an acquired neuropsychological syndrome with a different underlying source, since the system itself is not necessarily comparable in structure once development has gone awry (Isaacson, 1975). The issue of appropriate hemispheric specialization in learning-disabled children, for example, may be one of standard organization coupled with dysfunctional information transfer and/or intra- and interhemispheric allocation of resources, as Kershner discusses in Chapter 19. Alternatively, reading disability may be a function of unusual laterality patterns or speed of maturation. Bryden and Obrzut (Chapters 18 and 21, respectively) present empirical summaries on these issues in their chapters on reading skill and hemispheric specialization. Lateralization models offer possibilities for reading disabilities in particular. The division of poor readers into two types—those with a phonologically based difficulty and those with a visually based deficiency—is especially popular (Boder, 1973; Mitterer, 1982). It is easy to map these processes onto brain hemispheres, and there are many experimental studies doing so. It has also been demonstrated that reading-disabled children sometimes have visual-processing difficulties, sometimes have verbal problems, and sometimes have both. Although it would logically follow that the former two types have either right- or left-hemispheric unilateral deficits, respectively, no one has shown that, say, the visual deficits lie at the heart of the reading deficiency. In fact, as both Bryden and Obrzut note, the data concerning clear-cut relationships between laterality measures and learning disabilities are plagued with ambiguities. Both Bryden and Obrzut nevertheless remain optimistic. Bryden details the types of considerations that must be made in undertaking such studies, and Obrzut suggests some needed theoretical considerations. Other sources share this optimism. For example, Bakker (1984; see also Licht, 1987) has recently demonstrated, using an event-related brain potential paradigm, that some dyslexics show a right-hemisphere dominance while reading, and others a left-hemisphere dominance, and that these two groups differ on qualitative factors in their reading. This line of research appears promising, although the behavioral description of the reading difficulties bears little resemblance to the popular visual–phonological distinction. Clearly, the role of hemisphere-specific dysfunction in reading disability requires further clarification.

Individual differences in the pattern of cognitive skills are the focus of the remaining chapters in this section. Obviously, various patterns are available within the normal range. We usually think of a child's preference in thinking style as a strength, with this child being strong in verbal skills, that one in musical arts, the other in visual information processing, and so forth. It is not inconceivable, though, that there is some drawback to having a cognitive strength in that it may pull resources from other modes of thought. Gordon explores this notion that in normal children, the child with a pattern of strengths that is not in line with the common educational system is at a disadvantage.

Extreme patterns of strengths and weaknesses, however, more usually arise from clear deficits. Gibson (Chapter 17) presents a model of how profound deafness can influence apparent hemispheric organization, so that we must be careful about what we mean when we discuss brain organization in atypical populations. Similarly, Rourke and Fisk (Chapter 20) present their model of learning disability subtypes based on hemispheric dysfunction. The strength of these models is that they permit both theoretical and empirical extrapolation.

REFERENCES

Bakker, D. J. (1984). The brain as a dependent variable. *Journal of Clinical Neuropsychology, 6*(1), 1–16.

Benson, D. F. (1985). Alexia. In J. A. M. Frederiks (Ed.), *Clinical neuropsychology* (pp. 433–455). Amsterdam: Elsevier.

Boder, E. (1973). Developmental dyslexia: A diagnostic approach based on three atypical reading–spelling patterns. *Developmental Medicine and Child Neurology, 15,* 663–687.

Caramazza, A., & Zurif, E. (Eds.). (1978). *Language acquisition and language breakdown: Parallels and divergences.* Baltimore: John Hopkins University Press.

Ellis, A. (1984). *Reading, writing and dyslexia: A cognitive analysis.* London: Lawrence Erlbaum Associates.

Isaacson, R. L. (1975). The myth of recovery after early brain damage. In N. E. Ellis (Ed.), *Aberrant development in infancy.* London: Wiley.

Licht, R. (1987). *Reading disability subtypes: Cognitive and electrophysiological differences.* Manuscript, Paedogogical Institute of the Free University, Amsterdam.

Mitterer, J. O. (1982). There are at least two types of poor readers: Whole-word poor readers and recoding poor readers. *Canadian Journal of Psychology, 36,* 445–461.

Orton, S. T. (1937). *Reading, writing and speech problems in children.* New York: Norton.

18

Does Laterality Make Any Difference? Thoughts on the Relation between Cerebral Asymmetry and Reading

M. P. BRYDEN
University of Waterloo

In reading the popular press, one sometimes has the feeling that the realization that the two cerebral hemispheres have rather different functions is one of the major advances of the past decade. In particular, there are two major ways in which contemporary ideas of cerebral specialization have affected our thinking about educational policy. One is to argue that current educational practices neglect the right hemisphere, and must be altered to provide a better development of right-hemispheric functions. The other is to claim that particular individuals, by virtue of their abnormal cerebral lateralization, are at risk for some behavioral dysfunction, and to attempt to diagnose or remedy this dysfunction by dealing with the pattern of cerebral lateralization (see, for amplification, Chapter 8 by Harris, this volume).

The first argument depends on the assumption that the modal state of cerebral organization is somehow desirable and optimal. In general, the left hemisphere has been described as verbal, analytic, linear, and a serial processor of information, whereas the right hemisphere is considered to be spatial, nonverbal, holistic, a parallel processor, and "creative" (cf. Bradshaw & Nettleton, 1983; Bryden, 1982b). It should be recognized, however, that not all people are left-hemispheric for language or right-hemispheric for visuospatial skills (Bryden, Hecaen, & DeAgostini, 1983; Segalowitz & Bryden, 1983). Thus, although the majority of individuals are left-hemispheric for both language production and language perception, there are many exceptions to this, especially among left-handers. Similarly, most of us are right-hemispheric for certain nonverbal skills, such as visuospatial ones, but there are many exceptions. In particular, deviant cerebral organization seems to be more prevalent in women and in left-handers. However, the simple fact that a pattern of brain organization does not conform to the mode does not necessarily make it any worse. Likewise, it is not necessarily true that altering one's brain organization from amodal to modal will result in any improvement. This is potentially a very contentious issue, for it is often implied that women and/or left-handers are somehow inferior by virtue of the fact that their cerebral organization is less likely to conform to the modal pattern than that of men or right-handers (cf. Harris, 1985).

Although much has been written on the supposed benefits of educating the right hemisphere, the present chapter is not the place to provide a detailed review of this literature. Suffice it to say that there is remarkably little evidence for a biologically based "hemisphericity" as a general cognitive style (Beaumont, Young, & McManus, 1984; Ley & Kaushansky, 1985).

Rather, the present chapter will concentrate on the second supposed contribution of laterality research to education, namely the notion that people with abnormal patterns of lateralization are somehow deficient in certain cognitive skills, most notably those relevant to reading. Despite a number of critical reviews (Hiscock & Kinsbourne, 1982; Naylor, 1980; Young & Ellis, 1981), there remains a firm belief that developmentally dyslexic children have an abnormal pattern of lateralization. In fact, careful reviews by some researchers in the field (e.g., Corballis, 1983) suggest that poor readers are less likely to show the normal pattern of lateralization than are good readers.

The typical study involves comparing normal and poor readers on some behavioral task that consistently shows a lateral asymmetry in normal children and adults, such as a dichotic listening task, a visual half-field task, or a tactual dichhaptic task. If differences are found between the groups, then some relation between cerebral lateralization and reading ability is hypothesized. Problems arise because of poor selection of subjects, poor selection of a laterality measure, misapplied statistical analyses, or some combination of these factors. Thus, unfortunately, one can support almost any possible position by focusing on the right studies. Good evidence for this assertion appears in Best's (1985) excellent book on hemispheric function in children. In this book, different authors conclude that perceptual laterality is reduced in dyslexics (Gladstone & Best, 1985; Pirozzolo, 1985); that it is increased (Kershner, 1985); and that there are no systematic effects (Rudel, 1985).

THE BASIC DATA

Clearly, people have not agreed on how to assess the literature. Although there is no special reason for believing that one more review will clarify matters, a logical first step seems to be to try to make sense of the existing literature. A reasonably careful search led to 51 studies in which some relatively common behavioral measure of cerebral lateralization was related to reading ability in children, either by selecting defined groups of good and poor readers or by correlational techniques. The results of these studies are summarized in Tables 18-1 through 18-7. Of the 51 studies, 30 claim to show, to a greater or lesser extent, that poor readers are less lateralized than good readers. Of the remainder, 14 show no difference between groups, and 7 report that poor readers are more lateralized. A simple binomial test indicates that there are significantly more studies demonstrating weaker lateralization in poor readers than studies demonstrating greater lateralization ($p < .01$). Basically the same results are found with dichotic, visual, and dichhaptic techniques. Dichotic procedures are the most common, with 20 of 35 studies showing weaker lateralization in the poor readers, and only 5 showing greater lateralization. Of the visual half-field studies, 8 of 14 show weaker lateralization in poor readers, and 2 show greater lateralization, while both dichhaptic studies provide evidence for weaker lateralization in the poor readers. Thus, at least on the surface, Corballis's (1983) conclusion that poor readers are less lateralized than normal readers seems to be justified.

In previous writings, I have criticized those who assume that any test of perceptual laterality assesses only cerebral lateralization and is unaffected by other factors (Bryden, 1978, 1982a, 1982b). At its simplest, my argument has been that people adopt strategies to help them perform well on the tasks that we give them, and that these strategies may affect the balance of performance between left and right sides. If we do not understand how our subjects perform the tasks we set them, we may come to erroneous conclusions. As one example, subjects may realize that they are doing very poorly on left-ear items in a dichotic listening task, and decide to selectively attend and report the left-ear items. By recalling the left-ear items first, they must necessarily retain the right-ear items longer and subject them to output interference. By doing this, they may actually show a left-ear advantage (LEA) for verbal material, but this LEA should not be taken as evidence for right-

Table 18-1. Dichotic Listening Studies, Poor Readers Less Lateralized

Study	Subjects	Task	Results
Ayers, 1977	114 LD, B & G R & L, ages 6–10 48 normals	60 trials, CV pairs	LEA associated with poor auditory language scores; EA scores lower than in normal control group
Bakker, Smink, & Reitsma, 1973	1. 40 RH normals age 7, B & G	16 trials, 3 pairs; also 18 monaural	Best readers show smallest |EA|.
	2. 38 RH normals age 9, B & G	Monaural lists, 15 trials	Best readers show largest |EA|.
	3. 100 RH normals ages 7–11, B&G	Monaural lists, 18 trials	In young, best readers show smallest |EA|; in older, good readers give large |EA|.
Bryden, 1970	234 Grades 2, 4, 6 B & G, L & R hand	20 trials 2, 3 pairs digits	In boys, poor readers less likely to have EA same as handedness; in girls, true only for younger Ss.
Cermak, Drake, Cermak, & Kenney, 1978	47 RH boys, LD; 14 RH boys, normal	3 pairs digits also with tapping, 20 trials/cond.	Reduced EA in Ss with VIQ < PIQ; PIQ < VIQ
Hynd & Obrzut, 1981	90 LD B & G, ages 8–11; 90 matched normals	30 trials, CV pairs	Much reduced REA in LD, esp. in youngest (age 8) group
Leong, 1976	58 above-avg. readers, 58 dyslexics, all boys, ages 9–10	15 trials, digit lists, 2–4 pairs	Weaker REA in dyslexics, esp. on 3-pair lists
Mercure & Warren, 1978	30 normals, 27 "inadequate" readers B & G	60 trials, CV pairs	Normals give higher RE scores than poor readers.
Obrzut, Hynd, Obrzut, & Leitgeb, 1980	48 RH LD, B & G; 48 matched normals ages 7–12	30 trials, CV pairs	Reduced REA in LD, esp. in youngest group (ages 7–8.5)
Obrzut, Obrzut, Bryden, & Bartels, 1985	16 RH LD, B & G; 16 matched normals, ages 7.8–12.1	30 trials, CV pairs, free recall; 60 trials directed attn.	Reduced REA in LD in both free recall and directed attention
Orr, Mitterer, & Bryden, in preparation	19 normals, 51 poor readers Grade 3, B & G	60 trials, CV pairs, directed attn.	Poor readers have smaller |EA|; no differences between "recoding" and "whole word" poor readers.
Sadick & Ginsburg, 1978	175 normals, B & G ages 5–11	60 trials, CV pairs	Among Grade 2 (age 7) Ss, REA greater in poor readers. Overall, good readers have larger |EA| than poor readers.
Satz, Rardin, & Ross, 1971	20 dyslexic boys, 20 normals, ages 7–12	25 trials, 3 pairs digits	Reduced REA in poor readers
Satz & Van Nostrand, 1973	40 dyslexic, 40 normals	3 pairs digits	Reduced REA in poor readers
Sparrow & Satz, 1970	40 poor readers, 40 normals, ages 9–12, B & G	25 trials, 4 pairs digits	8% of normals and 2.8% of poor readers show LEA
Swanson & Mullen, 1983	24 LD boys, 24 normals, ages 8–13	12-word lists paired with white noise	LD generally have smaller REA, especially in older Ss (ages 11–13)

(*continued*)

Table 18-1 *(continued)*

Study	Subjects	Task	Results
Thomson, 1976	20 dyslexic, 20 normals, B & G ages 9–12	24 trials, lists of words or numbers	Reduced REA in dyslexics
Watson & Engle, 1982	34 poor readers, 36 normals, all boys, ages 7–15	24 trials each 3-pair words, numbers, 2-pair CVs; 60 trials, CV pairs	Poor readers, esp. younger, show reduced REA, but only with CV material.
Wellman & Allen, 1983	121 RH normals, ages 7–9	60 trials, CV pairs	20 best readers have bigger REAs than 20 worst readers.
Witelson & Rabinovitch, 1972	24 poor readers, 24 normals, ages 8–13	60 trials, 2 and 3 pairs of digits	LEA in poor readers; REA in normals
Zurif & Carson, 1970	14 poor readers, 14 normals, Grade 4 boys	10 trials, 3-pair digits	REA in normals, small LEA in poor readers

Table 18-2. Dichotic Listening Studies, Poor Readers Equally Lateralized

Study	Subjects	Task	Results
Abigail & Johnson, 1976	20 poor readers, 20 normals, ages 8.5–11	20 trials, 3-pair digits	No difference between groups in R–L score
Caplan & Kinsbourne, 1982	40 clinic poor readers, 40 normals, ages 7–18, B & G	60 trials, CV pairs	No differences on either EA or |EA|
Fennell, Satz, & Morris, 1983	208 boys, followed from 5.5 to 11 years	30 trials, 3-pair digits	No relation of EA at Grade 5 to WRAT reading
Hynd, Obrzut, Weed, & Hynd, 1979	48 LD, 48 normals, ages 7–12	30 trials, CV pairs	Overall REA, no interaction. Very small trend to less LEA in younger LD.
Koomar & Cermak, 1981	30 normals, 30 LD, ages 7–10	60 trials, of CV pairs, 20 trials of 3-pair digits	83% of both groups give REA on CVs; 70% of normals and 76% of LDs are REA on digit lists
McKeever & Van-Deventer, 1975	9 clinic dyslexics, 9 normals, all RH boys, ages 11–19	12 trials 3-pair digits	No group × ear interaction
Obrzut, Boliek, & Bryden, 1987	16 LD, RH; 16 RH normals, 16 LH normals, 16 RH bilinguals	CV pairs, 30 trials, free; 60 trials, directed attn.	LH give much smaller EA than others, but LD not significantly less than normals
Prior, Frolley, & Sanson, 1983	10 normals, 10 specific reading disability, 10 "backward" readers	Monitoring task, 80 targets per ear	No group differences in detection or RT
Witelson, 1977	85 dyslexic; 156 normal, all RH boys, ages 6–14	Lists of digits	Both groups show REA
Yeni-Komshian, Isenberg, & Goldberg, 1975	19 normals, 19 poor readers, ages 10–15, B & G	30 trials, 3-pair digits, ordered recall	REA overall, insignificantly larger in poor readers

Table 18-3. Dichotic Listening Studies, Poor Readers More Lateralized

Study	Subjects	Task	Results
Aylward, 1984	20 normals, 12 dyseidetics, 20 dysphonetics, 20 nonspecific poor readers	20 trials, 3-pair digits, ordered recall	Overall, poor readers show larger REAs, but no subgroup differences
Dermody, Mackie, & Katsch, 1983	15 normals, 15 poor readers, all boys, ages 10.5–13.5	60 trials, CV pairs, also 60 trials with 90-msec onset asynchrony	Greated REA in poor readers; greater lag effect in poor readers on asynchronous trials
Hynd, Obrzut, & Obrzut, 1981	23 normals, 23 LD, ages 9–13	30 trials, CV pairs	No correlation between dichotic LQ and reading achievement; LD group has larger LQ.
Obrzut, Hynd, Obrzut, & Pirozzolo, 1981	32 normals, 32 LD, ages 7–13	30 trials, CV pairs on each of free recall, attend left, attend right	On free recall, LDs show larger REAs; directed attention, LDs give larger REAs.
Richardson & Firlej, 1979	151 normals, all boys, 11–16	3 trials, 10 pairs of words	LEA correlates with good reading scores.

Table 18-4. Visual Hemifield Studies, Poor Readers Less Lateralized

Study	Subjects	Task	Results
Garren, 1980	80 boys, ages 8–10, divided by reading age	20 trials, bilateral words	Poor readers show LVF, good readers RVF.
Kershner, 1977	11 good readers, 10 poor readers, 12 gifted readers, age 10, B & G	20 trials, bilateral words	RVF effect greatest for gifted, least for poor readers
Marcel, Katz, & Smith, 1974	20 normals, 20 poor readers, ages 7:6–8:7, B & G	40 trials, unilateral words	RVF effect larger for good readers
Marcel & Rajan, 1975	40 normals, ages 7–9, B & G, split into good and poor readers	40 trials, unilateral words; also face recognition trials	Good readers have larger RVF for words. No sig. relation reading and face recognition.
McKeever & Van-Deventer, 1975	9 clinic dyslexics, 9 normals, all RH boys, ages 11–19	40 unilateral, 20 bilateral words; vocal RT to letters	Unilateral words: VF × group interaction. Bilateral words shows similar but smaller effect. Vocal RT, no differences.
Obrzut, Hynd, & Zellner, 1983	26 normals, 26 LD, all RH, B & G, ages 7–13	32 unilateral, 16 bilateral, 32 cued unilateral words	In all conditions, RVF effect reduced in LD
Olson, 1973	50 above-normal readers, 43 poor readers, ages 7–13, B & G	50 unilateral, 25 bilateral words	Younger (ages 8–9) poor readers without other deficits show no RFV on unilateral trials; otherwise, RVF throughout.
Pirozzolo & Rayner, 1979	18 normals, 18 poor readers, ages 10–14, RH boys	50 unilateral, 16 bilateral words, 24 unilateral faces	Words: Good readers show RVF, poor do not. Faces: LVF for both.

Table 18-5. Visual Hemifield Studies, Poor Readers Equally Lateralized

Study	Subjects	Tasks	Results
Aylward, 1984	20 normals, 12 dyseidetics, 20 dysphonetics, 20 nonspecific poor readers	20 trials, bilateral CVCs ordered recall	All groups show RVFs.
Davidoff, Beaton, Done, & Booth, 1982	12 adult illiterates, 12 adult normals, mean age 33; 12 normals, age 8, all males	72 trials; unilateral vertical CCCs, CVCs, and words	No differences in RVF or |VF|; adult normals show different serial position effects.
McKeever & Huling, 1970	10 normals, 10 poor readers, Grade 7	160 trials, unilateral words, half to each eye	Overall RVF, but no effect of eye or group
Vellutino, Bentley, & Phillips, 1978	36 normals, 36 poor readers, ages 7–8, 11–12	Learning to name Chinese characters; unilateral	RVF for all groups

Table 18-6. Visual Hemifield Studies, Poor Readers More Lateralized

Study	Subjects	Task	Results
Gross, Rothenberg, & Schottenfeld 1978	15 normals, 14 poor readers, ages 10–13.5; B & G	Duration thresholds for unilateral letters	Greater asymmetry for poor readers; also greater variance
Yeni-Komshian, Isenberg, & Goldberg, 1975	19 normals, 19 poor readers, ages 10–15, B & G	5-item lists of words or numbers presented in alternation to L or R and center	Poor readers better in RVF, good readers show no VF effect.

Table 18-7. Tactual Studies, Poor Readers Less Lateralized

Study	Subjects	Table	Results
Dalby & Gibson, 1981	15 normals, 15 dyseidetics, 15 dysphonetics, 15 nonspecifics, ages 9–12, RH boys	Unimanual direction perception	Normals, dyseidetics show LHA, nonspecifics and dysphonetics show no hand difference.
Witelson, 1977	85 dyslexic, 156 normal, all RH boys, ages 6–14	Dichhaptic form/ letter recognition	On forms, normals give LHA, dyslexics OHA; on letters, normals show trend to RHA, dyslexics show LHA.

Abbreviations used in Tables 18–1 through 18–7: Under "Subjects": B = boys, G = girls. RH = right handed; LH = left-handed; L & R handed = mixture of both. LD = learning-disabled, as defined by authors. Under "Task": CV = consonant–vowel nonsense syllables, usually involving stop consonants. "Pairs" involve a single item to each ear before report; "lists" involve several distinct items to each ear prior to recall. "Bilateral" presentation involves presentation of separate items in left and right visual fields simultaneously; "unilateral" presentation involves a single item in either left or right visual field. Under "Results": LEA = left-ear advantage; REA = right-ear advantage; |EA| = absolute ear advantage; EA = ear advantage. LVF = left visual field; RVF = right visual field; VF = visual field. LHA = left-hand advantage; RHA = right-hand advantage; OHA = no hand advantage.

hemispheric language. Only by properly controlling such strategies can we make any strong assertions about language lateralization.

Since there are a reasonably large number of dichotic studies, it seemed possible that one could isolate some factor that would account for the discrepant results. To accomplish this, the studies were classified according to seven distinguishing variables: (1) whether lists of digits or words or single consonant–vowel (CV) pairs were used; (2) whether the poor readers were formally classified as dyslexic, reading-disabled, or learning-disabled, or were simply the bottom of the normal classroom distribution; (3) whether the subjects were under 10 years of age, over 10, or both; (4) whether the sample of poor readers numbered more or less than 40; (5) whether left-handers were excluded or not; (6) whether the subjects were all boys or included both sexes; and (7) whether or not there were 60 or more dichotic trials. None of these factors has any compelling effect on the results, although there were slight trends in favor of finding that poor readers were less lateralized if younger subjects were used, if girls were included, if left-handers were included, and if a relatively large number of trials were used.

The variability of findings is clearly illustrated in the several papers by Obrzut and his colleagues. Despite using essentially the same selection procedure and basically similar dichotic tasks, different studies from this laboratory show widely different results. With a dichotic free-recall procedure, for example, Obrzut, Hynd, Obrzut, and Pirozzolo (1981) show greater lateralization in learning-disabled children, but Hynd, Obrzut, Weed, and Hynd (1979); Obrzut, Hynd, Obrzut, and Leitgeb (1980); and Obrzut, Obrzut, Bryden, and Bartels (1985) all show some evidence for weaker lateralization in learning-disabled children. The 1979 and 1980 studies also show that differences between normal and learning-disabled children are more pronounced in younger children, between 7 and 10 years of age. These two studies provide a rough reading-age control for the older learning-disabled children in the younger normals, but since the differences are primarily with the younger learning-disabled children, for whom there is no reading-age control, this does not really resolve the issue of whether the effects are due to reading level or to the categorization of the children as learning-disabled.

Although the reasons for the great discrepancy in findings in the dichotic literature is not immediately evident, if one ignores all the selection, procedural, and statistical variables that are involved, the general summary would at least lead one to believe that there are reasonable grounds for entertaining the hypothesis that poor readers are less lateralized than normal readers. Two questions immediately come to mind: Why should this be so, and how much faith can we have in the findings?

MODELS OF DISTURBED LATERALITY

There seem to be four basic reasons that one might expect to find abnormal patterns of cerebral lateralization in poor readers.

1. *A developmental lag:* Lenneberg (1967) had suggested that cerebral lateralization of language developed gradually over the first years of life, not reaching adult levels until puberty. On this argument, a weak lateralization is a sign of slow development, and poor readers are therefore people whose nervous systems have not developed at the normal rate. This is an optimistic view, in that one might expect such individuals to "grow out of it." However, current evidence on the development of lateralization does not support Lenneberg's hypothesis: There is little sign of any change in laterality with increasing age, at least from age 3 to adulthood (Bryden, 1982b; Bryden & Saxby, 1986; but see Kershner, 1985, for the argument that laterality actually decreases with age).

2. *A biological predisposition:* Poor readers are born with a damaged or poorly developed left hemisphere, so language is less clearly lateralized in these people. This might arise because of increased prenatal testosterone levels (Geschwind & Behan, 1982), some other prenatal developmental effect (Corballis, 1983), or a genetic cause. If it is genetic in origin, one might expect relatives of poor readers to manifest weak lateralization as well, although this hypothesis has not been adequately tested. This is a relatively pessimistic view, in that it is not clear what remedy would be applied.

3. *Linguistic deprivation:* Although the biological substrate for left-hemisphere language is normal, some experiential abnormality has led to its deterioration over time. Many poor readers also show auditory–linguistic deficits, and the failure to have normal language experience may prevent left-hemisphere language from becoming fixed, even though the appropriate substrate is there. If this is the case, one might look to enriching auditory experience as a remediation, or one might try to emphasize the visual rather than the auditory aspects of language (e.g., Rozin, Poritsky, & Sotsky, 1971).

4. *Interhemispheric communication problems:* The dichhaptic literature suggests that poor readers are also not as right-hemispheric for tactual form recognition as are normal children. Perhaps the involvement of the left hemisphere in putative right-hemisphere tasks results in a weakening of the left-hemispheric specialization for language. Again, if this were the case, an emphasis on the visuospatial basis of written language might prove an effective therapy.

CHOICE OF A LATERALITY MEASURE

In selecting a measure of cerebral lateralization, the researcher implicitly assumes that his or her measure reflects some aspect of cerebral functional asymmetry, rather than some other behavioral characteristic. Candidate measures have been reviewed in some detail by Bryden (1982b) and by Bradshaw and Nettleton (1983). In the literature on dyslexia, four measures have been the most popular: (1) handedness, (2) the dichotic REA, (3) dichhaptic asymmetry, and (4) visual half-field asymmetry. Let us consider the merits of these different approaches.

Handedness is simply a weak measure of cerebral function. It is true that virtually all right-handers are left-hemispheric for speech, but the majority of left-handers are as well (Segalowitz & Bryden, 1983). There is enough of a relationship between the two variables that a large sample of left-handers should differ from a large sample of right-handers in cerebral representation for language, but sample sizes of 100 or more are called for, and few studies employ such large numbers. Nevertheless, there is some evidence that dyslexia is associated with a high incidence of left-handedness in both targets and their relatives (Geschwind & Behan, 1982). At the same time, the possible relationship between handedness and dyslexia raises a serious problem for studies of perceptual laterality in poor readers. Our earlier review suggested that those dichotic studies that lumped left- and right-handers together were somewhat more likely to obtain evidence for reduced laterality in the poor readers. The problem then arises as to whether laterality is reduced because these children are poor readers or because they are left-handed. We really do not know what to expect, on an individual basis, from left-handers on a dichotic task. We know that as a group they should (and do) show a reduced laterality effect (cf. Bryden, 1986; Piazza, 1980). However, some left-handers are left-hemispheric for language and some are right-hemispheric, and we have no way of telling which is which (Segalowitz & Bryden, 1983). This makes it very difficult to interpret those studies that have included left-handers.

The visual laterality literature indicates that normal subjects identify words and letters more readily when they are exposed in the right visual field than when they appear in the left visual field (Bryden, 1982b). Such a task, however, is essentially a reading task, and one should feel uncomfortable about comparing the ability of good readers to read with the ability of poor readers on the same task. Many of the putative differences between good and poor readers may turn out to be simply reflections of the different reading abilities of the two groups. Some investigators have tried to escape this issue by using nonverbal tasks, where normal subjects typically exhibit a left visual-field advantage (LFA). There are two problems with such an approach. First, early reading may involve the acquisition of fine control over eye movements, and therefore good readers and poor readers may differ in fixation accuracy (Hochberg, 1970). Second, the use of a nonverbal laterality measure may assess *right*-hemisphere function, but not permit any statements to be made about language lateralization (cf. Bryden *et al.*, 1983). For these reasons, visual laterality studies with dyslexics should be viewed with caution.

Witelson (1977) has popularized the use of dichhaptic techniques, involving the simultaneous presentation of different shapes to the left and right hands. Here, shape perception generally yields a left-hand advantage in normal subjects, while letters may produce a right-hand advantage. Unlike the visual studies, the nonverbal effect is far more robust than the verbal one, perhaps because we rarely identify verbal material by touch. Again, we then seem to be assessing the functions of the right, rather than the left, hemisphere. Furthermore, it is difficult to control shifting of attention, the physical parameters of presentation, and the sequence of recall with dichhaptic presentation. The task is promising, but there is relatively little work with normal individuals, and it is a very time-consuming process to obtain stable data on individual subjects.

The most popular technique is that of dichotic listening, in which different sounds are presented simultaneously to the two ears. Most of the data regarding dyslexia involves the presentation of speech sounds, and by far the most common procedures are to present single pairs of CV syllables formed with the six stop consonants |*b*|, |*d*|, |*g*|, |*p*|, |*t*|, and |*k*| (Studdert-Kennedy & Shankweiler, 1970), or to employ lists of three or four pairs of digits or words (Kimura, 1961). Some years ago, I argued that dichotic list procedures permitted strategy and memory effects to exert a major influence (Bryden, 1978). To the extent that this is the case, group differences in the REA obtained with list procedures may not reflect group differences in cerebral lateralization. However, the difference in the REA between normal left- and right-handed groups is about the same for lists as it is for CV pairs (Bryden, 1983), so the controls for attentional and strategy effects may not be as crucial as I had thought. In any event, the dichotic task has been shown to be related to speech lateralization (Kimura, 1961) and can be administered without obvious artifact. It is perhaps the best choice of all the commonly used behavioral laterality measures. However, I would continue to argue that proper control over the deployment of attention is crucial. Although attention is sometimes controlled (e.g., Obrzut *et al.*, 1985; Obrzut, Boliek, & Bryden, 1987), more often the issue is ignored.

PROBLEMS WITH STATISTICAL MEASUREMENT

Probably the single most common finding in the literature on dichotic listening and reading ability is that good readers do better at the task than poor readers do. This simple difference leads to much grief in the interpretation of the data. It is conventional to enter the data into a mixed-design analysis of variance, with "ears" as a within-subjects factor and "reading level'' as a between-subjects factor, and to look for a significant interaction effect. Such an analysis operates on the difference between right- and left-ear scores and yields a significant effect if this difference is greater for one group than for the other. If overall performance is near the floor or the ceiling, however, then any difference between the ears will necessarily be small. In contrast, if performance is at an intermediate level, both large and small ear differences will be possible. I have argued (Bryden, 1982b) that this is why, for example, there is an apparent reduction in the REA with age in Kimura's (1963) developmental study (but cf. Kershner, 1985).

Many solutions have been offered to this problem (Bryden & Sprott, 1981; Marshall, Caplan, & Holmes, 1975; Repp, 1977); all involve the use of some laterality index whose value is essentially independent of overall performance level. Bryden and Sprott (1981), for example, recommended calculating a statistic based on the relative odds with which left- and right-side items are identified. In effect, this amounts to determining a signal detection ''d-prime'' for each side, and calculating the difference. Because the likelihood ratio calculated for each side approximates a normal distribution, the values of this statistic are not dependent on the total number of items correct. Along similar lines, Marshall *et al.* (1975) recommend the use of the proportion of total errors attributable to the left side for accuracy levels above 50%, and the proportion of correct responses attributable to the right side for accuracy levels below 50%. Since one is again concerned with the relative distribution of errors rather than the absolute difference in number of errors, this measure is largely independent of overall accuracy.

Despite the availability of such measures, however, few researchers make any use of laterality indices, or even seem to be aware of the problem.

SUBJECT SELECTION

Much of the initial research on laterality and reading ability seems to be based on the assumption that all poor readers are alike. Little attempt is made to classify different types of poor readers, despite the flood of research on different types of reading disability (Boder & Jannico, 1982; Doehring, Trites, Patel, & Fiedorowicz, 1981; Rutter, 1978; Satz & Morris, 1981). Some investigators have simply divided a normal classroom into those who are relatively good readers and those who are relatively poor (e.g., Bryden, 1970; Richardson & Firlej, 1979). Others have used children who have been referred to a clinic for reading or learning disabilities (e.g., McKeever & VanDeventer, 1975; Witelson, 1977) and still others have defined as poor readers those who are some specified number of years below grade level in terms of reading test score (Watson & Engle, 1982). Only a few studies have made any attempt to employ a differential diagnosis of different types of reading disability (e.g., Aylward, 1984; Dalby & Gibson, 1981; Prior, Frolley, & Sanson, 1983). None has used a reading-matched control as well as an age-matched control, although this is partially rectified by designs that use chronological age as a separate factor (e.g., Obrzut *et al.*, 1980).

SOME SUGGESTIONS

An examination of the literature on perceptual asymmetry and reading disability has provided some reasonable hints that good readers are more strongly lateralized than are poor readers. However, the experiments employ so many different procedures and yield such a diversity of results that it is quite unclear just what conclusions to accept. Given the lessons of the existing research, perhaps it is now possible to carry out a proper study of cerebral lateralization and developmental dyslexia. Such a study should have, at the very minimum, the following properties:

1. The reading-disabled group should be carefully selected, with an objective criterion for defining reading disability. This should include normal intelligence, evidence of adequate motivation through acceptable performance on some nonreading test of academic achievement, such as a mathematics test; and a reading level set at some reasonable level below age level, such as 2 years. By most hypotheses, one is not interested in showing that children of low intelligence or those who lack any interest in academic pursuits are different from those who are more academically inclined, but, rather, in determining whether or not a specific reading disability has anything to do with abnormal cerebral lateralization.

2. The poor reading group should be sufficiently well studied to permit some differential diagnosis of disability type. There are, for example, relatively simple tests to classify children according to Boder's categories of dyseidetic, dysphonetic, and mixed (Boder & Jannico, 1982; Camp & McCabe, 1977). There are already some suggestions that different types of poor readers show different patterns of lateralization (Dalby & Gibson, 1981; Pirozzolo & Rayner, 1979). It is certainly unreasonable to assume that all poor readers are alike. It is, however, not immediately evident which classification system will be more fruitful. As an alternative to the Boder classification, there is currently considerable interest in developmental analogues to the various forms of acquired dyslexia (cf. Ellis, 1985; Newcombe & Marshall, 1981) and in experimental analysis of the components of reading (cf. Mitterer, 1982).

3. Control subjects should include not only age- and IQ-matched normal readers, but also younger children matched for reading age (Backman, Mamen, & Ferguson, 1984). Admittedly, there is little evidence for any developmental shift in lateralization (Bryden & Saxby, 1986; but see Merola & Liederman, 1985), but one really wants to know whether any differences are driven by the deficit or by simple exposure to language.

4. Only right-handed subjects should be used, and careful measures of their hand preference and any evidence of familial sinistrality should be obtained. I would like to argue that left-handers should be included, since I think they represent an interesting subgroup, but until we know more about what is "normal" in sinistrals, it is impossible to detect what is abnormal. I fear that at the present time left-handers merely add noise to the data. Furthermore, it is a difficult task to find sufficient left-handers to constitute a group of reasonable size. In the long run, however, it may be very important to understand left-handed dyslexics, especially since Geschwind and Behan (1982) claim a higher incidence of both developmental dyslexia and immune disorders in left-handers.

5. Both boys and girls should be tested. Although there are more boys than girls diagnosed as developmentally dyslexic in North America (Finucci & Childs, 1981), there is some evidence that the etiology is different for boys than for girls. For instance, Lewitter, De Fries, and Elston (1980) have shown that a simple genetic model fits girls but not boys. Furthermore, the review of the existing literature suggests that one is somewhat more likely to find evidence for a reduced lateralization in studies that include both boys and girls.

6. The lateralization task should be carefully selected. For reasons outlined earlier, I am inclined to prefer a verbal dichotic listening task with directed attention, like that used by Obrzut *et al.* (1985). We understand the task reasonably well, know what to do to minimize the effects of subject's strategies, and have good control over the stimulus presentation. I would argue that visual half-field tasks are contaminated by one's knowledge

of reading, and that dichhaptic tasks are too difficult to control well. The dual-task methodology (Hiscock, 1985) offers an attractive alternative. In the typical dual-task experiment, subjects are asked to perform some simple and quantifiable manual task, such as tapping or dowel balancing, first with one hand and then with the other. They are then asked to do the same unimanual task again while engaged in some competing activity, such as reading or speaking. Typically, activities that engage the left hemisphere will disrupt right-hand activity more than they will affect left-hand activity, presumably because the resources of the left hemisphere are required for both activities. If poor readers are less lateralized than good readers, they should show more symmetrical interference patterns on such tasks (cf. Dalby & Gibson, 1981).

7. One should also administer some nonverbal lateralization task. Some of the evidence suggests a deficit in the right, rather than the left, hemisphere (e.g., Witelson, 1977), and few studies have made any attempt to assess it. One possibility is the tone localization task developed by Efron (Efron, Koss, & Yund, 1983; Gregory, Efron, Divenyi, & Yund, 1983). In this task, subjects hear two tones in succession, one higher in pitch than the other, at the left ear. Simultaneously, the same two tones, reversed in sequence, are heard at the right ear. The subject's task is to indicate whether he or she heard a ''high–low'' sequence or a ''low–high'' sequence. With a clearly discriminable but relatively small difference in frequencies, say 1,600 Hz and 1,800 Hz, right-handed subjects report hearing the tonal sequence that was presented to the left ear on the majority of trials. The Efron data suggest that this task generates a left-ear advantage in the same subjects in whom dichotic speech tasks produce a right-ear effect.

8. Use a laterality measure that is independent of overall level of accuracy, such as the lambda coefficient developed by Bryden and Sprott (1981). One of the most common findings is that the poor readers do not do as well at the task as do the good readers, and there must be some recognition of this difference in accuracy.

9. Consider group differences in degree of laterality as well as in direction. It may not be reasonable to assume that otherwise normal people with right-hemisphere language are different from those with left-hemisphere language. On the other hand, it seems quite plausible to suggest that people with bilateral language representation are different from those with unilateral language representation.

WHAT WOULD IT MEAN?

At present, the data on laterality and reading provide equivocal evidence in support of the contention that poor readers are less lateralized than are good readers. In the preceding paragraphs, we have offered some suggestions as to how one might carry out a more thorough test of this hypothesis. If we did so, and found more compelling evidence that poor readers were less lateralized, what would it mean?

A major clue to this may be found in the recent work of Gibson (Chapter 22, this volume). Employing a bimanual tactual laterality task, Gibson found that profoundly deaf children who had learned to read at or above the Grade 4 level showed a normal pattern of lateralization, whereas those who had failed to reach this level showed an abnormal pattern of lateralization. She has suggested that the failure to have normal auditory linguistic experience in early childhood has resulted in the degeneration of systems in the left hemisphere that would normally be responsible for linguistic processing, forcing other parts of the brain to take over the function. It is interesting to note that studies of young *language-impaired* children are virtually unanimous in showing a weaker lateralization in such individuals (Pettit & Helms, 1979; Rosenblum & Dorman, 1978; Sommers & Taylor, 1972; Springer & Eisenson, 1977; Williams, Keough, Fisher, Seymour, & Tanner, 1980). Not only do receptive language problems (deafness) produce a reorganization of cerebral function, but expressive problems do as well. Since speech perception and speech production are closely linked (Liberman & Mattingly, 1985), this should not be very surprising. Furthermore, Tallal, Stark, and Mellits (1985) have shown that language-impaired and normal children can be discriminated by a battery of tests assessing rapid temporal perception and production of auditory material. Since the left hemisphere has often been implicated in rapid sequential processing, failure on Tallal's tasks may be indicative of some specific left-hemisphere deficit. By this argument, early language deprivation will result both in the reorganization of cerebral function and in poor reading. Thus, some, but not all, poor readers should be expected to show poor lateralization.

AN ALTERNATIVE VIEW

Throughout this chapter, the emphasis has been on the dichotic listening procedure, for two reasons. First, there is far more literature using the dichotic procedure than any other approach, and this makes the search for regularities somewhat easier. Second, visual techniques often confound reading ability with the task itself. It is no great surprise if poor readers do not show a laterality effect if they also do not know the words being employed in the study. Nevertheless, it remains possible that any abnormalities of lateralization in poor readers are specific to the visual modality and would have to be tested with visual rather than auditory tasks. One way to avoid contamination with reading skills is to use a nonverbal task, such as a face recognition or line orientation task, but such tasks would presumably be measures of right-, not left-hemisphere function. An appropriate verbal task might be that employed by Saxby and Bryden (1985). They asked children to indicate whether or not two large letters, both lateralized to the same side, one capital and one in lower case, had the same name or not. Children showed a robust right-field superiority on this task, even in the earliest grades. Since most 1st-graders know the alphabet, this task may well provide a way of assessing left-hemisphere verbal functions with only a minimal contamination by reading skills. Even here, however, it would be wise to monitor eye movements carefully.

CONCLUSIONS

This review suggests that there is at least some fire in the smoke of reading ability and laterality. Although almost all possible results have been obtained at one time or another, the general pattern that appears is that poor readers are less lateralized for receptive language than are good readers. Although this may be true, compelling studies have not yet been done. The present chapter offers some guidelines as to how good experimentation might proceed in this area, and some tentative suggestions as to what it all might mean.

ACKNOWLEDGMENTS

Preparation of this chapter was aided in part by a Leave Fellowship from the Social Sciences and Humanities Research Council of Canada, and by a grant from the Natural Sciences and Engineering Research Council of Canada. I am indebted to Cheryl Gibson for her very insightful comments on an earlier draft of this chapter, and to Derek Besner, Valerie MacDonald, and John Obrzut for suggestions and encouragement.

REFERENCES

Abigail, E. R., & Johnson, E. G. (1976). Ear and hand dominance and their relationship with reading retardation. *Perceptual and Motor Skills, 43,* 1031–1036.

Ayers, A. J. (1977). Dichotic listening performance in learning-disabled children. *American Journal of Occupational Therapy, 31,* 441–446.

Aylward, E. H. (1984). Lateral asymmetry in subgroups of dyslexic children. *Brain and Language, 22,* 221–231.

Backman, J. E., Mamen, M., & Ferguson, H. B. (1984). Reading level design: Conceptual and methodological issues in reading research. *Psychological Bulletin, 96,* 560–568.

Bakker, D. J., Smink, T., & Reitsma, P. (1973). Ear dominance and reading ability. *Cortex, 9,* 301–312.

Beaumont, J. G., Young, A. W., & McManus, I. C. (1984). Hemisphericity: A critical review. *Cognitive Neuropsychology, 1,* 191–212.

Best, C. T. (Ed.). (1985). *Hemispheric function and collaboration in the child.* Orlando, FL: Academic Press.

Boder, E., & Jannico, S. (1982). *The Boder test of reading and spelling patterns: A diagnostic test for subtypes of reading disability.* New York: Grune and Stratton.

Bradshaw, J. L., & Nettleton, N. C. (1983). *Human cerebral asymmetry.* Englewood Cliffs, NJ: Prentice-Hall.

Bryden, M. P. (1970). Laterality effects in dichotic listening: Relations with handedness and reading ability in children. *Neuropsychologia, 8,* 443–450.

Bryden, M. P. (1978). Strategy effects in the assessment of hemispheric asymmetry. In G. Underwood (Ed.), *Strategies of information processing.* London: Academic Press.

Bryden, M. P. (1982a). The behavioral assessment of lateral asymmetry: Problems, pitfalls, and partial solutions. In R. N. Malatesha & L. C. Hartlage (Eds.), *Neuropsychology and cognition* (Vol. 2, pp. 44–54). The Hague: Martinus Nijhoff.

Bryden, M. P. (1982b). *Laterality.* New York: Academic Press.

Bryden, M. P. (1983). *Laterality: Studies of functional asymmetry in the intact brain.* Paper presented at the annual meeting of the Canadian Psychological Association, Winnipeg, Manitoba, June.

Bryden, M. P. (1986). Dichotic listening performance, cognitive ability, and cerebral organization. *Canadian Journal of Psychology, 40*(4), 445–456.

Bryden, M. P., Hecaen, H., & DeAgostini, M. (1983). Patterns of cerebral organization. *Brain and Language, 20,* 249–262.

Bryden, M. P., & Saxby, L. (1986). Developmental aspects of cerebral lateralization. In J. E. Obrzut & G. W. Hynd (Eds.), *Child Neuropsychology, Vol. 1: Theory and research* (pp. 73–94). Orlando, FL: Academic Press.

Bryden, M. P., & Sprott, D. A. (1981). Statistical determination of degree of laterality. *Neuropsychologia, 19,* 571–581.

Camp, B. W., & McCabe, L. (1977). *Denver reading and spelling test.* Unpublished manuscript, University of Colorado Medical Center.

Caplan, B., & Kinsbourne, M. (1982). Cognitive style and dichotic asymmetries of disabled children. *Cortex, 18,* 357–366.

Cermak, S. A., Drake, C., Cermak, L. S., & Kenney, R. (1978). The effects of concurrent manual activity on the dichotic listening performance of boys with learning disabilities. *American Journal of Occupational Therapy, 32,* 493–499.

Corballis, M. C. (1983). *Human Laterality.* New York: Academic Press.

Dalby, J. T., & Gibson, D. (1981). Functional cerebral lateralization in subtypes of disabled readers. *Brain and Language, 14,* 34–48.

Davidoff, J., Beaton, A. A., Done, D. J., & Booth, H. (1982). Information extraction from brief verbal displays: Half-field and serial position effects for children, normal and illiterate adults. *British Journal of Psychology, 73,* 29–39.

Dermody, P., Mackie, K., & Katsch, R. (1983). Dichotic listening in good and poor readers. *Journal of Speech and Hearing Research, 26,* 341–348.

Doehring, D. G., Trites, R. L., Patel, P. G., & Fiedorowicz, C. A. M. (1981). *Reading disabilities: The interaction of reading, language, and neuropsychological deficits.* New York: Academic Press.

Efron, R., Koss, B., & Yund, E. W. (1983). Central auditory processing: IV. Ear dominance—Spatial and temporal complexity. *Brain and Language, 19,* 264–282.

Ellis, A. W. (1985). The cognitive neuropsychology of developmental (and acquired) dyslexia: A critical survey. *Cognitive Neuropsychology, 2,* 169–205.

Fennell, E., Satz, P., & Morris, R. (1983). The development of handedness and dichotic ear listening asymmetries in relation to school achievement: A longitudinal study. *Journal of Experimental Child Psychology, 35,* 248–262.

Finucci, J. M., & Childs, B. (1981). Are there really more dyslexic boys than girls? In A. Ansara, N. Geschwind, A. Galaburda, M. Albert, & N. Gartrell (Eds.), *Sex differences in dyslexia* (pp. 1–10). Towson, MD: The Orton Dyslexia Society.

Garren, R. B. (1980). Hemispheric laterality differences among four levels of reading achievement. *Perceptual and Motor Skills, 50,* 119–123.

Geschwind, N., & Behan, P. (1982). Left-handedness: Association with immune disease, migraine, and developmental learning disorder. *Proceedings of the National Academy of Sciences (USA), 79,* 5097–5100.

Gladstone, M., & Best, C. T. (1985). Developmental dyslexia: The potential role of interhemispheric collaboration in reading acquisition. In C. T. Best (Ed.), *Hemispheric function and collaboration in the child* (pp. 87–118). Orlando, FL: Academic Press.

Gregory, A. H., Efron, R., Divenyi, P. L., & Yund, E. W. (1983). Central auditory processing: I. Ear dominance—A perceptual or attentional asymmetry? *Brain and Language, 19,* 225–236.

Gross, K., Rothenberg, S., & Schottenfeld, S. (1978). Duration thresholds for letter identification in left and right visual fields for normal and reading disabled children. *Neuropsychologia, 16,* 709–715.

Harris, L. J. (1985). Teaching the right brain: Historical perspective on a contemporary educational fad. In C. T. Best (Ed.), *Hemispheric function and collaboration in the child* (pp. 231–274). Orlando, FL: Academic Press.

Hiscock, M. (1985). Lateral eye movements and dual-task performance. In H. J. Hannay (Ed.), *Experimental techniques in human neuropsychology* (pp. 264–308). New York: Oxford University Press.

Hiscock, M., & Kinsbourne, M. (1982). Laterality and dyslexia: A critical review. *Annals of dyslexia, 32,* 177–226.

Hochberg, J. (1970). Attention in perception and reading. In F. A. Young & D. B. Lindsley (Eds.), *Early experience and visual information processing in perceptual and reading disorders* (pp. 219–230). Washington, DC: National Academy of Sciences.

Hynd, G. W., & Obrzut, J. E. (1981). Development of reciprocal hemisphere inhibition in normal and learning-disabled children. *Journal of General Psychology, 104,* 203–212.

Hynd, G. W., Obrzut, J. E., & Obrzut, A. (1981). Are lateral and perceptual asymmetries related to WISC-R and achievement test performance in normal and learning-disabled children? *Journal of Consulting and Clinical Psychology, 49,* 977–979.

Hynd, G. W., Obrzut, J. E., Weed, W., & Hynd, C. R. (1979). Development of cerebral dominance: Dichotic listening asymmetry in normal and learning-disabled readers. *Journal of Experimental Child Psychology, 28,* 445–454.

Kershner, J. R. (1977). Cerebral dominance in disabled readers, good readers, and gifted children: Search for a valid model. *Child Development, 48,* 61–67.

Kershner, J. R. (1985). Ontogeny of hemispheric specialization and relationship of developmental patterns to complex reasoning skills and academic achievement. In C. T. Best (Ed.), *Interhemispheric function and collaboration in the child* (pp. 327–360). Orlando FL: Academic Press.

Kimura, D. (1961). Cerebral dominance and the perception of verbal stimuli. *Canadian Journal of Psychology, 15,* 166–171.

Kimura, D. (1963). Speech lateralization in young children as determined by an auditory test. *Journal of Comparative and Physiological Psychology, 56,* 899–902.

Koomar, J. A., & Cermak, S. A. (1981). Reliability of dichotic listening using two stimulus formats with normal and learning-disabled children. *American Journal of Occupational Therapy, 35,* 456–463.

Lenneberg, E. (1967). *Biological foundations of language.* New York: Wiley.

Leong, C. K. (1976). Lateralization in severely disabled readers in relation to functional cerebral development and synthesis of information. In R. M. Knights & D. J. Bakker (Eds.), *The neuropsychology of learning disorders* (pp. 221–232). Baltimore, MD: University Park Press.

Lewitter, F. I., De Fries, J. C., & Elston, R. C. (1980). Genetic models of reading disability. *Behavior Genetics, 10,* 9–30.

Ley, R. G., & Kaushansky, M. (1985). The 4Rs: Readin', 'riting, 'rithmetic, and the right hemisphere. In A. A. Sheikh (Ed.), *Imagery and the education process.* Farmingdale, NY: Baywood.

Liberman, A. M., & Mattingly, I. G. (1985). The motor theory of speech perception revised. *Cognition, 21,* 1–36.

Marcel, A. J., & Rajan, P. (1975). Lateral specialization for recognition of words and faces in good and poor readers. *Neuropsychologia, 13,* 489–498.

Marcel, T., Katz, L., & Smith, M. (1974). Laterality and reading proficiency. *Neuropsychologia, 12,* 131–139.

Marshall, J. C., Caplan, D., & Holmes, J. M. (1975). The measure of laterality. *Neuropsychologia, 13,* 315–322.

McKeever, W. F., & Huling, M. D. (1970). Lateral dominance in tachistoscopic words recognitions of children at two levels of ability. *Quarterly Journal of Experimental Psychology, 22,* 600–604.

McKeever, W. F., & VanDeventer, A. D. (1975). Dyslexic adolescents: Evidence of impaired visual and auditory language processing with normal lateralization and visual responsibility. *Cortex, 11,* 361–378.

Mercure, R., & Warren, S. A. (1978). Inadequate and adequate readers' performance on a dichotic listening task. *Perceptual and Motor Skills, 46,* 709–710.

Merola, J. L., & Liederman, J. (1985). Developmental changes in hemispheric independence. *Child Development, 56,* 1184–1194.

Mitterer, J. O. (1982). There are at least two kinds of poor readers: Whole-word poor readers and recooding poor readers. *Canadian Journal of Psychology, 36,* 445–461.

Naylor, H. (1980). Reading disability and lateral asymmetry: An information processing analysis. *Psychological Bulletin, 87,* 531–545.

Newcombe, F., & Marshall, J. C. (1981). On psycholinguistic classifications of the acquired dyslexias. *Bulletin of the Orton Society, 31,* 29–46.

Obrzut, J. E., Boliek, C. A., & Bryden, M. P. (1987). *Dichotic listening with right-handed, left-handed, bilingual, and learning-disabled children.* Paper submitted to the International Neuropsychological Society meetings, Washington, DC, February.

Obrzut, J. E., Hynd, G. W., Obrzut, A., & Leitgeb, J. L. (1980). Time sharing and dichotic listening asymmetry in normal and learning-disabled children. *Brain and Language, 11,* 181–194.

Obrzut, J. E., Hynd, G. W., Obrzut, A., & Pirozzolo, F. J. (1981). Effect of directed attention on cerebral asymmetries in normal and learning-disabled children. *Developmental Psychology, 17,* 118–125.

Obrzut, J. E., Hynd, G. W., & Zellner, R. D. (1983). Attentional deficit in learning-disabled children: Evidence from visual half-field studies. *Brain and Cognition, 2,* 89–101.

Obrzut, J. E., Obrzut, A., Bryden, M. P., & Bartels, S. G. (1985). Information processing and speech lateralization in learning-disabled children. *Brain and Language, 25,* 87–101.

Olson, M. E. (1973). Laterality differences in tachistoscopic word recognition in normal and delayed readers in elementary school. *Neuropsychologia, 11,* 343–350.

Orr, C., Mitterer, J., & Bryden, M. P. Paper in preparation. Brock University, St. Catharine's, Ontario, Canada.

Pettit, J. M., & Helms, S. B. (1979). Hemispheric dominance in language disorders. *Journal of Learning Disabilities, 12,* 12–17.

Piazza, D. M. (1980). The influence of sex and handedness in the hemispheric specialization of verbal and nonverbal tasks. *Neuropsychologia, 18,* 163–176.

Pirozzolo, F. J. (1985). Neuropsychological and neuroelectric correlates of developmental reading disability. In C. T. Best (Ed.), *Hemispheric function and collaboration in the child* (pp. 309–326). Orlando, FL: Academic Press.

Pirozzolo, F. J., & Rayner, K. (1979). Cerebral organization and reading disability. *Neuropsychologia, 17,* 485–491.

Prior, M. R., Frolley, M., & Sanson, A. (1983). Language lateralization in specific reading retarded children and in backward readers. *Cortex, 19,* 149–163.

Repp, B. H. (1977). Measuring laterality effects in dichotic listening. *Journal of the Acoustical Society of America, 62,* 720–737.

Richardson, J. T. E., & Firlej, M. D. E. (1979). Laterality and reading attainment. *Cortex, 15,* 581–595.

Rosenblum, D. R., & Dorman, M. F. (1978). Hemispheric specialization for speech perception in language deficient kindergarten children. *Brain and Language, 6,* 378–389.

Rozin, P., Poritsky, S., & Sotsky, R. (1971). American children with reading problems can easily learn to read English represented by Chinese characters. *Science, 171,* 164–167.

Rudel, R. G. (1985). Hemispheric asymmetry and learning disabilities: Left, right, or in-between? In C. T. Best (Ed.), *Hemispheric function and collaboration in the child* (pp. 275–308). Orlando, FL: Academic Press.

Rutter, M. (1978). Prevalence and types of dyslexia. In A. L. Benton & D. P. Pearl (Eds.), *Dyslexia: An appraisal of current knowledge* (pp. 3–28). New York: Oxford University Press.

Sadick, T. L., & Ginsburg, B. E. (1978). The development of the lateral functions and reading ability. *Cortex, 14,* 3–11.

Satz, P., Morris, R. (1981). Learning disability subtypes: A review. In F. J. Pirozzolo & M. C. Wittrock (Eds.), *Neuropsychological and cognitive processes in reading* (pp. 109–141). New York: Academic Press.

Satz, P., Rardin, D., & Ross, J. (1971). An evaluation of a theory of specific developmental dyslexia. *Child Development, 42,* 2009–2021.

Satz, P., & Van Nostrand, G. K. (1973). Developmental dyslexia: An evaluation of a theory. In P. Satz & J. Ross (Eds.), *The disabled learner: Early detection and intervention* (pp. 121–148). Rotterdam: Rotterdam University Press.

Saxby, L., & Bryden, M. P. (1985). Left visual-field advantage in children for processing visual emotional stimuli. *Developmental Psychology, 21,* 253–261.

Segalowitz, S. J., & Bryden, M. P. (1983). Individual differences in hemispheric representation of language. In S. J. Segalowitz (Ed.), *Language functions and brain organization* (pp. 341–372). New York: Academic Press.

Sparrow, S. S., & Satz, P. (1970). Dyslexia, laterality, and neuropsychological development. In D. J. Bakker & P. Satz (Eds.), *Specific reading disability: Advances in theory and method* (pp. 41–60). Rotterdam: Rotterdam University Press.

Springer, S. P., & Eisenson, J. (1977). Hemispheric specialization for speech in language-disordered children. *Neuropsychologia, 15,* 287–293.

Sommers, R. K., & Taylor, M. L. (1972). Cerebral speech dominance in language-disordered and normal children. *Cortex, 8,* 224–232.

Studdert-Kennedy, M., & Shankweiler, D. (1970). Hemispheric specialization for speech perception. *Journal of the Acoustical Society of America, 48,* 579–594.

Swanson, H. L., & Mullen, R. C. (1983). Hemispheric specialization in learning disabled readers' recall as a function of age and level of processing. *Journal of Experimental Child Psychology, 35,* 457–477.

Tallal, P., Stark, R. E., & Mellits, E. D. (1985). Identification of language-impaired children on the basis of rapid perception and production skills. *Brain and Language, 25,* 314–322.

Thomson, M. E. (1976). A comparison of laterality effects in dyslexics and controls using verbal dichotic listening tasks. *Neuropsychologia, 14,* 243–246.

Vellutino, F. R., Gentley, W. L., & Phillips, F. (1978). Inter- versus intra-hemispheric learning in dyslexic and normal readers. *Developmental Medicine and Child Neurology, 20,* 71–80.

Watson, E. S., & Engle, R. W. (1982). Is it lateralization, processing strategies, or both that distinguishes good and poor readers? *Journal of Experimental Child Psychology, 34,* 1–19.

Wellman, M. M., & Allen, M. (1983). Variations in hand position, cerebral lateralization, and reading ability among right-handed children. *Brain and Language, 18,* 277–292.

Williams, H. G., Keough, V. A., Fisher, J. M., Seymour, C. J., & Tanner, M. G. (1980). Hemispheric specialization in normally and slowly developing children: A tachistoscopic and dichhaptic evaluation. *Perceptual and Motor Skills, 51,* 1187–1201.

Witelson, S. F. (1977). Developmental dyslexia: Two right hemispheres and none left. *Science, 195,* 309–311.

Witelson, S. F., & Rabinovitch, M. S. (1972). Hemispheric speech lateralization in children with auditory-linguistic deficits. *Cortex, 8,* 412–426.

Yeni-Komshian, G. H., Isenberg, D., & Goldberg, H. (1975). Cerebral dominance and reading disability: Left visual field deficit in poor readers. *Neuropsychologia, 13,* 83–94.

Young, A. W., & Ellis, A. W. (1981). Asymmetry of cerebral hemisphere function in normal and poor readers. *Psychological Bulletin, 89,* 183–190.

Zurif, E. B., & Carson, G. (1970). Dyslexia in relation to cerebral dominance and temporal analysis. *Neuropsychologia, 8,* 351–361.

19

Dual Processing Models of Learning Disability

JOHN R. KERSHNER
University of Toronto

The recent development of comprehensive models of interhemispheric information processing provides a new, albeit largely unrecognized, view into the possible neuropsychological basis of learning and reading (dyslexia) disability. Although the problematic relationship between laterality and learning disability is enriched, perhaps even unusually so, with competing theoretical notions (Hiscock & Kinsbourne, 1982), for the most part this field of research fails to address putative *brain mechanisms* that may subserve *interhemispheric processes*. Indeed, such an omission may be a serious shortcoming, especially in the face of empirical data suggesting a major role for interhemispheric processes in the etiology of developmental learning impairment (Badian & Wolff, 1977; Kershner, 1985; Kliepera, Wolff, & Drake, 1981; Wolff, Cohen, & Drake, 1984). The application of dual processing models to learning disability constitutes a novel and fundamentally different theoretical departure from mainstream laterality research with the learning disabled; consequently, only a few experimental studies from this persuasion have been reported (Kershner, Henninger, & Cooke, 1984; Swanson, 1986, 1987; Swanson & Mullen, 1983; Swanson & Obrzut, 1985).

My own interest in working with these models in an attempt to further our understanding of learning disabilities stems from three factors. Foremost among these motivating influences is a discontent with the almost exclusive devotion of laterality research to the theoretical question of whether or not learning-disabled children have adequate left cerebral lateralization for receptive linguistic processes (Orton, 1937). An important issue in its own right, the still unresolved, incomplete lateralization hypothesis and other closely related themes (Aaron, 1982; Bakker, 1979; Kershner, 1977; Witelson, 1977) have had an invigorating but, unfortunately, a narrowing influence on our conceptualizations of learning disability. Aside from high probability (Kershner, 1985) that there may be no difference between learning-disabled children and normal children in the way that lateralized processes are distributed structurally between hemispheres (see Obrzut, Obrzut, Bryden, & Bartels, 1985, for an opposing view), even if such a difference could be demonstrated reliably, it would do no more than beg the question (Naylor, 1980; Young & Ellis, 1981). In other words, confirmation in learning-disabled children of graded differences in the organization (structural lateralization) of cerebral functions would reveal nothing about how perceptual information is encoded, how much and what type of information can be activated from memory, or the efficiency of processing information relative to changing demands on capacity. Dual-processing models, on the other hand, are formulated to address the clear need for more formal, rule-based, and computational accounts, irrespective of where language processing is located, of the theoretical brain mechanisms that may subserve learning (Allen, 1983) and learning failure (Kershner, 1983). Stated simply, these models assume that lateralization is cognitive process.

My second reason for undertaking the present analysis is the unimpressive impact that our knowledge (or lack of knowledge) of lateralization has had on education for the learning disabled. This is not to say that neuropsychological thought, more generally speaking, has not been integrated successfully into educational practice (Evans, 1982; Hynd & Cohen, 1983; Rourke, Bakker, Fisk, & Strang, 1983) or even that promising developments are not occurring in the application of imaginative ideas about lateralization to instructional and theoretical issues. For instance, Rourke's (1982) bold attempt to forge a conceptual synthesis between left–right brain functions and Piagetian developmental stages stand out, and certainly the educational effects of direct hemispheric stimulation in dyslexic children reported by Bakker and Vinke (1985) are encouraging. Nevertheless, the evaluation literature as a whole on neuropsychologically based remedial programs shows invariably that these programs have not proved to be effective (Cummings, 1985; Kershner, Cummings, Clarke, Hadfield, & Kershner, 1986; Zarske, 1982). One of the long-standing problems with neuropsychologically inspired approaches to remediation is that they are indirect, focusing on processes that are claimed both to be lateralized and to be prerequisites of efficient learning. This orientation produces two negative consequences. As a precondition to educational instruction it becomes essential to know what processes and tasks are lateralized and where, and, second, considerable time is invested in unusual training activities and therapeutic practices requiring valuable time away from proven methods of direct instruction (Kershner *et al.*, 1986). In comparison, the dual-processing models discussed here not only are task-centered but also hold that, although the hemispheres differ in processing efficiency, most if not all tasks can be performed by either cerebral hemisphere. They are founded on formalizable principles of learning that can be applied to any task that requires information-processing skill. Thus, the dual-processing models to be discussed are unlike other neuropsychological approaches to remediation in that they have a potential for easy integration with orthodox forms of direct academic teaching. Finally, the overriding objective of these models is to explain how the cerebral hemispheres act together efficiently as a unit in performing multiple cognitive processes concurrently; these models assume that time-sharing demands on cognitive resources are the rule, not the exception. Such an orientation fits well with my working hypothesis that the coordination of interhemispheric functions may be a key neuropsychological dimension in the etiology of learning disabilities.

To summarize, dual-processing models of lateralization do not have as their primary focus such mainstream questions as: (1) what is lateralized, (2) how processes and tasks become lateralized or dyslateralized, or (3) whether or not the degree to which a hemisphere is specialized functionally has an important influence on human behavior. Rather, such a dual-processing perspective addresses the complex set of issue involved in conceptualizing how the hemispheres may work together, collaborate, and integrate their processes, and, in particular, how concurrently performed tasks and concurrently performed components of single tasks are carried out both within and between hemispheres.

THE MODELS

The two dual-processing models that I will discuss in this chapter have received the most formal development out of the field of possibilities and, consequently, are the subject of much current discussion and debate in cognitive neuroscience. One of these models is the *cerebral functional distance model* developed by Kinsbourne and his colleagues (Kinsbourne, 1981; Kinsbourne & Hicks, 1978; Kinsbourne & Hiscock, 1983), which is an outgrowth, refinement, and elaboration of Kinsbourne's selective activation theory of hemispheric processing (Kinsbourne, 1970, 1973, 1975). "Selective activation" is now subsumed as a limiting example of the more comprehensive functional distance model. This model, which I will refer to as the *neurological model* (NM), has a distinctive neurophysiological commitment. The second dual-processing model that is the topic of this chapter is the dual resource model advanced by Friedman and Polson and colleagues (Friedman & Polson, 1981; Friedman, Polson, Dafoe, & Gaskill, 1982; Herdman & Friedman, 1985). Friedman and Polson's conceptual framework was influenced considerably by Hellige and his co-workers (Hellige & Cox, 1976; Hellige, Cox, & Litvac, 1979; Hellige & Wong, 1983) and by Navon and Gopher's (1979) dissatisfaction with single-capacity models of divided attention and their subsequent argument for a multiple resources approach. The Friedman and Polson model owes a strong allegiance to cognitive psychology; I will refer to it as the *resource model* (RM).

The NM is based on a metaphor of the brain as a social network of specialized subprocessors where two or more tasks compete for interference-free operating space. The proximal origin of task interference is overcrowding or an absence of inhibitory barriers among subprocessors. However, birth and population control are not urban planning issues; it is not necessarily better to reside in Yellowknife than in Hong Kong. Overcrowding occurs when perceptual information, conceptual knowledge, or motor programs are poorly differentiated psychologically, which in brain space produces performance-expensive squabbling or interfering cross talk among subprocessors. Subprocessors become antagonistic neighbors with a potential for conflict as a combined function of their communication distance from one another in conceptual space and their actual topological locations in the brain. Geography, however, is secondary in importance to the excitatory and inhibitory spread of neuronal activation that occurs among subprocessors that are unprotected by inhibitory barriers. In the NM, therefore, the primary source of poor learning performance is *structural* interference between subprocessors in brain space as a result of inadequate conceptual differentiation among tasks. Finally, this community of subprocessors possesses three enduring political arrangements: (1) select subprocessors on the left are better equipped for linguistic processing; (2) the lateral gradient of attention is controlled by rightward- and leftward-orienting centers located in the left and right hemispheres, respectively; and (3) there is a natural rightward bias that facilitates information transfer between hemispheres from left to right.

The RM is based on a microeconomic metaphor. The brain is conceptualized as a two-vaulted repository of differently valued currencies that are paid out to tasks in a competitive marketplace where financial resources are in short supply. Each hemisphere is a separate resource pool with its own investment policy; each contains the same amount of potential currency for payout; no interbank loans are permitted; and, being undifferentiated, each cerebral hemisphere's resources are available for the universe of possible expenditures. The proximal cause of task interference is a bankruptcy in resource supplies. Bankruptcy occurs when there is a depletion in the supply of resources, brought about usually by tasks that overlap in resource demand. In the RM, therefore, the primary source of poor learning performance is *capacity* interference produced by difficult tasks imbued with a constellation of resource demands that exceed supply. Finally, in agreement with the NM but couched in economic terms, the RM assumes that verbal tasks are cheaper (requiring fewer resources) when performed primarily by the left hemisphere.

Each model suggests a very different metaphor, with markedly different operating principles, of how the brain works to achieve efficient levels of cognitive performance, and therefore each model has quite different implications for what may be the neuropsychological underpinnings of a learning disability. It is interesting, however, that although the NM and RM are undeniably incompatible on numerous theoretical claims, consideration of the major issues of contention between them serves to point up a limited number of pivotal neuropsychological issues that suggest, in turn, some fairly specific information-processing anomalies that may produce a learning disorder. On some issues, the two models converge in implicating a similar hypothetical brain dysfunction that may produce a learning disability; but they differ in their levels of analysis and terminology. On other issues, the models diverge to the extent that each advances a diametrically opposed view about what is, and what is not, an efficient pattern of neuronal organization.

In this chapter, I will attempt to show how a dialectical analysis of these models can be useful heuristically in arriving at novel and sophisticated conceptualizations of learning disabilities. My plan in the main text is to: (1) introduce the models in greater detail by describing four major issues of disagreement between them; (2) use these issues to generate hypothetical processing constraints that may be related to learning disabilities; (3) point out serious difficulties that one may encounter in attempts to test the models (retrospective data are notorious for their consistency with both models' explanatory frames of reference) but, nonetheless, propose potential ways in which the models might be tested; and (4) draw some tentative conclusions about the neuropsychology of learning disabilities based on an integration of my analysis with current research.

MAJOR ISSUES ON WHICH THE MODELS DISAGREE, AND LEARNING DISABILITY HYPOTHESES

On each of these issues I have taken the strategic approach that a learning disability may result if the brain actually works in close proximity to the claims of either model.

First Issue

1. Is the brain unified, in which case the hemispheres share resources, or are the hemispheres independent? My interpretation of the term "resource" in this context is that it refers to an energy substance not unlike neurophysiological arousal and that it is shared or not shared between hemispheres prior to and during the active engagement of processing.

The NM focuses on patterns of neuronal excitatory and inhibitory activation, permitting as much interchange in processing resources between as within hemispheres. Thus, a general implication is that a brain with hemispheres, either (1) not unified or (2) unified but not according to plan, may produce a learning disability.

The RM focuses on within-hemisphere competition for limited processing resources. The two hemispheres are claimed to constitute a dual-capacity system, with each hemisphere operating its own mechanisms, processes, and strategies independently, fueled by its own qualitatively different, nonsubstitutable, and limited resource supply. Although the mental productions that occur subsequent to initial encoding and elaborative processing can be shared, the hemispheres cannot share the raw processing energy that fires cognition. The hemispheres cannot share resources. Thus, a general implication is that a unified brain is abnormal and may produce a learning disability.

This issue presents us with two categories of hypotheses. The first is that learning disability may have something to do with the actual bridging structures that serve directly in interhemispheric processing. More specifically, the NM suggests that learning-disabled individuals may suffer from too much seepage between hemispheres in terms of spreading cortical arousal. If each hemisphere, by way of interhemispheric commissures, has the preprocessing arousal potential to innervate processes and to draw on processing energy in the other hemisphere, such preprocessing, interhemispheric coupling may be aberrant. For example, an atypical spread of activation between hemispheres in preparation for left-hemisphere, phonological processing would induce either excessive exitation or excessive inhibition of the right hemisphere. Excessive right-hemisphere excitation would (1) produce a poorly lateralized verbal response (notably, even though linguistic subprocessors may be represented asymmetrically in the left hemisphere) and (2) increase the risk for interfering cross talk emanating from an abnormally overactive right hemisphere. Abnormal inhibition of the right hemisphere during verbal processing would produce an asymmetrical response favoring the left hemisphere, but at the expense of any appreciable enhancement in absolute levels of left-hemisphere arousal due to the diffuse spread of activation. Indeed, the abnormally underaroused phonological subprocessors in the left hemisphere would be at increased risk for interference from cross talk, emanating in this case mostly from nonphonological subprocessors within the same hemisphere. Consequently, verbal tasks probably would show poorly lateralized performance as a result of an atypical spread of activation between hemispheres, irrespective of whether this was accompanied by excessive excitation or excessive inhibition of the right hemisphere.

Consideration of the RM on this point also suggests that a learning disability might be caused in two ways. If abnormal borrowing of resources takes place between hemispheres, then intrahemispheric processes may call up erroneously an atypical admixture of qualitatively diverse resources. Such a mixup would result in either (1) the use of the wrong (less efficient) resources for one or more task components or (2) the use of the correct resources but in the wrong proportions. In either occurrence, a predistribution mixup in the packaging and labeling of resources, even when coupled with a highly accurate schedule of paying out units of hemispheric resources to tasks, might overextend the capacity limits of one or both hemispheres before an efficient level of task performance could be reached. For example, if the optimal resource composition for the phonological component of a verbal task was estimated to be in the neighborhood of a 9:1, left–right ratio, then erroneously processing the phonological aspect of the task with all right-hemisphere resources (ratio of 0:10) or even with resources in an 8:2, left–right ratio would theoretically increase the likelihood of a verbal learning impairment due to inefficient phonological processing. Furthermore, the end effect of such excessive interhemispheric resource sharing on lateralized processing would coincide with the NM's expectations. Because higher yield, left-hemisphere processing would have the most to lose through packaging errors (even when followed by an accurate resource segregation and distribution plan) the most likely outcome of any deviation from a verbal task's optimal resource ratio would be a decrement in the degree of left-hemisphere superiority (lateralization).

Here, although each model uses very different explanatory constructs, each model suggests the same generic problem—too much preprocessing communication between hemispheres. The NM portrays this resource-sharing problem as one involving ungated neuronal cross talk between subprocessors or poorly controlled inhibitory innervation, whereas the RM does not permit an unambiguous neurological referent for a "leaky-resource" problem. In the RM, "resource sharing" is not defined operationally beyond its abstract theoretical connotations. The NM stresses the principal importance of structural interference and disallows capacity interference. RM processing is all about capacity interference, without specifying a role for structural interference. Nevertheless, the two models, taken together, point up the possibility for a categorically similar interhemispheric problem in sharing resources excessively.

In addition to the convergent likelihood for too much neuronal or resource collaboration between hemispheres, only the NM suggests that processing difficulties may be caused by too little hemispheric sharing of resources. Such a possibility is directly contradictory to the RM's characterization of the normally functioning hemispheres as uncharitable in resource sharing, even in their healthiest condition. Hence, this major point of contention between models—whether the hemispheres do or do not share resources—also suggests another brain dysfunction that may be of etiological significance to learning disabilities. Unlike the first hypothesis, however, this possibility draws on the incompatibility of the models on this issue. On the one hand, the RM maintains that interhemispheric fibers should perform primarily an insular function so that the hemispheres can act as independent processors; on the other hand, the NM suggests that if the brain is not unified sufficiently to facilitate easily the potential for preprocessing arousal exchange between hemispheres, then a learning disability may be the consequence. As an example, the core mechanism for attentional control in the NM resides in a finely tuned reciprocal balance between homologously linked subprocessors in each hemisphere, with excitatory activation in one hemisphere precipitating inhibitory impulses to the other hemisphere. In the absence of what amounts to left-hemisphere modulation over the right hemisphere when preparing for a verbal processing task, the right hemisphere would become an unconstrained source of potentially interfering intrahemispheric cross talk, upsetting the efficiency of its contribution to processing and lowering the ability to attend selectively to critical task dimensions. Again, the net effect on laterality would be consistent with the other possible processing difficulties that have been generated by a discussion of this first issue: As the liberated right hemisphere assumed a greater scope for unfettered processing, we could expect a decrement once again in left-hemisphere advantage, and a corresponding decrement in an overall processing efficiency.

The second category of hypotheses that can be generated by the first issue is related to questions of metacognitive control or the executive decisions (effortful and automatic) regulating and integrating the bihemispheric allocation of processing. Both models suggest that a less than ideal match between tasks and the brain processes that are committed to tasks can cause a learning problem; and, like the first set of hypotheses, each model implicates entirely different conceptual machinery.

According to the NM, in the unified brain, a single operator allocates processing to tasks from a single pool of resources on the basis of a complex interplay of structural and experiential factors. Learning disabilities could result feasibly from any number of management failures, ranging from the deployment of processes from the wrong hemisphere to the deployment of an inappropriate intrahemispheric strategy or even to the assignment of processes to irrelevant task features.

In contrast to NM's relatively simplified corporate structure, the RM's creation of two independent processing facilities in a semidivided brain, which shares products but not energy, necessitates the problematic operation of a twin executive and hierarchically ordered management. Qualitatively, the management responsibilities are much the same in both models, but in the RM the clerical workload doubles because resources are allocated to tasks independently by each hemisphere's manager. Additionally, because each hemisphere's products can be made available immediately to the other hemisphere, each manager has self-governing responsibilities over intrahemispheric allocation of raw materials and over the interhemispheric allocation of completed productions. Consequently, the risk of learning failure due to a misallocation of resources to processes or tasks is at least twofold in the RM, and the novel possibility is raised of a misallocation in sharing hemispheric products. Moreover, it would be an unnecessary semantic burden in the NM to make a distinction between effortful, resource-consuming processes and automatic, cost-free processes because both are operationalized in terms of the relative presence or absence of interfering cross talk and the potential need for an inhibitory barrier between subprocessors. Quite simply, automatic tasks are tasks that are 100% protected from cross talk.

The situation is quite different in the RM, where financial solvency is indexed by the volume of available capacity. Three kinds of tasks have been specified according to whether processing them can be controlled strategically and whether they are resource-expensive: (1) controlled, resource-expensive tasks; (2) automatic, resource-free tasks; and (3) mandatory, automatic, but resource-expensive tasks. The latter category is reserved for stimuli like written language, which has been shown to induce obligatory processing that also consumes resources. Learning disabilities might be caused by the misidentification of the category of a task or one of its components. Indeed, the potential for metacognitive mismanagement is greater in the RM as a consequence of its complex technical regulations and managerial hierarchy.

Second Issue

2. Can there be asymmetrical activation or is activation symmetrical?

The NM claims that one hemisphere can be aroused and activated selectively by subject and task parameters. Indeed, *the* foundational diachronic (developmental time) basis of hemispheric differences in function in the NM is an asymmetrical imbalance in patterns of neuronal activation. Thus, it is implied generally, quite independently of the functioning of interhemispheric commissures in resource sharing, that a learning disability may be produced by either (1) processing activation that is lateralized disproportionately or (2) processing activation that is perfectly symmetrical.

The RM claims that any increase in arousal or in processing activation in the normal brain is always symmetrical. The hemispheres cannot increment activity asymmetrically. Thus, a general implication is that asymmetrical activation is abnormal and may produce a learning disability.

It is important to mention that considerable physiological evidence has demonstrated that there can be differential arousal and activation patterns in hemispheric processing (Levy, 1983; Segalowitz & Gruber, 1977). However, because we are mixing metaphors in the present analysis, such data do not constitute unequivocal grounds for rejecting the RM claim against asymmetrical activation. It may be that activation will require a somewhat different operational definition in the two models or that the claim may have to be reduced to a weaker version that excludes restraints on activation but retains processing constraints on asymmetrical resource availability (with a potential for arousal and activation). However this turns out, it is still true that both the NM and RM suggest that abnormal asymmetries in hemispheric activation may cause learning problems. This issue presents the hypothetical notion that atypical arousal–activation during task engagement may be just as important as abnormal resources sharing in delineating the breadth of potential interhemispheric processing impairments. Such processing and postprocessing neuronal or cognitive activity implicates the combined functions of corticolimbic–brain stem activation pathways and the corpus callosum. However, both the NM and the RM imply much more intriguing possibilities than a mere state of underarousal or overarousal in learning disabilities. Both the NM and the RM concur in suggesting that learning disabilities may be correlated with a wide range of atypical hemispheric patterns of arousal–activation involving the relative overengagement or underengagement of one or the other hemisphere during task performance. Even though the NM permits asymmetrical activation and the RM does not, both models suggest that excessive lateralization may be undesirable and that performance on some tasks might suffer if the two hemispheres do not respond mutually in demanding learning situations, activating processes in both hemispheres.

In the NM, exaggerated unilateral processing would set off an atypical proliferation of intrahemispheric cross talk generated by the superengaged subprocessor(s) relative to the weakened strength of neighboring inhibitory barriers. As an illustration, overengagement of left-hemisphere phonological processing (pre or postlexical) would radiate potentially disruptive neuronal impulses into brain space that may be needed for orthographic or semantic processing or even for attentional or perceptual–motor processing demands. Of course, processing activity in the right hemisphere would also be curtailed abnormally.

In the RM, overall processing capacity would be effected negatively in direct proportion either to the degree to which resources were halved and made available only asymmetrically, or to the degree of half-brain engagement rather than whole-brain processing. Thus, although the RM takes an ultrastrong position on this issue, both models point to learning problems that may be related to an excessive reliance on the specialized processes of one hemisphere.

Conflict between models on this issue occurs because the NM implies, also, that it might be maladaptive in some situations should the hemispheres become yoked perfectly in activating together. Paired activation cannot be a problem in the RM. The RM in its present form allows only for asymmetries in performance output as equal amounts of resources from equally aroused and equally activated hemispheres are allocated to tasks. In the normally functioning brain of the RM there can be no asymmetries in processing activation per se. In contrast, according to the NM a learning problem might occur in situations that require unihemispheric processing if processing activity initiated in one hemisphere failed to reach a critical threshold, resulting in a nearly equal distribution of neuronal activity in the normally nonengaged hemisphere. I shall not elaborate on this possibility of dysfunction, however, because only a fine line distinguishes this "spread of activation" problem from the resource-sharing problem that was discussed earlier.

Thus, the question of the degree to which the hemispheres assume a more equal processing load during task engagement suggests a number of etiological mechanisms that may induce learning failure. Moreover, Tucker and Williamson (1984) have presented a multiple-factor hemispheric model of arousal–activation based on the attention control theory of Pribram and McGuinness (1975). Tucker and Williamson proposed that the right hemisphere functions primarily to augment the brain's phasic response to perceptual novelty, serving to increase information change and to reduce encoding redundancy. Operating in tandem, the left hemisphere is dedicated to the regulation of tonic activation processes, helping to decrease the rate of information change and to increase behavioral redundancy. Even though they do not specify if or where asymmetries in activation may happen, their formulation stresses the complementary but different functions of the two hemispheres, suggesting that any excessive imbalance in activity would be maladaptive. If Tucker and Williamson's formulation is correct in even its broad theoretical outlines—and they have synthesized an impressive wealth of evidence in its favor—then the arousal–activation dysfunctions suggested by the NM and the RM can be perceived within a rich, new field of interpretive implications.

Third Issue

3. Are hemispheric resources differentiated?

The NM says that brain space is a highly particularized network of task-dedicated processing resources. The guiding principles modulating energy flow are keyed to cross talk among topologically and conceptually linked subprocessors, and these principles are the same whether applied within hemispheres or between hemispheres.

The RM says that intrahemispheric resources are of one indistinguishable kind and that intrahemispheric resources are entirely substitutable among tasks and task components.

In effect, the NM implies that there are modular constraints that may limit subprocessor access to resources. Task interference, however, can come about only via structural interference from conflict among specific subprocessing units. Alternatively, the RM claims that resources are substitutable hydrokinetically within hemisphere (all tasks can compete without bias for the scarce resources that are available, but absolutely no sharing can take place between hemispheres). The RM does not deny the existence of specialized subprocessors for, say, phonological processing. It does deny that any process (e.g., phonological), or any processing routine (e.g., encoding), or any modality (e.g., visual) may have privileged access to a protected pool of resource supplies. Therefore, task interference in the RM is traceable to a capacity shortage and in the NM to a specific subprocessing mechanism.

The RM's challenging claim that resouces are undifferentiated has unsettling implications for long-standing trends in research and instruction in learning disabilities. The Zeitgeist has been consumed for some time in a search to identify a specific dysfunction in learning disabilities, be it phonological recoding, perceptual encoding, visual memory, or some other dysfunction. Despite a great deal of research, none of these possibilities has been confirmed as controversy surrounds each hypothesis. The current realization that not all learning-disabled children suffer from the same difficulty has freshened our search, but the philosophy and the focus are unchanged. Indeed, any claim for a subprocessor deficit is incompatible with the RM's portrayal of learning disorders as a capacity problem in the management of twin pools of undifferentiated resources.

Examination of this issue with respect to the two models suggests the diametrically opposite hypotheses that in learning disability, brain space either may be too differentiated (RM) or may not be differentiated enough (NM). In the case of overdifferentiation, the consequence would be that some resources would be protected from general use; all resources could not be shared, so to speak, on the open market, and tasks that might profit from more resources would not be able to draw them from a general supply pool. To illustrate this problem, if there were private resource pools for phonological processing, visual processing, and semantic processing, with the use of each reserved only to a specified category of task, task component, or level of processing, then a particularly taxing phonological task would be unable to tap into these other resource pools for help. In the case of too little differentiation, tasks would engage an overexpansive amount of brain space, producing interfering cross talk between tasks. On this issue, the models are completely at loggerheads, reflecting an irreconcilable difference that strikes at the core of the models.

Fourth Issue

4. Is task difficulty or task similarity the main obstacle to successful time sharing?

The NM has as its major operational principle that task similarity, which is isomorphic psychologically with the proximity of tasks in brain space (i.e., similar tasks are nearer), presents the greatest potential for interference in divided attention or dual-task performance. As tasks become less similar or greater differences are perceived and conceptualized between tasks and task components, the adjacent brain space between tasks is increased and, as inhibitory barriers are erected more easily between tasks, interfering neuronal cross talk is less likely to occur. Consequently, inhibition of spreading cortical activation is the sine qua non of the NM. This issue underscores *the* neuronal mechanism that possesses the greatest power for explaining developmental and individual differences in attentional ability and, perhaps, in bringing about a better understanding of brain dysfunction in learning disabilities. Task difficulty is of less importance than task similarity in producing interference because coping with task difficulty has less ecological validity. In other words, the priority given to task similarity reflects the biological priority of analytical processing in the growth of intelligence and abstract logic. The NM, also, makes further provision for facilitating in time sharing, especially when two tasks are compatible, or when they are performed in sequence rather than simultaneously, or when one or both tasks are fairly easy. In fact, Kinsbourne's selective activation principle was first advanced to account for hemispheric facilitation, or priming, effects. The cerebral functional distance model, which I am calling the NM, was advanced later to account for both priming and interference. According to the NM, shifts in arousal interact in Yerkes-Dodson law (1908) fashion with neuronal cross talk to influence dual-task performance. The Yerkes-Dodson principle is that tasks are performed best at moderate levels of arousal and less well at low and at high levels. In effect, the spillover of activation from one task to another can potentially raise arousal to a level that is more favorable or less favorable to successful dual-task performance. Advantageous cross-talk can be expected when tasks are compatible, easy, or performed sequentially instead of concurrently.

In the RM, an overlap in resource demand coupled with relative task difficulty is the key interference-producing factor in tasks that demand a division of attention. Task difficulty is the critical task–subject parameter because tasks compete for limited resources, and difficult tasks demand quantitatively more or better resources than do less difficult tasks. Dual-task performance suffers when there is an overlap in resource demand between tasks, and resources become scarce or are unavailable or are of an inferior kind (less efficient). Task similarity is downgraded in importance because similarity is defined by a task's resource composition, and in the RM there are only two kinds of resources, one affiliated with each cerebral hemisphere. As a result, most tasks will overlap in resource demand as tasks and task components are discriminated along a dichotomous dimension. Thus, similarity is only important operationally to the extent that similar tasks may require resources from the same hemisphere, raising the potential for an overlap in demand. Simply requiring resources from the same hemisphere, however, will not, by itself, produce interference. Rather, it is the total amount of resources demanded by tasks, regardless of the fact of their overlap, that is the critical variable—in other words, task difficulty. Also, although the RM was designed to account expressly for dual-task interference, it, too, can account for facilitation effects. Facilitation may occur in at least two ways, each a close parallel to dual-task facilitation in the NM. Dual-task facilitation occurs when tasks are not independent as they are performed conjointly. That is, a different task (less than the sum of the two) may be created when two tasks are combined, or two combined tasks may use some common intermediary process when performed concurrently. Second, if as Kahneman (1973) has argued, capacity is conceived of as a function of the mental effort expended in meeting the encoding demands of the task, then greater task demands will result in greater available capacity. According to the RM, capacity is a negatively accelerated, elastic function of the perceived demands of the task.

Finally, in both models interference can be produced additionally by concurrence costs—those costs that result when single-task to dual-task performance is not additive and a managerial cost is extracted. In RM terminology, of course, such a cost would be seen as a payroll expense, using up resource supplies; in NM terms, it would reflect the recruitment of a cross talk–producing subprocessor.

It appears that the salient difference between models in explaining dual-task performance is the association of each model's respective theoretical constructs with task similarity for the NM and with task difficulty for the RM. For instance, recalling dichotically presented stimuli that are phonologically confusing (e.g., *ba* and *da*) or semantically confusing (e.g., *dog* and *cat*) produces poorer memory performance than recalling stimuli that do not sound alike or do not belong to the same superordinate semantic category. According to the NM, it is the similarity of the stimuli that causes such poorer performance via the proximity of subprocessors in brain space. The addition of more distinguishing cues to the task (i.e., presenting left- and right-ear stimuli in different voices or at different levels of intensity, would decrease their similarity and, correspondingly, reduce interfering cross talk. In contrast, in the RM, rhyming or same-category stimuli demand similar resources, and it is the fact of their resource overlap coupled with the amount of resources consumed by the relative difficulty of the processing load that determines performance. Notably, reduced task similarity takes on significance in the RM only if it alters the resource composition of the task, and even then performance will be affected only to the extent that resource demand exceeds supply. In the RM, improved performance cannot occur unless tasks are made easier, demanding fewer resources.

Consideration of this issue offers quite different hypotheses about the interhemispheric mechanisms that may be significant etiologically in learning disabilities. This issue is similar to the third issue in that they both reflect a deep-seated theoretical contradistinction between models. The NM operationalizes and focuses on the reduction of interfering cross-talk to improve the distribution of attention in complex processing. Processing dysfunction may be produced by tasks being too similar. Alternatively, the RM operationalizes and focuses on reducing workload and on easing the competitive demand for scarce resources to improve attentional capacity. Processing dysfunction may be produced by tasks that overlap in resource demand and are overly difficult.

Summary of the Models

The NM, based on a social network metaphor, claims that the brain is a unified and differentiated community of neuronal subprocessors where tasks compete for functional brain space and the asymmetrically activated hemispheres share their resources. Capacity limits are not acknowledged. Interference between tasks occurs both within and between hemispheres when tasks encroach on the same conceptual space. Task interference is structural. Problem-free learning occurs to the extent that neuronal loci can function unimpeded by neighbors. The developmental priority is to make concurrently performed tasks less similar.

The RM, based on a microeconomic metaphor and using "resource" as an intervening, hypothetical construct, claims that the cerebral hemispheres are independent pools of undifferentiated resources that must be allocated to tasks by each hemisphere. Performance is capacity-limited. The hemispheres cannot be aroused asymmetrically. Interference occurs when there is competition for resources that are in short supply. Task interference is nonstructural. Problem-free learning occurs as long as tasks do not overlap in resource demand and the supply of capacity exceeds the demand for capacity. The developmental priority is to make tasks easier.

TESTING THE MODELS

Examination of published experiments is not very helpful in comparing the relative validity of the models. Insofar as many dual-task experiments have used laterality paradigms, both the NM and the RM would have made the same predictions. It just happens that the representation of tasks in opposite hemispheres also assures a wide separation of tasks in cerebral space, whereas the representation of tasks in the same hemisphere also assures that they are relatively nearer in cerebral space. For example, left-hand finger tapping and speaking are controlled primarily by the right and left hemispheres, respectively, whereas right-hand tapping and speaking are controlled by the same hemisphere (the left). A typical finding in dual-task experiments is for speaking (referred to as the *secondary* or *load* task) to have a relatively greater disruptive impact on right-hand tapping compared to left-hand tapping (tapping is referred to as the *primary* or *target* task). The usual explanation for this effect is that one task has a greater chance of interfering with the performance of another task whenever both tasks are programmed by the same hemisphere. Beyond that, it is impossible to infer a neuronal cross talk mechanism, as opposed to a scarce-capacity mechanism, because right-hand tapping and speech overlap in resource demand (RM) and also are in close proximity in between space (NM). Even if a trade-off could be demonstrated between the performance of target and load tasks as attention may be switched alternatively between them, one could not infer safely whether such a trade-off reflected competition for, on the one hand, scarce capacity or, on the other hand, scarce neuronal space as the inhibitory barrier between tasks encroached in seesaw fashion, favoring first one task and then the other. To make matter worse, there have not been any experiments reported where an attempt was made to untangle the issues separating these two models based on a priori predictions. Thus, at the moment, we have to rely wholly on post hoc interpretations, which, of course, must be considered with caution.

Two ways come to mind for testing the two models' competing theoretical ideas about how the normal brain works. It might be helpful to perform dual-task experiments in which there is a theoretical, a priori emphasis on what happens in the hemisphere not receiving the secondary or load task, rather than an emphasis on the overloaded hemisphere performing the conjoined tasks. Apart from both models' prediction of a general increase in arousal or capacity when shifting from a single task to a dual task, the two models make very different predictions about the parallel performance of the unloaded (single-task) hemisphere at the same point in time that the load hemisphere is engaged in performing the dual task. The NM is pessimistic, the RM optimistic. According to the NM, activation centered in the load hemisphere can be detrimental to processes in the unloaded hemisphere because (1) activation usually is asymmetrical, with homologous areas in the unloaded hemisphere likely to receive inhibitory signals across the corpus callosum, and (2) activation that is centered unilaterally in a totally unified brain has the potential to generate cross talk that may interfere with processes in the unloaded hemisphere. In marked contrast to this gloomy perspective on processing in the partner hemisphere while the load hemisphere is under strain, the RM maintains that the unloaded hemisphere will be more likely to show enhanced performance as the load hemisphere has to work harder. This prediction is based on two beliefs: (1) that the hemispheres are independent processors and (2) that as extra resources are demanded by one hemisphere (the load hemisphere), resources must be made available, if not activated, in equal amounts in the unloaded hemisphere.

Another approach to testing the models might be to vary the similarity of the load task independently of its difficulty. For example, the difficulty level of a load task consisting of a list of words to be remembered could be varied by changing the number of words on the list. It would also be possible to compile memory lists of words that varied along some dimension of similarity—for example, having some lists contain all rhyming words or all words from a similar semantic category. In this way the similarity and difficulty of a load task could be varied parametrically to test the NM prediction for a hemispheric interaction with similarity and the RM prediction for an interaction of hemisphere with task difficulty.

Such experimental approaches would begin to tease out the comparative validity of key theoretical notions held at variance by the two models. In the long term, these models promise to provide new insights into how the brain works as an integrated unit. At this time, however, both models are equally important for their intrinsic interest and heuristic value. Taken together, the NM and the RM have provided us with novel conceptualizations of how the brain may function, and both models have suggested specific brain mechanisms that may be dysfunctional in learning and reading disability.

SUMMARY AND DISCUSSION

Table 19-1 contains the list of potential neuropsychological processing dysfunctions that may produce learning problems. The list was generated by my analysis of key theoretical issues that divide the NM and the RM. Each of these factors may be related hypothetically to any number of learning difficulties. Because most research in this area has been done with dyslexic children, however, I shall now summarize my conclusions in reference to developmental reading disability or dyslexia.

Excessive Resource Sharing and Excessive Unilateral Activation

The first two possibilities are derived from the questions of whether the hemispheres share processing resources (energy) and whether subsequent hemispheric arousal–activation can occur unilaterally. Both issues implicate to some extent the combined functions of the

Table 19-1. Possible Learning Disability Dysfunctions

Dysfunction	Model
1. Too much resource sharing	Both
2. Overactivation of one hemisphere	Both
3. Too little sharing of resources and/or products	Both
4. Metacognitive misallocation of resources	Both
5. Hemispheric underdifferentiation	NM
6. Hemispheric overdifferentiation	RM
7. Dysfunction due to task similarity	NM
8. Dysfunction due to task difficulty	RM

neocortical commissures and brain stem arousal–activation circuits, and the NM and the RM concur in suggesting (1) that the hemispheres in the learning disabled may share resources too easily and (2) that the hemispheres of the learning disabled may not respond mutually to demanding cognitive tasks that should engage bihemispheric arousal–activation mechanisms in deep levels of processing. In the first event, there is excessive collaboration between hemispheres during preprocessing as the hemispheres draw on the brain's processing resources, with arousal in one hemisphere spreading too readily to the other hemisphere. In the second event there is an exaggerated imbalance in hemispheric task engagement, with unilateral activation correlated too strongly with contralateral suppression. It is important to note that the first event biases against lateralized processing, producing an *ostensible* duplication in hemispheric processes, whereas the second event promotes lateralized processing, producing an *apparent* deduplication of hemispheric processes. Learning-disabled children may suffer from one, both, or neither of these problems, but it is highly significant to recognize that these hypothetical processing dysfunctions have nothing whatsoever to do with the argument about whether dyslexic children are or are not lateralized; each of these eventualities is produced by situation-specific and task-specific information-processing demands on abnormal interhemispheric arousal–activation functions.

Regarding the first point, if resource sharing can be excessive and if it is unrelated to structural lateralization, one would expect dyslexic children compared to normals either to be lateralized equally or to fail to display the same degree of left-hemisphere specialization for language under relatively simple, free-recall, dichotic listening tasks that make no special demands on arousal–activation mechanisms.[1] Indeed, a review of the dichotic literature shows some cautious support for this idea. Equivalent lateralization in disabled and normal children has been reported with digits (Obrzut, 1979; Watson & Engle, 1982), with word pairs (Prior, Frolley, & Sanson, 1983), and with CV syllables (Hynd, Obrzut, Weed, & Hynd, 1979; Obrzut, Hynd, & Obrzut, 1983; Obrzut, Hynd, Obrzut, & Pirozzolo, 1981). These results are inconsistent with the belief that learning disabled children are dyslateralized structurally. In a more recent study, Obrzut *et al.* (1985) reported that dyslexic children compared to normals failed to show the same degree of right-ear advantage on a simple, CV syllable free-recall task. Obrzut *et al.* (1985) interpreted their findings as support for the earlier notion that dyslexic children are (1) less lateralized structurally and (2) suffering from a left-hemisphere dysfunction. A review of the pooled, dichotic research, however, coupled with my present analysis, demonstrates that the Obrzut *et al.* (1985) findings can be interpreted entirely differently. Both the NM and the RM suggest that such results (1) can occur in dyslexic children whose hemispheres are lateralized normally and (2) can reflect a task-specific overflow in interhemispheric processing (each hemisphere too easily accessing processing resources or innervating processes in the other hemisphere) rather than a left-hemisphere dysfunction. Research supporting this contention more directly has been reported. Milberg, Whitman, and Galpin (1981), using a dichotic procedure that was designed to produce moderate error rates, reported that dyslexic children compared to controls used a temporal recall strategy regardless of presentation rate, showing an inability to inhibit verbal stimuli from the unattended ear. At the same time that the dyslexics were reporting a greater number of intrusion errors, they maintained an equal degree of lateralization (difference between attended ears) compared to the nondisabled controls. Also, Dermody, Mackie, and Katch (1983) reported that poor readers (not clearly dyslexic) compared to normals showed an exaggerated lag effect in dichotic listening. Using an easy, single-paired CV identification task in which one member of each stimulus pair was presented either 500 msec or 1,000 msec in advance of the other CV stimulus, they found that the poor readers excelled in reporting delayed syllables. In fact, the poor readers showed a better hemispheric response than did the normals (who also showed the lag effect) but only after their opposite hemisphere had been stimulated. Therefore, these theoretical and empirical considerations, taken together, would seem to mandate a more cautious interpretation of any research that reports less lateralization in dyslexics. Both models suggest a competing interpretation. The NM and the RM converge in suggesting that dyslexics may suffer from a surplus in interhemispheric resource sharing—a problem that is unrelated to questions of hemispheric specialization.

Regarding the second point (failure of the hemisphere to activate mutually in task processing), both models concur in pointing up the theoretical possibility for the existence of cognitive constraints that may result from an inability to process perceptual inputs, or to engage conceptual processing and retrieval mechanisms, bihemispherically. Research consistent with this hypothesis has shown that when dichotic testing was made more demanding by instructions to report only from the right ear in otherwise easy CV discrimination tasks, dyslexic children actually produced a greater right-ear advantage in comparison to normals (Obrzut *et al.*, 1981, 1983). One study using the same paradigm failed to replicate this effect (Obrzut *et al.*, 1985). However, if the NM and the RM are accurate in their basic assertion that perceptual asymmetries reflect dynamic human information-processing characteristics and not a fixed, structural feature of the mind, then some inconsistencies in research are to be expected until we are able to identify and to control the increased number of variables that can affect lateralized processing and our laterality measures. Further tentative support for the abnormal unilateral activation hypothesis comes from studies that have found a left-ear advantage in dyslexics when they were precued to report CV syllables from the left ear (Obrzut *et al.*, 1981, 1985) and when they were required to recall strings of dichotic digits in writing rather than repeating them orally (Kershner *et al.*, 1984). One interpretation of these effects is that the increased right-hemisphere demands of the experimental tasks (attending left and visual processing) may have engaged the right hemisphere at the expense of important left-hemisphere verbal processing. In fact, the dyslexic children may have been unable, in the face of dual hemispheric processing demands, to maintain a normal level of parallel processing in both hemispheres. More reliable (not post hoc) support for the unilateral activation hypothesis has been found by Swanson and his colleagues in a series of investigations into hemispheric, semantic memory processes in reading-disabled children (Swanson, 1986, 1987; Swanson & Mullen, 1983; Swanson & Obrzut, 1985). After varying the encoding instructions and the linguistic organization of word lists (semantic, phonemic, graphemic) presented dichotically, Swanson reported (1) that there were no reliable differences in laterality between groups in the absence of word feature, orienting strategies; (2) that dyslexics were more diffuse in attempts at activating selected word features in long-term memory; and (3) that dyslexics were less flexible in oriented processing, failing to activate bihemispheric word knowledge structures independently of the activated hemisphere. In summing up this series of provocative studies, Swanson (in press, b) concluded that the primary information-processing disturbance in poor readers appeared to be their inefficiency in coordinating bihemispheric resources relative to encoding, elaborative activation, and retrieval demands placed on semantic memory.

Therefore, there is more than ample theoretical and empirical evidence to suggest that dyslexics may be lateralized equally, lateralized poorly, and—perhaps at the same time—lateralized too much. Structural features of brain lateralization have no bearing on this characterization of dyslexia. Both models concur in suggesting that an arousal–activation dysfunction in dyslexics may either deplete the potential for lateral processing or overly engage one hemisphere under high-demand processing.

Too Little Sharing of Resources and/or Products

The third possibility, derived from the first issue, is suggested only by the NM at the resource level but is also suggested by both models at the product level. The hypothesis for too little resource (energy) sharing as an etiological factor in dyslexia has a long history, stemming from the work of Geschwind and colleagues (Geschwind, 1962). Although this idea runs counter to the suggestive evidence already discussed in favor of an excess of resource sharing in dyslexia, Rudel (1980); Vellutino, Scanlan, and Bentley (1983); and Gladstone and Best (1985) have presented cogent arguments for variations of this theme, but at a level of processing that includes products as well as energy. In general, they suggest that dyslexia may be functionally equivalent to a hemispheric disconnection syndrome. Gladstone and Best (1985) presented a carefully researched argument in favor of this proposition in which they noted that many characteristics of dyslexics are similar to those of commissurotomy and acallosal patients. An important point in considering data that might address this issue is that early childhood failure of the development of the corpus callosum might produce an abnormal bihemispheric representation of functions that in the normal brain are laterally represented (Levy, 1985). Levy's detailed analysis of callosal function suggests that one of the many functions of the callosum is progressively to inhibit hemispheric processes for which there are duplicate programs in the other hemisphere. Hence, we are confronted with the implication that whenever dyslexic children demonstrate poorly lateralized performance, it may be caused either by (1) a task-invariant absence of hemispheric specialization if a callosal dysfunction has prevented the interhemispheric coupling necessary to inhibit duplicate processes or (2) a task-dependent lack of lateralized processing in the event that a callosal dysfunction promotes excessive interhemispheric sharing. Research evidence to support more directly the hypothesis for an absence of interhemispheric connections in dyslexia is not available. The few studies that have been reported with this issue in mind have not supported it (Broman, Rudel, Helfgott, & Krieger, 1985; Vellutino *et al.*, 1983); but it was assumed, perhaps erroneously, that the dyslexics were lateralized normally, and, moreover, testing procedures failed to yield reliable lateral differences in the normal control groups. Therefore, in view of the theoretical arguments in its favor combined with a serious paucity of research, we have to consider the possibility that dyslexics may suffer from too little sharing between hemispheres, and, by implication, that they may be less lateralized because of it.

Metacognitive Misallocation of Resources

Both models agree in pointing up the importance of metacognitive supervision in interhemispheric processing. Unfortunately, we do not have a sophisticated research strategy to test for resource allocation difficulties per se as etiological or correlated factors in dyslexia. Such factors may have played a covert role in every one of the studies that we have discussed. To illustrate a study that begs for a metacognitive interpretation, Larry Morton and I (Kershner & Morton, submitted) found that two separate cohorts of learning-disabled children compared to normal controls were poorer in dichotic digit and CV syllable recall regardless of whether they were instructed to recall selectively from the left or from the right ear. There were no laterally differences between groups in free recall. Thus, the disabled children were underlateralized when attending right in what was presumably a left-hemisphere task; but the same children were overlateralized when attending left, which presumably is a task requiring considerable bihemispheric processing. We interpret this to mean that the learning-disabled children may have poorer control over the allocation of both left-hemisphere resources and bihemispheric resources. However, any number of resource sharing, unilateral activation or attentional factors may also be implicated. All we can say with confidence is that there are solid theoretical reasons but only suggestive research evidence for the proposition that dyslexics may have poor regulation over allocating hemispheric processes to tasks.

Hemispheric Differentiation, Task Similarity, and Task Difficulty

The last four possibilities in Table 19-1 (5, 6, 7, and 8) reflect salient theoretical points on which the RM and the NM are in strong disagreement. At this time, we do not have research with normals or with learning-disabled children that would provide substantive grounds for a useful discussion. Sadly, there is not a single laterality experiment with learning-disabled children that cannot be interpreted easily within each framework. We need research with learning-disabled children that pits one model's view against the other's. Dyslexia in the NM might involve a failure in perceptual and cognitive analysis correlated with poorly differentiated mapping of events in brain space. In the RM, it might involve poor returns for effortful amounts of expended energy drawn from difficult-to-access resource pools. It is hoped that each of these very different conceptualizations of dyslexia will be useful in untangling the web of mystery that continues to surround this disorder.

CONCLUSIONS

A consideration of the four theoretical issues, taken from a comparison of the NM and the RM in the context of current research in dyslexia, has produced a set of theoretically grounded working hypotheses about the neuropsychology of the disorder. It is suggested that dyslexia may be related to an interhemispheric dysfunction involving corticolimbic, brain stem activation and the neocortical commissures. This is not to deny that left-hemisphere dysfunction may also play a role in some, if not all, types of dyslexia. The present analysis offers a resolution to a major dispute in the literature over whether dyslexics are or are not poorly lateralized. It is suggested that dyslexics may show poorly lateralized performance under low task demand or arousal, but that the same children may show exaggerated unihemispheric processing in situations entailing high cognitive demand. Whether their poorly lateralized performance is a result of hemispheres that are less specialized (produced by an interhemispheric disconnection) or of hemispheric nonindependence in processing (produced by ungated interhemispheric exchange) is unknown. Thus, an outstanding issue is whether there is too much or too little interplay between hemispheres in dyslexia. In addition, metacognitive control over intrahemispheric and interhemispheric allocation of processing is proposed as an important component that needs to be taken into consideration in fully appreciating the dyslexic's information processing problems.

In summary, interhemispheric laterality problems in dyslexia may be produced by (1) a disconnection-like syndrome coupled with a state of less specialization, (2) unbridled resource sharing, (3) unbalanced arousal–activation, and (4) metacognitive mismanagement. Overall, the RM and the NM have much in common in suggesting similar neuropsychological problems underlying dyslexia. Nevertheless, they also suggest diametrically opposed theoretical mechanisms for carrying out successful learning in the intact brain. Thus, each model provides a theoretically unique but cohesive and comprehensive paradigm for basic research into these issues. Our knowledge about learning disabilities can only be enriched as a result.

ACKNOWLEDGMENT

I would like to thank Alinda Friedman and Marcel Kinsbourne for the major scholarly contributions that they have made in originating and developing these ideas and for their helpful comments on an earlier draft. Of course, I take entire responsibility for this characterization of their models and for this application of the models to developmental learning disabilities. This chapter is dedicated to reducing the gulf between neuropsychology and cognitive psychology.

NOTE

1. Dichotic listening research provides the most compelling data base to address issues of lateralized processing in learning disabilities. The usual procedure is simultaneously to project dissimilar verbal stimuli (e.g., words or digits) to the two ears and to observe whether recall is better from the left or the right ear. A right-ear advantage is interpreted as an indication of linguistic superiority of the left cerebral hemisphere. This inference is based on the notions that (1) the left hemisphere is preprogrammed when activated differentially for attending selectively to the right side of space, (2) the contralateral pathways are prepotent over ipsilateral (same ear–same hemisphere) auditory pathways, and (3) in most right-handed people the left hemisphere is specialized for linguistic processing.

REFERENCES

Aaron, P. (1982). The neuropsychology of developmental dyslexia. In R. Malatesha & P. Aaron (Eds.), *Reading disorders: Varieties and treatments* (pp. 5–67). Toronto: Academic Press.

Allen, M. (1983). Models of hemispheric specialization. *Psychological Bulletin, 93,* 73–104.

Badian, N., & Wolff, P. (1977). Manual asymmetries of motor sequencing in reading disability. *Cortex, 13,* 343–349.

Bakker, D. (1979). Hemispheric differences and reading strategies: Two dyslexias? *Bulletin of the Orton Society, 29,* 84–100.

Bakker, D., & Vinke, J. (1985). Effects of hemisphere-specific stimulation on brain activity and reading in dyslexics. *Journal of Clinical and Experimental Neuropsychology, 7,* 505–525.

Broman, M., Rudel, R., Helfgott, E., & Krieger, J. (1985). Inter- and intrahemispheric processing of visual and auditory stimuli by dyslexic children and normal readers. *International Journal of Neuroscience, 26,* 27–38.

Cummings, R. (1985). *An evaluation of the Tomatis Listening Training Program.* Unpublished doctoral dissertation, University of Toronto.

Dermody, P., Mackie, K., & Katch, R. (1983). Dichotic listening in good and poor readers. *Journal of Speech and Hearing Research, 26,* 341–348.

Evans, J. (1982). Neuropsychologically based remedial reading procedures: Some possibilities. In R. Malatesha & P. Aaron (Eds.), *Reading disorders: Varieties and treatments* (pp. 371–388), Toronto: Academic Press.

Friedman, A., & Polson, M. (1981). Hemispheres as independent resource systems: Limited-capacity processing and cerebral specialization. *Journal of Experimental Psychology: Human Perception and Performance, 7,* 1031–1058.

Friedman, A., Polson, M., Dafoe, C., & Gaskill, S. (1982). Dividing attention within and between hemispheres: Testing a multiple resources approach to limited-capacity information processing. *Journal of Experimental Psychology: Human Perception and Performance, 8,* 43–68.

Gladstone, M., & Best, C. (1985). Developmental dyslexia: The potential role of interhemispheric collaboration in reading acquisition. In C. Best (Ed.), *Hemispheric function and collaboration in the child* (pp. 87–118). Toronto: Academic Press.

Geschwind, N. (1962). The anatomy of acquired disorders of reading. In J. Money (Ed.), *Reading disability: Progress and research needs in dyslexia.* Baltimore, Johns Hopkins Press.

Hellige, J., & Cox, P. (1976). Effects of concurrent verbal memory on recognition of stimuli from the left and right visual fields. *Journal of Experimental Psychology: Human Perception and Performance, 2,* 210–221.

Hellige, J., Cox, P., & Litvac, L. (1979). Information processing in the cerebral hemispheres: Selective hemispheric activation and capacity limitations. *Journal of Experimental Psychology: General, 108,* 251–279.

Hellige, J., & Wong, T. (1983). Hemispheric-specific interference in dichotic listening: Task variables and individual differences. *Journal of Experimental Psychology: General, 112,* 218–239.

Herdman, C., & Friedman, A. (1985). Multiple resources in divided attention: A cross-model test of the independence of hemispheric resources. *Journal of Experimental Psychology: Human Perception and Performance, 11,* 40–49.

Hiscock, M., & Kinsbourne, M. (1982). Laterality and dyslexia: A critical view. *Annals of Dyslexia, 32,* 177–225.

Hynd, G., & Cohen, M. (1983). *Dyslexia,* Toronto: Grune and Stratton.

Hynd, G., Obrzut, J., Weed, W., & Hynd, C. (1979). Development of cerebral dominance: Dichotic listening asymmetry in normal and learning-disabled children. *Journal of Experimental Child Psychology, 28,* 445–454.

Kahneman, D. (1973). *Attention and effort.* Englewood Cliffs, NJ: Prentice-Hall.

Kershner, J. (1977). Cerebral dominance in disabled readers, good readers, and gifted children. Search for a valid model. *Child Development, 48,* 61–67.

Kershner, J. (1983). Laterality and learning disabilities: Cerebral dominance as a cognitive process. *Topics in Learning and Learning Disabilities, 3,* 66–74.

Kershner, J. (1985). Ontogeny of hemispheric specialization and relationship of developmental patterns to complex reasoning skills and academic achievement. In C. Best (Ed.), *Hemispheric function and collaboration in the child* (pp. 327–360). Toronto: Academic Press.

Kershner, J., Cummings, R., Clarke, K., Hadfield, A., & Kershner, B. (1986). Evaluation of the Tomatis Listening Training Program with Learning Disabled Children. *Canadian Journal of Special Education, 2,* 1–32.

Kershner, J., Henninger, P., & Cooke, W. (1984). Written recall induces a right hemisphere linguistic advantage for digits in dyslexic children. *Brain and Language, 21,* 105–122.

Kershner, J., & Morton, L. (submitted). Effects of arousal, attention, and stimulus type on speech lateralization in reading disabled and non-disabled children.

Kinsbourne, M. (1970). The cerebral basis of asymmetries in attention. *Acta Psychologia, 33,* 193–201.

Kinsbourne, M. (1973). The control of attention by interaction between the cerebral hemispheres. In S. Kornblum (Ed.), *Attention and performance IV* (pp. 239–256). Toronto: Academic Press.

Kinsbourne, M. (1975). The mechanism of hemispheric control of the lateral gradient of attention. In P. Rabbitt & S. Dornic (Eds.), *Attention and performance V* (pp. 81–97). Toronto: Academic Press.

Kinsbourne, M. (1981). Single channel theory. In D. Holding (Ed.), *Human skills* (pp. 124–139). Chichester, Sussex: Wiley.

Kinsbourne, M., & Hicks, R. (1978). Functional cerebral space: A model for overflow, transfer and interference effects in human performance. In J. Requin (Ed.), *Attention and performance VII* (pp. 345–363). Toronto: Wiley.

Kinsbourne, M., & Hiscock, M. (1983). Asymmetries of dual-task performance. In J. Hellige (Ed.), *Cerebral hemispheres asymmetry* (pp. 255–334). New York: Praeger.

Kliepera, C., Wolff, P., & Drake, C. (1981). Bimanual co-ordination in adolescent boys with reading retardation. *Developmental Medicine and Child Neurology, 23,* 617–625.

Levy, J. (1983). Individual differences in cerebral hemisphere asymmetry: Theoretical issues and experimental considerations. In J. Hellige (Ed.), *Cerebral hemisphere asymmetry* (pp. 465–497). New York: Praeger.

Levy, J. (1985). Interhemispheric collaboration: Single-mindedness in the asymmetric brain. In C. Best (Ed.), *Hemispheric function and collaboration in the child* (pp. 11–31) Toronto: Academic Press.

Milberg, V., Whitman, R., & Galpin, R. (1981). Selective attention and laterality in good and poor readers. *Cortex, 17,* 571–582.

Navon, D., & Gopher, D. (1979). On the economy of the human-processing system. *Psychological Review, 86,* 214–255.

Naylor, H. (1980). Reading disability and lateral asymmetry: An information-processing analysis. *Psychological Bulletin, 87,* 531–545.

Obrzut, J. (1979). Dichotic listening and bisensory memory skills in qualitatively diverse dyslexic readers. *Journal of Learning Disabilities, 12,* 24–34.

Obrzut, J., Hynd, G., & Obrzut, A. (1983). Neuropsychological assessment of learning disabilities: A discriminant analysis. *Journal of Experimental Child Psychology, 35,* 46–55.

Obrzut, J., Hynd, G., Obrzut, A., & Pirozzolo, F. (1981). Effect of direct attention on cerebral asymmetries in normal and learning disabled children. *Developmental Psychology, 17,* 118–125.

Obrzut, J., Obrzut, A., Bryden, M., & Bartels, S. (1985). Information processing and speech lateralization in learning-disabled children. *Brain and Language, 25,* 87–101.

Orton, S. (1937). *Reading, writing and speech problems in children.* New York: Norton.

Pribram, K., & McGuinness, D. (1975). Arousal, activation, and effort in the control of attention. *Psychological Review, 82,* 116–149.

Prior, M., Frolley, M., & Sanson, A. (1983). Language lateralization in specific reading retarded children and backward readers. *Cortex, 19,* 149–163.

Rourke, B. (1982). Central processing deficiencies in children: Toward a developmental neuropsychological model. *Journal of Clinical Neuropsychology, 4,* 1–18.

Rourke, B., Bakker, D., Fisk, J., & Strang, J. (1983). *Child neuropsychology,* New York: Guilford Press.

Rudel, R. (1980). Learning disability-diagnosis by exclusion and discrepancy. *Journal of the American Academy of Child Psychiatry, 19,* 547–569.

Segalowitz, S., & Gruber, F. (1977). *Language development and neurological theory.* New York: Academic Press.

Swanson, H., (1983). Hemispheric specialization in learning disabled readers' recall as a function of age and level of processing. *Journal of Experimental Child Psychology, 35,* 457–477.

Swanson, H. (1986). Do semantic memory deficiencies underlie learning disabled readers' encoding processes? *Journal of Experimental Child Psychology, 41,* 461–488.

Swanson, H. (1987). The combining of multiple hemispheric resources in learning disabled and skilled readers' recall of words: A test of three information processing models, *Brain and Cognition, 6,* 41–55.

Swanson, H., & Obrzut, J. (1985). Learning disabled readers' recall as a function of distinctive encoding, hemispheric processing and selective attention. *Journal of Learning Disabilities, 18,* 409–418.

Tucker, D., & Williamson, P. (1984). Asymmetric neural control systems in human self-regulation. *Psychological Review, 91,* 185–215.

Vellutino, F., Scanlan, D., & Bentley, W. (1983). Interhemispheric learning and speed of hemispheric transmission in dyslexic and normal readers: A replication of previous results and additional findings. *Applied Psycholinguistics, 4,* 209–228.

Watson, E., & Engle, R. (1982). Is it lateralization, processing strategies, or both that distinguishes good from poor readers? *Journal of Experimental Child Psychology, 34,* 1–19.

Witelson, S. (1977). Developmental dyslexia: Two right hemispheres and no left? *Science, 195,* 309–311.

Wolff, P., Cohen, C., & Drake, C. (1984). Impaired motor timing control in specific reading retardation. *Neuropsychologia, 22,* 587–600.

Yerkes, R., & Dodson, J. (1908). The relation of strength of stimulus to rapidity of habit formation. *Journal of Comparative and Neurological Psychology, 18,* 459–482.

Young, A., & Ellis, A. (1981). Asymmetry of cerebral hemispheric function in normal and poor readers. *Psychological Bulletin, 89,* 183–190.

Zarske, J. (1982). Neuropsychological intervention approaches for handicapped children. *Journal of Research and Development in Education, 15,* 66–75.

20

Subtypes of Learning-Disabled Children: Implications for a Neurodevelopmental Model of Differential Hemispheric Processing

BYRON P. ROURKE
University of Windsor

JOHN L. FISK
Henry Ford Hospital

INTRODUCTION

This chapter was designed as a summary of our attempts to address some issues pertaining to one aspect of the study of different subtypes of learning-disabled children. Specifically, we attempt herein to deal with the evidence that we have gathered to date regarding differences in the developmental progression and manifestation of learning disabilities that appear to be related primarily to deficiencies in linguistic processing, as opposed to those that appear to have their origins in nonverbal processing deficits. In so doing, we have framed these findings within the context of a developmental neuropsychological model (Rourke, 1982) that has been formulated on the basis of some of our earlier investigations, and which has been instrumental in guiding our more recent empirical efforts. Some notes regarding the basic aims of this model may be beneficial at this point.

Aims of the Model

The Rourke (1982) model derives from a theoretical position (Goldberg & Costa, 1981) that constitutes a comprehensive attempt to deal with the differentiation and integration of left- and right-hemispheric neuropsychological systems. Rourke's extension of this model was an attempt to deal with some of the basic developmental dimensions and ramifications of the Goldberg and Costa formulation. It was designed specifically to address issues relating to the etiology of developmental disabilities, including those usually labeled "learning disabilities."

One cornerstone of the Rourke (1982) position is that the notion of learning disabilities should be conceived and dealt with in the widest possible human sense. It maintains that a model that purports to deal adequately with the manner in which central processing deficiencies hamper learning in the developing child must take into consideration, encompass, and explain *all* aspects of the child's developmental (learning) demands. For example, within the framework of this model, it is as important to deal adequately with the vicissitudes of social learning as it is to address issues relating to reading disability; problems in graphomotor learning, listening skill development, mechanical arithmetic, social sensitivity, orientation in terms of time and place, and the multitude of developmental learning demands that the child must face become grist for the model's mill. As the chapter proceeds, we hope that it will become clearer why this perspective is important; we also attempt to explain some of its particular aspects during this brief exposition.

Format of the Chapter

This chapter has a very straightforward format. First, we review the results of studies carried out in our laboratory that were designed to shed some light on the neuropsychological skills and abilities of selected subtypes of learning-disabled youngsters. This review concentrates on the investigations that are germane to the focus of this book: those that deal with aspects of the neurodevelopmental dimensions of left- and right-hemispheric processing. The next section deals with the socioemotional implications of the patterns of information-processing abilities and deficits that have been demonstrated in these subtypes of learning-disabled children. Finally, we attempt to provide some theoretical structure for these findings by integrating them within the Rourke (1982) model. Before embarking on this task, however, we would be remiss were we not to acknowledge the seminal contributions of Helmer Myklebust to our efforts in this area.

Helmer R. Myklebust

Much of what will be explained herein represents some specifications and elaborations of material contained within a chapter authored by Myklebust (1975). Although our own efforts in this area of investigation (e.g., Rourke, 1975; Rourke & Telegdy, 1971; Rourke, Young, & Flewelling, 1971) were proceeding simultaneously with Myklebust's studies, it is abundantly clear that his very insightful clinical observations antedated some of our own analyses, especially with respect to the specification of the academic and social manifestations of the child suffering from a "nonverbal learning disability." Indeed, a careful reading of his aforementioned chapter in conjunction with the material that follows would be of considerable value for the thoughtful investigator. Now, for our review.

PATTERNS OF ABILITIES AND DEFICITS OF SELECTED SUBTYPES OF LEARNING-DISABLED CHILDREN

Except where specifically noted to the contrary, the subjects employed in the series of investigations to be reviewed herein met a fairly standard definition for children with learning disabilities (Rourke, 1975, 1978). That is, these children

1. Were markedly deficient in at least one school subject area
2. Obtained WISC Full Scale IQs within the roughly normal range
3. Were free of primary emotional disturbance
4. Had adequate visual and auditory acuity
5. Lived in homes and communities where socioeconomic deprivation was not a factor
6. Had experienced only the usual childhood illnesses
7. Had attended school regularly since the age of 5½ or 6 years
8. Spoke English as their native language

The first study in this series (Rourke, Young, & Flewelling, 1971) was designed to assess the relationships between Verbal Intelligence Quotient (VIQ) and Performance Intelligence Quotient (PIQ) discrepancies on the Wechsler Intelligence Scale for Children (WISC; Wechsler, 1949) on the one hand and selected verbal, auditory–perceptual, visual–perceptual, and problem-solving abilities on the other. Three groups, each containing 30 learning-disabled children, were formed on the basis of the relationship between their VIQ and PIQ scores on the WISC. Group 1 (HP–LV) consisted of subjects whose PIQ was at least 10 points higher than their VIQ; Group 2 (V = P) was composed of subjects with VIP and PIQ within 4 points of each other; and the members of Group 3 (HV–LP) had VIQ values at least 10 points higher than their PIQ. All subjects fell within a Full Scale WISC range of 79 to 119 and an age range of 9 to 14 years; there were no significant differences in either WISC Full Scale IQ or age between the three groups.

As expected, the performance of the HV–LP group was superior to that of the HP–LV group on those tasks that involved verbal, language, and auditory–perceptual skills: Peabody Picture Vocabulary Test (PPVT; Dunn, 1965); Aphasia Screening, Speech-Sounds Perception, and Seashore Rhythm Tests (Reitan & Davison, 1974); Reading, Spelling, and Arithmetic subtests of the Wide Range Achievement Test (WRAT; Jastak & Jastak, 1965). The differences on all but the PPVT were statistically significant. The performances of the HP–LV group were, as expected, superior to those of the HV–LP group on tasks that primarily involve visual–perceptual skills: Trail Making Test (TMT), Part A, and Target Test (Reitan & Davison, 1974). Also as expected, the performances of the V = P group occupied positions roughly intermediate between those of the other two groups over most of the dependent measures. Although the discrepancy was not statistically significant, the HP–LV group did somewhat better than the HV–LP group on the Category Test (Reitan & Davison, 1974).

Of particular importance in the present context were two additional findings. First, the HV–LP group did well on the TMT, Part B, relative to Part A, whereas the HP–LV group did poorly on TMT, Part B, relative to Part A. It appeared probable that the subjects in the HV–LP group performed better on TMT, Part B, relative to the TMT, Part A, because, though relatively deficient in the visual–perceptual abilities necessary for success on both parts of the TMT, they were relatively more adept at the complex verbal and symbolic abilities necessary for success on TMT, Part B.

Second, an a posteriori comparison of the Reading, Spelling, and Arithmetic subtests of the WRAT within each of the three groups indicated a striking difference between Reading and Spelling (high) on the one hand and Arithmetic (low) on the other hand for the HV–LP group. Although no such statistically significant differences in performance on these three subtests of the WRAT were present in either of the other two groups, there was an opposite trend evident in the performance of the HP–LV group on these WRAT measures—that is, a tendency toward higher performance on the WRAT Arithmetic subtest relative to performance on the WRAT Reading and Spelling subtests.

Clearly, the results of this investigation indicated that, in older (9- to 14-year-old) children, the WISC VIQ–PIQ relationship is a far more important consideration with regard to learning disabilities than is general level of psychometric intelligence (i.e., Full Scale IQ). Indeed, although we did not emphasize this point at the time, it appeared that the groups of learning-disabled children formed on the basis of WISC VIQ–PIQ discrepancies might very well constitute unique subtypes within the learning-disabled population. This appeared to be so not only for independent measures of verbal, auditory–perceptual, and visual–spatial abilities, but also for patterns of performance on the Reading, Spelling, and Arithmetic subtests of the WRAT. Subsequent examinations of all these dimensions have demonstrated that this seems, in fact, to be the case (see Fletcher, 1985).

Since these groups of learning-disabled children with different configurations of VIQ–PIQ discrepancies exhibited patterns of performance that might suggest differential impairment of skills ordinarily thought to be subserved primarily by one or other of the two cerebral hemispheres, it was thought advisable to carry out a subsequent investigation including dependent variables that might shed some additional light on this question.

Thus, three groups of subjects who exhibited patterns of VIQ–PIQ discrepancies virtually identical to those of the Rourke *et al.* (1971) investigation were selected in order to compare their performances on motor and psychomotor tasks that allowed for separate assessments of right-hand and left-hand efficiency (Rourke & Telegdy, 1971). The motor and psychomotor tasks used were chosen in terms of what seemed to be varying degree of two dimensions: (1) complexity and (2) the visual–spatial skills necessary for success. Thus, the dependent measures ranged from relatively simple motor tasks (e.g., strength of grip, speed of tapping) to relatively complex psychomotor tasks (e.g., timed placement of grooved pegs into holes). The 45 male learning-disabled subjects (15 in each of the HP–LV, V=P and HV–LP groups) selected for study were between the ages of 9 and 14 years, and their WISC Full Scale IQs fell within the range of 85 to 115. There were no statistically significant differences between the groups in terms of age or WISC Full Scale IQ.

The performances of these groups on 25 measures indicated clear superiority of the HP–LV group on most measures of complex motor and psychomotor abilities, regardless of the hand employed. The clearest separation of the groups was observed on the most complex psychomotor measure (Grooved Pegboard Test; Klove, 1963); on this task, the differences were evident for both right- and left-hand trials, with the following pattern of relative superiority between the groups obtaining: HP–LV > V=P > HV–LP. There were nonsignificant trends in evidence favoring the right-hand over the left-hand performances of the HV–LP group on the Finger Tapping (Reitan & Davison, 1974) and Tactual Performance (Reitan & Davison, 1974) Tests, with the opposite pattern of right-hand and left-hand results for the HP–LV group. These findings, in addition to the superior performance of the HP–LV over the HV–LP group on the Location component of the Tactual Performance Test (Reitan & Davison, 1974) offered support for one of the alternative hypotheses of the study, that is, that the HP–LV group, because of relative superiority in visual–perceptual skills, would do better than the HV–LP group on tasks involving complex visual–motor coordination and spatial visualization and memory. Although expectations involving differential hand superiority of the HP–LV and HV–LP groups were not supported, the results were considered consistent with the view that WISC VIQ–PIQ discrepancies reflect the differential integrity of the two cerebral hemispheres in older children with learning disabilities.

At this point in our research program, it was clear that older (9- to 14-year-old) learning-disabled children did not constitute a homogeneous group. Indeed, simply separating them for study on the basis of WISC VIQ–PIQ differences suggested strongly that one subtype within this group (HV–LP) seemed to be relatively efficient at tasks thought to be subserved primarily by the left cerebral hemisphere (e.g., speech-sounds discrimination), whereas another subtype (HP–LV) appeared to be much more efficient at tasks thought to be subserved primarily by the right cerebral hemisphere (e.g., visual–spatial tasks). In addition, the consequences of this separation of the groups for levels and patterns of performance in reading, spelling, and arithmetic appeared to be important. Before pursuing the implications of the latter, however, we felt it necessary to investigate the correlates of

VIQ–PIQ discrepancies among younger children with learning disabilities. It was thought that some developmental implications regarding the emerging abilities and deficits of learning-disabled children might be revealed thereby.

In this study (Rourke, Dietrich, & Young, 1973), 82 5- to 8-year-old learning-disabled children were divided into three groups using virtually the same criteria as those employed in the Rourke *et al.* (1971) and Rourke and Telegdy (1971) investigations. The children had WISC Full Scale IQs ranging from 79 to 120; there were no significant differences between the groups with respect to age and Full Scale IQ. The study employed as dependent variables measures within the following two categories: (1) the verbal, auditory–perceptual, visual–perceptual, and problem-solving tests similar to those employed in the Rourke *et al.* (1971) study; and (2) the motor and psychomotor tests similar to those employed by Rourke and Telegdy (1971).

In contrast to the findings of Rourke *et al.* (1971) and Rourke and Telegdy (1971), there were few significant differences in performance evident among the three groups in the Rourke *et al.* (1973) study. However, the pattern of group differences on the PPVT, WRAT, Speech-Sounds Perception Test, Seashore Rhythm Test, Category Test, and Target Test closely resembled that obtained by Rourke *et al.* (1971). The only statistically significant differences evident among the motor and psychomotor measures indicated superiority of the HP–LV over the HV–LP group on selected aspects of the Mazes (Klove, 1963), Grooved Pegboard, and Tactual Performance Tests. Given the large number of comparisons carried out, the latter differences may have emerged by chance.

Although the pattern of performances on the verbal and auditory–perceptual measures was of interest because of its similarity to results obtained with older learning-disabled children, the absence of any strong indications of motor and psychomotor patterns and the relatively large variability of performances across the majority of measures at this age level suggested strongly that meaningful developmental patterns would be difficult to determine with these data. What appeared clear was that there was an emerging differentiation of abilities in learning-disabled children similar to that seen with great regularity in normal children. In addition, this progressive differentiation of abilities appeared to be accompanied by an emerging differentiation of selective deficits in these subtypes of learning-disabled youngsters. (For extensive treatments of the implications of these emerging patterns for concepts of developmental lag versus deficit and the concept of "psychic edema," the interested reader is referred to Rourke, 1976, and Rourke, 1983, respectively).

Another implication of the results of the series of studies reviewed to this point was that further investigation of the differential integrity of left- and right-hemispheric systems as these relate to patterns of abilities and deficits in various subtypes of learning-disabled children would best be accomplished by in-depth study of the 9- to 14-year-old group. Hence, the next studies in this series focused on this age group, with special attention to the patterns of WRAT Reading, Spelling, and Arithmetic performances noted in our aforementioned investigations.

In the first of these investigations, Rourke and Finlayson (1978) attempted to determine whether children who exhibited specific patterns of WRAT Reading, Spelling, and Arithmetic performances would also exhibit predictable patterns of neuropsychological abilities and deficits. In this study, learning-disabled children between the ages of 9 and 14 years were divided into three groups (15 subjects in each group) on the basis of their patterns of performance in reading and spelling tasks relative to their level of performance in arithmetic. The subjects in Group 1 were uniformly deficient in reading, spelling, and arithmetic. Group 2 was composed of subjects whose arithmetic performance, although clearly below age expectation, was significantly better than their performances in reading and spelling. The subjects in Group 3 exhibited normal reading and spelling and markedly impaired arithmetic performance. Although all three groups performed well below age expectation in arithmetic, the performances of Groups 2 and 3 were superior to that of Group 1; Groups 2 and 3 did not differ from one another in their impaired levels of arithmetic performance. The three groups were equated for age and WISC Full Scale IQ.

The three groups' performances on 16 dependent measures, chosen in the light of the results of previous studies in this series (e.g., Rourke *et al.*, 1971), were compared. The results of this investigation may be summarized as follows: (1) the performances of Groups 1 and 2 were superior to those of Group 3 on measures of visual–perceptual and visual–spatial abilities (e.g., WISC Block Design, Target Test); and (2) Group 3 performed at superior levels to Groups 1 and 2 on measures of verbal and auditory–perceptual abilities (e.g., WISC Vocabulary, Speech-Sounds Perception Test). In the context of the results of the previous studies in this series, it was notable that all subjects in Group 1 had a lower VIQ than PIQ, that 14 of the 15 subjects in Group 2 had a lower VIQ than PIQ (one subject had equivalent VIQ and PIQ), and that all subjects in Group 3 had a higher VIQ than PIQ. It is clear that Groups 1 and 2 performed in a fashion very similar to that expected of groups of older children with learning disabilities who exhibit the WISC HP–LV pattern, and that Group 3 performed in a manner expected of older children with learning disabilities who exhibit the WISC HV–LP pattern (Rourke *et al.*, 1971).

If there is reason to believe that WISC VIQ–PIQ discrepancies may be associated with or reflect the differential integrity of the two cerebral hemispheres in older children with learning disabilities, as has been suggested here, then it would appear that the basis on which the groups were chosen in the Rourke and Finlayson (1978) study may also reflect this difference. At the very least, the results of the latter investigation would be consistent with the view that the subjects in Group 3 may be limited in their performance because of compromised functional integrity of the right cerebral hemisphere, and that the subjects in Groups 1 and 2 were suffering from the adverse effects of relatively dysfunctional left-hemispheric systems. These inferences were felt to be reasonable because the subjects in Group 3 did particularly poorly *only* in those skills ordinarily thought to be subserved primarily by the right cerebral hemisphere, whereas the subjects in Groups 1 and 2 were markedly deficient *only* in those skills ordinarily thought to be subserved primarily by the left cerebral hemisphere.

Also of importance in the present context was the fact that the two groups of subjects who had been equated for deficient arithmetic performance (Groups 2 and 3) exhibited vastly different performances on verbal and visual–spatial tasks. These differences were clearly related to their *patterns* of reading, spelling, and arithmetic rather than to their *levels of performance* in arithmetic per se. Indeed, although the WRAT Reading, Spelling, and Arithmetic subtest scores of Group 2 were in no case significantly superior to those of Group 3, the performances of Group 2 were significantly superior to those of Group 3 on all of the measures of visual–perceptual and visual–spatial skills (WISC Picture Completion, Picture Arrangement, Block Design, and Object Assembly; Target Test) employed in this investigation. More generally, it seemed reasonable to infer that the neurocognitive bases for the impaired arithmetic performances of Groups 2 and 3 differed markedly: Whereas subjects in the Group 2 subtype would appear to experience difficulty in mechanical arithmetic because of "verbal" deficiencies, subjects of the Group 3 subtype would be expected to encounter difficulties with mechanical arithmetic as a direct result of deficiencies in "visual–spatial" abilities. Indeed, a qualitative analysis of the errors made by these two subtypes of learning-disabled youngsters suggested very strongly that this is, in fact, the case (see Rourke & Strang, 1983; Strang & Rourke, 1985b).

The methodological implications of such findings for research in children's learning disabilities is quite clear: Were subjects from Groups 2 and 3 combined to form a single group defined as "disabled in arithmetic" for the purpose of parametric investigation, comparisons of measures of central tendency between such a combined group and a group performing at a normal level in arithmetic would severely distort and mask the very marked differences in verbal and visual–spatial abilities exhibited by these two learning disability subtypes. In addition, it would appear to be the case that children of these two subtypes require quite different modes of educational intervention in order to make academic progress in their areas of deficiency (Rourke, Bakker, Fisk, & Strang, 1983; Rourke & Strang, 1983; Strang & Rourke, 1985b).

Before proceeding to a discussion of the next investigation in this series, it would be well to point out the reasons for excluding Group 1 from an in-depth analysis in conjunction with this group of studies. Our reasons for this relate to the specific aims of this chapter and to the fact that Group 1 appears to be made up of several discrete subtypes of learning-disabled children (Fisk & Rourke, 1979). An adequate treatment of the implications of the latter issue for our current discussion would take us too far afield.

Following the Rourke & Finlayson (1978) study, we decided to determine whether these same three groups of 9- to 14-year-old learning disabled subjects would differ in predictable ways on measures of motor, psychomotor, and tactile–perceptual skills. In this investigation (Rourke & Strang, 1978), we were particularly interested to determine if there were any evidence that might be adduced thereby to support a view that these children were suffering from differential impairment of functional systems thought to be subserved primarily by structures and systems within the left or the right cerebral hemisphere. We hoped to accomplish this through an analysis of the right- and left-hand performances of these groups of right-handed learning-disabled children on selected motor, psychomotor, and tactile–perceptual measures.

The motor tests included the Finger Tapping Test and the Strength of Grip Test (Reitan & Davison, 1974). The psychomotor measures included the time measures for the Maze Test, the Grooved Pegboard Test, and the Tactual Performance Test. The tests for tactile–perceptual disturbances were those described in Reitan and Davison (1974), as follows: Finger Agnosia, Finger-Tip Number-Writing Perception, and Coin Recognition. A summary score that included all errors on the latter tests for tactile–perceptual disturbances for each hand was derived for use in this study. The principal results of this investigation and their implications for the current discussion are as follows.

There were no statistically significant differences between or among the groups on the (simple) motor measures over and above those that would be expected to be exhibited by the exclusively right-handed children employed in this study. The expected superiority of performances for Groups 1 and 2 over those of Group 3 were clearly in evidence on two of the (complex) psychomotor measures (Maze and Grooved Pegboard Tests). Differential hand superiority was found between the groups only on the Tactual Performance Test. Groups 1 and 3 displayed a pattern of poor left-hand performance relative to right-hand performance on this measure, whereas the exact opposite pattern was exhibited by Group 2. The left-hand performance of Group 2 was significantly superior to that of Groups 1 and 3. In line with the patterns evident for the Maze and Grooved Pegboard Tests, the performances of Groups 1 and 2 on the "both hands" measure of the Tactual Performance Test was superior to that of Group 3. Finally, comparisons favoring the performances of Groups 1 and 2 over those of Group 3 on the composite tactile–perceptual measure were significant for both the right and left hands. There was also a tendency evident among subjects in Group 3 for their right-hand performance to be superior to that with the left hand.

Thus, it was demonstrated that learning-disabled children in Group 3 have marked deficiencies relative to Groups 1 and 2 in some psychomotor and tactile–perceptual skills. In addition, comparisons of these results with the norms available for these tests (Knights & Norwood, 1980) indicated that the performances of Group 3 fell well below age expectation on these measures, whereas the performances of Groups 1 and 2 were well within normal limits.

The very marked discrepancy between the performances of Groups 2 and 3 on the Tactual Performance Test would offer clear support for the hypothesis regarding differential hemispheric integrity for these two groups that was advanced in connection with the Rourke and Finlayson (1978) study. Confining our discussion to the performances of Groups 2 and 3 in the two studies under consideration, it is clear that Group 2 scored lower than expected on measures of abilities ordinarily thought to be subserved primarily by systems within the left cerebral hemisphere, and much better (in an age-appropriate fashion) on measures of abilities ordinarily thought to be subserved primarily by right-hemispheric systems; the opposite state of affairs obtained in the case of learning-disabled children of the Group 3 subtype.

A comparison of the results of the Rourke and Strang (1978) study with those of Rourke and Finlayson (1978) is especially important in the case of Group 3. The particular pattern that emerged for this group is one that is somewhat analogous to that seen in the Gerstmann syndrome (Benson & Geschwind, 1970; Kinsbourne & Warrington, 1963). That is, the children in Group 3 exhibited the following: outstanding deficiencies in arithmetic (within a context of normal reading and spelling); visual–spatial orientation difficulties, including right–left orientation problems; general psychomotor incoordination, including problems that would fall under the rubric of "dysgraphia"; and impaired tactile–discrimination abilities, including finger agnosia. At the same time, it must be emphasized that the patterning of abilities and deficits exhibited by children in Group 3 would appear to be most compatible with relatively deficient *right*-hemispheric systems rather than with deficient *left*-hemispheric systems as advanced by Benson & Geschwind (1970).

The results of the Rourke and Finlayson (1978) and the Rourke and Strang (1978) investigations would appear to have significant and widespread import for the academic and social remediation of such children (see Strang & Rourke, 1985a, and the next section of this chapter) and for the determination of subtypes of learning-disabled youngsters (Fletcher, 1985; Rourke, 1983; Rourke & Strang, 1983; Strang & Rourke, 1985b). Rather than deal with these implications at this juncture, however, it would be instructive to consider the results of the last two studies in this series—one dealing with the concept-formation and problem-solving abilities of 9- to 14-year-old Group 2 and 3 children (Strang & Rourke, 1983); the other, with the determination of the verbal, visual–spatial, psychomotor, and tactile–perceptual capacities of 7- to 8-year-old Group 1, 2, and 3 children (Ozols & Rourke, 1988; Ozols & Rourke, *in preparation*).

In the Strang and Rourke (1983) investigation, 9- to 14-year-old Group 2 and 3 children (15 in each group) were chosen in a fashion virtually identical to that employed in the two studies just reviewed. They were equated for age and WISC Full Scale IQ (range: 86–114). The dependent measures employed in this study included the number of errors on the six subtests of the Halstead Category Test (Reitan & Davison, 1974) and the total number of errors scored on the entire test. The form of the Category Test used for children 9 to 15 years of age includes 6 subtests and 168 items. The sixth subtest includes only review items from subtests 2, 3, 4, and 5 in a randomly ordered fashion. The Category Test is a relatively complex concept-formation measure involving nonverbal abstract reasoning, hypothesis-testing, and the ability to benefit from positive and negative informational feedback. The most important results of this study were the following.

As predicted, Group 3 scored significantly higher on the Category Test total errors score than did children in Group 2. Furthermore, the level of performance of Group 3 children on this measure was approximately one standard deviation below age expectation (Knights & Norwood, 1980), whereas Group 2 children performed in an age-appropriate manner. An analysis of performances on the subtests of the Category Test revealed that the performance of Group 2 was significantly superior to that of Group 3 on the final three subtests (4, 5, and 6). It is notable that subtests 4 and 5 of the Category Test are those that are most complex in terms of their requirements for visual–spatial analysis, and that subtest 6 requires incidental memory for the previously correct solutions. The latter is one measure of the child's capacity to benefit from experience with the task.

These results were expected in view of the previously documented deficiencies exhibited by Group 3 children that we thought would have interfered with the normal development of the higher-order cognitive skills presumably tapped by this test. Our reasoning was as follows. It would seem highly likely that the majority of children in Group 3 have suffered since birth from the ill effects of their neuropsychological deficiencies (i.e., bilateral tactile–perceptual impairment; bilateral psychomotor impairment; and, poorly developed visual–perceptual–organizational abilities). In terms of the theory regarding the development of intellectual functions formulated by Piaget (1954), one would expect that these deficiencies would have a negative effect on the successful acquisition of "higher order" cognitive skills for which they are prerequisites. Specifically, Piaget has suggested that the behavioral acquisitions and developments during the first 2 years of life (the sensorimotor stage of development) underlie the successful acquisition of cognitive skills at later stages. Piaget's description of what he considered to be significant sensorimotor activities serves to highlight the importance of tactile–perceptual, psychomotor, and visual–perceptual–organizational functions for the infant and young child. Since Group 3 children are particularly deficient in these neuropsychological functions (and probably have been so since birth), it would seem highly probable that they have not benefited as much as have most children from the sensorimotor period of development. Furthermore, their cognitive operations, particularly those that are not regulated easily by language functions (e.g., higher order analysis, organization, and synthesis), would also be expected to be deficient.

Finally, in a developmental neuropsychological model modified and extended by Rourke (1982) to account for information-processing deficiencies in children, an underlying principle states that the formation of constructs and concepts is dependent on right-hemispheric systems for their content. Since the bulk of the evidence accumulated in our previous studies regarding the neuropsychological status of Group 3 children suggested strongly that they have underdeveloped or deficient right-hemispheric systems, it seemed reasonable to hypothesize that the concept-formation abilities of Group 3 children would be somewhat underdeveloped, particularly when the content for the concept is primarily novel and nonverbal. It is clear that comparisons of the performance of Group 3 children with age-based norms offered support for this hypothesis. A comparison of Group 3 performance with that of Group 2 also offered support for the principal elements of this theoretical model.

The essentially intact Category Test performance of Group 2 would suggest strongly that language and thought, as Piaget suggested, are quite distinct. Group 2 youngsters, although deficient in many aspects of linguistic and auditory–perceptual functioning, performed at normal levels on this very complex test of nonverbal concept formation and problem solving. Apart from some difficulties exhibited on subtest 1 (which involves the *reading* of Roman numerals), they performed well within age expectations on the other subtests. They also exhibited a much better developed capacity to benefit from experience with this task than did the Group 3 children. Finally, they showed considerable capacity to deal effectively and adaptively with the novel problem-solving, hypothesis-testing, and cognitive flexibility requirements of the Category Test.

In terms of the Rourke (1982) model, these well-developed abilities are thought to reflect the functioning of intact right-hemispheric systems, whereas the deficiencies in linguistic and auditory–perceptual skills exhibited by Group 2 are inferred to reflect deficits in left-hemispheric systems. The fact that there is absolutely no evidence of impairment in tactile–perceptual, visual–spatial–organizational, and psychomotor skills in Group 2 children would suggest that their course through the sensorimotor period of intellectual development described by Piaget would be expected to have been normal. Even though afflicted with fairly obvious difficulties in the development and elaboration of psycholinguistic skills, their development of higher order cognitive processes seems to have proceeded without complication.

In order to summarize the results of the studies of 9- to 14-year-old children in Groups 2 and 3 reviewed to this point, we have included Figure 20-1, which illustrates the major findings of the Rourke *et al.* (1971), Rourke and Telegdy (1971), and Strang and Rourke

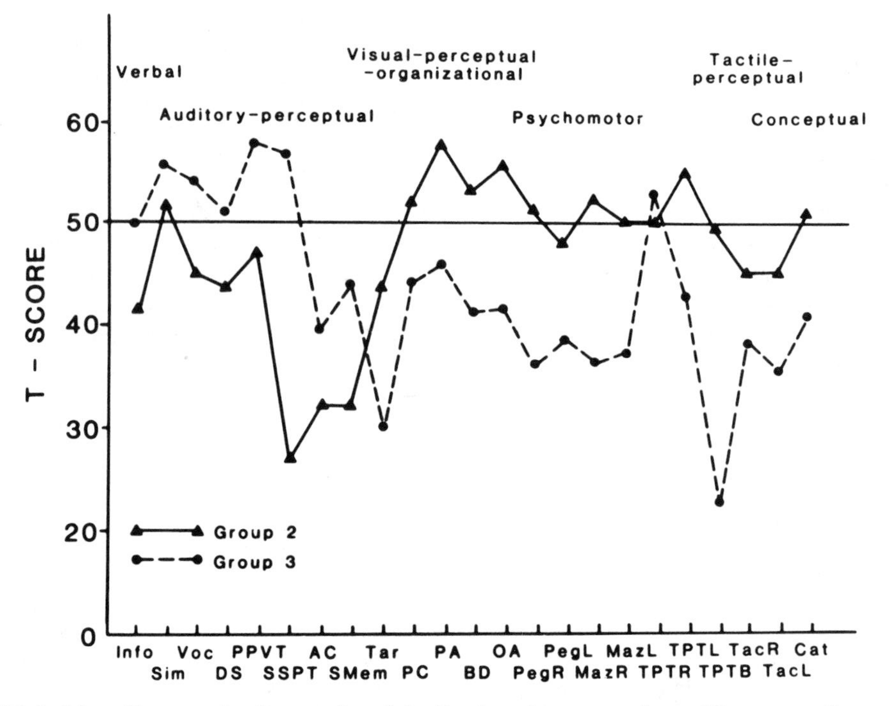

Figure 20-1. Mean T scores for Groups 2 and 3. Good performance: above 50; poor performance: below 50. Abbreviations: Info, WISC Information; Sim, WISC Similarities; Voc, WISC Vocabulary; DS, WISC Digit Span; PPVT, Peabody Picture Vocabulary Test; SSPT, Speech-Sounds Perception Test; AC, Auditory Closure Test; SMem, Sentence Memory Test; Tar, Target Test; PC, WISC Picture Completion; PA, WISC Picture Arrangement; BD, WISC Block Design; OA, WISC Object Assembly; PegR, Grooved Pegboard—Right Hand; PegL, Grooved Pegboard—Left Hand; Maz R Maze Test—Right Hand; Maz L, Maze Test—Left Hand; TPT R, Tactual Performance Test—Right Hand; TPT L, Tactual Performance Test—Left Hand; TPT B, Tactual Performance Test—Both Hands; TacR, Tactual–perceptual abilities—Right Hand; TacL, Tactual-perceptual abilities—Left Hand; Cat, Category Test. Reprinted by permission from "Arithmetic Disability Subtypes: The Neuropsychological Significance of Specific Arithmetical Impairment in Childhood" by J. D. Strang and B. P. Rourke, 1985, in *Neuropsychology of Learning Disabilities: Essentials of Subtype Analysis,* edited by B. P. Rourke, New York: Guilford Press.

(1983) investigations. In Figure 20-1, the *T* score means are structured in such a way that average performance for the particular age group in question, according to the Knights and Norwood (1980) norms, is represented by $T = 50$, with a standard deviation (S.D.) of 10. Thus, a *T* score of 60 represents a level of performance that is one S.D. above the mean, whereas a *T* score of 40 represents a score that is one S.D. below the mean for the particular age group. This use of *T* scores allows direct comparisons to be made among the various tests in a type of profile analysis, which would not be possible if raw scores were used.

As can be seen in Figure 20-1, the deficiencies, relative to age-based norms, exhibited by Group 2 children are virtually confined to the "verbal" and especially the "auditory–perceptual" areas. On the other hand, Group 3 children exhibit deficiencies in a wide variety of visual–perceptual–organizational, psychomotor, tactile–perceptual, and conceptual areas. Their problems with the Auditory Closure Test and the Sentence Memory Test may be a reflection of their difficulties in dealing with novel tasks (Auditory Closure) and their problems in understanding and utilizing semantic/meaningful content as a memory aid (Sentence Memory), as would be expected in terms of the Rourke (1982) model.

Finally, the results of a recent investigation that employed almost all of the aforementioned measures in the investigation of Group 1, 2, and 3 children between the ages of 7 and 8 years (Ozols & Rourke, 1988, in preparation) yielded results quite compatible with those obtained in the studies of 9- to 14-year-old children. However, as in the Rourke *et al.* (1973) study of 6- to 8-year-old children who were assigned to groups on the basis of their patterns of WISC VIQ–PIQ discrepancies, the results were not as clear-cut as were those evident for older learning-disabled children. In addition, it was not possible to measure higher order concept-formation abilities in an adequate fashion in these younger children, who are, in Piaget's terms, still functioning within the stage of concrete operational thought.

This completes our survey of the levels and configurations of neuropsychological abilities and deficits exhibited by Group 1, 2, and 3 children. For a summary of validation studies of these subtype comparisons from other laboratories, the interested reader is referred to Fletcher (1985). We turn now to an examination of the socioemotional correlates and ramifications of these characteristic patterns.

SOCIOEMOTIONAL AND PERSONALITY DIMENSIONS OF SUBTYPES OF LEARNING-DISABLED CHILDREN

Thus far we have developed several important points regarding the neuropsychological abilities of learning-disabled children. First, studies in our laboratory have demonstrated that WISC VIQ–PIQ discrepancies constitute sensitive indices of differing patterns of performance across a wide range of neuropsychological dimensions, including psychomotor, tactile–kinesthetic, visual–spatial, linguistic, and higher order concept-formation skills and abilities. Second, we have demonstrated that specific patterns of neuropsychological abilities and deficits are also predictable on the basis of patterns of performance on the WRAT Reading, Spelling, and Arithmetic subtests. In short, we have illustrated the manner in which both sets of measures are sensitive to the heterogeneity in neuropsychological abilities displayed by specific subtypes of learning-disabled children. Moreover, we have proposed that specific patterns of (1) academic achievement and (2) WISC VIQ–PIQ scores are reflections of the differential integrity of left- and right-hemispheric systems in these subtypes of learning-disabled children.

It is clear that training in academic and related skills constitutes one of the most important developmental demands for children between the ages of 6 and 16 years, at least in western European and North American societies; learning to cope with the social and interpersonal demands of home, school, and community environments constitutes a no less important dimension of every child's development. It seems to us ironic that so much neuropsychological research is devoted to the former set of demands and so little to the latter. Furthermore, it is our opinion that the generalizations and conclusions drawn in the very limited literature on the neuropsychology of socioemotional functioning in children is, at best, primitive, and, at worst, downright misleading (see Rourke, in press, for a review).

For example, with regard to the learning-disabled child, popular wisdom suggests that pressure for academic success from parents and teachers, accompanied by repeated school failure, produces a discouraged, if not frankly neurotic, child whose self-image is permanently distorted. Indeed, some investigators (e.g., Black, 1974; Halechko, 1977; Zimmerman & Allebrand, 1965) have gone so far as to maintain that learning-disabled children exhibit a particular cluster of frankly pathological socioemotional characteristics. However, as we have proposed previously (Rourke & Fisk, 1981), there is evidence to suggest that learning-disabled children are heterogeneous with respect to socioemotional functioning. In this section, we review a series of investigations conducted in our laboratory that was specifically designed to explore this hypothesis and some of its implications.

In a direct attempt to examine the heterogeneity hypothesis, Porter and Rourke (1985) selected 100 learning-disabled children between the ages of 5 and 15 years for study. These subjects met the usual exclusionary criteria that have been used in most of our previous investigations. In this study, the *Q* factor analysis algorithm was utilized to analyze the clinical scales of the Personality Inventory for Children (PIC; Wirt, Lachar, Klinedinst, & Seat, 1977). The PIC is composed of 600 true–false questions relating to the child's behavior, attitudes, and interpersonal relations. It can be scored for 3 validity or response-style scales (Lie, F, and Defensiveness); 1 general screening scale (Adjustment); 12 clinical scales (Achievement, Intellectual Screening, Development, Somatic Concern, Depression, Family Relations, Delinquency, Withdrawal, Anxiety, Psychosis, Hyperactivity, and Social Skills); and 17 supplemental scales (Adolescent Maladjustment, Aggression, Asocial Behavior, Cerebral Dysfunction, Delinquency Prediction, Ego-Strength, Excitement, Externalization, Infrequency, Internalization, Introversion–Extraversion, K, Learning Disability Prediction, Reality Distortion, Sex Role, Social Desirability, and Somatization).

Examination of the mean PIC profile for the total sample revealed that, for 100 learning-disabled children, the Intellectual Screening scale was significantly elevated (i.e., T score > 70) and that only the Achievement scale approached this level. These scale elevations would be expected in any sample of learning-disabled children. Of greater interest was the finding that those clinical scales specifically designed to evaluate socioemotional functioning were within normal limits. Had Porter and Rourke chosen to carry out no further analysis, they would have been justified in concluding that learning-disabled children are not particularly prone to socioemotional difficulties. However, the results of the subsequent *Q* factor analysis suggested a very different interpretation of these data.

This analysis yielded four interpretable factors that accounted for 69.5% of the common variance. Subjects with factor loadings $> .50$ on a single factor scale were identified and composed into 4 groups (77 subjects in all). Multivariate analyses of variance revealed significant differences across the 4 subtypes overall ($p < .01$) as well as on 28 of the 33 individual PIC scales. Bearing in mind that interpretation of PIC protocols remains a somewhat inexact science (or art), the following subtype descriptions were formulated.

The largest subtype, comprising approximately one-half of the classified subjects, was characterized by minimal clinical scale elevations and between-scale variations, indicating that this group of subjects was relatively well adjusted in terms of their socioemotional functioning. A second subtype, comprising approximately one-quarter of the sample, exhibited marked elevations on 5 of the clinical scales and moderate elevations on 6 of the other clinical scales. As a group, these children appeared to be rather seriously disturbed from a socioemotional standpoint. A third subtype, composed of approximately 15% of the subjects, was characterized by scale elevations typically seen in children diagnosed as "hyperkinetic." Indeed, this profile was virtually identical to that described by Breen and Barkley (1984) in their investigation of the PIC profile of so-called hyperactive children. A final subtype, comprising somewhat less than 10% of the classified subjects, exhibited a marked elevation on only one scale, Somatic Concern. This protocol suggests roughly normal socioemotional functioning, accompanied by a variety of somatic complaints on the part of the child; it is also possible that this represents the reports of "overprotective" mothers who express elevated concern regarding their children's physical well-being.

With respect to the last subtype, further analysis of the classified subjects (Pohlman, 1983) using stepwise discriminant function analysis employing 4 PIC Factor Scales, revealed a lack of differentiation between subtype 1 (normals) and subtype 4 (Somatic Concern). Pohlman noted that these two subtypes were virtually identical on all clinical scales except Somatic Concern and that their identification in the Porter and Rourke (1985) study may have been an artifact of the method of analysis employed.

In any case, the results of the Porter and Rourke (1985) investigation constitute a formidable challenge to the view that learning-disabled children are relatively uniform in terms of their socioemotional characteristics. Furthermore, one must question the notion that learning disability, broadly defined, constitutes a sufficient condition to produce emotional disturbance. Although obviously one cannot ignore the possibility that learning-disabled children confront a very different interpersonal environment than do their normally achieving peers, it would seem that many children defined as learning disabled perform competently in many aspects of day-to-day adaptive functioning. Clinically, we have examined a number of learning-disabled children of relatively advanced age who, despite having experienced years of frustration in their attempts to perform well in the classroom, were relatively intact in terms of their emotional status.

None of the foregoing implies that learning-disabled children are necessarily free of socioemotional difficulties. Indeed, the Porter and Rourke study indicates that, for certain learning-disabled children, the socioemotional dimension is a salient concern. In this regard, the results of studies in our laboratory (Strang, 1981; Strang & Rourke, 1985a) have shown that children with poor visual–spatial skills within a context of well-developed linguistic abilities exhibit PIC profiles similar to that of the emotionally disturbed subtype identified in the Porter and Rourke (1985) study. This finding suggests that children exhibiting visual–spatial and other associated nonverbal deficits are prone to behavioral disturbances even in family and community situations that are typically judged as psychologically healthy. These same studies (Strang, 1981; Strang & Rourke, 1985a) also demonstrated that children characterized by poor verbal and language-related skills and relatively well developed visual–spatial abilities exhibited PIC profiles not unlike that of the "normal" subjects identified by Porter and Rourke.

All of this suggests that there is a very important link between ability structure and socioemotional functioning, at least in some types of learning-disabled children. Since, as we have clearly demonstrated, the WISC VIQ–PIQ discrepancy is a sensitive index of ability structure in learning-disabled youngsters, it follows that such a measure might also be predictive, at least to some degree, of the emotional status of such children. To test this hypothesis, Fisk, Fuerst, and Rourke (in preparation) cluster-analyzed PIC data obtained from 132 learning-disabled children between 6 and 12 years of age. These subjects were selected so as to comprise 3 separate subgroups of 44 subjects each, as follows: Group HP–LV, whose WISC PIQ exceeded VIQ by at least 10 points; Group V = P, whose WISC VIQ–PIQ discrepancy was no more than 3 points in either direction; and Group HV–LP, whose WISC VIQ exceeded PIQ by at least 10 points. Each subgroup was composed of 22 males and 22 females in two age categories (6–8 years and 9–12 years), with age equated across the three groups at each age categorization.

The results of this analysis yielded four interpretable clusters. Three of these appeared to be virtually identical to those identified in the Porter and Rourke (1985) study: namely, a normal group (18 subjects), an emotionally disturbed group (26 subjects), and a group classified as hyperactive (16 subjects). One relatively unique cluster (21 subjects) was characterized by several scale elevations consistent with that typically seen in children who are considered to be mildly anxious and/or depressed. Thus, in large part these results cross-validated the Porter and Rourke findings.

The most interesting aspect of this study was the evaluation of how the subject selection criteria, namely WISC VIQ–PIQ discrepancies, related to the four PIC clusters. Of the 18 subjects comprising the "normal" cluster and the 21 subjects comprising the "mild anxiety/depressive" cluster, only 2 subjects (1 in each cluster) were from the HV–LP group. In contrast, 12 of the 26 subjects in the "emotionally disturbed" cluster and 10 of the 16 subjects in the "hyeractive" cluster were from the HV–LP group. Roughly 65% of the HP–LV and V = P subjects who were classified fell within the "normal" and "mild anxiety/depressive" clusters, whereas 35% of the subjects in these two groups fell within the "emotionally disturbed" and "hyperacitve" clusters. The approximate corresponding percentages for the HV–LP subjects who fell within each of these two combined cluster classifications were 8% ("normal" and "mild anxiety/depressive") and 92% ("emotionally disturbed" and "hyperactive").

These results are consistent with the earlier findings of Strang (1981) that learning-disabled children with relatively deficient visual–spatial–organizational skills are more likely to be described by parents as emotionally or behaviorally disturbed. In contrast, normal subjects, at least as mirrored by PIC profiles, were almost exclusively drawn from children who exhibited relatively well developed visual–spatial abilities within the context of poor psycholinguistic and language-related skills. Although the results of this study have not yet been cross-validated, it would seem reasonable to propose that WISC VIQ–PIQ discrepancy is a sensitive marker of socioemotional disturbances in at least some types of learning-disabled children.

To the best of our knowledge there have been no published investigations dealing with the extent to which patterns of academic performance might constitute a similar index, although studies to evaluate this relationship are currently underway in our laboratory. For example, a very recent investigation (Stewart, 1986) designed to evaluate the relationship between specific patterns of academic performance on the Wide Range Achievement Test (Jastak & Jastak, 1965) and adaptive behavior as measured by the Vineland Adaptive Behavior Scales (VABS; Sparrow, Balla, & Cichetti, 1984) is germane to this line of investigation. Stewart found that children with average or above-average scores on the WRAT Reading and Spelling subtests in conjunction with deficient performances on the WRAT Arithmetic subtest exhibited significant elevations on the VABS Maladaptive Behavior Scale as compared with children who were uniformly deficient on all three of the WRAT Reading, Spelling, and Arithmetic subtests. These results were especially intriguing in view of the fact that the former group was superior to the latter in the Communication domain, as measured by the VABS.

The studies described thus far do not address the question of what sort of mechanism might account for the social and emotional problems exhibited by children with nonverbal learning disabilities. On the basis of clinical observation, we would hypothesize that failure to attend to and interpret correctly nonverbal social clues (e.g., body postures, gestures, facial expressions, etc.) might interfere with the performance of such children in many social situations. Indeed, an experimental investigation by Ozols and Rourke (1985) offered some support for this hypothesis.

In this investigation, Ozols and Rourke compared two groups of learning-disabled children on four exploratory measures of social sensitivity. One group exhibited a pattern of relatively poor auditory–perceptual and language-related skills within the context of well-developed visual–spatial abilities, whereas the second group exhibited the opposite pattern of abilities and deficits. The results revealed that children in the language-disorder group performed more effectively than did those in the visual–spatial disorder group on tasks requiring nonverbal responses. In contrast, tasks requiring verbal responses yielded exactly the opposite results. This data indicates that social awareness and responsiveness varies markedly for these two groups of learning-disabled children, probably as a function of the task demands of the situation. Another implication of these data is that the information-processing skills of learning-disabled children are quite important with respect to at least some dimensions of socioemotional behavior.

Although obviously we are in no position to provide a definitive description of the relationship between socioemotional characteristics and ability structure in this population of children, the studies described thus far do offer some directions with respect to testable hypotheses. For example, it may be that impaired visual–spatial abilities and deficits in tactile–perceptual, psychomotor, and concept-formation abilities shown to be related thereto (Rourke & Finlayson, 1978; Rourke & Strang, 1978; Strang & Rourke, 1983) constitute a sufficient condition for the development of some sort of emotional and/or behavioral disturbance. Conversely, it would seem appropriate to propose that impaired psycholinguistic and language-related functioning do not constitute sufficient conditions for the genesis of socioemotional disturbance.

Further research dealing with these important questions is clearly indicated. Indeed, the potential implications of such research with respect to the treatment of behavioral and/or emotional disturbance in learning-disabled children may be profound. For example, we would question the wisdom, let alone the cost-effectiveness, of embarking on "insight-oriented" or "talking" therapies with emotionally disturbed children and adults of the type characterized by poor visual–spatial and related concept-formation deficits. The overlearned, rote verbal skills of such patients often make them appealing candidates for such forms of therapy. In point of fact, however, our experience indicates that pursuing such a therapeutic avenue is counterproductive. Of particular interest from a theoretical perspective is the support for the working hypothesis of this series of investigations that such therapeutic failures offer: viz., that particular patterns of neuropsychological abilities and deficits have a differential impact, not only on learning and information processing in the academic milieu, but also on efforts at adaptation in ambient social situations.

THEORETICAL IMPLICATIONS

The Rourke (1982) model is organized in terms of five principles, as follows:

1. There is an ontogenetic progression from the salience of right-hemisphere functions to that of left-hemisphere functions.

2. The evident change in children's conceptualizations from global to specific is a reflection of the right- to left-hemisphere ontogenetic development.
3. The development of right-hemisphere systems is a prerequisite for the adequate development of left-hemisphere systems.
4. In the normal course of affairs in the formation of constructs and concepts, right-hemisphere systems provide the content for concepts, whereas left-hemisphere systems are particularly geared to their articulation, elaboration, and stereotypic application.
5. Diminished access to or disordered functioning of right-hemisphere systems is especially debilitating with respect to the development of adaptive skills.

The results of the studies reviewed in this chapter would seem to provide fairly strong support for some of these principles and some deductions therefrom. This would seem to be especially the case with respect to principles 3, 4, and 5. For example, it would be consistent with these principles that the speech and language development of Group 3 (HV–LP) children would be in some ways limited: The lack of meaningful content in their linguistic productions; the impoverished pragmatics of their typical discourse; and the circumlocutions, repetitions, and illogicality of their speech and language behavior would be consistent with the view that, although they are capable of generating in a stereotypical fashion much verbal behavior, the pragmatics of their linguistic performances suffer because of lack of access to or disordered functioning of those right-hemispheric systems that are capable of providing the content for concepts. It is as though their left-hemispheric systems developed without the benefit of access to those aspects of right-hemispheric processing capabilities that would serve to bolster the content and pragmatics of the final products of their linguistic performances.

On the other hand, Group 2 (HP–LV) children appear to perform as though right-hemispheric systems are functioning well, but as if those left-hemispheric systems that are geared to the articulation, elaboration, and stereotypical application of concepts are dysfunctional. Their superior performances on such measures as the Category Test and the subtests of the Performance section of the Wechsler scales would suggest strongly that concept formation, strategy generation, hypothesis-testing, and the capacity to modify ongoing cognitive activity adaptively in the presence of appropriate informational feedback are developing in an age-appropriate fashion. This would also be consistent with the view that such abilities and skills can develop reasonably well even in the absence of intact left-hemispheric systems.

Moreover, the different patterns of abilities and deficits exhibited by these two subtypes of learning-disabled children would seem to bear strong relationships to both their academic and their social learning penchants and potentials. Whereas Group 2 children would be expected to experience considerable difficulty with all scholastic endeavors because of their impaired facility with various aspects of language and linguistic competence, there would appear to be no necessary relationship between such impaired linguistic skills and deficiencies in socioemotional functioning. This is not to say that such children cannot turn out to be emotionally disturbed; indeed, many do. What is important in the present context is that there seems to be no *necessary* relationship between linguistic disturbance and emotional disturbance. Put another way, language deficiency would not appear to be a *sufficient* condition for deviant personality development.

Group 3 (HV–LP) children, though relatively adept at many linguistic functions and at word recognition and spelling, also encounter considerable problems in the academic milieu; these are typically seen most clearly in the area of mechanical arithmetic and in some types of graphomotor performances. Other, only slightly less obvious, deficiencies are usually noted in the areas of reading comprehension, natural science, and a host of other academic skill areas that require age-appropriate judgment and reasoning. In addition, these children suffer from very marked social learning difficulties. Their failures to deal effectively with cause-and-effect relationships, social cues, novel problem situations, personal social distance (territoriality), facial and emotional recognition, prosodic cues, humor, time durations, and a host of related deficiencies render them all but social outcasts in most social milieux by the time they reach early adolescence. This state of affairs tends to become more exaggerated with the passage of time, especially in the areas of fine psychomotor coordination, problem solving, strategy generation, and higher order concept formation (Rourke, Fisk, & Strang, 1986; Rourke, Young, Strang, & Russell, 1985). In our view, these developmental deficiencies continue and worsen in their effects because of the progressive degeneration of right-hemispheric systems. In this connection, it may very well be the case that lack of access to these systems—possibly as a result of impaired or impoverished interhemispheral connections—serves to promote their degeneration through disuse. This last point requires a degree of elaboration that would go far beyond the scope of this chapter (see Rourke, 1987, for an extended treatment of this and related issues).

For now, we wish simply to emphasize the point that neurodevelopmental differences in the acquisition and elaboration of new descriptive systems would appear to be related to the differential integrity of left- and right-hemispheric systems, and that this state of affairs can and does lead to quite distinct modes of information-processing capabilities that have markedly different implications for adaptation at all stages of ontogenetic development.

REFERENCES

Benson, D. F., & Geschwind, N. (1970). Developmental Gerstmann syndrome. *Neurology, 20,* 293–298.

Black, F. W. (1974). Self-concept as related to achievement and age in learning disabled children. *Child Development, 45,* 1137–1140.

Breen, M. J., & Barkley, R. A. (1984). Psychological adjustment in learning disabled, hyperactive, and hyperactive/learning-disabled children as measured by the Personality Inventory for Children. *Journal of Clinical Child Psychology, 13,* 232–236.

Dunn, L. M. (1965). *Expanded manual for the Peabody Picture Vocabulary Test.* Minneapolis: American Guidance Services.

Fisk, J. L., Fuerst, D., & Rourke, B. P. (in preparation). *Examination of the relationship between WISC VIQ-PIQ discrepancies and the Personality Inventory for Children.*

Fisk, J. L., & Rourke, B. P. (1979). Identification of subtypes of learning-disabled children at three age levels: A neuropsychological, multivariate approach. *Journal of Clinical Neuropsychology, 1,* 289–310.

Fletcher, J. M. (1985). External validation of learning disability typologies. In B. P. Rourke (Ed.), *Neuropsychology of learning disabilities: Essentials of subtype analysis* (pp. 187–211). New York: Guilford Press.

Goldberg, E., & Costa, L. D. (1981). Hemisphere differences in the acquisition and use of descriptive systems. *Brain and Language, 14,* 144–173.

Halechko, A. D. (1977). Self-esteem and perception of parental behavior in children with learning disabilities. *Dissertation Abstracts International, 38,* 359B. (University Microfilms No. 77-15, 246.)

Jastak, J. F., & Jastak, S. R. (1965). *The Wide Range Achievement Test.* Wilmington, DE: Guidance Associates.

Kinsbourne, M., & Warrington, E. K. (1963). The developmental Gerstmann syndrome. *Archives of Neurology, 8,* 490–501.

Klove, H. (1963). Clinical neuropsychology. In F. M. Forster (Ed.), *The medical clinics of North America.* New York: Saunders.

Knights, R. M., & Norwood, J. A. (1980). *Smoothed normative data on the neuropsychological test battery for children.* Ottawa, Ontario: Author.

Myklebust, H. R. (1975). Nonverbal learning disabilities: Assessment and intervention. In H. R. Myklebust (Ed.), *Progress in learning disabilities* (Vol. 3, pp. 85–121). New York: Grune and Stratton.

Ozols, E. J., & Rourke, B. P. (1985). Dimensions of social sensitivity in two types of learning-disabled children. In B. P. Rourke (Ed.), *Neuropsychology of learning disabilities: Essentials of subtype analysis* (pp. 281–301). New York: Guilford Press.

Ozols, E. J., & Rourke, B. P. (1988). Characteristics of young learning-disabled children classified according to patterns of academic achievement: Auditory–perceptual and visual–perceptual abilities. *Journal of Clinical Child Psychology, 17,* 44–52.

Ozols, E. J., & Rourke, B. P. (in preparation). Characteristics of young learning-disabled children classified according to patterns of academic achievement: Motor, psychomotor, and tactile–perceptual abilities.

Piaget, J. (1954). *The construction of reality in the child.* New York: Basic Books.

Pohlman, C. L. (1983). *PIC factor scales: An investigation of broad-band dimensions of psychopathology among personality subtypes of learning-disabled children.* Unpublished master's thesis, University of Windsor.

Porter, J. E., & Rourke, B. P. (1985). Socioemotional functioning of learning-disabled children: A subtypal analysis of personality patterns. In B. P. Rourke (Ed.), *Neuropsychology of learning disabilities: Essentials of subtype analysis* (pp. 257–279). New York: Guilford Press.

Reitan, R. M., & Davison, L. A. (Eds.). (1974). *Clinical neuropsychology: Current status and applications.* Washington, DC: Winston.

Rourke, B. P. (1975). Brain–behavior relationships in children with learning disabilities: A research program. *American Psychologist, 30,* 911–920.

Rourke, B. P. (1976). Reading retardation in children: Developmental lag or deficit? In R. M. Knights & D. J. Bakker (Eds.), *Neuropsychology of learning disorders: Theoretical approaches* (pp. 125–137). Baltimore, MD: University Park Press.

Rourke, B. P. (1978). Reading, spelling, arithmetic disabilities: A neuro-psychologic perspective. In H. R. Myklebust (Ed.), *Progress in learning disabilities* (Vol. 4, pp. 97–120). New York: Grune and Stratton.

Rourke, B. P. (1982). Central processing deficiencies in children: Toward a developmental neuropsychological model. *Journal of Clinical Neuropsychology, 4,* 1–18.

Rourke, B. P. (1983). Reading and spelling disabilities: A developmental neuropsychological perspective. In U. Kirk (Ed.), *Neuropsychology of language, reading, and spelling* (pp. 209–234). New York: Academic Press.

Rourke, B. P. (Ed.). (1985). *Neuropsychology of learning disabilities: Essentials of subtype analysis.* New York: Guilford Press.

Rourke, B. P. (1987). Syndrome of nonverbal learning disabilities: The final common pathway of white-matter disease/dysfunction? *Clinical Neuropsychologist, 1,* 209–234.

Rourke, B. P. (in press) Socio-emotional disturbances of learning-disabled children. *Journal of Consulting and Clinical Psychology.*

Rourke, B. P., Bakker, D. J., Fisk, J. L., & Strang, J. D. (1983). *Child neuropsychology: An introduction to theory, research, and clinical practice.* New York: Guilford Press.

Rourke, B. P., Dietrich, D. M., & Young, G. C. (1973). Significance of WISC Verbal–Performance discrepancies for younger children with learning disabilities. *Perceptual and Motor Skills, 36,* 275–282.

Rourke, B. P., & Finlayson, M. A. J. (1978). Neuropsychological significance of variations in patterns of academic performance: Verbal and visual–spatial abilities. *Journal of Abnormal Child Psychology, 6,* 121–133.

Rourke, B. P., & Fisk, J. L. (1981). Socioemotional disturbances of learning disabled children: The role of central processing deficits. *Bulletin of the Orton Society, 31,* 77–88.

Rourke, B. P., Fisk, J. L., & Strang, J. D. (1986). *Neuropsychological assessment of children: A treatment-oriented approach.* New York: Guilford Press.

Rourke, B. P., & Strang, J. D. (1978). Neuropsychological significance of variations in patterns of academic performance: Motor, psychomotor, and tactile–perceptual abilities. *Journal of Pediatric Psychology, 3,* 62–66.

Rourke, B. P., & Strang, J. D. (1983). Subtypes of reading and arithmetical disabilities: A neuropsychological analysis. In M. Rutter (Ed.), *Developmental neuropsychiatry* (pp. 473–488). New York: Guilford Press.

Rourke, B. P., & Telegdy, G. A. (1971). Lateralizing significance of WISC Verbal–Performance discrepancies for older children with learning disabilities. *Perceptual and Motor Skills, 33,* 875–883.

Rourke, B. P., Young, G. C., & Flewelling, R. W. (1971). The relationships between WISC Verbal–Performance discrepancies and selected verbal, auditory perceptual, and problem-solving abilities in children with learning disabilities. *Journal of Clinical Psychology, 27,* 475–479.

Rourke, B. P., Young, G. C., Strang, J. D., & Russell, D. L. (1985). Adult outcomes of central processing deficiencies in childhood. In I. Grant & K. M. Adams (Eds.), *Neuropsychological assessment in neuropsychiatric disorders: Clinical methods and empirical findings* (pp. 244–267). New York: Oxford University Press.

Sparrow, S. S., Balla, D. A., & Cicchetti, D. B. (1984). *The Vineland Adaptive Behavior Scales; A revision of the Vineland Social Maturity Scale by Edgar A. Doll.* Circle Pines, MN: American Guidance Services.

Stewart, M. L. (1986). *The adaptive behavior characteristics of learning-disabled children classified by patterns of academic achievement.* Unpublished master's thesis, University of Windsor.

Strang, J. D. (1981). *Personality dimensions of learning-disabled children: Age and subtype differences.* Unpublished doctoral dissertation, University of Windsor.

Strang, J. D., & Rourke, B. P. (1983). Concept-formation/non-verbal reasoning abilities of children who exhibit specific academic problems with arithmetic. *Journal of Clinical Child Psychology, 12,* 33–39.

Strang, J. D., & Rourke, B. P. (1985a). Adaptive behavior of children with specific arithmetic disabilities and associated neuropsychological abilities and deficits. In B. P. Rourke (Ed.), *Neuropsychology of learning disabilities: Essentials of subtype analysis* (pp. 302–328). New York: Guilford Press.

Strang, J. D., & Rourke, B. P. (1985b). Arithmetic disability subtypes: The neuropsychological significance of specific arithmetic impairment in childhood. In B. P. Rourke (Ed.), *Neuropsychology of learning disabilities: Essentials of subtype analysis* (pp. 167–183). New York: Guilford Press.

Wechsler, D. (1949). *Wechsler Intelligence Scale for Children.* New York: Psychological Corporation.

Wirt, R. D., Lachar, D., Klinedinst, J. K., & Seat, P. D. (1977). *Multidimensional description of child personality: A manual for the Personality Inventory for Children.* Los Angeles: Western Psychological Services.

Zimmerman, I. L., & Allebrand, G. N. (1965). Personality characteristics and attitudes toward achievement of good and poor readers. *Journal of Educational Research, 57,* 28–30.

21

Deficient Lateralization in Learning-Disabled Children: Developmental Lag or Abnormal Cerebral Organization?

JOHN E. OBRZUT
University of Arizona

This chapter reviews the data on perceptual asymmetries in learning-disabled children and attempts to draw inferences regarding the developmental implications of brain lateralization. The intent is to provide some perspective on laterality mechanisms as assessed by noninvasive techniques in a group of children who have presumed neurodevelopmental anomalies. The major question addressed is whether deficiencies experienced by learning-disabled children in academic tasks are due to developmental lags or to abnormal brain organization.

HISTORICAL PERSPECTIVE OF LEARNING DISABILITIES

Interest in the relationship between learning disabilities and neurological factors has existed since the late 1800s, but systematic study of this relationship has only taken place within the last several decades.

Regardless of the particular label used to describe this condition, the assumption held is that deficiencies in cognitive tasks such as reading and language skills have been attributed to an abnormal or weak pattern of lateralization (Orton, 1937). This assumption has been tested in numerous studies, most of which have not shown conclusive evidence to substantiate this claim. However, these studies have usually contained serious methodological flaws such as inadequate sampling procedures and improper use of statistical designs, lack of sophisticated research techniques and equipment, and inadequate or unreliable operational definitions of the learning disability syndrome (Bryden, 1982).

One of the major reasons for the lack of conclusive evidence in this line of inquiry is that, although there is an enormous volume of literature available on the topic of brain asymmetry and lateralization of function, relatively few of these studies have used well-defined samples of learning-disabled children. The heterogeneous nature of these samples selected in most research does not allow for valid generalization across studies. Additionally, sample selection for laterality studies has included individuals from school as well as clinic/hospital settings. Children chosen from the latter institutions are often very different (i.e., more severe) in their presenting symptomatology. Thus, the results from these populations are inconsistent with the results of studies that use school populations. Learning-disabled groups drawn from school populations have generally been selected on the basis of criteria for placement in special education classes according to federal and state guidelines. A multidisciplinary team including a certified school psychologist participates in the child's diagnosis and resulting special class placement. In order to qualify, the student must have demonstrated average intellectual potential (Wechsler Intelligence Scale for Children—Revised [WISC-R] IQ>80); evidence a processing deficit in reception, discrimination, association, organization/integration, retention, or application of information; and exhibit a 2-year achievement deficit on one or more standardized individual achievement tests such as the Woodcock Reading Mastery Test or the Key Math Diagnostic Test.

Laterality and Learning Disabilities

Cerebral lateralization is of considerable interest when it is related to a presumed anomalous population such as the learning disabled. In general, learning-disabled children have been thought to exhibit characteristics similar to those found in neurologically impaired individuals. Specifically, from his review of the literature, Corballis (1983) suggests that learning-disabled children's poor academic performance on cognitive tasks, such as reading, could be the result of an abnormal or weak pattern of lateralization (p. 171). Thus, the study of lateral preference patterns via performance on tests of perceptual asymmetries in learning-disabled children may elucidate the relationship between cerebral organization and academic achievement. Further, if one attributes cognitive deficits to abnormal cerebral lateralization, then it remains to be determined whether the weak lateralization is the result of developmental delay or of basic structural differences in brain organization.

The following material reviews evidence for lateralization as determined by motor and perceptual functions in learning-disabled children to examine whether this lateralization differs from that of normal control subjects. Laterality techniques, hypotheses, and research findings relative to learning-disabled groups are discussed.

Lateral Preference Research

Laterality has been studied extensively through indirect methods or behavioral techniques. One behavioral technique involves motor preference as measured by handedness, eyedness, and footedness. The other primary technique involves the measurement of perceptual asymmetries via dichotic listening, visual half-field presentation, and verbal–manual time sharing. By using these measures of motor preference and perceptual asymmetries, inferences about cerebral dominance (i.e., lateralization) for language function can be made.

Early studies of lateral preference related deficits in academic achievement to poorly established handedness, eyedness, and footedness in learning-disabled children, but only handedness has received more than a cursory examination. It is often assumed that deficits found in learning-disabled children on measures of handedness are reflective of poorly established functional laterality. Thus, if a child is left-handed and learning-disabled, it is thought that the left-handedness reflects the fact that language abilities have been lateralized to the right cerebral hemisphere. However, the relation between handedness and cerebral organization is very weak and it is difficult to interpret a difference between left- and right-handedness in terms of differences in cerebral organization (Bryden & Saxby, 1986). For example, it has been shown from the study of aphasic patients that approximately two-thirds of all left-handers are lateralized to the left cerebral hemisphere for speech function, as are the majority of right-handed individuals (Annett, 1975).

With regard to handedness, it has often been concluded that learning-disabled children demonstrate weak preferences and that left-handers are often poor readers (Kinsbourne & Hiscock, 1978). However, according to a comprehensive survey conducted by Hardyck and Petrinovitch (1977), there is little evidence to support the notion that left-handers are poor readers. In support of these authors, Heim and Watts (1976) failed to find that left-handers do less well than right-handed counterparts on cognitive measures relating to verbal, visuospatial, and numerical reasoning. In fact, left-handers performed significantly better than right-handers on the numerical reasoning measure. In a study of 5- to 14-year-olds, McCormick (1978) found no overall difference in hand preference in normals as compared with children who were experiencing learning, emotional, and behavioral problems.

Other well-controlled studies have examined lateral preference patterns in relation to performance on measures of cognitive ability in children (Hardyck, Petrinovitch, & Goldman, 1976; Kaufman, Zalma, & Kaufman, 1978; Ullman, 1977). Clearly, there is little or no relationship between handedness and poor achievement on cognitive tasks. It has been argued elsewhere that investigating cerebral lateralization indirectly through handedness may well overestimate the small correlation between handedness and language lateralization (Segalowitz & Bryden, 1983). Thus, the best evidence regarding laterality and cerebral organization is derived from studies that have used more direct noninvasive measures of central language processing with learning-disabled children.

Dichotic listening and visual half-field techniques have been used primarily to investigate this hemispheric organization. Although these research techniques have accounted for most of the experimental/behavioral methodology, other methods, such as hemispheric verbal–manual time sharing (Dalby & Gibson, 1981; Hughes & Sussman, 1983; Obrzut, Hynd, Obrzut, & Leitgeb, 1980), have also been employed as noninvasive techniques to examine lateralization of language.

DICHOTIC LISTENING

The dichotic listening technique has been used extensively in the assessment of lateralized language abilities. This technique was originally conceived by Broadbent (1956) as an experimental paradigm to investigate a mechanical model of memory. The procedure involves presenting paired stimuli simultaneously to each ear. Stimuli used in research include digits, words, consonant–vowel (CV) syllables, and sentences. The stimuli reported by the subject will usually provide evidence of an "ear effect," where a greater proportion of the dichotic stimuli are correctly reported favoring one ear.

Working with normal adult subjects, Kimura (1961a, 1961b) demonstrated that the majority of right-handed subjects correctly identified more stimuli presented to the right ear when the stimuli were verbal, and more stimuli presented to the left ear when the stimuli were nonverbal. Since this initial work, the dichotic listening technique has been employed in many experiments as a measure of speech lateralization for both adults and children. Whereas early research used the dichotic listening task to examine brain-damaged adults (Kimura, 1961a, 1961b; 1963, 1967), more recent focus has been directed at observing whether normal cerebral asymmetry exists in children with disorders of learning. Most normal (right-handed) children report right-ear stimuli more accurately than left. This right-ear advantage (REA) is thought to reflect left-hemisphere representation for language. However, studies using the dichotic listening paradigm with reading/learning-disabled populations have not produced a consistent pattern of findings.

A summary of the main results of all studies that report data on left–right ear asymmetry for reading/learning-disabled groups, regardless of type of dichotic response required, is presented in Table 21-1. The methodological problems in these studies are numerous, with perhaps the greatest difficulty being the lack of an agreed-on operational definition of the learning disability syndrome. In spite of this problem, however, the di-

Table 21-1. Summary of Results of Studies on Verbal Dichotic Tests in Reading/Learning-Disabled Children

Study	Subjects	Stimuli	Response	Score	Results
Bakker, Smink, & Reitsma, 1973	Experiment I: 7 yr old, n=40, B & G	3 pairs of digits	FR	Number correct per ear	Positive relation between ear dominance and reading ability at 9–11 yr of age. In younger subjects, negative relation between ear dominance and reading. Conclusions suggest gradual increasing of lateralization.
	Experiment II: 8–9 yr old, n=38, B & G	30 series of 5 digits	FR	Number correct per ear	
	Experiment III: 7–11 yr old, n=100 B & G	6 series of 4 digits, 8 series of 5 digits, 4 series of 6 digits	FR	Number correct per ear	
Bryden, 1970	7, 9, 11, yr old, n=152, B & G	2 & 3 pairs of digits	FR	Side of greater accuracy	Only about 58% of the 7-year-old group showed greater right- than left-ear scores, and this proportion increased with age. No sex difference.
Hynd & Obrzut, 1981	7–12 yr old, n=90, G & B	30 pairs of CVs	FR	Mean number correct per ear	REA for normals & LDs. LDs performance was poorer than normals.
Hynd, Obrzut, Weed, & Hynd, 1979	7–12 yr old, n=96, G & B	30 pairs of CVs	FR	Mean number correct per ear	REA for normals and LDs. LD performance was quantitatively lower than normals.
McKeever & Van Deventer, 1975	11–18 yr old, n=18, B	Experiment II: 3 pairs of digits	FR	Number incorrect per ear	REA for normals and dyslexics, but normals performed significantly better.
Mercure & Warren, 1978	8–10 yr old, n=57, B & G	60 pairs of CVs	FR	Mean number correct per ear	REA for normals and inadequate readers, but normals performed significantly better.
Obrzut, 1979	2nd & 4th graders, n=144, B	2 & 3 pairs of digits	FR	Number correct per ear	REA for normals and 3 dyslexic groups. Alexic and dysphonetic LD groups had poorer performance than normals and dyseidetic subjects.
Obrzut, Hynd, & Obrzut, 1983	9–12 yr old, n=46, G & B	30 pairs of CVs	FR, DR, DL	Mean number correct per ear per condition	REA for normals. Attentional bias evident in DR & DL conditions for LDs.
Obrzut, Hynd, Obrzut, & Leitgeb, 1980	7–11 yr old, n=96, G & B	30 pairs of CVs	FR	Mean number correct per ear	REA for normals & LDs but LD performance quantitatively lower than normals.
Obrzut, Hynd, Obrzut, & Pirozzolo, 1981	7–13 yr old, n=64, G & B	30 pairs of CVs	FR, DL, DR	Mean number correct per ear per condition	REA for normals and LDs. No REA for LDs in DL condition.
Obrzut, Obrzut, Bryden, & Bartels, 1985	7–12 yr old, n=32, G & B	30 pairs of CV syllables	FR, DR, DL	Mean number correct per ear per condition	REA observed for normal subjects. Weaker REA for LD in FR and no REA in directed attention.
Sadick & Ginsburg, 1978	5–6 yr old, n=81; 7 yr old, n=68; 8–11 yr old, n=26	60 pairs of CVs	FR	Mean number correct per ear	Small L–R ear difference in 7-yr-old good readers. Significant difference found in ear advantage in 8–11-yr-old good readers. Relationship between reading ability and language lateralization exists, but it is negative and age-dependent.

Study	Subjects	Stimuli	Response	Score	Results
Satz, Rardin, & Ross, 1971	7–8, 11–12 yr old, $n = 20$, B	3 pairs of digits	FR	Percentage correct per ear	Both age groups showed REA.
Sparrow & Satz, 1970	9–12 yr old, $n = 80$, B	4 pairs of digits	FR	Number correct per ear	REA for normals and dyslexics, but 4 times as many dyslexics had LEA (28% vs. 8%).
Springer & Eisenson, 1977	8 yr & older, $n = 20$, B & G	30 pairs of CVs	FR	Mean number correct per ear	REA for normals and language-disordered, but normals performed significantly better. Size of ear asymmetry inversely related to severity of linquistic impairment.
Witelson, 1976	6–14 yr old, $n = 245$, G & B	2 & 3 pairs of digits	FR	Number correct per ear	REA observed for each age-sex subgroup.
Witelson & Rabinovitch, 1972	8–13 yr old, $n = 48$, B & G	2 & 3 pairs of digits (3 different rates)	FR	Number correct per ear	No significant REA in the LD or normal group
Yeni-Komshian, Isenberg, & Goldberg, 1975	10–15 yr old, $n = 38$, B & G	3 pairs of digits	FR	Mean number correct per ear	REA for normals and poor readers, but normals performed significantly better.
Zurif & Carson, 1970	4th-graders, $n = 28$, B & G	3 pairs of digits	FR	Number correct per ear	Normal readers showed REA while dyslexics were more accurate in reporting LE stimuli.

Abbreviations: DL (directed left-ear report); DR (directed right-ear report); Abbreviations: B (boys); FR (free recall); G (girls); LD (learning-disabled); REA (right-ear advantage)

chotic listening paradigm has produced several viable hypotheses concerning the relationship between cerebral laterality and learning disabilities. Hypotheses such as incomplete cerebral dominance, maturational lag, and attentional bias for learning disabilities have been advocated.

Incomplete Dominance Hypothesis

The incomplete cerebral dominance hypothesis is similar to the verbal–nonverbal model earlier proposed by Kimura (1967). This model suggests that the superiority of each ear for verbal or nonverbal material reflects the functional specialization of the contralateral hemisphere (see Witelson, 1977, for a review). Early studies with learning-disabled children were conducted by Zurif and Carson (1970) and Witelson and Rabinovitch (1972). These authors reported that the normal children demonstrated a REA that bordered on statistical significance, whereas the dyslexic group exhibited a slight tendency to recall more material accurately from the left ear than from the right ear. Thus, although some support was provided for the incomplete cerebral dominance theory of dyslexia, the results are limited in theoretical significance by the marginality of the effects.

Bryden (1970) and Sparrow and Satz (1970) did not find significant differences in right-ear superiority between good and poor readers. Other researchers have demonstrated a significant REA for both normal and learning-disabled groups using dichotic lists of numbers or words (e.g., Leong, 1976; McKeever & Van Deventer, 1975; Witelson, 1976; Yeni-Komshian, Isenberg, & Goldberg, 1975). For example, McKeever and Van Deventer

(1975) compared a small sample of dyslexic ($N=9$) and normal ($N=9$) male adolescents (mean age 13.7 years) on the dichotic task and found that although both the dyslexic and the control children demonstrated a significant right-ear effect (left-hemisphere) for language, the dyslexics recalled less material from both sides of space than did the normals.

The results of these studies of an auditory nature tend to contradict the hypothesis that learning-disabled children are not as well lateralized for language functioning as are normal control children. Therefore, it may be proposed that there is little support for the hypothesis that the nature of dysfunction in learning-disabled children is incomplete lateralization that directly affects intellectual or cognitive processes. It is more likely that language is lateralized in both normal and learning-disabled children, but that the efficiency of the language processor is less functional in learning-disabled children and may represent one aspect of a more general maturational lag (Obrzut & Hynd, 1981).

The Maturational Lag Hypothesis

The basic notion underlying the maturational lag hypothesis stems from the work of Lenneberg (1967) who contended that the left hemisphere becomes increasingly specialized for language during development. Therefore, in normal children, between-hemisphere differences in language mediation should increase as the child advances in age (Rourke, Bakker, Fisk, & Strang, 1983). Translating this to dichotic listening performance, one should expect to find that the dichotic REA for verbal material increases with age during the primary school years. As Bryden and Saxby (1986) conclude, although there have been a few reports of a gradually increasing right-ear effect (e.g., Larsen, 1984; Satz, Bakker, Teunissen, Goebel, & Van der Vlugt, 1975), it is now generally agreed that there are no systematic changes in either the magnitude or the incidence of a right-ear effect in children in the age range 5 to 14 (cf. Berlin, Hughes, Lowe-Bell, & Berlin, 1973; Bryden & Allard, 1981; Geffen, 1976, 1978; Goodglass, 1973; Hynd & Obrzut, 1977; Saxby & Bryden, 1984). This theory also predicts a lag in the maturation of the central nervous system (CNS) in learning-disabled children. In essence, learning-disabled children experience a delay of left-hemispheric specialization that may have a negative impact on their ability to acquire normal age-related cognitive skills.

Bakker and associates (Bakker, 1973; Bakker, Smink, & Reitsma, 1973; Bakker, Teunissen, & Bosch, 1976) as well as Satz and colleagues (Satz & Van Nostrand, 1972; Sparrow & Satz, 1970) have argued that there is a relationship between developmental dyslexia and degree of lateralization only among older dyslexic children. The theory predicts that motor, perceptual, and linguistic functions become successively important in learning to read, and lateralize to the dominant left hemisphere at different stages of development. From this theory, these researchers hypothesized that visual–motor and auditory–visual integration skills that presumably develop earlier would be delayed in younger dyslexic readers, while linguistic skills that develop later would be more delayed in older dyslexic children. This theory, of course, is based on the assumption that speech processes become more completely lateralized with increasing age.

Satz, Rardin, and Ross (1971) used the dichotic listening task in a cross-sectional study of younger (7–8 years) and older (11–12 years) dyslexic boys matched for age, sex, race, and IQ, with normal reader control groups. The results indicated that although a significant REA (left-hemisphere) was found in both groups of dyslexic children as well as in normals, the magnitude of the REA was significantly greater in the older normal group as compared with the older dyslexic group. No differences in magnitude were found between younger normals and dyslexics. This finding led the authors to conclude that the brain becomes increasingly lateralized with age but that this process does not occur as rapidly in dyslexic readers as it does in normal readers.

The studies in Holland conducted by Bakker and his associates (Bakker, 1973; Bakker *et al.*, 1973, 1976) have also reported patterns consistent with the theory that normal children have well-established cerebral lateralization, whereas dyslexics are lateralized like their younger normal counterparts. Further support for a developmental delay in dyslexic children comes from Witelson (1976) and Sadick and Ginsberg (1978). These studies found that good readers displayed a consistent decrease in ambilaterality and a consistent increase in magnitude of the REA with increasing age. In contrast, poor readers displayed little evidence of a shift in ambilaterality with age.

It is difficult to accept a theory that postulates a developmental lag in the establishment of cerebral lateralization when there is little convincing evidence that there are any systematic changes in cerebral lateralization with age (see Bryden, 1982, for a review). It is interesting to note that differences between normal and dyslexic children have been reported less frequently when single pairs of CV syllables, such as stop consonants, have been employed in dichotic studies (see Mercure & Warren, 1978; Springer & Eisenson, 1977). However, methodological problems, such as poor selection criteria employed in sampling, complicate any clear understanding of the results. Recently, a series of studies using well-defined groups of learning-disabled children and normal counterparts have been carried out by Obrzut and his associates (Hynd & Obrzut, 1981; Hynd, Obrzut, Weed, & Hynd, 1979; Obrzut, Hynd, Obrzut, & Leitgeb, 1980; Obrzut, Hynd, Obrzut, & Pirozzolo, 1981) in an attempt to investigate the developmental hypothesis.

In a representative study by Hynd *et al.* (1979), the magnitude of the dichotic right-ear advantage was assessed in 48 normal and 48 learning-disabled children matched according to age, gender, and handedness. The subjects were divided into two groups: a younger group of 24 children (mean age = 8.3 years) and an equally large group of older children (mean age = 10.6 years). All subjects were clinically diagnosed as learning-disabled according to state and federal guidelines as described earlier.

Table 21-2 presents the number of correctly reported CV syllables summed for each ear according to developmental levels for both the normal and the learning-disabled children. The results indicated that although both the normal and the learning-disabled children

Table 21-2. Mean Number of Correctly Reported CV Syllables for Each Ear by the Normal and Learning-Disabled Children

			Left ear		Right ear	
Subject group	Developmental level (age range)	N	$\bar{X}$	S.D.	$\bar{X}$	S.D.
Learning disabled	Younger (7 yr 0 mo to 9 yr 6 mo)	24	10.21	2.67	11.83	3.31
	Older (9 yr 7 mo to 11 yr 11 mo)	24	8.38	3.56	12.67	5.32
Normal	Younger (7 yr 0 mo to 9 yr 6 mo)	24	11.67	3.56	14.17	4.59
	Older (9 yr 7 mo to 11 yr 11 mo)	24	10.58	2.60	14.79	2.61

Source: Reprinted with permission from "Development of Cerebral Dominance: Dichotic Listening Asymmetry in Normal and Learning Disabled Children" by G. W. Hynd, J. E. Obrzut, W. Weed, and C. R. Hynd, 1979, *Journal of Experimental Child Psychology, 28,* pp. 445–454.

Note: A total source of 30 was possible for each ear.

reported a significant REA, $F(1,92) = 22.29$, $p < .001$), a significant difference existed between the two groups, $F(1,92) = 36.75$. More important, no significant developmental effect or interactions were noted. The authors concluded that no developmental lag or delay existed between normal and learning-disabled children in terms of lateralized language processing. The authors went on to suggest that any differences between these groups of children were attributable to differences in selective attention that resulted in a higher rate of guessing among the learning-disabled children. These results raise serious question about the idea that learning-disabled children do not display the same *degree* of cerebral language lateralization as normal children.

In summary, although most of the studies using older dyslexic children and normal reader controls have reported that both groups demonstrate the REA (left-hemisphere), the dyslexic children perform at a degraded level in comparison to their normal counterparts. These findings were interpreted, for example, by Bakker *et al.* (1976), Leong (1976), and Satz (1976) as support for a developmental lag theory of dyslexia. Other researchers, such as Witelson (1976), interpret their cross-sectional data as indicating a disorder in left-hemispheric functioning for speech in dyslexic children. Finally, the studies conducted by Hynd *et al.* (1979), Hynd and Obrzut (1981), and Obrzut *et al.* (1980, 1981) do not support the notion that cerebral lateralization increases with age. These studies suggest that lateralized language capabilities exist in normal children from ages 6 through 12. Furthermore, it appears that these lateralized language asymmetries do not develop after age 6, nor are they affected by gender. The findings also indicate that differences in lateralized language processes between normal and learning-disabled children are not due to delayed cerebral dominance but, rather, are likely due to attentional deficiencies in the learning-disabled children. As Bryden (1982) suggests, the differences between normals and dyslexics could be attributed to differences in the strategies that subjects adopt for performing the task rather than to differences in cerebral lateralization.

Attentional Bias Hypothesis

Following this line of thinking, Kinsbourne (1970) earlier proposed an alternative hypothesis of functional asymmetry. His model of lateral functioning states that the REA results from a selective arousal of the left hemisphere for verbal activity. The expectation of a verbal task selectively activates the left hemisphere, which causes a shift in attention toward the right side of space (i.e., language activity would lead to a tendency to turn the head and eyes to the right). Kinsbourne's model emphasizes situational variables of selectivity, attention, planning, and related factors. Even the expectancy for verbal input would serve to activate the left hemisphere and bias attention to the right side. Conversely, a set for nonverbal stimuli would activate the right hemisphere and bias attention to the left side.

In an effort to test the attentional hypothesis, the role of directed attention in dichotic listening performance has been examined (Dean & Hua, 1982; Geffen, 1978; Hiscock & Kinsbourne, 1980; Obrzut *et al.*, 1981). However, the only data gathered on a learning-disabled population were reported by Obrzut *et al.* (1981). In an attempt to minimize or control for the effects of variability in selective attention, these researchers employed a prestimulus cueing paradigm with a group of 32 learning-disabled children matched with 32 normal children. The matched pairs ranged in age from 7 years 6 months to 13 years 2 months and were divided into two age levels. The dichotic stimuli consisted of 30 pairs of synthesized consonant–vowel (CV) syllables. After a free-recall condition, a prestimulus cueing procedure was used. Each child was told to listen carefully and report only stimuli received in the one (target) ear.

The number of correctly reported dichotic CV syllables by group, age level, and condition is reported in Table 21-3. In the free-recall condition, both groups clearly demonstrated a significant REA, $F(1,60)=60.83$, $p<.001$. No developmental effect existed. When attention was directed to the left perceptual field (left ear), however, an interaction, $F(1,60)=17.14$, $p<.001$, between subject group and ear effect was found. The normal children did not shift their ear effect, but the learning-disabled subjects dramatically reversed their ear effect, showing a strong LEA. When attention was directed toward the stimuli presented to the right ear, a similar interaction was found, $F(1,60)=57.85$, $p<.001$, in that whereas both groups of children showed a REA, the learning-disabled children could increase the magnitude of the between-ear difference. From these results, it appears that learning-disabled children show attentional biases on a dichotic task if asked to direct attention toward the stimuli presented to a targeted ear. Although their performance generally was deficient when total accuracy was examined, the learning-disabled children were able to increase correct recognition of left- and right-ear presentations on cue from the examiner. The authors suggested that learning-disabled children probably do not suffer from developmental delays but, rather, from a defect in callosal functioning that interferes with their ability to process verbal information simultaneously (Obrzut *et al.*, 1981).

Additional evidence for the validity of these findings was obtained in a follow-up study conducted by Obrzut, Hynd, and Obrzut (1983). The directed dichotic task was administered as part of a comprehensive neuropsychological assessment battery to a matched population of 23 normal and 23 learning-disabled children. The matched pairs ranged in age from 9 years 1 month to 13 years 1 month. The stepwise discriminant function analysis illustrated that both of the directed dichotic tasks contributed the most of 13 neuropsycho-

Table 21-3. Mean Number of Correctly Reported Dichotic CV Syllables by Group, Age Level, and Condition

	Listening condition					
			Direction			
	Free recall		Left		Right	
Subject group/ age level	Left	Right	Left	Right	Left	Right
Normal						
Younger						
Mean	10.56	13.31	11.38	13.69	10.94	14.19
S.D.	1.86	2.39	3.16	3.00	2.41	1.91
Older						
Mean	11.06	13.81	10.88	13.19	11.06	13.88
S.D.	1.48	2.51	1.36	1.94	2.08	2.42
Learning-disabled						
Younger						
Mean	9.56	13.63	12.44	9.13	6.56	19.81
S.D.	1.75	1.46	3.54	2.96	1.67	2.54
Older						
Mean	8.88	13.44	11.94	9.69	6.56	18.50
S.D.	2.73	3.76	3.19	3.32	3.20	5.06

Source: Reprinted with permission from "Effect of Directed Attention on Cerebral Asymmetries in Normal and Learning Disabled Children" by J. E. Obrzut, G. W. Hynd, A. Obrzut, and F. J. Pirozzolo, 1981, *Developmental Psychology, 17*, pp. 118–125.

Note: Age range for younger group = 7.42–10.41 years, for older group = 10.42–13.17 years.

logical measures to the significant group separation. Normal children demonstrated a right-ear advantage (REA) in all conditions: free recall, directed left, directed right. Learning-disabled children, however, appeared susceptible to attentional biases on both directed conditions when compared with their free-recall performance. When attention was directed to the right ear, they dramatically increased their REA; when it was directed to the left ear, a left-ear advantage (LEA) was found. In contrast, normal children were not influenced by directed attention, as they were better able to report verbal information from the right ear while simultaneously attending to the left ear. This finding reflects the inherent REA and is consistent with the structural hypothesis predicting that the left hemisphere is prewired for language. When attention was directed, the learning-disabled children performed as if there were minimal interaction between the two cerebral hemispheres in processing the dichotic stimuli. Thus, the inclusion of the directed dichotic task was supportive of Kinsbourne's (1975) attentional biases theory and may be an important construct useful in the classification of learning disabilities.

Kinsbourne and Hiscock (1981) have suggested that the ability of the language-dominant hemisphere to mediate linguistic material verbally develops with a concurrent suppression of the (nondominant) right hemisphere. The results of the last two studies have indicated that, perhaps, in normal children, the mechanism of suppression of information from the nondominant hemisphere is established. Thus, the normal children cannot willingly attend to verbal stimuli with facility in an incompatible perceptual field. In contrast, the learning-disabled children, because of a failure of the linguistic information to be shared efficiently across the corpus callosum, have not established a mechanism for reciprocal inhibition and divide or direct attention to stimuli presented in either perceptual field.

Further efforts are needed to extend the theoretical and clinical implications of this research. For example, the work related to subtype analysis may shed some light on discrepancies found with auditory perceptual asymmetries. Until quite recently, researchers tended to view learning-disabled populations as homogeneous entities (Benton, 1975). However, the effort to identify subtypes of learning/reading-disabled children has been quite successful (e.g., Boder, 1973; Doehring, Hoshko, & Bryans, 1979; Fisk & Rourke, 1979; Mattis, French, & Rapin, 1975; Pirozzolo & Campanella, 1981; Satz & Morris, 1981). Most of these researchers have obtained data to demonstrate at least two types of disabled readers, those with auditory–linguistic problems and those with visuospatial problems. Perhaps not all poor readers would show weak lateralization or attentional biases, but only those who manifest certain deficiencies in expressive or receptive language (Bryden, 1982).

Some support for this hypothesis was found by Obrzut (1979), who employed the dichotic listening task with Boder's (1973) subtypes of dysphonetics and dyseidetics. He found that poorer auditory lateralization was characteristic of those readers with greater auditory–linguistic deficits (dysphonetic) than of those with visuospatial deficits (dyseidetics). However, no attempt was made to examine attentional factors with these groups of disabled readers. Clearly, the need is to examine ear effects of lateralized attention on carefully matched subtypes of learning/reading-disabled children.

VISUAL HALF-FIELD

The visual half-field (VHF) technique also has been employed as an experimental behavioral index of cerebral asymmetry. This technique involves the tachistoscopic presentation of verbal or spatial stimuli to either the right or the left visual field for unilateral presentations, or to both visual fields simultaneously for bilateral presentations. Stimuli perceived in the left VHF are processed in the right cerebral hemisphere; stimuli perceived in the right VHF are processed in the left cerebral hemisphere. The typical results of such lateralized tachistoscopic procedures reveal that normal subjects identify words and letters readily in the right VHF (left hemisphere) (Kimura, 1966), while nonverbal stimuli, such as faces and geometric forms, are recognized better in the left VHF (right hemisphere) (Kimura & Durnford, 1974).

Several studies with reading/learning-disabled children that have attempted to investigate the issue of left-hemisphere specialization for language functions utilizing lateral tachistoscopic presentation of linguistic stimuli are presented in Table 21-4. As with the dichotic listening literature, however, results have been inconsistent. For example, McKeever and Huling (1970) compared the performance of 10 normal children to that of 10 poor readers on the unilateral tachistoscopic presentation of four-letter nouns. Both groups demonstrated a significant right visual half-field advantage (RVHF) (left hemisphere). Thus, this study provides little support for the theory of incomplete or delayed cerebral dominance for speech in the reading disabled. Although other studies demonstrated that both reading-disabled and control children have an RVHF advantage (Bouma & Legein, 1977; Kershner, 1977; Marcel, Katz, & Smith, 1974; Marcel & Rajan, 1975; McKeever & Van Deventer, 1975), the poor readers showed a lesser degree of asymmetry in reporting words and letters.

For instance, Marcel, Katz, and Smith (1974) presented five-letter verbs and concrete nouns, horizontally displayed, to either the left or the right visual field. The groups of good and poor readers each consisted of 10 boys and 10 girls of approximately 8 years of age. No control for IQ, neurological impairment, sensory handicap, and/or emotional problems was reported. The results indicated that although a significant RVHF asymmetry (left hemisphere) was found in both the good and poor reader groups, the RVHF superiority was much attenuated in the poor readers. The authors concluded that good readers process linguistic data more asymmetrically than poor readers and were more in favor of a cerebral lateralization explanation of the results. A replication study conducted by Marcel and Rajan (1975) lends further support to such a conclusion.

McKeever and Van Deventer (1975) used both unilateral and bilateral tachistoscopic procedures with 9 dyslexic and control children ranging in age from 11 to 18 years (mean age = 12.9 years). Based on their results, McKeever and Van Deventer (1975) concluded that their older dyslexics possessed clear left-hemisphere language lateralization. The findings of a reduced RVHF on the unilateral task suggest that these dyslexic readers may have a dysfunction of the left hemisphere.

Kershner (1977) also used a bilateral presentation procedure with a group of 12 high-IQ gifted readers, 11 good readers, and 10 dyslexic readers. Although all reader groups demonstrated a significant RVHF (left-hemisphere) advantage, the gifted and good readers demonstrated a significantly higher RVHF score than did the dyslexic group. Although the dyslexic group reported more LVHF (right-hemisphere) stimuli than both the gifted and the good readers, a significant difference was reached only with the gifted reader group. The author also found that when he controlled for reading ability between the gifted and dyslexic reader groups, the cerebral dominance effect was eliminated. This led Kershner (1977) to conclude that reading impairment is related to hemispheric differences in processing reading material. The use of horizontally displayed words makes it possible that the overall RVHF superiority is influenced not only by cerebral lateralization but also by directional scanning factors. Perhaps these dyslexic readers use inefficient strategies of scanning and encoding words, rather than displaying poor cerebral lateralization.

Table 21-4. Summary of Results of Lateral Tachistoscopic Procedures with Linguistic Stimuli in Reading/Learning-Disabled Children

Study	Subjects	Stimuli	Response and score	Results
Bouma & Legein, 1977	9–14 yr old, $n=40$, B & G	23 lower-case letters, 48 familiar Dutch words. 3 stimuli: letters isolated, letters embedded between Xs, 2 × 24 words/WRD/ equally distributed over 3 lengths	Verbal recall. Percentage correct per condition.	Dyslexics and normals did equally well on isolated letters; dyslexics did poorer on embedded letters and words.
Kershner, 1977	10 yr old, $n=33$, G & B	4-letter familiar words, H, U	Verbal recall. Number of words correct per field.	Poor readers were inferior in RVF performance when compared with gifted and good readers. Poor readers produced higher LVF scores and lower VF difference.
Marcel, Katz, & Smith, 1974	7–8 yr old, $n=20$, G & B	5-letter familiar words, H, U	Verbal recall. Number of words and letters correct per field.	RFV obtained for both socres. Boys showed greater RFV.
Marcel & Rajan, 1975	7–9 yr old, $n=20$, G & B	5-letter familiar words, H, U	Verbal recall. Number of words and letters correct per field.	RVF obtained for both scores. No sex difference.
McKeever & Huling, 1970	13 yr old, $n=10$	4-letter familiar nouns, H, U	Verbal recall. Number of words correct per field.	RVF obtained. 8/10 subjects showed greater right field accuracy.
McKeever & Van Deventer, 1975	11–18 yr old, $n=18$, B	4-letter familiar words, H, U, Bi	Verbal recall. Number of words and letters correct per field, per condition.	Older dyslexics showed normal RVF dominance. In VRT to letter stimuli, dyslexics showed significantly faster RVF than LVF.
Obrzut, Hynd, & Zellner, 1983	7–13 yr old, $n=52$, G & B	4-letter familiar words, H, U, Bi	Nonverbal recall (pointing). Mean number correct per condition, per visual field.	RVF obtained for normals. LDs obtained RVF in unilateral condition but made visual and acoustical errors under bilateral condition.
Witelson, 1977	6–14 yr old, $n=86$, B	Pairs of same or different, upper-case, vertically arranged letters, U	Distinguish same or different. Number of pairs correct per field.	RVF obtained only in 6–7-yr-old subgroup.
Yeni-Komshian, Isenberg, & Goldberg, 1975	10–13 yr old, $n=19$, G & B	Experiment 1: Arabic digits, U Experiment 2: words (numbers), vertically arranged, U	Verbal recall. Percentage correct.	No RVF obtained.

Abbreviations: B (boys); Bi (bilateral); G (girls); H (horizontal); LD (learning disabled); LVF (left visual field); RVF (right visual field); U (unilateral); VRT (visual reaction time)

A similar question is raised when analyzing the results of another study conducted by Yeni-Komshian *et al.* (1975). These authors presented arabic numerals and vertically oriented words serially, with the first, third, and fifth words lateralized to one side, and the second and fourth words centered at fixation. The 19 poor readers and 19 good readers ranged in age from 10.6 to 13.4 years (mean age = 12.8). The results indicated that the poor readers showed a larger RVHF superiority (left hemisphere) for both numerals and words than did the good readers. This finding led the authors to conclude that the poor readers were more lateralized than the good readers. The good readers, however, did not produce a reliable RVHF (left-hemisphere) asymmetry. The effect found occurred largely because accuracy in the LVHF was much lower for poor readers than for good readers. The results, taken together, led the authors to suggest further that poor readers experience a right-hemispheric processing deficit or that interhemispheric processing is deficient in these readers. Because the task requires a shifting of attention from center to periphery, with the pattern being different for left and right visual-field presentations, it is possible that the poor readers have some specific form of processing deficit in the right hemisphere.

Witelson (1976) employed the unilateral tachistoscopic presentation of unfamiliar figures of people along with a dichotomous tactual stimulation test with nonsense shapes in order to study right-hemisphere superiority for spatial processing. The children were 85 right-handed boys of normal intelligence, ranging in age from 6 to 14 years, with a delay in reading achievement of 2.5 grade levels. The normal readers were 156 right-handed boys, also in the same age and IQ range.

The unilateral presentation of pictures of people required each child to view two pictures in either the left or the right visual field. The subjects were asked to indicate whether the stimuli were the same or different. Because the right hemisphere is specialized for spatial processing, the hypothesis was that the spatial stimuli (figures) would be better perceived when presented to the left visual half-field. As predicted, Witelson (1976) found that the normal readers showed a significant LVHF (right-hemisphere) superiority, whereas the dyslexic readers demonstrated a nonsignificant trend in the same direction. Additionally, whereas both groups showed reduced RVHF (left-hemisphere) scores, the dyslexic reader group showed a reduced LVHF (right-hemisphere) superiority as compared to the normal reader group. These findings led Witelson (1976) to conclude that whereas normal readers demonstrate the typical right-hemisphere specialization for visual–spatial processing, dyslexic readers either lack right-hemisphere spatial processing or function with bilateral spatial representation.

On the nonverbal dichotomous tactual-stimulation task, subjects were required to feel two different nonsense shapes simultaneously for 10 seconds, one with each hand. The subject was then required to choose those two stimuli from a visual display of six shapes. After 10 trials were administered, accuracy for each hand was analyzed. On this task, if the right hemisphere is more effective in processing spatial information, left-hand scores would be significantly higher than right-hand scores. Witelson (1976) reported that both groups showed greater left-hand (right-hemisphere) scores than right-hand scores. In addition, Witelson (1976) reported a highly significant interaction between reading groups and hand, with the dyslexic children demonstrating a slight right-hand advantage. Witelson's data also indicated that whereas left-hand superiority for younger dyslexic children (aged 5–9 years) was similar to that found in normal readers, older dyslexic children (aged 10–14 years) displayed a right-hand superiority. It appears, then, that differences between the two reading groups are more marked at later stages of development.

Taken together, the result of the tachistoscopic and dichotomous tactual stimulation tests in this study seem to suggest that right-hemisphere spatial processing is deficient in the dyslexics and that they may possess a bilateral representation of spatial functions. This bilateral spatial representation interferes with the processing of linguistic functions normally dependent on the left hemisphere. However, as Bryden (1982) suggests, Witelson's procedure does not provide any control over subjects' deployment of attention during the 10-second trial. Thus, the results may be more indicative of differences in attentional strategies between the reader groups rather than of differences in cerebral specialization.

Recently a study was designed to control for attentional effects and to determine the laterality difference in VHF performance between a group of carefully matched learning-disabled and normal controls (Obrzut, Hynd, & Zellner, 1983). Twenty-six learning-disabled children were matched with 26 normal children on the basis of gender, age, and handedness. The matched pairs (7 female, 14 males) ranged in age from 7 years 4 months to 13 years 1 month.

The stimulus materials consisted of eight sets of three four-letter words, including a target word (BEAR), a visually confusable feature word (DEAR), and an acoustically confusable word (FARE). Each subject was administered 32 unilateral word presentations, and 32 unilateral-cued word presentations. For the unilateral-cued condition, the subject was told the field (left or right) in which the word would be shown. Threshold exposure durations were 20 msec for both unilateral conditions and 40 msec for bilateral presentations. These exposure durations served to control for any possible directional-scanning artifact that may have confounded an estimate of cerebral asymmetry.

As can be seen by referring to Figure 21-1, the normals demonstrated a superior RVHF (left-hemisphere) advantage across all conditions, whereas the learning-disabled showed the expected RVHF (left hemisphere) advantage only in the unilateral-cued condition. In both the unilateral and bilateral conditions, the learning-disabled children recognized a greater number of stimuli presented to the left visual field (right hemisphere).

This result would appear to support the incomplete lateralization hypothesis of Orton (1937). Evidence against this hypothesis, however, comes from the fact that although learning-disabled children favored the left field over the right field under unilateral and bilateral presentations, these children did demonstrate the RVF superiority for word recognition under the directed-cueing condition. Because of this finding, Obrzut, Hynd, and Zellner (1983) concluded that the differences in performance do not lie solely in the functional asymmetry of the visual–verbal processor of the left hemisphere, but in the ability to direct

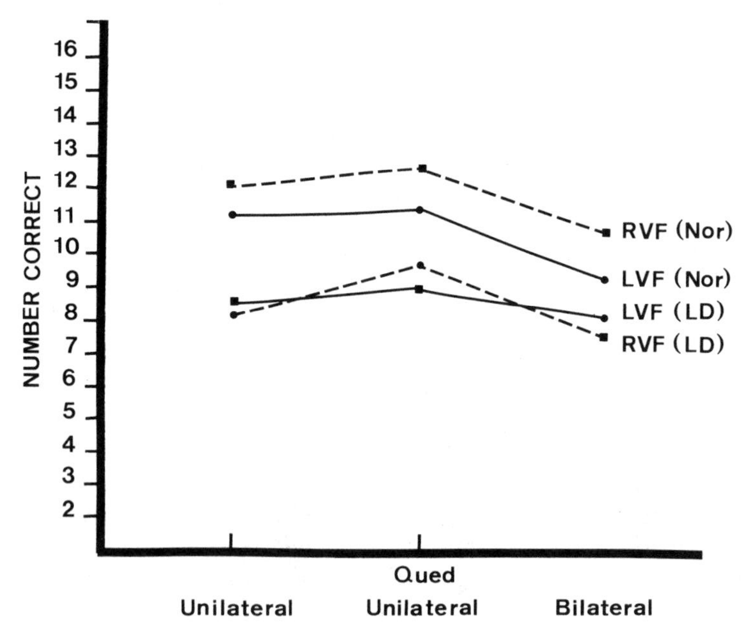

Figure 21-1. Mean number correct for the learning disabled and normal subjects by visual field and condition. Reprinted with permission from "Attentional Deficit in Learning-Disabled Children: Evidence from Visual Half-Field Asymmetries" by J. E. Obrzut, G. W. Hynd, and R. D. Zellner, 1983, *Brain and Cognition, 2,* 89–101.

attention alternately from one field to the other. Similar shifts in perceptual asymmetries due to directed cueing were shown using a dichotic listening paradigm (Obrzut *et al.*, 1981; Obrzut, Hynd, & Zellner, 1983).

It appears that structured cueing (i.e., by directing subjects' attention to stimuli) can modify laterality test outcome to a greater extent with learning-disabled children than with normal subjects. From the more recent work accomplished with both dichotic listening and visual half-field procedures, it is likely that learning-disabled children have brain activation patterns that are susceptible to attentional effects that are not found in normal children. The differences in degree of lateralization often found between reading/learning-disabled children and normal children may be strongly influenced by individual differences in processing strategies.

VERBAL–MANUAL TIME SHARING

Another behavioral assessment technique using motor output is the time-sharing paradigm. Time sharing is a type of experiment that contrasts the subjects' ability to perform concurrent activities when they are programmed in the same hemisphere (e.g., speaking and right manual activities) and when they are programmed in separate hemispheres (speaking and left manual activities). The consequence of this effect of "hemisphere sharing" appears to be competition and "cross talk" between incompatible timing mechanisms hierarchically organized in the brain (Kinsbourne & Cook, 1971). Unlike the strictly auditory and visual perceptual phenomena used in dichotic and tachistoscopic studies, this technique makes use of motor concomitants of lateralized cerebral processes that may allow for a more sensitive measure of developmental trends in lateralized function.

In normals, researchers such as Kinsbourne and McMurray (1975), using kindergarten children, and White and Kinsbourne (1980), using children 3 to 12 years of age, have generally found that children tap their fingers more slowly while simultaneously verbalizing, than when tapping without concurrent verbalization. Although the concurrent verbalization diminished the tapping rate of both hands, the right-hand tapping rate was lower than the left-hand tapping rate. Piazza (1977) also found that when the concurrent tasks were divided into verbal and nonverbal, the verbal task showed greater interference on the right-hand tapping (left-hemisphere) rate, whereas the nonverbal task has a greater effect on the left-hand tapping (right-hemisphere) rate.

Only recently have researchers employed the verbal–manual time-sharing technique as an index of aspects of hemisphere specialization. Table 21-5 summarizes a few such studies involving reading/learning-disabled children and their normal counterparts. One such study by Cermak, Cermak, Drake, and Kenney (1978) used a dichotic listening task concurrently with a manual tapping task with three groups of learning-disabled children and a normal control group. The authors concluded that various subtypes of the learning disabled are differentially lateralized and differentially affected by the facilitative–inhibitory effects of concurrent hemispheric activities.

Obrzut *et al.* (1980) also employed a time-sharing procedure with a group of 48 learning-disabled children and 48 normal children matched according to age, gender, and handedness. All subjects ranged in age from 7 years 0 months to 11 years 10 months. The learning-disabled children demonstrated at least average intelligence (WISC-R IQ > 80) and were delayed at least 2 years in achievement. All children preferred the use of their right hand for normal activities. The normal control children had average to above-average intelligence and were reading at or above their grade placements. In order to examine developmental trends in cerebral speech lateralization, subjects in both groups were divided

Table 21-5. Summary of Results of Studies on Verbal-Manual/Time-Sharing Tasks with Reading/Learning-Disabled Children

Study	Subjects	Stimuli	Score	Results
Cermak, Cermak, Drake, & Kenney, 1978	8–13-yr-old, $n = 61$, B	Verbal: 3 pairs of digits Manual: Finger tapping	Mean difference in ear report	3 types of LDs (based on WISC profiles) showed differential lateralization and were differentially affected by time sharing tasks.
Dalby & Gibson, 1981	9–12-yr-old, $n = 60$, B	Verbal: Animal names Spatial: Colored progressive matrices Manual: Finger tapping	Percentage change in tapping	Lateralization of verbal and/or spatial function differed among reading—disabled groups. (dysphonetic and dyseidetic)
Hughes & Sussman, 1983	4–7-yr-old, $n = 24$, G & B	Verbal: Speaking Manual: Finger tapping	Percentage change in tapping	All language concurrent tasks produced tapping reductions for both hands for both LDs and normals.
Obrzut, Hynd, Obrzut, & Leitgeb, 1980	7–11-yr-old, $n = 96$, G & B	Verbal: Animal names Manual: Finger tapping	Mean difference in tapping	Condition I: Normals outperformed LDs. Both had strong RH laterality tapping rate. Increased with age. Condition II: Showed asymmetry of interference for both groups.

into three age levels of 16 children each. The authors found that learning-disabled children were shown to tap slower than normals and had significantly greater magnitudes of concurrent task interference. Figure 21-2 represents the percentage decrease in tapping rate for the right and left hands. As shown by this figure, the right-hand decrement exceeds the left-hand decrement at all age levels in normal and learning-disabled children. Upon closer inspection of the data, however, it appears that the decrement for both hands revealed robust interference effects (right hand = 69%; left hand = 68%). Although the claim is made that these dual-task results support left-hemisphere language lateralization in both groups of children at all developmental levels, this effect may not be as strong when right-hemisphere interference exhibited during the verbal concurrent task is considered.

Dalby and Gibson (1981) used a time-sharing paradigm that involved verbal and spatial tasks concurrently in the assessment of 45 boys classified into three reading-disabled subtypes according to the Boder (1973) classification system. It was hypothesized that different types of reading disability would be associated with different patterns of lateralized brain function. Their results indicated that although the control group showed the typical left lateralization of language and right lateralization of spatial functions, the reading-disabled groups demonstrated atypical lateralization. Dysphonetic readers, who presumably make nonphonetic reading/spelling errors, showed bilateral representation of both verbal and spatial functions; dyseidetic readers, who presumably do not respond to words as gestalts, showed bilateral verbal representation and right lateralization of spatial functions; and the nonspecific readers, who make phonetically acceptable errors and respond to gestalts, showed left language lateralization and bilateral spatial representation. These results confirmed the authors' hypothesis that patterns of cerebral organization vary across types of reading disability.

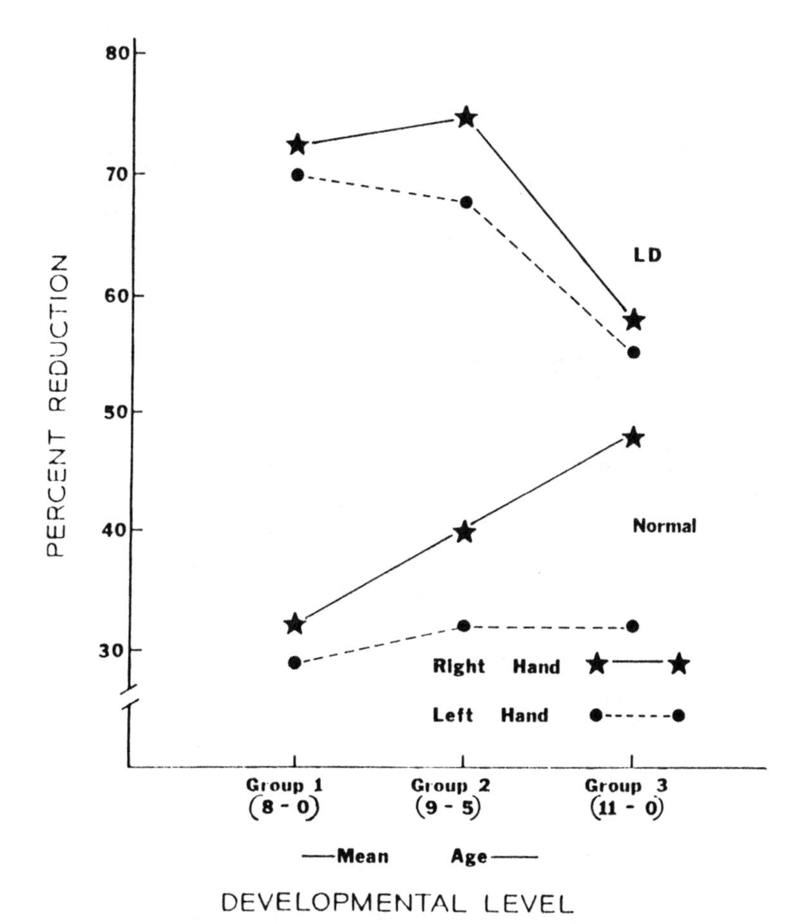

Figure 21-2. Mean reduction in right-hand and left-hand tapping rate, relative to the control condition, when the concurrent task was recitation of animal names. Reprinted with permission from "Time-Sharing and Dichotic Listening Asymmetry in Normal and Learning-Disabled Children" by J. E. Obrzut, G. W. Hynd, A. Obrzut, and J. L. Leitgeb, 1980, *Brain and Language, 11,* 181–194.

In a final study, Hughes and Sussman (1983) used a time-sharing technique to assess language lateralization in 12 language-disordered children and 12 normal children (7 male and 5 female in each group). The authors found that all language concurrent tasks produced tapping reductions (greater interference effects) for both hands for both groups. This was in contrast to previous studies, which show percentage reduction scores greater for the right-hand concurrent conditions than for the left-hand concurrent conditions (Obrzut *et al.,* 1980; White & Kinsbourne, 1980). For this study, the effect of the time-sharing paradigm worked in the opposite direction for these language-disordered children who showed reduced verbal output in place of reduced finger tapping. Thus, there were no significant main effects for group or hand with the dependent variable of percentage reduction scores. In fact, the mean percentage reduction scores for both groups were very similar. This finding led the authors to conclude that the time-sharing "paradigm does not serve as an adequate behavioral index for language lateralization in children, regardless of whether they are language-disordered or not" (p. 60). It is likely, however, that the consistent display of robust asymmetrical right-hand tapping disruptions shown by adults, along with the more modest effects shown by learning-disabled children, may be related to the amount of verbal output during concurrent conditions. That is, when subjects produce fewer syllables, as with language-disordered children, there seems to be less of a difference in percentage reduction scores between experimental and control groups.

It appears that although the time-sharing procedure has produced mixed results with child populations, it is of potential value in assessing cerebral organization. However, experimental variables such as the linguistic tasks employed, careful subject selection, and more control over verbal output with and without concurrent tapping need to be implemented.

CURRENT INVESTIGATION IN LATERALITY

From this review, it is clear that performance differences could be attributed to methodological problems inherent in the behavioral procedure employed, rather than to differences in cerebral lateralization. It is also likely that asymmetrical performance is affected by differences in processing strategy and experimental factors, that is, selective attention, rather than to differences in cerebral lateralization alone. Perhaps learning-disabled children use inefficient strategies of processing and encoding words, which is generally interpreted as a display of poor cerebral organization. Unfortunately, there have been very few studies that controlled for variation in processing strategies between normal and learning-disabled children. In fact, Morris, Bakker, Satz, and Van der Vlugt (1984) concluded, for example, that the data derived from recall of dichotic lists are essentially meaningless for making inferences about cerebral lateralization.

In an effort to control for these experimental or strategy effects, some recent studies have attempted to investigate the role of attention and its relation to cerebral processing in learning-disabled children. For example, Obrzut, Obrzut, Bryden, and Bartels (1985) found that whereas learning-disabled children shift their attention more readily than normal children, the learning disabled did not appear to be ''biased'' attenders when analyses were conducted on individual subjects. Additional experimental factors have also been found to influence the magnitude of the REA in dichotic listening. Recently, Hynd, Snow, and Willis (1986) showed that, at least in adults, dichotic listening accuracy was significantly increased when visual–spatial orientation was directed to the right or the left side of space, thereby reflecting the hemispheric bias suggested by Kinsbourne (1972).

To delineate further the effect of attentional bias on children's dichotic listening performance, Obrzut, Boliek, and Obrzut (1986) administered four types of dichotic stimuli (words, digits, CV syllables, and melodies) in three experimental conditions (free recall, directed left, and directed right) to a sample of high academically performing children. Figure 21-3 shows the mean percentage left- and right-ear stimuli correctly reported for each condition and type of verbal stimuli.

As can be seen in this figure, whereas the expected REA for words and CV syllables was found under free recall, the directed conditions produced varied results depending on the nature of the stimuli. Directed condition had no effect on recall of CV syllables but had a dramatic effect on recall of digits. Word stimuli and directed condition interacted to produce an inconsistent pattern of perceptual asymmetries. These findings appear to support the hypothesis that perceptual asymmetries can be strongly influenced by the type of stimulus material used and the effect of the attentional strategy employed.

Finally, the extent to which hemispatial position and directed verbal attention affects the REA in dichotic listening performance of children is currently being investigated (Boliek, Obrzut, & Shaw, in press). Preliminary results indicate that various attentional strate-

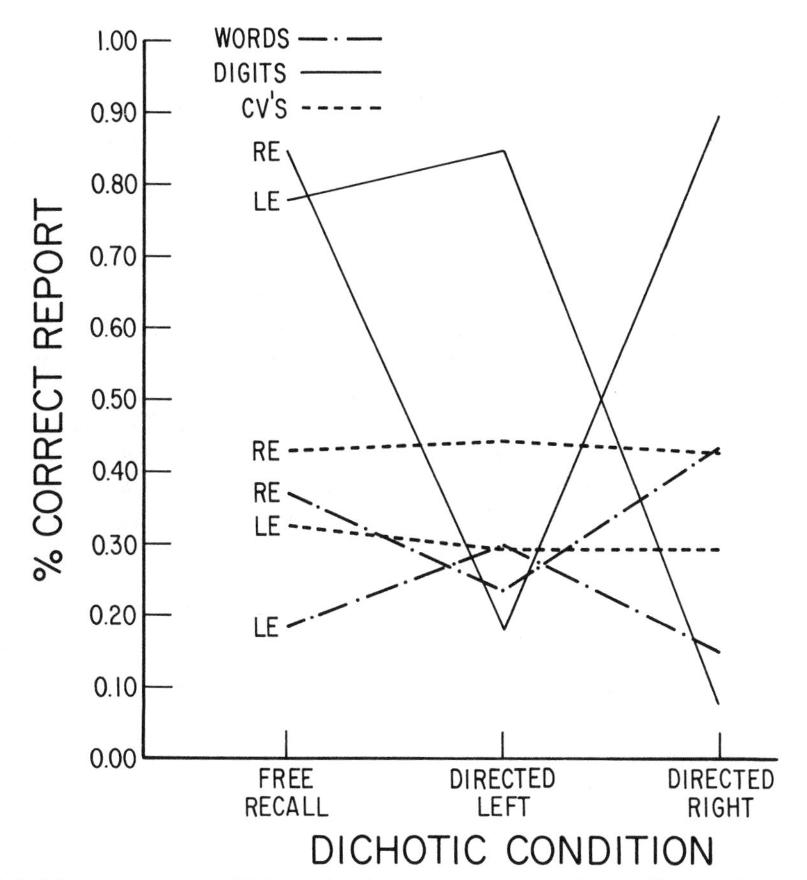

Figure 21-3. Mean percentage of left- and right-ear correct report by condition and verbal stimulus type.

gies and stimulus types can influence children's perceptual laterality. In addition, learning-disabled children appear to present a laterality structure that is more susceptible to these environmental influences (attentional strategies) than is that of children without processing deficits.

CONCLUSIONS

It has often been suggested that learning-disabled children display a deficient pattern of lateralization, which results in their inability to acquire adequate academic skills. Two competing hypotheses have been advanced to account for this weakness in lateralization: a developmental lag hypothesis and an abnormal cerebral organization hypothesis. The developmental lag hypothesis suggests that the learning disabled lag behind their normal counterparts in the development of verbal–linguistic skills necessary for the reading task. Thus, language has not fully lateralized to the left hemisphere, leading to weak asymmetries on tests of perceptual laterality. The competing hypothesis suggests that dysfunction in the structure of cerebral organization, either prenatally or during early postnatal development, has led to abnormal cerebral organization. In this review, results from auditory, visual, and concurrent verbal–manual asymmetry techniques have basically indicated that the developmental lag hypothesis is quite untenable. Since learning-disabled children demonstrated deficit performance (weak lateralization) on tasks involving all modalities, I am in agreement with Corballis (1983), that abnormal cerebral organization may underlie the learning disability syndrome. However, better techniques and longitudinal studies are needed to validate this hypothesis.

It must also be concluded from the present review that many factors other than cerebral asymmetry can affect performance on the tasks used to assess lateralization. Whereas an attempt is being made, as noted earlier, to address some of the deficiencies in studies cited in this chapter, more work must be accomplished in an effort to separate experimental effects from effects due to cerebral organization. For example, future research should further control task parameters and strategies used by children in performing dichotic listening tasks so that the developmental course and mechanisms underlying dichotic listening performances can be better identified. Thus, the issue of whether all verbal tasks measure the same underlying REA could be addressed. It may be necessary to introduce more neurological variance by using left-handers or perhaps bilinguals. The dichotic task should carefully control task stimuli, attentional and memory factors, and the spatial attentional and memory factors, and the spatial orientation of the subject. Finally, as Bryden and Saxby (1986) suggest, the measurement of dichotic listening performance should permit some statistical statement to be made about individual subjects and be independent of overall performance (see Bryden & Sprott, 1981). Even partial accomplishment of the preceding will begin to expand our limited knowledge regarding the nature and mechanisms underlying brain lateralization in children.

REFERENCES

Annett, M. (1975). Hand preference and the laterality of cerebral speech. *Cortex, 11,* 305–328.

Bakker, D. J. (1973). Hemispheric specialization and stages in the learning to read process. *Bulletin of the Orton Society, 23,* 15–27.

Bakker, D. J., Smink, T., & Reitsma, P. (1973). Ear dominance and reading ability. *Cortex, 9,* 301–312.

Bakker, D. J., Teunissen, J., & Bosch, J. (1976). Development of laterality reading patterns. In R. M. Knights & D. J. Bakker (Eds.), *The neuropsychology of learning disorders: Theoretical approaches.* Baltimore, MD: University Park Press.

Benton, A. L. (1975). Developmental dyslexia: Neurological aspects. In W. J. Friedlander (Ed.), *Advances in neurology* (Vol. 7). New York: Raven Press.

Berlin, C. I., Hughes, L. F., Lowe-Bell, S. S., & Berlin, H. L. (1973). Dichotic right ear advantage in children 5 to 13. *Cortex, 9,* 393–401.

Boder, E. (1973). Developmental dyslexia: A diagnostic screening procedure based on three characteristic patterns of reading and spelling. In B. Bateman (Ed.), *Learning disorders.* Seattle, WA: Special Child Publications.

Boliek, C. A., Obrzut, J. E., & Shaw, D. (in press). The effects of hemispatial and asymmetrically focused attention on dichotic listening with normal and learning-disabled children. *Neuropsychologia.*

Bouma, H., & Legein, C. P. (1977). Foveal and parafoveal recognition of letters and words by dyslexics and average readers. *Neuropsychologia, 15,* 69–80.

Broadbent, D. E. (1956). Successive responses to simultaneous stimuli. *Journal of Experimental Psychology, 8,* 145–152.

Bryden, M. P. (1970). Laterality effects in dichotic listening: Relations with handedness and reading ability in children. *Neuropsychologia, 8,* 443–450.

Bryden, M. P. (1982). *Laterality: Functional asymmetry in the intact brain.* New York: Academic Press.

Bryden, M. P., & Allard, F. A. (1981). Do auditory perceptual asymmetries develop? *Cortex, 17,* 313–318.

Bryden, M. P., & Saxby, L. (1986). Developmental aspects of cerebral lateralization. In J. E. Obrzut & G. W. Hynd (Eds.), *Child neuropsychology* (Vol. 1, pp. 73–94). Orlando, FL: Academic Press.

Bryden, M. P., & Sprott, D. A. (1981). Statistical determination of degree of laterality. *Neuropsychologia, 19,* 571–681.

Cermak, S. A., Cermak, L. S., Drake, D., & Kenney, R. (1978). The effect of concurrent manual activity on the dichotic listening performance of boys with learning disabilities. *American Journal of Occupational Therapy, 32,* 493–499.

Corballis, M. C. (1983). *Human laterality.* New York: Academic Press.

Dalby, J. R., & Gibson, D. (1981). Functional cerebral lateralization in subtypes of disabled readers. *Brain and Language, 14,* 34–48.

Dean, R. S., & Hua, M. (1982). Laterality effects in cued auditory asymmetries. *Neuropsychologia, 20,* 685–690.

Doehring, D. G., Hoshko, I. M., & Bryans, B. N. (1979). Statistical classification of children with reading problems. *Journal of Clinical Neuropsychology, 1,* 5–16.

Fisk, J. L., & Rourke, B. P. (1979). Identification of subtypes of learning-disabled children at three age levels: A neuropsychological, multivariate approach. *Journal of Clinical Neuropsychology, 1,* 289–310.

Geffen, G. (1976). Development of hemispheric specialization for speech perception. *Cortex, 12,* 337–346.

Geffen, G. (1978). The development of the right ear advantage in dichotic listening with focused attention. *Cortex, 14,* 11–17.

Goodglass, H. (1973). Developmental comparison of vowels and consonants in dichotic listening. *Journal of Speech and Hearing Research, 16,* 744–752.

Hardyck, C., & Petrinovitch, L. F. (1977). Left handedness. *Psychological Bulletin, 84,* 385–404.

Hardyck, C., Petrinovitch, L. F., & Goldman, R. D. (1976). Left handedness and cognitive deficit. *Cortex, 12,* 266–279.

Heim, A. W., & Watts, K. F. (1976). Handedness and cognitive bias. *Quarterly Journal of Experimental Psychology, 28,* 355–360.

Hinshelwood, J. (1895). Wordblindness and visual memory. *Lancet, 2,* 1564–1570.

Hiscock, M., & Kinsbourne, M. (1980). Asymmetries of selective listening and attention switching in children. *Developmental Psychology, 16,* 70–82.

Hughes, M., & Sussman, H. M. (1983). An assessment of cerebral dominance in language-disordered children via a time-sharing paradigm. *Brain and Language, 19,* 48–64.

Hynd, G. W., & Obrzut, J. E. (1977). Effect of grade level and sex on the magnitude of the dichotic ear advantage. *Neuropsychologia, 15,* 689–692.

Hynd, G. W., & Obrzut, J. E. (1981). Development of reciprocal hemispheric inhibition in normal and learning-disabled children. *Journal of General Psychology, 104,* 203–212.

Hynd, G. W., Obrzut, J. E., Weed, W., & Hynd, C. R. (1979). Development of cerebral dominance: Dichotic listening asymmetry in normal and learning disabled children. *Journal of Experimental Child Psychology, 28,* 445–454.

Hynd, G. W., Snow, J., & Willis, W. G. (1986). Visual–spatial orientation, gaze direction and dichotic listening asymmetries. *Cortex. 22,* 313–317.

Kaufman, A. S., Zalma, R., & Kaufman, W. L. (1978). The relationship of hand dominance to the motor coordination, mental ability, and right–left awareness of young normal children. *Child Development, 49,* 885–888.

Kershner, J. R. (1977). Cerebral dominance in disabled readers, good readers and gifted children: Search for a valid model. *Child Development, 48,* 61–67.

Kinsbourne, M. (1970). The cerebral basis of lateral asymmetries in attention. *Acta Psychologica, 33,* 193–201.

Kinsbourne, M. (1972). Eye and head turning indicates cerebral lateralization. *Science, 176,* 539–541.

Kinsbourne, M. (1975). The mechanism of hemispheric control of the lateral gradient of attention. In P. M. A. Rabbit & S. Dornic (Eds.), *Attention and performance V* (pp. 118–132). New York and London: Academic Press.

Kinsbourne, M., & Cook, J. (1971). Generalized and lateralized effect of concurrent verbalization on a unimanual skill. *Quarterly Journal of Experimental Psychology, 23,* 341–343.

Kinsbourne, M., & Hiscock, M. (1978). Cerebral lateralization and cognitive development. In *Education and the Brain,* Seventy-Seventh Yearbook of the National Society for the Study of Education (Chapter VI, pp. 169–222).

Kinsbourne, M., & Hiscock, M. (1981). Cerebral lateralization and cognitive development: Conceptual and methodological issues. In G. W. Hynd & J. E. Obrzut (Eds.), *Neuropsychological assessment and the school-age child: Issues and procedures* (pp. 125–166). New York: Grune and Stratton.

Kinsbourne, M., & McMurray, J. (1975). The effects of cerebral dominance on time sharing between speaking and tapping by preschool children. *Child Development, 46,* 240–242.

Kimura, D. (1961a). Some effects of temporal-lobe damage on auditory perception. *Canadian Journal of Psychology, 15,* 156–165.

Kimura, D. (1961b). Cerebral dominance and the perception of verbal stimuli. *Canadian Journal of Psychology, 15,* 166–171.

Kimura, D. (1963). Speech lateralization in young children as determined by an auditory test. *Journal of Comparative and Physiological Psychology, 56,* 899–902.

Kimura, D. (1966). Dual functional asymmetry of the brain in visual perception. *Neuropsychologia, 4,* 275–285.

Kimura, D. (1967). Functional asymmetry of the brian in dichotic listening. *Cortex, 3,* 163–178.

Kimura, D., & Durnford, M. (1974). Normal studies on the function of the right hemisphere in vision. In S. J. Diamond & J. F. Beaumont (Eds.), *Hemisphere function in the human brain* (pp. 55–81). London: Elek Science.

Larsen, S. (1984). Developmental changes in the pattern of ear asymmetry as revealed by a dichotic listening task. *Cortex, 20,* 5–18.

Lenneberg, E. H. (1967). *Biological foundations of language.* New York: Wiley.

Leong, C. K. (1976). Lateralization in severely disabled readers in relation to functional cerebral development and synthesis of information. In R. M. Knights & D. J. Bakker (Eds.), *Neuropsychology of learning disorders: Theoretical approaches* (pp. 221–231). Baltimore, MD: University Park Press.

Marcel, T., Katz, L., & Smith, M. (1974). Laterality and reading proficiency. *Neuropsychologia, 12,* 131–139.

Marcel, T., & Rajan, P. (1975). Lateral specialization for recognition of words and faces in good and poor readers. *Neuropsychologia, 13,* 489–497.

Mattis, S., French, J. H., & Rapin, I. (1975). Dyslexia in children and young adults: Three independent neuropsychological syndromes. *Developmental Medicine and Child Neurology, 17,* 150–163.

McCormick, D. P. (1978). Right–left orientation and writing hand in children referred for neurodevelopmental assessment. *Perceptual and Motor Skills, 46,* 1175–1180.

McKeever, W. F., & Huling, M. D. (1970). Lateral dominance in tachistoscopic word recognition of children at two levels of ability. *Quarterly Journal of Experimental Psychology, 22,* 600–604.

McKeever, W. F., & Van Deventer, A. D. (1975). Dyslexic adolescents: Evidence of impaired visual and auditory language processing with normal lateralization and visual responsivity. *Cortex, 11,* 361–378.

Mercure, R., & Warren, S. A. (1978). Inadequate and adequate readers' performance on a dichotic listening task. *Perceptual and Motor Skills, 46,* 709–710.

Morris, R., Bakker, D., Satz, P., & Van der Vlugt, H. (1984). Dichotic listening ear asymmetry: Patterns of longitudinal development. *Brain and Language, 22,* 49–66.

Obrzut, J. E. (1979). Dichotic listening and bisensory memory skills in qualitatively diverse dyslexic readers. *Journal of Learning Disabilities, 12,* 304–314.

Obrzut, J. E., Boliek, C. A., & Obrzut, A. (1986). The effect of stimulus type and directed attention on dichotic listening with children. *Journal of Experimental Child Psychology, 41,* 198–209.

Obrzut, J. E., & Hynd, G. W. (1981). Cognitive development and cerebral lateralization in children with learning disabilities. *International Journal of Neuroscience, 14,* 139–145.

Obrzut, J. E., Hynd, G. W., & Obrzut, A. (1983). Neuropsychological assessment of learning disabilities: A discriminant analysis. *Journal of Experimental Child Psychology, 35,* 46–55.

Obrzut, J. E., Hynd, G. W., Obrzut, A., & Leitgeb, J. L. (1980). Time-sharing and dichotic listening asymmetry in normal and learning-disabled children. *Brain and Language, 11,* 181–194.

Obrzut, J. E., Hynd, G. W., Obrzut, A., & Pirozzolo, F. J. (1981). Effect of directed attention on cerebral asymmetries in normal and learning disabled children. *Developmental Psychology, 17,* 118–125.

Obrzut, J. E., Hynd, G. W., & Zellner, R. D. (1983). Attentional deficit in learning-disabled children: Evidence from visual half-field asymmetries. *Brain and Cognition, 2,* 89–101.

Obrzut, J. E., & Obrzut, A., Bryden, M. P., & Bartels, S. G. (1985). Information processing and speech lateralization in learning disabled children. *Brain and Language, 25,* 87–101.

Orton, S. T. (1937). *Reading, writing and speech problems in children.* New York: Norton.

Piazza, D. M. (1977). Cerebral lateralization in young children as measured by dichotic listening and finger tapping tasks. *Neuropsychologia, 15,* 417–425.

Pirozzolo, F. J., & Campanella, D. J. (1981). The neuropsychology of developmental speech disorders, language disorders, and learning disabilities. In G. W. Hynd & J. E. Obrzut (Eds.), *Neuropsychological assessment and the school-age child: Issues and procedures* (pp. 167–191). New York: Grune and Stratton.

Rourke, B. P., Bakker, D. J., Fisk, J. L., & Strang, J. D. (1983). *Child neuropsychology: An introduction to theory, research, and clinical practice.* New York: The Guilford Press.

Sadick, T. L., & Ginsberg, B. E. (1978). The development of the lateral functions and reading ability. *Cortex, 14,* 3-11.

Satz, P. (1976). Cerebral dominance and reading disability: An old problem revisited. In R. M. Knights & D. J. Bakker (Eds.), *The neuropsychology of learning disorders: Theoretical approaches*. Baltimore: University Park Press.

Satz, P., Bakker, D. J., Teunissen, J., Goebel, R., & Van der Vlugt, H. (1975). Developmental parameters of the ear asymmetry: A multivariate approach. *Brain and Language, 2,* 171–185.

Satz, P. & Morris, R. (1981). Learning disability subtypes: A review. In F. J. Pirozzolo & M. C. Wittrock (Eds.), *Neuropsychological and cognitive processes in reading* (pp. 109–141). New York: Academic Press.

Satz, P., Rardin, D., & Ross, J. (1971). An evaluation of a theory of specific developmental dyslexia. *Child Development, 42,* 2009–2021.

Satz, P., & Van Nostrand, G. K. (1972). Developmental dyslexia: An evaluation of a theory. In P. Satz & J. J. Ross (Eds.), *The disabled learner* (pp. 46–62). Lisse: Swets and Zeitlinger.

Saxby, L., & Bryden, M. P. (1984). Left-ear superiority in children for processing auditory emotional material. *Developmental Psychology, 20,* 72–80.

Segalowitz, S. J., & Bryden, M. P. (1983). Individual differences in hemispheric representation of language. In S. J. Segalowitz (Ed.), *Language functions and brain organization*. New York: Academic Press.

Sparrow, S., & Satz, P. (1970). Dyslexia, laterality and neuropsychological development. In D. J. Bakker and P. Satz (Eds.), *Specific reading disability: Advances in theory and method.* Rotterdam: Rotterdam University Press.

Springer, S. P., & Eisenson, J. (1977). Hemispheric specialization for speech in language-disordered children. *Neuropsychologia, 15,* 287–293.

Ullman, D. G. (1977). Children's lateral preference: Frequency and relationships with achievement and intelligence. *Journal of School Psychology, 15,* 36–43.

White, N., & Kinsbourne M. (1980). Does speech output control lateralize over time?: Evidence from verbal-manual time-sharing tasks. *Brain and Language, 10,* 215–223.

Witelson, S. F. (1976). Abnormal right hemisphere specialization in developmental dyslexia. In R. M. Knights & D. J. Bakker (Eds.), *Neuropsychology of learning disorders: Theoretical approaches.* Baltimore: University Park Press.

Witelson, S. F. (1977). Early hemisphere specialization and interhemisphere plasticity: An empirical and theoretical review. In S. J. Segalowitz & F. A. Gruber (Eds.), *Language development and neurological theory* (pp. 213–287). New York: Academic Press.

Witelson, S. F., & Rabinovitch, M. S. (1972). Hemispheric speech lateralization in children with auditory–linguistic deficits. *Cortex, 8,* 412–426.

Yeni-Komshian, G. H., Isenberg, D., & Goldberg, H. (1975). Cerebral dominance and reading disability: Left visual field deficit in poor readers. *Neuropsychologia, 13,* 83–94.

Zurif, E. F., & Carson, G. (1970). Dyslexia in relation to cerebral dominance and temporal analysis. *Neuropsychologia, 8,* 351–361.

22

The Impact of Early Developmental History on Cerebral Asymmetries: Implications for Reading Ability in Deaf Children

CHERYL GIBSON
E. C. Drury School for the Hearing Handicapped, Milton, Ontario

Deaf children provide a unique opportunity to explore cerebral specialization for linguistic ability and it relationship to early developmental history. When children are born profoundly deaf, they are not able to detect their own speech, or the speech of others, without a hearing aid. Some profoundly deaf children are never able to detect speech, even with a hearing aid. Since it is still generally true that the average deaf child is diagnosed at approximately 2 years of age, they would therefore experience 2 years of auditory deprivation. The auditory deprivation literature (see Kyle, 1978, for a review) has suggested that a critical period exists for the normal development of the auditory cortex, in much the same way that it appears to exist for the visual cortex. Thus, auditory deprivation in the first 2 years of life could have a profound impact on the cerebral lateralization of speech and language.

CEREBRAL ASYMMETRY IN DEAF CHILDREN: A REVIEW OF THE LITERATURE

A variety of approaches have been used to determine whether deaf children develop the same pattern of cerebral asymmetries as hearing children. Since the auditory channel is clearly inappropriate for profoundly deaf children, a majority of the research has focused on the visual and tactile channels. Unfortunately, these investigations have done little to clarify the impact of deafness on cerebral organization. A great deal of confusion has arisen as a result. This chapter will first present a review of the literature (see Table 22-1 for a summary). It will then introduce a possible explanation for this confusion and will conclude by presenting an experimental investigation of cerebral asymmetry in deaf children.

Before discussing the literature in detail, however, it might be helpful to clarify some of the terms that are used to discuss hearing loss. A hearing loss is often reported as the threshold where a pure tone is detected, averaged over three frequencies (500, 1,000, and 2,000 Hz). In this chapter, this is expressed as the hearing level in decibels (dB HL) with reference to the 1969 ANSI standards. A moderate loss consists of a threshold between 45 and 70 dB on a pure tone test. A loss would be considered severe in the 70- to 90-dB range and profound if greater than 90 dB. People are usually unable to hear their own speech, without a hearing aid, if the loss is greater than 85 dB (Risberg & Martony, 1972). There is also a marked dropoff in speech intelligibility after 90 dB.

Both pure tone and speech reception tests (SRTs) are used to establish the degree of loss. For the speech reception test, the children are given a list of two-syllable words, and their SRT is the intensity at which they get 50% correct. Some of the children in the 90-

Table 22-1. Results of Studies of Cerebral Asymmetry in Deaf Children

Author	Loss	Subjects	Stimuli	Response	Results
		A. Words			
Kelly & Tomlinson-Keasey, 1977	56 dB	8–10 yr D, $N=39$	High image words; low image words; unilateral; 100 msec exposure	Reaction time	LVF+ for high image words
Kelly & Tomlinson-Keasey, 1981		8 yr H, $N=30$	High image words; Low image words; unilateral; 100 msec exosure	Reaction time	RVF+ low image words for hearing children
	85 dB	10 yr D, $N=30$			LVF+ high image words for deaf
Manning *et al.*, 1977		17 yr H, $N=16$	4-letter words & masking stimuli; bilateral; 20 msec exposure	Hearing reported word verbally deaf used fingerspelling	RVF+ for hearing students
	65–75 dB	17 yr H/H, $N=8$			RVF+ for H/H group
	50–60 dB	17 yr H/H, $N=7$			
	85 dB	17 yr D, $N=16$			
	85 dB	17 yr 0–2, $N=10$			RVF+ for 0–2 group
	85 dB	17 yr 3–8, $N=7$			
Phippard, 1977		17–23 yr H, $N=10$	Letters; unilateral; variable exposures, 50% recognition rate	Identify & point to letter	RVF+ for hearing Ss
		11–15 yr H, $N=30$			
	70 dB	12–19 yr D (TC), $N=28$			LVF+ for Oral, no difference TC group
		12–16 yr D (Oral), $N=10$			
Scholes, 1979		College age H, $N=9$	Pictures, unilateral, 100-msec exposure	Indicate if letter occurred in name of object	RVF+ for hearing Ss
	70 dB	16.3 yr D, $N=13$, skilled			No difference for deaf
	62 dB	16.8 yr D, $N=13$, unskilled			
Vargha-Khadem, 1983		13–18 yr H, $N=16$	4-letter nouns, bilateral 85-msec exposure	Point to correct word from all words	RVF+ for hearing Ss
	80 dB	12–17 yr D $N=16$			No difference for deaf
		B. Sign or fingerspelling			
Manning *et al.*, 1977		As above	Signs, bilateral, 30-msec exposure	Sign response	No significant VF difference
		high school students H, $N=12$		Match signs to pictures	
	80 dB	High school students D, $N=24$			

Author	Loss	Subjects	Stimuli	Response	Results
Virostek & Cutting, 1979		22 yr H (signers), $N=8$	Fingerspell letters, numbers, hand shapes; unilaterally, 100-msec exposure	Write "S" if shape is same & "D" if different	RVF+ for Ss who signed for fingerspelled letters
		32 yr H (no sign), $N=16$			
	?	17 yr D, $N=8$			
Vargha-Khadem, 1983		12–18 yr H (know ASL), $N=10$	Static signs, moving signs, bilateral	Point to correct sign from picture of sign	LVF+ for static signs for hearing
		13–18 yr H, $N=12$		A person signed 4 words, Ss had to pick correct signs	RVF+ for moving signs, naive signers
		13–20 yr H, $N=16$			
	80 dB	12–17 yr D, $N=16$			No difference for deaf
			C. Nonverbal		
Kelly & Tomlinson-Keasey, 1981		See above	Concrete pictures, abstract pictures	Reaction time	No difference for hearing Ss
	See above				Deaf faster LVF
Manning *et al.*, 1977	See above	See above	Shapes	Point to correct shape	No difference for hearing or deaf
Virostek & Cutting, 1979	See above	See above	Shapes	Write "S" if shape is same & "D" if different	LVF+ for hearing and deaf
Phippard, 1977	See above	See above	Line orientation	Pointing response	LVF+ hearing, LVF+ oral, no difference TC
Vargha-Khadem, 1983	See above	See above	Face identification	Point to correct face	LVF+ hearing, RVF+ deaf
			D. Tactile		
LaBreche *et al.*, 1977		17.2 yr H, $N=24$	Witelson's shapes; letters; bilateral	Point to shape: fingerspell letter; write letter	RH advantage in hearing group with letters first, no other difference
	85 dB	15.3 yr D, $N=24$			
Cranney & Ashton, 1982		6–8 yr H, $N=32$	Witelson's shapes; unilateral	Indicate if second shape same as first	LH advantage, 8-year-old hearing, no other differences
	65 dB	9–10 yr D, $N=16$			
		24 yr H, $N=32$			
Vargha-Khadem, 1982		12–16 yr H, $N=16$	3 letter words; Witelson's shapes; bilateral	Point to 2 words	RH advantage for words, no difference for shapes
	80 dB	?D, $N=16$			
Gibson & Bryden, 1984		10 yr H, $N=20$	Letters; shapes; bilateral	Point to letters or shapes	RH+ for letters, LH+ for shapes for hearing Ss
	90 dB	10 yr D, $N=19$			LH+ for letters for deaf

(continued)

Table 22-1 (*continued*)

Author	Loss	Subjects	Stimuli	Response	Results
		E. EEG			
Neville, 1977	90 dB	9–13 yr H, $N=16$ 9–13 yr D, $N=15$	Pictures of common objects; unilateral	Choose that object from 5 others, record ERP	No difference behavioral data, right hemisphere+for hearing (ERP) Left-hemisphere advantage for signing deaf No asymmetry for nonsigning deaf
		F. Concurrent tapping			
Ashton & Beasely, 1982	75 dB	5–12 yr H, $N=20$ 5–12 yr D, $N=20$	Say "dog," "cat," "baa, baa"; solve puzzle; control tapping	Tapping rate	RH decrease for verbal material in hearing; both decrease in deaf; no difference in puzzle
Marcotte & LaBarba, 1985	70 dB	3–14 yr H, $N=50$ 5–14 yr D, $N=20$	Say "dog," "cat," "baa, baa," "how are you?"; control tapping	Tapping	RH decrease during verbalization for hearing; both hands decrease for deaf

Abbreviations: D = deaf; H = hearing; H/H = hard of hearing; LH (left hand); LVF+ = left visual field advantage; RH (right hand); RVF+ = right visual field advantage.

to 100-dB range can understand speech, but few children in the 100-dB range can understand speech. In experiments with deaf children, then, if it is crucial to select children who did not have any early auditory input, especially exposure to speech, it is necessary to select children with a loss of at least 90 dB. It may also be important to be aware of the extent of their ability to understand speech, as measured by their SRT.

Visual Studies

LINGUISTIC STIMULI: WORDS OR LETTERS

The first study of deaf children using a visual half-field technique was reported by Kelly and Tomlinson-Keasey (1977). They presented high-imageability nouns from the Paivio list (Paivio, Yuille, & Madigan, 1968) and low-imageability words (articles, conjunctions, and adverbs) to 39 hearing-impaired children between the ages of 8 and 10 years. The children had hearing losses ranging upward from 56 dB. A word was presented to one visual field, followed by a second word projected to the same visual field. The children were asked to decide whether the words were the same or different and to respond by pressing a button. The authors reported a significant left-visual-field (LVF) advantage for the high-imageability words using a reaction time measure. Unfortunately, there was no significant difference between the hemifields for the low-imageability words. There was no control group, and the authors did not report whether the children understood any of the words.

In 1981 Kelly and Tomlinson-Keasey reported another visual study that appears to be identical to the 1977 study, but with a control group added. There were 30 deaf and 30 hearing children between the ages of 8 and 11. The deaf children had hearing losses of 85 dB or more. The data from this experiment are difficult to interpret, but it appears that the deaf children responded significantly faster for the high-imageability words in the LVF, while the hearing were significantly faster for low-imageability words in the right visual field (RVF). There was a significant interaction between groups and hemifield, suggesting that the deaf and the hearing respond differently to stimuli in the left and right visual fields. Thus, whereas the normal pattern of asymmetry was observed in the hearing for low-imageability words, the deaf demonstrated the opposite effect for high-imageability words.

This difference between the deaf and hearing was not replicated by Manning, Goble, Markman, and LaBreche (1977) when they used a bilateral presentation. They not only compared hearing and deaf adolescents but also examined the age of onset of the hearing loss, and different degrees of loss. They used four-letter words in two-word pairs, followed by a masking stimulus. They found that the hearing students had a significant RVF advantage for the words, which was the expected pattern. The deaf subjects were divided into five groups, depending on the age of onset and the degree of loss, but a significant advantage was found for only two of the groups. The hard-of-hearing group (loss between 65 and 75 dB), and the students who had lost their hearing between birth and 2 years, had a significant RVF advantage. However, the congenitally deaf group, the other hard-of-hearing group (50 to 60 dB), and the group who became deaf between the ages of 3 and 8 all had a tendency toward an RVF advantage, although it was not significant. They suggested that the within-group variability obscured the results. The small size of each group (n = 7 to 10), probably also contributed to the equivocal results.

Phippard (1977) also investigated different subgroups within the deaf population. She compared deaf adolescents from a Total Communication program to students from an Oral program. The hearing loss of the students in these groups was at least 70 dB. Two hearing control groups were used in addition to the deaf groups. The stimuli consisted of lowercase letters, which were presented unilaterally. Afterward the subjects had to identify each stimulus from the entire set of stimuli. The hearing group had a significant RVF advantage for the letters, but the Oral group had a significant LVF advantage for the same material. The Total Communication group was equally accurate in both visual fields. Phippard suggested that the Orally trained group relied on visual encoding rather than on linguistic encoding for this task. She also suggested that the Total Communication group may not have used linguistic encoding or may have had bilateral language representation. It is possible that the two groups differed on the degree of hearing loss in addition to educational placement, and this might also have contributed to the difference between the groups. For example, although Phippard did not comment on this, the students in the Oral group may have had a less severe loss than the students in the Total Communication group.

Scholes and Fischler (1979) hypothesized that deaf subjects who were linguistically skilled would perform differently on a laterality task than would linguistically unskilled deaf subjects. The subjects were classified as skilled if they were able to understand passive sentences. The subjects were matched on numerous other variables such as IQ, age, and hearing loss. A control group of hearing college students was also used. In this experiment, pictures of common objects were presented centrally, and were followed by a letter, which was presented unilaterally. The subjects had to indicate if the letter occurred in the name of the object. The hearing subjects were significantly faster when the letters were presented to the RVF. The two deaf groups did not differ from each other and did not perform differently in the two visual fields. This suggests several possibilities: The task may not have been sensitive to differences in linguistic skills; the criterion to determine linguistic competence may not have been valid; both hemispheres may be involved in processing visually presented verbal material for all deaf subjects, regardless of their language ability.

While Scholes and Fischler (1979) had suggested that linguistic ability was important in determining cerebral asymmetry, Vargha-Khadem (1983) investigated the possibility that specific experience with sign language might be important. In her study, the deaf students ranged in age from 12 to 17 and had a hearing loss of 80 dB or more. The hearing subjects had studied sign language for at least one year and ranged in age from 13 to 18. The hearing subjects showed the expected RVF advantage for words, but the deaf did not show a difference between the visual fields. Vargha-Khadem suggested that the individual deaf student did show a consistent visual-field superiority but that this could favor either the right or the left. This consistent pattern for cerebral asymmetry disappeared in the group data.

In summary, a number of different approaches have been used to determine if deaf children have a normal pattern of cerebral asymmetry. In the one experiment where words were presented unilaterally, the hearing subjects demonstrated an RVF advantage and the deaf an LVF advantage (Kelly & Tomlinson-Keasey, 1977, 1981). When words were presented bilaterally (Manning *et al.*, 1977; Vargha-Khadem, 1983), the hearing subjects again had a RVF advantage but the deaf were inconsistent. When letters were presented unilaterally (Phippard, 1977; Scholes & Fischler, 1979), the results were even more inconsistent for the deaf, but the hearing groups again displayed the normal RVF pattern of cerebral asymmetry. This inconsistency suggests at least two possibilities. The deaf groups may differ on some important but uncontrolled variables, or the visual technique may not be appropriate for use with deaf children. Since Beggs, Breslaw, and Wilkinson (1982) have demonstrated that many deaf children have abnormal eye movement patterns during reading, this latter possibility should be taken seriously, and it should not be assumed that the deaf and the hearing would respond to visual stimuli in the same manner. It may be that a visual technique is inappropriate for this population.

LINGUISTIC STIMULI: SIGNS OR FINGERSPELLING

Several authors have explored cerebral asymmetry for linguistic stimuli using either sign language or fingerspelling. Again, the results have been very inconsistent.

Manning *et al.* (1977) included signs in the previously discussed experiment. Signs were presented bilaterally to both groups. Since both hearing and deaf groups could sign, the subjects signed their response. There was no significant visual-field difference for either group. A second experiment was designed to try to encourage linguistic processing by having the subjects match the signs to pictures. These signs were presented bilaterally to 24 deaf adolescents (hearing loss greater than 85 dB) and 12 hearing high school students. They reported a significant visual field by stimulus interaction such that words were perceived more accurately in the RVF and signs in the LVF by the deaf subjects. The hearing subjects in this experiment were not used in the sign condition. Presumably the signs were being coded linguistically; yet they appeared to be processed in the right hemisphere. This suggests that there is either a bilateral representation of language in the deaf, or the signs were not being coded linguistically.

While some authors have suggested that linguistic skill or age of onset might be important determinants of cerebral asymmetry, Virostek and Cutting (1979) hypothesized that the use of sign language was a critical variable. They presented either fingerspelled letters, fingerspelled numbers, or illegitimate hand shapes to three different groups. One group was composed of deaf adolescents, a second group contained college students who knew sign language, and the last group contained hearing subjects who could not sign. The only significant result occurred for the two signing groups, who had a RVF advantage for fingerspelled letters. Since the performance of the deaf and hearing was very similar, these authors concluded that auditory experience was not crucial for cerebral lateralization.

Vargha-Khadem (1983) also presented signs as stimuli, but she included both moving and static signs. She hypothesized that the left hemisphere is presumably specialized for complex motor sequences rather than language, and therefore the sequential component of moving signs was of critical importance. When static signs were presented to hearing subjects who were fluent in ASL, a significant LVF advantage was obtained. However, when moving signs were presented bilaterally to hearing subjects, a RVF advantage was obtained by those who knew sign language, and also by hearing subjects who did not know sign language. The deaf adolescents, who received both static and moving signs, did not show any visual-field asymmetries. She reported that, individually, the deaf subject has a consistent visual-field superiority, but this could be biased toward either the right or the left. In fact, she reported that all the subjects who had a LVF advantage and therefore, presumably, a right-hemisphere language representation, also had poor speech, whereas those who had left-hemisphere language representation had good speech. The group data, however, obscured these differences.

In summary, manual linguistic stimuli elicit a RVF advantage in hearing subjects. However, a LVF advantage for static signs was found in one group of hearing subjects who were proficient in ASL. The deaf were inconsistent when treated as a group, although individually they tended to have a consistent visual-field asymmetry. Again, this suggests that some major subject or task variables were not controlled or that the visual task was not appropriate for these subjects.

NONVERBAL STIMULI

A number of the previously mentioned investigators also included nonverbal stimuli in their studies, but few were successful in eliciting significant visual-field asymmetries in either the hearing or the deaf group. For example, Kelly and Tomlinson-Keasey (1977, 1981) used both concrete and abstract pictures. The concrete pictures were examples of high-imageability words on Paivio's list, and the abstract pictures were "nondescript visuals." These authors reported that a visual-field asymmetry did not occur in the hearing group, although they appear to suggest that a LVF advantage occurred in the deaf group. Two studies reported that shapes did not elicit a visual-field asymmetry in either the hearing or the deaf (Manning *et al.,* 1977; Virostek & Cutting, 1979).

Two studies, however, did report a significant LVF advantage for traditionally right-hemisphere tasks. Phippard (1977) found that a line orientation task elicited a LVF advantage in the hearing and Oral deaf group but that no visual asymmetry was evident in the Total Communication group. Vargha-Khadem (1983) used a face identification task and reported a LVF advantage for the hearing subjects and a RVF advantage for the deaf. The inconsistent responding of the deaf again suggests that some important variables may not have been controlled.

Tactile Studies

The visual studies have revealed that deaf children respond in a very inconsistent manner to visual stimuli. Beggs *et al.* (1982) suggested that abnormal eye movement patterns occur in deaf children during a reading task. This raises the possibility that visual tasks may be inappropriate for this population. Some authors have attempted to circumvent this issue by using a tactile task. Since the major sensory pathway for light touch and pressure is contralateral, it is assumed that information presented to the right hand is first processed by the left hemisphere, and information to the left hand by the right hemisphere.

LaBreche, Manning, Goble, and Markman (1977) used a tactile technique to determine the cerebral asymmetry for linguistic and nonlinguistic stimuli in deaf adolescents. The deaf students had hearing losses of at least 85 dB. The hearing subjects were volunteers from a local high school who had learned to fingerspell. Nonsense shapes first employed by Witelson (1974), and letters, were presented bilaterally. For the nonsense shapes, the subjects responded by pointing to a response board. In the letter condition, they either fingerspelled the letter or wrote their response. The authors reported a significant right-hand advantage for shapes for the hearing group, but only for the group exposed to the letter condition first. Witelson had reported a left-hand advantage, and thus these authors were unable to replicate Witelson's findings. There were no other significant differences. They concluded that early environmental differences did not influence cerebral asymmetry for shapes; however, these conclusions were based on negative findings.

A similar finding was reported by Cranney and Ashton (1982), who also used Witelson's shapes. They presented the shapes unilaterally, and the subject had to indicate if a second shape was the same or different. They included two groups of hearing children (mean ages of 8 and 6) and one group of deaf children (mean age of 9) along with a group of adults (mean age of 24). Although most of the deaf children had a loss of at least 90 dB, one child had a loss of 65 dB. They found a left-hand advantage only in the 8-year-old hearing group; none of the other groups had any significant differences between the hands. The only difference between the deaf and hearing subjects indicated that the deaf children were more accurate. It appears that these authors were also unable to replicate Witelson's results—that is, hearing subjects did not demonstrate the expected asymmetry effect—and these conclusions are therefore based on negative results.

Vargha-Khadem (1982) used a unique bilateral tactile presentation of words and reported a significant right-hand advantage in both hearing and deaf groups. She presented three-letter words, one letter at a time, and Witelson's nonsense shapes to deaf and hearing adolescents. The deaf had a hearing loss of at least 80 dB. The deaf were significantly less accurate than the hearing, but both groups had a right-hand advantage for the words. The nonverbal shapes elicited no differences between the hands for either group.

The most recent tactile experiment was reported by Gibson and Bryden (1984). They presented letters and shapes to 10-year-old hearing and deaf children. The deaf children had hearing losses of at least 90 dB. The hearing children were more accurate on the right hand for the verbal material and on the left hand for the nonverbal material. There was also a significant hand × group × task interaction such that the deaf had a left-hand advantage for the verbal condition while the hearing had a right-hand advantage.

In summary, only two of the tactile experiments reported a significant difference between the hands for deaf children. Both of these (Gibson & Bryden, 1984; Vargha-Khadem, 1982) used a bilateral presentation and verbal stimuli. In these experiments, the deaf performed the same as the hearing in one experiment and showed a reversal in the other. The deaf did not show any hand advantage for the nonverbal shapes in any of the experiments.

EEG Studies

The only EEG study of deaf children has been reported by Neville (1977) using 9- to 13-year-old deaf and hearing children. Pictures of common objects were presented unilaterally, and the children were asked to choose that object from five other objects. Both behavioral and EEG measures were collected. Although there were no significant differences with the behavioral data, the ERP results indicated right-hemisphere superiority for hearing children. The signing deaf children exhibited a left-hemisphere dominance on this task, but the nonsigning deaf children displayed no asymmetry.

Concurrent Tapping

One other type of lateral asymmetry experiment was reported. A concurrent tapping task was used by Ashton and Beasley in 1982. On this task, deaf and hearing 5- to 12-year-olds were asked to say either "dog-cat" or "baa-baa" repeatedly, while tapping. The nonverbal task required the children to solve an embedded-figures puzzle, while tapping. Both groups showed a greater right-hand decrement on the verbal task, but the deaf also showed a left-hand decrement. There was no significant difference for either the hand or group on the nonverbal task.

A dual-task paradigm was also used by Marcotte and LaBarba (1985). They used verbal stimuli similar to the Ashton and Beasley stimuli, but with an additional condition in which the children said, "How are you?" There were 50 hearing children (ages 3 to 14) and 20 deaf children (ages 5 to 14). The deaf children had a hearing loss of 70 dB or greater. All the children were right-handed. They reported a significant hand × task interaction for the hearing subjects, such that the tapping rate of the right hand decreased during verbalization. There was, however, no significant interaction between hand and task for the deaf children; in fact, there was a decline in both hands. They also report a significant hearing status × task interaction. They argue that their data demonstrate bilateral control of speech production for the deaf and left-hemisphere control in the hearing. They also report that there were no developmental changes in either group.

SOME CONCLUSIONS ABOUT CEREBRAL ASYMMETRY IN THE DEAF

Although these data appear to be very confusing, it is possible to determine if the hearing and deaf subjects perform in the same way on a laterality task by examining the significance of the interactions. For example, if a significant task × hemifield × group interaction occurs, we know that the hearing and deaf groups are performing differently on that particular task.

When the visual data are analyzed in this way, 80% (4 out of 5 cases) reported a significant interaction between the hearing and the deaf groups. Several authors did not report their data in terms of interactions, and these were excluded from the above analyses. When the tactile data are analyzed, 66% (2 out of 3 cases) reported a significant interaction indicating that the deaf and hearing perform differently on tactile tasks. In terms of the EEG data, Neville reported a significant interaction such that the activation of the hemispheres was different for the hearing and the deaf. The Ashton and Beasley concurrent tapping experiment did not report that the interaction was significant, although they suggested that the deaf and the hearing performed differently on the task. The Marcotte and LaBarba paper also reported that the deaf and the hearing performed differently, but they did find a significant interaction. Thus, the general tendency in the data suggests that the deaf and the hearing perform differently on a variety of cerebral asymmetry tasks.

The one experiment in the visual literature that did not find a significant difference was reported by Vargha-Khadem (1983). Although she found significant interactions on several tasks, the "word" task did not reach significance. She reported that the within-group differences appeared to reduce the overall group mean, although the individual subjects appeared to have reliable patterns of cerebral asymmetry. For example, the deaf subjects who used sign language appeared to have right-hemisphere language, and the subjects who used speech appeared to have left-hemisphere language. Since the subjects who had a hearing loss of 80 to 90 dB were technically hard of hearing, the inclusion of this group introduced a confound that could have obscured the results for the deaf subjects.

A discrepancy between the deaf and the hearing was also reported in two tactile experiments. Gibson and Bryden (1984) reported that the deaf and hearing children performed differently on this task, and Vargha-Khadem (1982) found a right-hand advantage for both the hearing and the deaf groups. In Vargha-Kadem's experiment, three-letter words were presented bimanually, and the subjects had to pick the correct word from a choice of six words. There were several difficulties with this experiment. The deaf and hearing groups differed on IQ (with the deaf being lower) and 38% of the hearing group performed at ceiling level. The accuracy of the deaf group was significantly lower. A cutoff of 80 dB on a pure tone measure was used (again, this includes a group with a severe rather than a profound loss). The Gibson and Bryden (1984) experiment, in which a difference was found between the deaf and the hearing, used a bimanual letter task. There was no significant difference in accuracy between the groups, and a cutoff of 90 dB was used to select the deaf students.

In summary, then, a significant interaction between the task, the group, and the hemifield occurred on 80% of the visual tasks and 66% of the tactile tasks. The experiments that did not report a significant interaction included hard-of-hearing students and therefore had not controlled an important variable. Thus, it appears that deaf and hearing subjects appear to perform differently on cerebral asymmetry tasks when the major variables are controlled.

If deaf children do exhibit a different pattern of cerebral asymmetry as a result of early auditory deprivation, then it is important to determine which aspects of the auditory experience are crucial. For example, the speech signal might provide the critical information that creates a bias toward left-hemisphere dominance language, but so might the syntactic component of language or the motor control of speech. Some authors (e.g., Corballis, 1983) have also argued that the left hemisphere is specialized for sequential skills and this may be the crucial variable.

The following experiment was designed to determine if sequential information processing was a critical component for the development of cerebral asymmetry in deaf children. It also examined the reading ability of deaf children to determine if an abnormal pattern of cerebral asymmetry is related to the inability of the average deaf child to learn to read.

CEREBRAL ASYMMETRY AND READING ABILITY: AN EXPERIMENT

It has been reported that only 10% of 18-year-old deaf students can read at or above Grade 8 (Trybus & Karchmer, 1977). In addition, the average reading comprehension level for 16- to 18-year-old deaf students is Grade 3.5 to 4. This level has been reported in several countries, using a variety of tests. It appears that the greatest difference between the deaf and the hearing occurs at the level of the transition to skilled reading, which normally takes place at Grade 4. Furth (1966) defined minimal reading competence as greater than a Grade 4.9 reading level, and he reported that only 12% of deaf students reached that level.

By the 4th grade, in normal readers, many of the subskills of the reading process become automatic, which frees more cognitive capacity for comprehension (Gibson & Levin, 1976). Reading, then, becomes an interactive information-processing procedure, driven by the information in the text and augmented by the reader's knowledge of the world. The average deaf child is unable to pass this boundary and learn to read for meaning.

Although there are a variety of explanations for this discrepancy between the reading ability of deaf and hearing children, there are few real answers that account for this persistent finding. The intransigence of the problem, and the consistent finding that the degree of hearing loss is important, suggests that the major limitation to proficiency may occur at the biological level. In addition, the review of the cerebral asymmetry research suggested that deaf and hearing children appear to have different patterns of cerebral asymmetry.

It is often stated that sequential information processing is a major characteristic of the left hemisphere, and spatial processing of the right. We might hypothesize that deaf children are limited in their reading ability because they are tied to a right-hemisphere process during reading. The following experiment examined cerebral asymmetry in deaf children using sequential and spatial stimuli. These stimuli were presented in the tactile modality, and the results were then correlated with reading ability.

There were 204 subjects in the entire group. The following information was collected on most of these students: age, sex, IQ, pure tone loss, Speech Reception Threshold (SRT), socioeconomic status (SES), age of onset, and reading comprehension.

A number of these variables were found to be correlated with reading ability. Specifically, IQ ($r = .30$, $p = .001$, $n = 165$), hearing loss ($r = .21$, $p = .002$, $n = 164$), and SES ($r = -.18$, $p = .01$, $n = 162$) were correlated with reading, such that a child with a high IQ, with a less severe loss, and from a family at the managerial level tended to have a higher score on the reading comprehension test (Stanford Achievement Test—Hearing-Impaired Version).

In addition, a tactual measure of cerebral asymmetry was available for 24 of these students. For the tactual experiment, the subjects placed both their hands on a box and positioned their fingers over eight small holes. A solenoid was situated under each hole, and these could be activated to touch each finger in either a sequential or a spatial pattern. For the sequential pattern, one finger on each hand was stimulated, followed by a second finger on each hand. The subjects were required to report the order of the stimuli by pressing a microswitch, which was adjacent to each hole, in that same order. For the spatial pattern, two fingers on one hand and one finger on the other hand were stimulated at the same time, and the subjects had to report the spatial pattern.

One measure of reading is the ability to read for meaning. It may be that deaf children who are able to read for meaning would have a different pattern of cerebral laterality than those who do not. Since a previous experiment (Gibson & Bryden, 1984) had indicated a reversal in laterality on a verbal task, it could be possible that the students who could read for meaning might have the typical pattern of left-hemisphere bias for sequential information, and those who could not would show a reversal.

Furth used the Grade 4.9 level to indicate minimal reading ability, but others have used every value between Grade 2 and Grade 10. The often cited level of Grade 4 (Gibson & Levin, 1976) was used for this experiment, and a somewhat arbitrary figure of Grade 4.5 was chosen as the cutoff point. The use of a Grade 4.5 cutoff point resulted in a more conservative estimate, compared to Furth's Grade 4.9 estimate of reading competence.

Thus, students who could read for meaning (greater than Grade 4.6) and those who could not (less than Grade 4.5) were compared on the laterality task. A difference score was calculated (right hand–left hand). The good readers had a sequential laterality score of +13.91, and the poor readers had a score of −4.16. These means were significantly different on a *t*-test ($p = .02$, $t = 2.49$, df = 21). Thus the students who could read for meaning had a normal pattern of laterality (right hand better than left hand), and those who could not read for meaning had a reversed pattern. In fact, all the students who could read for meaning had a normal pattern of laterality (right hand better than left).

In addition, hearing loss was significantly correlated with the sequential laterality score ($r = .51$, $n = 24$, $p = .005$), such that students who could not detect speech were more likely to have a reversed pattern of laterality. Thus, students who could read for meaning tended to have a normal pattern of laterality and were more likely to be able to detect speech.

NEUROPSYCHOLOGICAL MODELS OF LANGUAGE

There are two major models of language organization that could account for the inability of the deaf to read. The Wernicke-Geschwind model (cf. Kolb & Whishaw, 1980) would suggest that when a written word is visualized, the primary visual association areas would receive that information. This is then transmitted to the angular gyrus, which evokes the corresponding auditory form in Wernicke's area. Wernicke assumed that if deaf people learned to read, this area would not be in the circuit.

There have been many criticisms of this model, and these generally revolve around the issue of the rigid localization of function that was proposed. For example, Kolb and Whishaw (1980) report that receptive and expressive speech disorders are found in all aphasic patients, and thus language production and reception are not as specifically localized as the model suggests.

A somewhat different model of language organization has been proposed by Ojemann (1983). He suggests that language is dependent on two basic systems. There appears to be a perisylvian sequencing–phoneme–decoding system that is surrounded by a short-term memory system. Language functions appear at the interface of these two systems. Thus, the same cortical areas appear to control the sequencing of motor movements (especially orofacial) and the decoding of speech sounds. By this model, then, there is a common area for speech decoding and production. In addition, he postulates that a single mechanism (such as precise timing) may be the common denominator for both of these functions.

Support for Ojemann's model has been provided by Tallal (1985) in her series of studies of language-impaired children. She found that language-impaired children had difficulty with auditory sequencing, such that they could not detect (or produce) rapidly changing speech sounds, and this deficit disrupted the normal development of speech and language in these children.

With deaf children, then, it is possible that the inability to detect and produce certain speech sounds may alter the neurological substrate for language. Some support for this speculation comes from a study of babbling development in hearing-impaired infants by Stoel-Gammon and Otomo (1986). They reported that babbling development not only decreased in quantity but also differed in quality from that of hearing infants. There is some evidence that the prenatal environment may set the stage for later hemispheric development and the absence of auditory stimulation may reduce the typical left-hemisphere bias for speech (see Turkewitz, Chapter 4, this volume). Thus, if the production of speech sounds can be seen as a measure of the development of a basic structure of language, then deaf children differ from hearing children at a very early age. Since reading is dependent on language, an altered neurological substrate could have a detrimental effect on the ability of deaf children to learn to read.

The present study found that both normal cerebral organization and the ability to detect speech were related to the ability to read. That is, the deaf students who had a normal pattern of cerebral organization for sequential information, and who could detect speech were better readers. Thus, the data from the present experiment were consistent with Ojemann's model. The association between motor sequencing, speech decoding, and reading, which Ojemann has postulated and which appeared in this study, appears to have a neurological base. This, in turn, suggests that early developmental history could have a profound impact on neurological organization in young children and on reading ability in school-age children.

CONCLUSION

In conclusion, the confusion about cerebral asymmetries in deaf children is more apparent than real. It appears that deaf and hearing children perform differently on many different cerebral asymmetry tasks, and that this relationship is clearer when hard-of-hearing children are excluded from the experiments. Hearing loss, then, is an important variable that must be controlled; a minimum hearing loss of 90 dB should be maintained as the cutoff level.

In addition, a crucial component of the early auditory environment appears to be the ability to attend to sequential information. The normal bias towards a left-hemisphere dominance for linguistic tasks may reflect the salience of sequential information, which is inherent in speech and verbal language. When a child is not exposed to this critical component in the first few years of life, or prenatally, the appropriate neural substrate for language may not develop, and this in turn may not only interfere with the development of a verbal language but also the development of advanced reading skills. Thus, early developmental history appears to have a profound impact on the development of brain lateralization.

ACKNOWLEDGMENTS

Financial support for this research was provided by a grant from the National Sciences and Engineering Research Council of Canada to Dr. M. P. Bryden. I am grateful to Dr. Bryden for many helpful suggestions about this chapter. I would also like to thank the staff and students at the E. C. Drury School for the Hearing Handicapped for their cooperation and assistance.

REFERENCES

Ashton, R., & Beasely, (1982). Cerebral laterality in deaf and hearing children. *Developmental Psychology, 18*(2), 294–300.

Beggs, W. D. A., Breslaw, P. I., & Wilkinson, P. I. (1982). Eye movements and reading achievement in deaf children. In R. Grover & P. Fraisse (Eds.), *Cognition and eye movements.* Amsterdam: North Holland and Berlin Deutscher Veerlag der Wissenschafter.

Corballis, M. C. (1983). *Human laterality.* New York: Academic Press.

Cranney, J., & Ashton, R. (1982). Tactile spatial ability: Lateralized performance of deaf and hearing groups. *Journal of Experimental Child Psychology, 34,* 1–19.

Furth, H. G. (1966). *Thinking without language.* New York: Free Press.

Gibson, C., & Bryden, M. P. (1984). Cerebral laterality in deaf and hearing children. *Brain and Language, 23,* 1–12.

Gibson, E. J., & Levin, H. (1976). *The psychology of reading.* Cambridge, MA: MIT Press.

Kelly, R. R, & Tomlinson-Keasey, C. (1977). Hemispheric of deaf children for processing words and pictures visually to the hemispheres. *American Annals of the Deaf,* December, pp. 525–533.

Kelly, R. R., & Tomlinson-Keasey, C. T. (1981). The effect of auditory input on cerebral laterality. *Brain and Language, 13,* 67–77.

Kolb, B., & Whishaw, I. Q. (1980). *Human neuropsychology.* San Francisco: Freeman.

Kyle, J. G. (1978). The study of auditory deprivation from birth. *British Journal of Audiology, 12,* 37–39.

LeBreche, T. M., Manning, A. A., Goble, W., & Markman, R. (1977). Hemispheric specialization for linguistic and nonlinguistic tactual perception in a congenitally deaf population. *Cortex, 13,* 184–194.

Manning, A. A., Goble, W., Markman, R., & LaBreche, T. (1977). Lateral cerebral differences in the deaf in response to linguistic and nonlinguistic stimuli. *Brain and Language, 4,* 309–321.

Marcotte, A. C., & LaBarba, R. C. (1985). Cerebral lateralization for speech in deaf and normal children. *Brain and Language, 26,* 244–258.

Neville, H. (1977). Electroencephalographic testing of cerebral dominance in normal and congenitally deaf children: A preliminary report. In S. Segalowitz & F. A. Gruber (Eds.), *Language development and neurological theory.* New York: Academic Press.

Ojemann, G. (1983). Brain organization for language from the perspective or electrical stimulation mapping. *Behavioral and Brain Sciences,* 189–230.

Paivio, A., Yuille, J. C., & Madigan, S. A. (1968). Concreteness, imagery, and meaningfulness values for 925 nouns. *Journal of Experimental Psychology, 76,* 1–25.

Phippard, D. (1977) Hemifield differences in visual perception in deaf and hearing subjects. *Neuropsychologia, 15,* 555–561.

Risberg, A., & Martony, J. (1972). A method for the classification of audiograms. In G. Font (Ed.), *International symposium on speech communication and profound deafness,* A. G. Bell Association.

Scholes, R. J., & Fischler, I. (1979). Hemispheric function and linguistic skill in the deaf. *Brain and Language, 7,* 336–350.

Stoel-Gammon, C., & Otomo, K. (1986). Babbling development of hearing-impaired and normally hearing subjects. *Journal of Speech and Hearing Disorders, 51,* 33–41.

Tallal, P. (1985). Neuropsychological research approaches to the study of central auditory processing. *Human Communication Canada,* 9(4), 17–22.

Trybus, R., & Karchmer, M. (1977). School achievement scores of hearing impaired children: National data on achievement status and growth patterns. *American Annals of the Deaf Directory of Programs and Services, 122,* 62–69.

Vargha-Khadem, F. (1982). Hemispheric specialization for the processing of tactual stimuli in congenitally deaf and hearing children. *Cortex, 18,* 277–286.

Vargha-Khadem, F. (1983). Visual field asymmetries in congenitally deaf and hearing children. *British Journal of Developmental Psychology, 1,* 375–387.

Virostek, S., & Cutting, J. E. (1979). Asymmetries for Ameslan handshapes and other forms in signers and nonsigners. *Perception and Psychophysics,* 26(6), 505–508.

Witelson, S. F. (1974). Hemispheric specialization for linguistic and nonlinguistic tactual perception using a dichotomous stimulation technique. *Cortex, 10,* 3–17.

Index